Contemporary Nephrology

Volume 5

Contemporary Nephrology

Editors-in-Chief: SAULO KLAHR • St. Louis, Missouri
SHAUL G. MASSRY • Los Angeles, California

Contemporary Nephrology

Volume 5

Edited by

Saulo Klahr, M.D.
Washington University School of Medicine
St. Louis, Missouri

and

Shaul G. Massry, M.D.
University of Southern California School of Medicine
Los Angeles, California

PLENUM MEDICAL BOOK COMPANY
NEW YORK AND LONDON

ISBN-13: 978-1-4612-8103-0   e-ISBN-13: 978-1-4613-0829-4

DOI: 10.1007/978-1-4613-0829-4

Softcover reprint of the hardcover 1st edition 1989

© 1989 Plenum Publishing Corporation
233 Spring Street, New York, N.Y. 10013

Plenum Medical Book Company is an imprint of Plenum Publishing Corporation

Contributors

Luis Baez, M.D. • Hematology Section, Medical Service, Veterans Administration Hospital, University of Puerto Rico School of Medicine, San Juan, Puerto Rico 00936

Julio E. Benabe, M.D. • Renal Section, Veterans Administration Hospital, University of Puerto Rico School of Medicine, San Juan, Puerto Rico 00936

William M. Bennett, M.D. • Department of Medicine, Oregon Health Sciences University, Portland, Oregon 97201

Sylvia L. Betcher, M.D., Ph.D. • Division of Nephrology, Department of Internal Medicine, Medical College of Virginia, Virginia Commonwealth University, Richmond, Virginia 23298-0160

Stephen Brennan, M.D. • Renal Section, Department of Medicine, Baylor College of Medicine, Houston, Texas 77030

E. C. Cameron, M.D. • Division of Nephrology, Vancouver General Hospital, and University of British Columbia, Vancouver, British Columbia, Canada V5Z 1M9

Vito M. Campese, M.D. • Division of Nephrology, LAC/USC Medical Center, Los Angeles, California 90033

Cindy L. Corpier, M.D. • Renal Section, Baylor College of Medicine, The Methodist Hospital, Houston, Texas 77030

Calvin U. Cotton, M.D. • Department of Physiology and Biophysics, University of Texas Medical Branch, Galveston, Texas 77550

William G. Couser, M.D. • Division of Nephrology, University of Washington, Seattle, Washington 98195

Norman P. Curthoys, Ph.D. • Department of Microbiology, Biochemistry, and Molecular Biology, University of Pittsburgh, Pittsburgh, Pennsylvania 15261

Garabed Eknoyan, M.D. • Renal Section, Department of Medicine, Baylor College of Medicine, Houston, Texas 77030

Lee W. Henderson, M.D. • Extramural Grant Research, Baxter Healthcare Corporation, Renal Therapy Division, Round Lake, Illinois 60073

H. David Humes, M.D. • University of Michigan Medical School, and Veterans Administration Medical Center, Ann Arbor, Michigan 48105

Ali A. Khraibi, M.D. • Departments of Physiology and Biophysics, and Medicine, Mayo Medical School, Mayo Foundation, Rochester, Minnesota 55905

Franklyn G. Knox, M.D., Ph.D. • Departments of Physiology and Biophysics, and Medicine, Mayo Medical School, Mayo Foundation, Rochester, Minnesota 55905

Neil A. Kurtzman, M.D. • Department of Internal Medicine, Texas Tech University Health Sciences Center, Lubbock, Texas 79430

Melvin E. Laski, M.D. • Department of Internal Medicine, Texas Tech University Health Sciences Center, Lubbock, Texas 79430

Bradley J. Maroni, M.D. • Renal Division, Emory University Medical School, Atlanta, Georgia 30322

Manuel Martinez-Maldonado, M.D. • Medical Service, Veterans Administration Hospital, University of Puerto Rico School of Medicine, San Juan, Puerto Rico 00936

Larry B. Melton, M.D. • Department of Medicine, Harvard Medical School, and Beth Israel Hospital, Boston, Massachusetts 02115

Joseph M. Messana, M.D. • University of Michigan Medical School, and Veterans Administration Medical Center, Ann Arbor, Michigan 48105

William E. Mitch, M.D. • Renal Division, Emory University Medical School, Atlanta, Georgia 30322

Luis Reuss, M.D. • Department of Physiology and Biophysics, University of Texas Medical Branch, Galveston, Texas 77550

Anton C. Schoolwerth, M.D. • Division of Nephrology, Department of Internal Medicine, Virginia Commonwealth University, Richmond, Virginia 23298-0160

Terry B. Strom, M.D. • Department of Medicine, Harvard Medical School, and Beth Israel Hospital, Boston, Massachusetts 02115

Wadi N. Suki, M.D. • Renal Section, Baylor College of Medicine, The Methodist Hospital, Houston, Texas 77030

Roger A. L. Sutton, M.D. • Division of Nephrology, Vancouver General Hospital, and University of British Columbia, Vancouver, British Columbia, Canada V5Z 1M9

Preface

Volume 5 of *Contemporary Nephrology* summarizes major advances in 15 different areas of nephrology. As in previous volumes the different chapters constitute updates in both basic and clinical aspects of the discipline contributed by individuals with in-depth expertise in their respective areas. We are grateful to the authors for their outstanding contributions to this fifth volume.

Drs. Reuss and Cotton review in Chapter 1 new advances in our understanding of water transport in epithelial tissues responsive to antidiuretic hormone. In Chapters 2 and 3 Dr. Knox and Dr. Schoolwerth and their associates summarize respectively new information in the areas of renal hemodynamics and electrolyte excretion, and renal metabolism. Chapter 4, written by Drs. Laski and Kurtzman, updates recent developments in the regulation of acid–base balance in health and disease. Chapter 5, contributed by Drs. Sutton and Cameron, provides the reader with a detailed account of progress in the area of mineral metabolism. In Chapter 6, Dr. Campese examines the contribution of sodium, calcium, and neurogenic factors in the pathogenesis of essential hypertension. The immunological aspects of renal disease are clearly discussed by Dr. Couser in Chapter 7. New developments in this field are emphasized and should provide the reader with a clear understanding of the direction in which this field is moving. Drs. Humes and Messana (Chapter 8) discuss selected areas in which new developments have occurred in our understanding of acute renal failure and toxic nephropathy. Special emphasis is given to the nephrotoxicity of aminonucleoside antibiotics and cyclosporine. Chapters 9 (Drs. Corpier and Suki) and 10 (Dr. Martinez-Maldonado and associates) discuss, respectively, the effects of certain systemic diseases on the kidney, and recent advances in our understanding of Alport's syndrome as well as a detailed account of the electrolyte and metabolic disorders seen with certain tumors. New developments related to the uremic syndrome are discussed by Drs. Brennan and Eknoyan in Chapter 11. Dr. Mitch, one of the major contributors to the field of nutrition in renal disease, and Dr. Maroni summarize advances in this area during the last two years in Chapter 12. Advances in the field of dialysis and transplantation are covered by Dr. Henderson, and Drs. Melton and Strom in Chapters 13 and 14. Finally, Chapter 15, written by Dr. Bennett, updates the metabolism of drugs in renal failure and provides rational guidelines for the use of a number of drugs in the setting of renal failure.

As the explosion of information accelerates, we expect that the summaries of advances in different areas of nephrology provided by *Contemporary Nephrology* will help the reader keep abreast of developments in areas of the subspecialty that are outside his/her immediate area of interest. Again, suggestions and criticisms on the part of our readership regarding this volume are encouraged.

Saulo Klahr, M.D.
Shaul G. Massry, M.D.

St. Louis and Los Angeles

Contents

Chapter 2
Renal Hemodynamics and Sodium Chloride Excretion
Ali A. Khraibi and Franklyn G. Knox

Chapter 3
Renal Metabolism
Anton C. Schoolwerth, Sylvia L. Betcher, and Norman P. Curthoys

Chapter 4
Acid–Base Physiology and Pathophysiology
Melvin E. Laski and Neil A. Kurtzman

Chapter 5
Mineral Metabolism
Roger A. L. Sutton and E. C. Cameron

Chapter 6
Sodium, Calcium, and Neurogenic Factors in the Pathogenesis of Essential Hypertension
Vito M. Campese

Chapter 7
Immunologic Aspects of Renal Disease
William G. Couser

Chapter 8
Acute Renal Failure and Toxic Nephropathy
H. David Humes and Joseph M. Messana

Chapter 9
The Kidney in Systemic Disease
Cindy L. Corpier and Wadi N. Suki

Chapter 10
Congenital Disorders of the Kidneys and Tumors: Alport's Syndrome and Electrolyte and Metabolism Disorders in Apudomas
Julio E. Benabe, Luis Baez, and Manuel Martinez-Maldonado

Chapter 11
The Uremic Syndrome
Stephen Brennan and Garabed Eknoyan

Chapter 12
Nutrition in Renal Disease
Bradley J. Maroni and William E. Mitch

Chapter 13
Dialysis
Lee W. Henderson

Chapter 14
Renal Transplantation
Larry B. Melton and Terry B. Strom

Chapter 15
Drugs and the Kidney
William M. Bennett

Water Transport across ADH-Sensitive Epithelia

Luis Reuss and Calvin U. Cotton

1. Introduction

Several epithelia are virtually water-impermeable under at least certain physiological or experimental conditions. In the mammalian urinary pathway examples include all segments of the renal tubule beyond the bend of the loop of Henle and all segments of the urinary tract from the renal pelvis to the urethra. In amphibia, epithelial preparations that exhibit a very low osmotic water permeability (P_{os}) under control conditions include the anuran epidermis and urinary bladder (e.g., of frog and toad). Under the action of a variety of peptide hormones collectively named antidiuretic hormones (ADHs), some of these epithelia increase their water permeability dramatically. In the presence of a favorable transepithelial difference in osmotic pressure, this change in permeability results in water reabsorption and is one of the major mechanisms of water conservation. Epithelia sensitive to ADH include the cortical and medullary collecting ducts of the mammalian kidney, the frog and toad urinary bladders and epidermis, and others. In mammals, both the thin and the thick ascending loop of Henle and also the epithelia of the urinary tract distal to the papillary duct do not respond to ADH with an increase in osmotic water permeability. However, salt transport by the thick ascending loop of Henle is sensitive to ADH.

In this chapter we will review recent advances in our understanding of the

LUIS REUSS and CALVIN U. COTTON • Department of Physiology and Biophysics, University of Texas Medical Branch, Galveston, Texas 77550.

mechanisms of water transport, and its regulation, in ADH-sensitive epithelia. The recent results will be considered within the context of older mechanistic studies. Basic aspects of the biophysics of water transport and isosmotic transepithelial transport were reviewed by us in a previous volume of this series[1] and will be mentioned only briefly here. Before discussing specific details, we think that it will be useful to provide an overview of the theme, in which we summarize current views pertaining to water transport in ADH-sensitive epithelia, both in the control state and during the action of the hormone.

2. A Working Hypothesis

2.1. The Control Condition

The rate-limiting barrier for water transport in ADH-sensitive epithelia is the apical (luminal) barrier, represented by the parallel arrangement of the apical membrane of the epithelial cells and the tight junctions. The mechanism of the low basal osmotic water permeability is unclear. Since in artificial membranes (pure lipid bilayers) the osmotic water permeability is quite variable, depending on lipid composition, it is likely that the lipid composition of the membrane accounts for the low oil/water partition coefficient of water, and hence for its low permeability by solubility–diffusion. The basolateral membrane of the epithelial cells has a high P_{os} both in the absence and in the presence of ADH.

2.2. The Action of ADH

ADH causes an increase in P_{os} that appears to be localized to the apical cell membrane (i.e., the effect is not on the junctions). Phenomenologically speaking, the end result of the action of ADH is to alter the properties of the apical membrane in a way consistent with the appearance of narrow aqueous pores which are permeable to water only. The alternative possibility of an increase in P_{os} mediated by an increase in membrane fluidity is unlikely, based on lack of effect of the hormone on the diffusive permeability to other nonelectrolytes.

Freeze-fracture and thin-section electron microscopic studies show generally excellent correlation between the hydrosmotic effect of ADH and the fusion of cytoplasmic tubules with the apical membrane. The tubules are lipid vesicles containing particles that upon fusion are partly transferred (by lateral diffusion) to the surface apical membrane. The particles are organized in aggregates and presumed to be transmembrane proteins whose presence would account for the porelike behavior of the aqueous pathway.

The mechanism of action of ADH involves generation of 3′,5′-cyclic adenosine monophosphate in the target cells, activation of protein kinase, cytoskeletal phosphorylation, and profound modifications of the cytoskeleton and the ultrastructure of the cells. Since the putative pores preexist in a cytoplasmic pool, ADH is believed to permit their insertion.

The magnitude and direction of the osmotic gradient and/or the resulting water flow and intracellular factors such as pH and pCa have important permissive and/or modulating roles in the effect of ADH. Under maximum ADH effect, structures distal to the apical membrane can become rate-limiting to osmotic water transport. Eventually, the water transport pathway is removed by endocytosis.

In the body of this chapter we will discuss (1) the biochemical aspects of the action of ADH, (2) the biophysics of osmotic water transport, (3) the evidence for pores in epithelia under the hydrosmotic action of ADH, including the unstirred-layer complications, the evidence against an effect on membrane fluidity, the changes in cell structure and volume, and the arguments against a paracellular pathway, (4) the evidence for pore insertion, and (5) the role of the cytoskeleton and modulating factors in the onset and cessation of the effect of ADH.

3. Biochemical Aspects of the Mechanism of Action of ADH

The biochemical pathways by which antidiuretic hormones alter the permeability properties of responsive epithelial cells is similar to that described for other hormone systems. Antidiuretic hormone binds to a specific receptor, which in turn interacts with adenylate cyclase and stimulates the production of cAMP. Elevation of intracellular cAMP levels activates a cAMP-dependent protein kinase, which in turn phosphorylates proteins. Eventually, the cAMP levels are reduced by intracellular phosphodiesterases. Little is known about either the final events (phosphorylation or dephosphorylation of specific proteins) or the regulation of the cascade of events that is ultimately responsible for the changes in cell membrane solute and water permeability. We will review the relevant information on each of the steps in the pathway and some of the mechanisms by which the process is modulated.

3.1. ADH Receptors

Antidiuretic hormone receptors have been divided into two classes, V_1 and V_2, based on the relative affinities for ADH analogs and whether their effects are mediated by stimulation of adenylate cyclase (V_2) or by changes in intracellular Ca^{2+} and phospholipid metabolism (V_1). V_1 receptors have been identified in vascular smooth muscle cells and hepatocytes, whereas V_2 receptors are typical of target cells with hydrosmotic response, namely, renal cells and amphibian skin and urinary bladder. Over 100 ADH analogs have been synthesized; some are partial agonists and some are antagonists. Reasonably specific V_1 receptor antagonists have been described; however, the V_2 receptor antagonists are less specific.[2,3] Recently, Mann et al.[4] reported on eight ADH antagonists that inhibited the ADH-stimulated water flux in toad urinary bladder with half-maximal concentrations in the range of 5×10^{-9} M to 3×10^{-7} M. A photoreactive analog of ADH with agonist properties has also been studied[5] and may prove useful for isolation and characterization of V_2 receptors. Kirk et al.[6] used a fluorescent ADH analog to identify the basolateral membrane of principal cells of rabbit cortical collecting duct as the site of action of ADH. Studies concerned with the synthesis, regulation, and degradation of ADH receptors have not been undertaken.

3.2. Adenylate Cyclase

Orloff and Handler[7] provided the first evidence that the ADH-induced increase in water, Na^+, and urea permeability was mediated by the second messenger cAMP. They found that exogenous cAMP, but not 5'-AMP increased the osmotic water permeability and stimulated Na^+ transport across the toad urinary bladder epithelium. Furthermore, theophylline, an inhibitor of phosphodiesterase, had a similar effect. Handler et al.[8] subsequently reported that ADH and theophylline stimulated the formation of cAMP in toad urinary bladder. Grantham and Burg[9] found the ADH and cAMP increased osmotic water permeability and Na^+ absorption in isolated, perfused rabbit cortical collecting duct. Later, the introduction of microanalytical methods made it possible to measure adenylate cyclase activity in individual nephron segments. Imbert et al.[10] demonstrated ADH-dependent adenylate cyclase activity in medullary and cortical thick ascending limb, as well as in branched, cortical, and medullary collecting ducts. Proximal convoluted tubule, thin descending limb, and distal convoluted tubule had no measurable ADH-stimulated adenylate cyclase activity. At the time of these studies, an effect of ADH on thick ascending limb had not yet been identified. Subsequent investigations demonstrated that ADH stimulates salt absorption by the medullary thick ascending segment of the loop.[11,12] Additional evidence for the role of adenylate cyclase in the epithelial response to ADH was provided by DeSousa and Grosso,[13] who demonstrated that forskolin, an agent that directly stimulates adenylate cyclase, induced a rapid, reversible, dose-dependent increase in osmotic water permeability in toad urinary bladder.

3.3. Cyclic AMP-Dependent Protein Kinase and Protein Phosphorylation

The effects of elevation of intracellular cAMP are thought to be mediated by activation of cAMP-dependent protein kinase. Dousa and Barnes[14] reported that ADH increased cAMP-dependent protein kinase activity in bovine renal medulla, and Schlondorff and Franki[15] made the same observation in toad urinary bladder. Functional roles for protein phosphorylation in ADH-sensitive epithelia have not been delineated. DeLorenzo et al.[16] and Ferguson and Twite[17] found cAMP-dependent dephosphorylation of a 50-kD membrane-associated protein (protein D) in toad bladder. In contrast, Shimada et al.[18] identified three proteins (73, 30, and 12 kD) whose phosphorylation was enhanced by cAMP in toad urinary bladder. Phosphorylation of specific cytoskeletal proteins is an attractive hypothesis for the hydrosmotic effect of ADH.[19] However, there is no direct experimental evidence supporting this possibility.

3.4. Modulators of the Hydrosmotic Response

The pathway outlined in the preceding sections is clearly of central importance for the expression of ADH's effects; however, a variety of modulators have been proposed.

3.4.1. Calcium and Calmodulin

Morphologic and electrophysiologic studies have implicated exocytosis and endocytosis in the hydrosmotic response to ADH. Consequently, the role of calcium has been the subject of many investigations. Indirect evidence for a role for Ca^{2+} includes: (1) elevation of serosal solution $[Ca^{2+}]$ tends to decrease the response to ADH[20]; (2) quinidine, which is thought to increase intracellular free Ca^{2+} concentration, inhibits ADH and cAMP-induced increases in osmotic water permeability in toad urinary bladder[21]; (3) the calcium ionophores A23187 and X537A both inhibit ADH and cAMP-stimulated water flow.[22] In spite of the indirect evidence that suggests a role for intracellular Ca^{2+} in the response to ADH, experiments with a calcium-sensitive dye (Quin 2) in toad urinary bladder dissociated cells failed to detect ADH-induced changes in intracellular free Ca^{2+} concentration.[23] The authors concluded that changes in the sensitivity of proteins to intracellular Ca^{2+}, rather than changes in Ca^{2+} activity, may be important in the effect of ADH. Intracellular calcium-binding proteins, in particular calmodulin, have been implicated in many Ca^{2+}-dependent processes.

Ausiello and Hall[24] examined the regulation of ADH-stimulated adenylate cyclase activity by calmodulin in cultured LLC-PK$_1$ cells. These cells are reported to respond to ADH with an increase in cAMP; however, it is unclear whether the hormone elicits a hydrosmotic response in these cells. Ausiello and Hall found that exogenous, purified calmodulin stimulated adenylate cyclase activity, but only in the presence of high Ca^{2+} (>130 μm). Furthermore, calmodulin increased the ADH-stimulated adenylate cyclase activity at Ca^{2+} concentrations of 230 μm and higher. The significance of these observations must be questioned in light of the much lower intracellular Ca^{2+} concentrations reported for most cells (<1 μm).[25] Grosso et al.[26] found that the calmodulin inhibitor trifluoperazine (TFP) prevented the ADH or cAMP-induced hydrosmotic response in toad urinary bladder. Furthermore, addition of TFP to ADH-prestimulated bladders rapidly attenuated the osmotic response. Amitriptyline and harmaline also blocked ADH or cAMP-induced increase in osmotic water permeability, presumably via the same mechanism as TFP. The existence of membrane-associated and cytosolic calmodulin was also reported in toad bladder.[26] In the same preparation, however, these authors found that purified bovine brain calmodulin failed to activate adenylate cyclase, soluble phosphodiesterase, or Ca^{2+}–Mg^{2+}–ATPase activity. In rabbit cortical collecting duct, Dillingham et al.[27] demonstrated that TFP and W-7 (another calmodulin antagonist) inhibited ADH-induced changes in water permeability.

Interpretation of the results with so-called "specific" calmodulin antagonists is difficult since a number of nonspecific effects of these inhibitors have been described.[28] In addition, there is an apparent contradiction between the inhibition of the hydrosmotic effect of ADH by maneuvers expected to elevate intracellular Ca^{2+} and the presumed role of calmodulin activation of the hydrosmotic response. The precise roles of calcium and calmodulin as physiologically relevant modulators of the actions of ADH remain to be established.

3.4.2. Protein Kinase C

Regulation of the activity of protein kinase C has been suggested as an important mechanism for the modulation of a number of transport processes. Two groups of investigators have studied the role of protein kinase C in the regulation of water permeability in toad urinary bladder.[29,30] Both groups found that phorbol myristate acetate (PMA), which can substitute for diglyceride as an activator of protein kinase C, increased baseline water permeability when added to the mucosal bathing solution. However, the magnitude of the increase in water permeability elicited by subsequent addition of ADH was reduced. Exposure to PMA from the serosal side did not alter basal water permeability, but the response to ADH was partially inhibited.[29,30] In contrast, the increase in water permeability elicited by 8-Br-cAMP, isobutyl-methyl-xanthine, or forskolin was not inhibited by PMA. Although the magnitude of the inhibition was small, these results suggest that at least one step in the pathway leading to the hydrosmotic effect of ADH is affected by activation of protein kinase C.

3.4.3. Prostaglandins

Grantham and Orloff[31] suggested that prostaglandins (PGE) are endogenous modulators of ADH action, based on the observation that a low concentration of PGE_1 inhibited ADH-stimulated water flow in toad urinary bladder.[32] Subsequent studies with cAMP, arachidonic acid, and inhibitors of prostaglandin biosynthesis led investigators to conclude that PGE inhibits the actions of ADH by interfering with ADH-induced cAMP generation.[33-35]

Several studies have demonstrated that collecting duct cells and interstitial cells from renal medulla synthesize prostaglandins in response to ADH, perhaps via activation of a cellular acylhydrolase.[36-38] Although a role for PGE_2 as an endogenous modulator of the ADH-induced increase in water permeability is difficult to establish, the work of Zusman et al.[39] supports this possibility. They found that ADH stimulates the production of prostaglandins in toad urinary bladder. Although cAMP and theophylline mimic the effect of ADH on water permeability, neither agent altered PGE synthesis, which indicates that the action of ADH on prostaglandin metabolism is direct and not mediated by its hydrosmotic effect. Furthermore, in vivo administration of indomethacin, an inhibitor of cyclooxygenase and hence of prostaglandin synthesis, enhances ADH-induced water reabsorption in the dog[40] and rat[41] and in humans.[42] The mechanism by which PGE_1 inhibits ADH-stimulated cAMP accumulation is not known.

3.4.4. Inhibitors of the Hydrosmotic Response

A large number of agents with diverse pharmacologic actions inhibit, to a varying extent, the hydrosmotic response in ADH-sensitive tissues (see Table I). These compounds may be divided into two broad classes: agents that inhibit the ADH-dependent, but not the cAMP-induced, increased in osmotic water permeability, and agents that block the hydrosmotic response elicited by either ADH or cAMP. The period of exposure, side of exposure (mucosal, serosal, or both), and extent of the inhibition vary; therefore, the specific references provided in the table should be consulted for details.

4. Biophysics of Osmotic Water Flow

It is quite clear that transepithelial water flow in ADH-sensitive tissues is osmotic in nature, i.e., is driven by a transepithelial difference in osmotic pressure. This has been shown in isolated preparations of frog skin, toad urinary bladder, and mammalian renal collecting ducts. In addition, the results to date support the conclusion that water transport in the presence of ADH and a difference in osmotic pressure across the tissue is transcellular. Finally, as will be discussed in detail in

Table 1. Inhibitors of the Hydrosmotic Response[a]

Inhibitors	Stimulus		References
	ADH	cAMP	
General anesthetics (methohexital, halothane, methoxyflurane)	I	—	Levine et al., 1976
Metabolic inhibitors (rotenone, dinitrophenol, methylene blue)	I	—	Hays et al., 1979[44]
Prostaglandin E_2	I	—	Orloff and Zusman, 1978[45]
Atrial natuiretic factor	I	—	Dillingham and Anderson, 1986[46]
Ionophores (A23187, X537A)	I	—	Taylor et al., 1987
Quinidine	I	I	Lorenzen et al., 1987
Microtubule inhibitors (colchicine, vinblastine, nocodazole)	I	I	Svelto and Lippe, 1978[47]
Cytochalasin B	I	I	DeSousa et al., 1974[48]
Glutaraldehyde	I	I	Eggena, 1983[49]
Monensin	I	I	Mendoza and Thomas, 1982[50]
Silver	I	I	DeSousa and Grosso, 1985
Calmodulin antagonists (triflouperazine, W-7)	I	I	Gross et al., 1982 Dillingham et al., 1986
Protein synthesis inhibitors (cycloheximide, puromycin)	I	I	Hoch et al., 1988[51]
Vanadate	I	I	DeSousa and Grosso,, 1979[52]

[a]ADH = antidiuretic hormone (oxytocin, arg-vasopressin, etc.). cAMP = cyclic adenosine 3′, 5′-monophosphate (8 bromo-cAMP, forskolin, theophylline). I = inhibition of the hydrosmotic response elicited by the stimulus. — = no inhibition of the response elicited by the stimulus.

Section 5.2, it is also clear that in the unstimulated state, that is, in the absence of ADH, the rate-limiting water transport barrier is the apical cell membrane.

In principle, osmotic water flow can occur across the lipid moiety of the bilayer, by a process referred to as *solubility–diffusion,* or via specialized pores in the membrane, likely to be proteins, by *bulk flow* if the pores are relatively wide, or by a process called *single-file diffusion,* if the pores are narrow. In the case of solubility–diffusion, water is transported across the membrane independently, with no interaction (frictional or otherwise) with other transported substances. In brief, water permeation obeys the independence principle and can be described by the formalisms of simple (nonmediated) diffusion. In the case of bulk flow, the movement of water across the membrane is via an aqueous pathway that in principle allows also for permeation of other molecules. Water molecules can interact among themselves and with solute molecules within the pore (viscous interactions), and the translocation across the membrane does not obey the independence principle. Under these conditions, the water flow can be described by Poiseuille's law or similar formulations, rather than by diffusion. In addition, solute and water fluxes can be coupled (see Section 4.5). In the case of single-file diffusion, only one water molecule can traverse a cross-section of the pore at any time; i.e., water molecules cannot slip past each other. In this situation, the independence principle is not obeyed, because in order for a water molecule to enter the pore all water molecules must move forward. The process requires a formal treatment different from either simple diffusion or bulk flow.

In all three cases, near equilibrium, i.e., for small driving forces, the volume flow is linearly related to the driving force:

$$J_v = L_p(\Delta P - \Delta \pi) \qquad (1)$$

where J_v is the volume flow (volume·area^{-1}·time^{-1}), L_p is the hydraulic permeability coefficient of the membrane, and ΔP and $\Delta \pi$ are the differences in hydrostatic and osmotic pressure, respectively. The L_p is usually expressed in cm·sec^{-1}·(osmoles/kg)$^{-1}$.

The single most important argument used to explain the mechanism of osmotic water flow has been to compare the osmotic and diffusive water permeabilities. Hence, in the following sections we will briefly discuss the biophysical bases for such comparison for each of the three cases just defined, and then we will address the complications created by the presence of unstirred layers. For further details, the reader should consult the recent reviews by Finkelstein[53] and Reuss and Cotton.[1]

4.1. Water Transport by Solubility–Diffusion

As briefly stated earlier, in this transport process water moves from the solution into the membrane lipid, and across this phase to the other aqueous solution. Net water transport by this mechanism requires a net driving force across the membrane, i.e., $\Delta P - \Delta \pi \neq 0$. Consider the case in which osmotic water flow is driven only by a difference in impermeant solute concentration (and hence $\Delta\pi$) across the membrane (i.e., $\Delta P = 0$). The differences in osmotic pressure are related to differences in solute concentrations, according to van't Hoff's law: $\pi = RTC_s$, where R and T are the gas constant and the absolute temperature, respectively, and C_s is the molar concentration of solute particles. The reason for the water flow in such a situation is that the water chemical potentials (μ_w) on both sides of the membrane differ. Excess of solute in the "concentrated" side decreases the water chemical potential on that side relative to that in the "dilute" solution. The water chemical potential (μ_w) is given by $\mu_w = \mu_w{}^\circ + RT\ln X_w + P\bar{V}_w$ (where $\mu_w{}^\circ$ is the standard chemical potential, X_w is the water mole fraction, i.e., moles of water/(moles of water + moles of solute), P is the hydrostatic pressure, and $\bar{V}_w$ is the partial molar volume of water). At constant temperature and hydrostatic pressure, there is a greater probability for water molecules to cross the membrane from the dilute solution into the concentrated solution than in the opposite direction, simply because X_w is greater in the dilute solution. As evident from the equation, a net driving force could also be provided by a net difference in hydrostatic pressure across the membrane or, more generally, by any condition in which $\Delta P - \Delta\pi \neq 0$. The osmotic water permeability of the lipid membrane is described by[53]

$$P_{os} = \frac{D_w^m \beta_w \bar{V}_w}{d\bar{V}_{oil}} \qquad (2)$$

where D_w^m is the water diffusion coefficient in the membrane, β_w is the oil/water water partition coefficient, d is the membrane thickness, and $\bar{V}_{oil}$ is the partial molar volume of the membrane lipid.

The diffusional water permeability (P_{dw}) of a lipid membrane, estimated from the tracer water flux, is described by exactly the same equation.[1,53] Hence, for the case of solubility–diffusion, the permeability ratio is unity, i.e.,

$$P_{os}/P_{dw} = 1 \qquad (3)$$

4.2. Water Transport via Aqueous Pores

The driving force for net water flow through membrane pores can be hydrostatic or osmotic. In both cases, it is ultimately due to differences in water chemical potential, as in the case of solubility–diffusion. It is intuitively obvious that a difference in hydrostatic pressure between the extremes of the pore will cause a difference in water chemical potential favoring the flux from the high-pressure side. When the driving force is only a difference in osmotic pressure, the mechanism is not obvious. Let us assume for simplicity that the solute does not penetrate the pore, and that at time = 0 the pore is filled with pure water and the two aqueous phases are instantaneously changed from pure water to solutions at different concentrations. Immediately, water will tend to exit the pore at both ends (because the water chemical potential is decreased in the solutions by the presence of solute) and the water flux toward the concentrated solution will be greater. The pressure *within the pore* will decrease, and a pressure gradient will be established such that a negative pressure will exist inside the pore, with a lower value at the end of the pore facing the high-concentration solution. At the steady state, the differences in concentrations of the solutions result in a steady pressure gradient which drives viscous flow through the pore. In the case of relatively large aqueous cylindrical pores of length L and radius r, with a density of n pores per unit area, and if the solute does not penetrate the membrane, the water flow is described by Poiseuille's law, derived to describe water flow in thin capillaries:

$$J_v = \frac{n(\Pi)r^4}{8L\eta} \Delta P \tag{4}$$

where η is the viscosity of water and the symbol (Π) has been used to denote the constant $3.1415 \ldots$, to avoid confusion with π = osmotic pressure.

The osmotic permeability of the porous membrane (neglecting both water permeation via the lipid bilayer and diffusive water flow via the pores, P_{os}') is described by

$$P_{os}' = \frac{n(\Pi)r^4 RT}{8L\eta \bar{V}_w} \tag{5}$$

The above treatment is generally valid for pores of radius equal to or greater than ca. 15 nm.[54] For smaller pores, no satisfactory theory exists, but a simulation study by Levitt[55] suggests that the Poiseuille formulation provides a satisfactory description. (See also Finkelstein[53] and Reuss and Cotton.[1])

The diffusional water permeability of the porous moiety of the membrane is given by

$$P_{dw} = \frac{n(\Pi)r^2 D_w}{L} \tag{6}$$

where the area for tracer water diffusion is equal to the cross-sectional area of pores $[n(\Pi)r^2]$ and D_w is the water self-diffusion coefficient (in the membrane, tracer water diffuses in the water-filled pores).

Considering both "viscous" and "diffusive" modes of osmotic water flow, the ratio of permeability coefficients is

$$P_{os}/P_{dw} = \frac{RT}{8\eta D_w \bar{V}_w} r^2 + 1 \tag{7}$$

where the 1 comes from the contribution of the diffusive water flow through the pores. The pore size can be in principle determined from this relationship. At 25°C, $[RT/(8\eta D_w \bar{V}_w)]$ is $8.04 \cdot 10^{-14}$ cm^{-2}, and therefore

$$r^2 = [(P_{os}/P_{dw}) - 1]/8.04 \cdot 10^{-14} \tag{8}$$

4.3. Water Transport via Narrow (Single-File) Pores

Single-file transport of water or solute across pores is defined by the restriction that the transported molecules cannot pass each other inside the pore. It is intuitively obvious that in the case of water, single-file transport will take place if the pore diameter is less than twice the diameter of the water molecule, but other factors can result in single-file behavior in pores of somewhat larger dimensions.

The derivations of equations describing single-file transport are beyond the scope of this review. The interested reader should consult the reference material quoted by Finkelstein.[53] The osmotic water permeability of a membrane containing single-file pores is given by

$$P_{os} = \frac{n\bar{v}_w kTN}{\gamma L^2} \tag{9}$$

where $\bar{v}_w$ is the volume per water molecule, k is the Boltzmann constant ($=R/N_A$, where N_A is Avogadro's number), N is the number of water molecules in the pore, and γ is the frictional coefficient per water molecule.

The diffusive water permeability of the same membrane is described by*

$$P_{dw} = \frac{n\bar{v}_w kT}{\gamma L^2} \tag{10}$$

and therefore the ratio of permeabilities is equal to the number of water molecules in the pore:

$$P_{os}/P_{dw} = N \tag{11}$$

4.4. Effects of Unstirred Layers

Unstirred layers are layers of fluid near the interface between a surface and the solution, which are not mixed with the bulk solution. Transport of water and solute in these layers is exclusively by diffusion. Unstirred layers can cause both transient and steady-state differences in solute concentration with respect to the well-mixed bulk solutions. The presence of unstirred layers in series with biologic membranes can cause significant errors in the experimental determinations of both P_{dw} and P_{os}, which can lead to incorrect conclusions about the existence of water-permeable pores in the membrane.

Measurements of the apparent P_{dw} of a membrane and the adjacent unstirred layers will yield a result that includes the unstirred layers as series barriers for diffusion. Their "permeability" is directly proportional to the water self-diffusion

---

*In the review by Reuss and Cotton,[1] there is a typographical error in the corresponding equation [equation (22)]: The denominator should read γL^2 instead of dL^2.

coefficient and inversely proportional to the unstirred layer thicknesses, as shown in the next equation:

$$\frac{1}{P_{dw}^0} = \frac{1}{P_{dw}} + \frac{1}{D_w/\delta_1} + \frac{1}{D_w/\delta_2}$$

(12)

where P_{dw}^0 is the measured value, P_{dw} is the true permeability of the membrane, D_w is the water self-diffusion coefficient, and δ_1 and δ_2 are the unstirred layer thicknesses, respectively.

Equation 12 can be solved for P_{dw}^0. For the simple case of $\delta_1 = \delta_2 = \delta$,

$$P_{dw}^0 = \frac{1}{1 + P_{dw} (2\delta/D_w)} P_{dw}$$

(13)

showing that for any value of $\delta > 0$ the true diffusive water permeability will be underestimated.

The presence of unstirred layers can also cause errors in the experimental determination of P_{os}. A typical experiment could be to measure either the transient or the steady-state change in J_v induced by imposing a difference in the osmotic pressure of the two solutions. For instance, we can start with a membrane bathed with NaCl at the same concentration on both sides and add sucrose to one solution only. The first complication introduced by the unstirred layer is that the change in osmolality at the membrane surface will not be instantaneous, but will have a time course dependent on both the rate of mixing of the bulk solution and the time necessary for diffusion in the unstirred layer.[56] In addition, the water flow induced by the osmotic gradient will influence the time course of the osmolalities at both membrane surfaces. At the steady state, when most published transepithelial measurements have been made, the osmotic water flow causes "concentration" of the NaCl side, and "dilution" of the NaCl + sucrose side, so that the true $\Delta\pi$ is less than that calculated from the osmolalities of the bulk solutions. The steady-state solute concentration at the membrane surface (for the "diluted" side) is given by

$$C_m = C_b \exp(-v\delta/D_s)$$

(14)

and for the "concentrated" side is

$$C_m = C_b \exp(v\delta/D_s)$$

(15)

where C_m and C_b are the solute concentrations at the membrane surface and in the bulk solution, respectively, v is the flow velocity of water (perpendicular to the membrane surface), and D_s is the diffusion coefficient of either solute in water.

This treatment is a simplified one. If one or more solutes are permeable, their permeability must be considered.[57,58] In addition, structural considerations are of importance in the case of biological membranes and particularly in the case of epithelia. Note that the magnitude of the effect of the unstirred layer on C_m/C_b depends on the flow velocity of water, which is equal to flow divided by surface area. Hence, when water flow is restricted, as one might expect in elements of small cross-sectional area, such as microvilli, lateral intercellular spaces, and other slitlike and tubelike structures, a large error in the estimate of P_{os} results from the high value of v. This error may be much larger than in the case of a planar membrane bounded by unstirred layers without structural restrictions for water flow.[57]

In most cases, the effects of unstirred layers in the estimation of water permeability coefficients are to underestimate both, with a larger error in P_{dw} than in P_{os}. Therefore, if unstirred layers are present and not taken into account, the apparent ratio P_{os}/P_{dw} can be greater than unity even if the sole mechanism of water transport is solubility–diffusion, which may cause the investigator to conclude incorrectly on the existence of aqueous pores in the membrane.

4.5. Solvent Drag

When a porous membrane is exposed on both sides to identical concentrations of a pore-permeating solute, inducing net water flow by an osmotic and/or a hydrostatic pressure difference will cause a net solute flux in the same direction as the water flow. This happens in the absence of a nominal (i.e., bulk solution) concentration difference or a membrane voltage (a pertinent consideration in the case of ions). The net solute flux has been attributed to frictional interactions between solvent and solute inside the pores: the solvent "drags" the solute. For flow governed by Poiseuille's law, if the solute concentrations are the same in both solutions, the solute flux is described by

$$J_s = J_v \, C_s \, (1 - \sigma_s) \tag{16}$$

where J_s is the net solute flux, J_v is the volume flow, C_s is the solute concentration, and σ_s is the solute reflection coefficient (whose value is zero if the solute is as permeant as water and unity if the solute is impermeant).

Frequently, the demonstration of an association between J_v and J_s under experimental conditions similar to those described above has been considered a strong argument for the existence of pores in the membrane. However, if there are unstirred layers in the system, the water flow will cause changes in solute concentration at the membrane surfaces, as described by equations (14) and (15). Therefore, if the membrane is permeable to the solute, a net solute flux will occur, which is entirely diffusional, and not necessarily via a pore. The net solute flux in this case would be caused by the differences in C_s at the two membrane surfaces, given by equations (14) and (15):

$$J_s = P_{ds} \, C_s \, [\exp(v\delta/D_s) - \exp(-v\delta/D_s)] \tag{17}$$

For example, such a mechanism could operate in a membrane in which osmotic water flow is by solubility–diffusion and solute transport is either by diffusion or by a carrier-mediated process. The phenomenon described has been called "pseudo solvent drag."[58] Lack of consideration of this mechanism has sometimes precipitated premature claims of pore-mediated osmotic water flow.[1]

5. Experimental Bases for the Pore Hypothesis of Water Permeation

5.1. Studies Based on Measurements of Transepithelial Osmotic Water Flow

The first experimental evidence in favor of pores accounting for osmotic water flow in ADH-sensitive epithelia was obtained from studies in frog and toad skin.[59] These data were based on measurements of steady-state transepithelial tracer water flux and osmotic water flow. It was found that ADH causes a large increase in P_{os} and a modest increase in P_{dw}, with a large value of P_{os}/P_{dw}. Similar observations were made in toad urinary bladder.[60] Since the value of the permeability ratio must increase with pore radius [see equation (8)], it was reasonably concluded that water permeation is via pores; ADH either enlarges the pores or opens up larger new pores. The radius of the putative pores was calculated by Andersen and Ussing.[61]

The complications produced in such experiments by the existence of unstirred layers were first pointed out by Dainty.[62] He concluded that P_{os}/P_{dw} is overestimated because P_{dw} is underestimated (see Section 4.4). Dainty and House[63] found that the rate of stirring of the bathing solution did, in fact, affect the measurement of P_{dw}, but nevertheless ADH increased P_{os} and had virtually no effect on P_{dw}. The conclusion of water permeation via pores was in principle supported by these results, but increasing the stirring rate does not reduce the thickness of the anatomic unstirred layer present on the basolateral side of amphibian epithelia such as skin or urinary bladder. In fact, Hays and Franki[64] found in toad urinary bladder under the action of ADH that P_{os}/P_{dw} falls with stirring.

Because of these results, in the early seventies the pore hypothesis was discredited and investigators in the field turned to examine the possibility that water permeation in ADH-sensitive epithelia could be by solubility–diffusion and that the hydrosmotic effect of the hormone could be by increasing the fluidity of the membrane. This possibility was proposed from studies in both rabbit cortical collecting duct[65] and toad urinary bladder.[66] The change in membrane fluidity elicited by ADH could be by modifications in bilayer composition and/or structure.[53]

The main argument against osmotic water flow by solubility–diffusion is the lack of parallelism between the effects of ADH on water and nonelectrolyte permeability.[67,68] In artificial lipid bilayers, changes in membrane fluidity elicited by a variety of experimental perturbations result in proportional changes in the permeability for water and liposoluble nonelectrolytes,[67] whereas in the toad urinary bladder ADH causes a 50-fold increase in P_{os} with virtually no change in non-electrolyte permeability.[66,68] These observations, which appear to be inconsistent with the possibility of solubility diffusion, account for the rebirth of the pore hypothesis in the mid-seventies.

Recent studies of the biophysics of water permeation in ADH-sensitive epithelia have provided increasing evidence in support of the hypothesis of narrow (single-filing) pores. An early argument was the fact that in the toad urinary bladder ADH increases P_{os}, but has virtually no effect on the permeabilities of most small hydrophilic nonelectrolytes.[69] This observation was initially difficult to interpret because, in addition to its effect on P_{os}, ADH increases the permeability of urea and small amides (formamide, acetamide), a result consistent with the possibility of a common permeation pathway for water and these molecules. This possibility was ruled out by the elegant experiments of Levine and associates, who demonstrated that in toad urinary bladder phloretin inhibits solute permeability but not water permeability,[70] whereas general anesthetics have the opposite effect, namely, to inhibit water permeability without affecting solute permeability.[43] These results indicate clearly that the ADH-dependent water and solute permeation pathways must be separate. In the cortical collecting duct, the case for a narrow pore is even stronger, because ADH appears to increase only water permeability.[71,72] In toad urinary bladder epithelium, the ADH-induced "water pore" has an electrical conductance four orders of magnitude lower than that of the gramicidin A pore, which indicates an extremely low ion permeability.[73] A sizable, although small, proton permeability was measured by Gluck and Al-Awqati,[74] but these results have been disputed by Parisi *et al.*[75] In any event, the ionic permeability of the putative pores is anomalously low compared to that of well-studied single-file pores such as gramicidin A.[53] One explanation is the possibility that the ADH-induced pores are longer, narrower, or lined by walls of lower dielectric constant. Alternatively, the low ionic permeability could be due to net charges of opposite sign at the pore ends.[53]

In summary, in the sixties and seventies the two major advances in this field were (1) to rule out solubility–diffusion as the major or sole mechanism of osmotic water flow in ADH-stimulated epithelia, on the basis of measurements of the permeability of lipophilic nonelectrolytes, and (2) to provide evidence supporting the idea of a water permeation pathway with the characteristics of a single-file (narrow) pore; the latter conclusion was based on measurements of permeabilities of hydrophilic nonelectrolytes in ADH-stimulated preparations.

Recent studies in toad urinary bladder epithelium have reexamined the question of the value of P_{os}/P_{dw} taking into consideration unstirred layer effects (Table II). Parisi and Bourguet[77] used methanol, a substance with a high oil/water partition coefficient, to assess the apparent unstirred layer thickness, assuming that the cell membrane resistance to transepithelial diffusion of methanol is negligible, compared to that imposed by the unstirred layers. Levine *et al.*[80] used maximum concentrations of both ADH and the pore-forming polyene antibiotic amphotericin B to elevate the water permeability of the luminal membrane and

Table II. Transpithelial Osmotic (P_{os}) and Diffusive (P_{dw}) Water Permeabilities in ADH-Sensitive Epithelia[a]

Preparation	USL Correction	$P_{os}/10^{-4}$ cm·s^{-1}	$P_{dw}/10^{-4}$ cm·s^{-1}	$\Delta P_{os}/\Delta P_{dw}$	References
CCT	n-Butanol	6	5	—	Schafer and Andreoli[76]
CCT + ADH	n-Butanol	178	14	19.1	Schafer and Andreoli[76]
FUB	Methanol	3	1	—	Parisi and Bourguet[77]
FUB + ADH (12 min)	Methanol	146	17	9.4	Parisi and Bourguet[77]
TUB	Amphotericin B	2	1	—	Levine et al.[78]
TUB + ADH	Amphotericin B	41	2	17.1	Levine et al.[78]
CCT	None	5	—	—	Kirk et al.[79]
CCT + ADH	None	170	—	—	Kirk et al.[79]

[a]CCT = rabbit cortical collecting duct. TUB = toad urinary bladder. FUB = frog urinary bladder. ADH = antidiuretic hormone (vasopressin in Refs. 76, 78, and 79; oxytocin in Ref. 77). $\Delta P_{os}/\Delta P_{dw}$ = ratio of the changes in permeabilities coefficients elicited by ADH. Values are rounded means.

assumed that the remaining resistance to water diffusion was entirely attributable to elements in series with the native apical membrane. Parisi and Bourguet found a P_{os}/P_{dw} of about 9, whereas in the experiments of Levine et al.,[78] the corresponding value was 17. The latter authors also performed an important validating experiment: They measured the value of P_{os}/P_{dw} after treating the tissue with amphotericin B, whose effects on water and ion permeation have been well characterized in artificial membranes. In the toad bladder, P_{os}/P_{dw} was 3.7, which compares well with the 3.0 value found in lipid bilayers doped with amphotericin B. Interestingly, fixation of the frog urinary bladder epithelium with a low concentration of glutaraldehyde preserves the ADH-induced water permeability. Under these conditions, the ADH-dependent P_{os}/P_{dw} ratio remains unchanged; after fixation of unstimulated bladders, treatment with amphotericin B resulted in a P_{os}/P_{dw} of 3.1.[81]

The complications introduced by series resistances in assessments of P_{dw} have also been recognized by investigators working on mammalian cortical collecting duct.[76,82] Correcting for these effects by measuring the permeability to the lipophilic probe n-butanol, a P_{os}/P_{dw} of 7.5 has been calculated, in reasonable agreement with the values in toad urinary bladder epithelium. As pointed out by Finkelstein,[53] this calculation is difficult because P_{dw} is dominated by the series resistance, which makes the estimated true apical membrane diffusive water permeability uncertain. Regardless of these limitations and differences, the conclusion of a value of P_{os}/P_{dw} significantly greater than unity appears to be solid. In conjunction with the exclusion of hydrophilic nonelectrolytes from the pathway, these results suggest that osmotic water flow in ADH-stimulated epithelia is via narrow, single-file pores. If P_{os}/P_{dw} is in fact 17,[78] it would mean that the pore must accommodate 17 water molecules (see equation (11)]. The required dimensions are 50 Å in length and 2 Å in diameter. Arguments to be presented later in this chapter suggest, however, that a simple model of parallel narrow pores does not fully account for the observations.

5.2. Studies of Osmotic Water Permeability of Single Cell Membranes

The difficulties involved in obtaining reliable transepithelial water transport data are overwhelming, as illustrated in the preceding section. Recent technical developments have permitted direct measurements of osmotic water permeability of single cell membranes. In the case of epithelial cells retaining the epithelial architecture, two such methods are available: high-resolution optical techniques[83-87] and electrophysiologic techniques.[88,89] To our knowledge, the latter method has not been applied to ADH-responsive epithelia.

It is generally accepted that the limiting barrier for transepithelial osmotic water flow in ADH-responsive epithelia in the absence of hormone is apical (for review, see Hebert and Andreoli[72]). Transmission electron-microscopic studies[90,91] and light microscopy of living cortical collecting tubules[76] showed that luminal hypotonicity causes cell swelling only in ADH-treated preparations, whereas lowering the osmolality of the bathing solution caused swelling either in the presence or in the absence of the hormone. Furthermore, Schafer et al.[92] found that luminal hypertonicity, which increases junctional permeability, caused a much smaller water flow than the one induced by ADH, although the luminal hypertonicity makes the junctional complexes leaky to urea. This and other results suggest that the ADH-induced increase in P_{os} involves the apical membranes of the principal cells. Although ADH might have a junctional effect, this does not seem to be necessary or sufficient.

The details of the cellular alterations elicited by osmotic water flow in ADH-treated cortical collecting duct have been subject of an interesting recent controversy. Kirk et al.[93] used differential interference contrast microscopy to study isolated rabbit cortical collecting ducts in the absence of ADH and at room temperature. They found that reducing the bath osmolality from 290 to 190 mosM caused rapid swelling that was maintained for at least 20–30 min. The change in cell volume was ca. 90% of that calculated for ideal osmometric behavior. The swelling was due to bulging of the cells into the lumen, with no changes in the outside diameter of the tubule or in the width of the lateral intercellular spaces. Nuclei and mitochondria were swollen. In ADH-treated preparations, reducing the osmolality of the luminal solution to 130 mosM caused lumen-to-bath osmotic water flow, as expected, and also sustained increases in the volume of the cells and the width of the lateral intercellular spaces, by 28 to 78%, respectively.[79] In contrast with the observations in cells swollen by bath hyposmolality, cytoplasmic vacuoles formed slowly during the response to ADH and hypotonic luminal solution and persisted for a long time. The vacuoles, which were observed also in early electron-microscopic studies of cortical[90] and medullary collecting ducts,[94] form only when there is water flow in the absorptive direction. Kirk et al.[79] concluded that the vacuoles are a slowly filling compartment connected with the transepithelial pathway for osmotic water flow and estimated that during maximal ADH stimulation the hydraulic conductivities of the opposing cell membranes are nearly equal. A limitation in their analysis is that they neglected to consider two important complicating factors, namely, the small subepithelial compartment in series with the cell membranes, bounded by basolateral and basement membranes, and the unstirred layers. Cell swelling and cytoplasmic dilution have also been observed in toad urinary bladders treated with ADH and exposed to a dilute luminal solution.[95]

The possibility has been raised that the vacuoles signify the existence of a preferential transcellular water transport pathway which would prevent or limit detrimental dilution of the cytoplasm. In addition, it is possible that cell swelling plays a role in controlling apical membrane water permeability by feedback regulation.[96,97] In contrast with the studies in cortical collecting duct summarized below, in toad urinary bladder optical-sectioning techniques have shown changes in cell volume in response to alterations of luminal osmolality in ADH-treated tissues.[98] Mucosal solution hyperosmolality caused rapid cell shrinkage, which was followed by regulatory volume increase. Surprisingly, the magnitude of the shrinkage was larger than expected for an ideal osmometric response, although the serosal bathing solution was isosmotic. The presence of a thick serosal unstirred layer complicates the interpretation of these results, but the large shrinkage reported is difficult to reconcile with a situation in which both cell membranes have similar osmotic water permeabilities (see Cotton et al.[99]).

Strange and Spring[100,101] used optical-sectioning techniques to measure cell volume changes in rabbit cortical collecting tubules studied at 37°C in a laminar-flow chamber. In contrast with the studies of Kirk et al.,[79] they found virtually no detectable changes in cell volume of principal or intercalated cells after treatment with ADH and exposure to a 130-mosM luminal solution, although the epithelial thickness (i.e., the height of the cells) did increase. Strange and Spring[100,101] calculated that during maximal stimulation with ADH, the cell membrane P_{os} ratio (basolateral : apical) was about 7 (expressed per unit of tubule length, i.e., not corrected for true membrane surface area). This is consistent with the lack of cell swelling because, according to these results, the apical membrane of ADH-stimulated cells remains rate-limiting for osmotic water flow. Strange and Spring concluded that the increase in cell height observed under these experimental conditions is due not to increased cell volume, but to swelling of the lateral intercellular spaces and the space between basal cell membrane and tubule basement membrane. Such a swelling can be explained by the smaller area of basement membrane (compared to basolateral membrane) and its finite hydraulic resistance. The water flowing across the cells accumulates in the subepithelial space, causing a small elevation in hydrostatic pressure which accounts for both water flow across the basement membrane and deformation of the cells. Strange and Spring[101] believe that the "cytoplasmic vacuoles" described in earlier publications are really these extracellular pockets of fluid. Finally, Kirk et al.[93] and Strange and Spring[100] differ also in their observations pertaining to cell volume regulation after swelling by basolateral hypotonicity, although there was a significant difference in experimental conditions. Whereas Strange and Spring observed volume regulatory decrease at 37°C, Kirk et al. saw no regulation at 25°C.

Kirk[102] reexamined the question of vacuole formation by high-resolution differential interference contrast microscopy and by use of a fluorescent probe for basolateral fluid-phase endocytosis. Vacuoles were again observed in principal cells, and to a lesser extent in intercalated cells. They were 1–3 μm in diameter, appeared within 10 min of the ADH/osmotic challenge, and shrank and disappeared within 60–90 min of the onset of the hydrosmotic response, while the preparation was still exposed to ADH and the hyposmotic luminal solution. Kirk argued for the intracellular location of the vacuoles on two grounds: (1) Elimination of the osmotic gradient at the peak of vacuole formation causes very slow collapse, an observation inconsistent with an extracellular location, and (2) during formation, the vacuoles could be loaded with lucifer yellow, which remains trapped for as long as 30 min after dye removal. Kirk concluded that the vacuoles are intracellular and form by endocytosis at the basolateral membrane.

It is difficult to reconcile these two sets of observations, particularly because it is unclear at what time the observations of Strange and Spring[101] were made. Apparently, the measurements were carried out at 1–2 min (as in Strange and Spring[100]). If such were the case, there is no necessary incompatibility of the data pertaining to vacuoles: The phase observed by Strange and Spring could simply precede the one described by Kirk. Perhaps more important from both biophysical and physiologic points of view is whether during stimulation with ADH and P_{os} values of apical and basolateral membranes are nearly equal or differ by a factor of 7. Estimates of P_{os} are extremely difficult with optical techniques, which simply do not have an appropriate time resolution. Application to this problem of the electrophysiologic techniques that we have developed to study isosmotic transport[56,89,99] might prove useful. Table III

Table III. Cell Membrane Osmotic Water Permeability (P_{os}) in ADH-Sensitive and ADH-Insensitive Epithelia[a]

Preparation	Method	$P_{os}/\mu m.sec^{-1}$ Apical	Basolateral	References
TUB	A	0	—	Kachadorian et al.[98]
TUB + ADH	A	210	—	Kachadorian et al.[98]
CCT, PC	A	20	66	Strange and Spring[100b]
CCT, PC + ADH	A	92	74[c]	Strange and Spring[100b]
CCT, IC	A	25	62	Strange and Spring[100b]
CCT, IC + ADH	A	86	61[c]	Strange and Spring[100b]
PT	A	1300[d]	1400–5500	Gonzalez et al.[103,104] Carpi-Medina et al.[105,106]; Welling et al.[85]
NGB	A	600	1200	Persson and Spring[107]
NGB	B	400–640	460–900	Zeuthen[88]; Cotton et al.[99]

[a]TUB = toad urinary bladder. CCT = rabbit cortical collecting duct. PT = rabbit proximal tubule. NGB = *Necturus* gallbladder. PC = principal cell. IC = interrelated cell. ADH = antidiuretic hormone. Methods of cell volume measurements were optical (A) or electrophysiologic (B). Values are rounded means.
[b]The values of Strange and Spring were corrected for the true membrane surface area.
[c]Tubule lumen filled with oil.
[d]Tubule immersed in oil bath.

summarizes the results of measurements of cell membrane P_{os} in both ADH-sensitive and ADH-insensitive epithelia.

5.3. The Pathway for Water Permeation

Chevalier et al.[108] made the crucial observation that in frog urinary bladder, treatment with oxytocin resulted in appearance of intramembrane particle (IMP) aggregates in the apical membrane, identified by freeze-fracture electron microscopy. This result was confirmed and extended by several groups of investigators. Kachadorian et al.[109] pointed out that the particle aggregates have distinct organization and occur in antidiuretic hormone–stimulated toad urinary bladder epithelium, but not in unstimulated preparations. Kachadorian and associates[110] also showed that the area density of aggregates correlates well with the osmotic water permeability, an observation that has been confirmed repeatedly (for review, see Wade[111]). Brown et al.[112] showed the appearance of aggregates in hormone-treated toad skin, nd Harmanci et al.[113] found them in mammalian collecting tubule. Taken together, these results support the notion that the aggregates are the sites of water permeation. On the basis of a freeze-fracture study combined with chemical labeling, Chevalier et al.[114] suggested that the IMPs are glycoproteins.

Later, it was shown that particles indistinguishable from those seen in the apical membrane of ADH-stimulated cells are present in cytoplasmic tubular structures.[115,116] These tubules, which can be studied by specialized electron-microscopic techniques, fuse with the apical membrane upon stimulation with ADH, and the number of fusion events correlates with the number of aggregates transferred to the apical membrane.[117] The fusion has also been demonstrated by measurements of the apical membrane electrical capacitance, which increases by 10–30% (depending on the experimental conditions) with ADH stimulation.[118–121] This measurement is perhaps the most reliable indication of a sizable increase in effective apical membrane area during ADH stimulation, which constitutes an important argument pertaining to the location of the water transport sites (see below).

The ADH-induced fusion has been exhaustively studied in recent years. The likely sequence of events has been very well summarized in the excellent review by Hays et al.[122]

In the resting cell, the tubules, identified by transmission, scanning, and freeze-fracture electron microscopy, have a diameter of ca. 0.1 µm and a length of ca. 0.9 µm. They are positioned in most cases near the apical membrane, parallel to its surface.[123] Their ends are shaped as segments of sphere and coated with clathrin. The particles in the tubule wall are arranged in helical arrays. Finally, the sides of the tubules exhibit protuberances, which may correspond to fusing or exiting vesicles. Filaments connect the ends and sides of the tubules to the cytoskeleton. It is possible that these connections play roles in both anchoring and motility of the tubules.

With ADH stimulation, tubule fusion and appearance of aggregates in the apical membrane are evident by about 2.5 min. Maxima for both number of aggregates and osmotic water flow are reached in about 20 min.[124] In response to ADH stimulation, the tubules tilt upward, especially when they are located in the middle level of the apical region of the cell. The basal anchorage, via microfilaments, is retained during fusion.[123] Labeling experiments with horseradish peroxidase and colloidal gold suggest that during the action of ADH there is a dynamic process of fusion and detachment.[117,125−127] This is certainly the case in the presence of an osmotic gradient. The individual cycles probably last 15 min or less.[128] After ADH removal, the label is transferred from the tubules to multivesicular bodies and other vesicles.[117,129] Other tubules appear to return to the "resting," horizontal position, becoming available for the next ADH-induced fusion cycle.

Regardless of these major developments, as pointed out by Hays et al.,[122] a number of questions remain, including the duration of fusion events; the number of aggregates delivered per individual fusion; the mechanisms of tubule fusion and detachment; the rates of generation, disappearance, and reutilization of tubules; the tubular "reserve" and supply; and the mechanisms of tubule motion. Needless to say, these are questions at the very core of some of the major current unresolved problems in cell biology.

The question of whether the IMP aggregates suffice to account for the P_{os} elicited by ADH in toad urinary bladder epithelium has been the subject of interesting quantitative analyses by Wade[111,130] and by Levine et al.[78,80] (see also Finkelstein[53]). The essential question is whether water transport takes place via the aggregates in the apical membrane alone or via these and those contained in the tubules as well. The latter possibility raises the interesting issue of a dual barrier to water transport, namely, the tubule length, which would constitute the equivalent of an unstirred layer, and the pores themselves. We summarize here the calculation outlined by Levine et al.[78] Assuming that all the water-transporting pores are in the apical surface, the area of membrane available for each pore can be calculated from the apical membrane P_{os} during ADH ($5 \cdot 10^{-2}$ cm/sec, Levine et al.[80]) and the density of aggregates ($10^8/cm^2$, Kachadorian et al.[131]). It follows that the P_{os} per aggregate is $5 \cdot 10^{-10}$ cm³/sec. Assuming a P_{os}/pore equal to that of the gramicidin channel ($3 \cdot 10^{-14}$ cm³/sec), the number of water pores per aggregate is $2 \cdot 10^4$, and since the area of membrane occupied per aggregate is 10^{-2} μm² (Kachadorian et al.[110]), the area available for each pore is 50 Å², which means a center-to-center distance of 8 Å. Since the inside diameter of the pore is 4 Å, the wall thickness would be less than 2 Å, which is unrealistic.

The total area of aggregates in the apical membrane is insufficient to account for P_{os} on the basis of pores in parallel, but the area could be sufficient if a series-parallel model is assumed, such as the "showerhead" model described by Levine et al.[78] The model divides the pore in two segments in series: a long, wide channel (stem) in series with an arrangement of numerous short and narrow single-file pores (contained in the cap). Possible dimensions are as follows: for the stem: length = 50 Å, radius = 20 Å, and for the cap: radius = 200 Å, number of pores = 500, pore radius = 2 Å. Six showerheads fit in the area of one aggregate. The model is conceptually similar to the dual-barrier hypothesis proposed about 30 years ago.[61,69,132]

An alternative possibility to account for the discrepancy between measured P_{os}

and apical membrane aggregate area is that the aggregates in the fused tubules contribute to water permeation. In a way, the wall of these tubules, because of the fusion process, is a functional part of the apical membrane and in principle can contribute significantly to the apical membrane P_{os} because of the high density of aggregates. The magnitude of the change in membrane capacitance suggests that a large number of tubules effectively communicate with the mucosal compartment at any time during the action of ADH. Including fused tubules, Wade[111] estimates the total area of aggregates to correspond to at least 5% of the total apical membrane area, a fraction adequate to account fully for the P_{os} value in ADH. In contrast with the surface membrane, the tubule carries with it a series resistance to diffusion, i.e., the tubule lumen. Therefore, P_{os}/P_{dw} will have a high value (greater than unity) for the entire membrane (or the tissue) even if for the single pore the value of the ratio is unity.[78]

This picture is complicated further by recent observations indicating a high frequency of fusion events in unstimulated toad and frog urinary bladders.[133] It was observed that in the absence of ADH fusion, images are smaller and that the hormone increases not only the number of fusions but also their size.

6. Role of the Cytoskeleton and Modulation of the Hydrosmotic Effect of ADH

It has been proposed that the transfer of cytoplasmic aggregates to the apical membrane may be a quantal process analogous to the exocytosis characteristic of stimulus–secretion coupling observed in many different types of cells.[134] In each case, fusion of intracellular vesicles or granules with the plasma membrane and consequent release of the intravesicular contents has been reported. Similarly, the ADH-induced increase in water permeability is accompanied by exocytosis. Masur et al.[135,136] and Gronowicz et al.[125] suggested a role for exocytosis in the effect of ADH on toad urinary bladder epithelium based on three sets of observations: (1) "omega figures" resulting from fusion of intracellular granules with the apical membrane, (2) depletion of subapical granules and the appearance of their contents (glycoproteins) on the apical surface, and (3) a net addition of membrane to the apical surface. Endocytosis, occurring later in the hydrosmotic response, was demonstrated by the presence of horseradish peroxidase (HRP), a fluid-phase marker, in cytoplasmic vesicles of cells exposed to HRP on the apical side during ADH treatment.[125] Additional evidence for endocytosis was the decrease in apical membrane surface area (compared to the ADH-induced increase) after the eventual reversal of the ADH-induced increase in water permeability.

Microtubules and microfilaments play a crucial role in exo- and endocytosis, probably by facilitating interactions between the membranes of the cytoplasmic structures functioning as reservoirs of transporters, on one hand, and the apical membrane, on the other. The reservoirs in this case contain packed membrane transporters, instead of secretory products. An interesting observation consistent with this view is that in toad skin basolateral depolarization elicited by raising the K^+ concentration of the external solution produces both the appearance of apical membrane IMPs and an increase in P_{os}.

There is abundant evidence for a major role of the cytoskeleton in the processes of insertion and removal of aggregates and also in modulating the hydrosmotic effect of ADH, but the details of the links between the changes in water permeability, the observed membrane fusion and retrieval, and the role of the cytoskeleton are not completely understood. In fact, these relationships are strongly suggested by available results, but direct proof of cause–effect relationships is still lacking. A role for the cytoskeleton in the action of ADH was initially proposed by Taylor et al.[137] and supported by observations from a number of laboratories (for reviews, see De Sousa,[134] Pearl and Taylor,[19] Wade,[111] and Hays et al.[122]). Drugs active on microtubules (colchicine, vincristine) or microfilaments (cytochalasins) decrease water flow stimulated by ADH, without effects on Na^+ transport. In addition, colchicine and methohexital inhibit the increase in capacitance elicited by ADH.[119,120] As pointed out by Wade,[111] the interpretation of these results is somewhat complicated because colchicine has effects on prostaglandin synthesis,[138] which is certain to have a modulatory role on the hydrosmotic effect of ADH (see above). Furthermore, with both colchicine and cytochalasin B the number of aggregates and the membrane capacitance are decreased, but the latter agent does not reduce fusion events, which suggests an effect at a step distal to the fusion. These observations suggest that the role of the cytoskeleton in mediating and/or modulating the action of ADH is complicated.

The cytoskeleton is a highly cross-linked structure. Intracellular pCa and pH, and possibly other factors, control gel–sol transitions (the gel state being characteristic of a high degree of cross-linking). Ausiello and Hartwig[139] have hypothesized that ADH, via generation of cAMP and activation of protein kinase, produces phosphorylation of actin-binding protein, which ultimately causes a reduction in cross-linking of the cortical actin network. A concomitant elevation of intracellular calcium activates villin (an actin-severing protein), with the same end effect, causing morphologic alterations of the apical region of the ADH-responsive cells. The literature pertaining to the cytoskeletal aspects of the action of ADH has been reviewed in detail by Ausiello et al.[140] In the presence of ADH, an osmotic gradient from mucosa to serosa produces cell swelling and radical changes in shape and cytoskeletal structure, which are reversible and do not damage organelles. The cell acquires an "ice cream cone" shape by bulging of the apical membrane, which has been interpreted as a local gel–sol transformation.[139,141] DiBona[142] showed that with ADH the distribution of actin, assessed with the fluorescent probe NBD-phallacidin, changes. This accompanies the change in cell shape. In contrast, if a similar degree of swelling is elicited by serosal hypotonicity, there is organelle damage.[143,144] The difference has been taken to indicate that the hormonal effect and/or the pattern of absorptive water flow alter specifically the apical cytoskeleton and cause a different kind of "dilution" of the cytoplasm.

Cytochalasin B inhibits the effect of ADH,[145,146] but has no effect on cell geometry in the absence of an osmotic gradient. If the tissue is pretreated with ADH and then fixed with glutaraldehyde before the osmotic gradient is imposed, cytochalasin B has no effect on water flow.[147] Cytochalasin B also alters the number of aggregates, but this has been only shown to occur in the presence of an osmotic gradient.[148] There is, therefore, a strong possibility that the apical cytoskeleton has a role in the hydrosmotic response to ADH independent of the effect of the hormone on the apical membrane P_{os}. DiBona[142] has concluded that swelling requires cytoskeletal alterations which cause low-resistance pathways for water flow across the cytoplasm. Such pathways have not been identified optically in living tissues.[79,144,149,150]

In summary, a working hypothesis is that in ADH-sensitive cells in the unstimulated state the apical cytoskeleton is a resistive barrier to water flow because of an extensively cross-linked actin network. With ADH, cross-linking decreases, fragmenting and shortening proteins are activated, a gel–sol transition takes place, and the water flow is allowed. The necessary proteins exist in apical regions of toad urinary bladder and cortical collecting duct cells.[140] In cortical collecting duct during ADH-induced water flow there is swelling of the principal cells, with apical rounding and widening of the lateral intercellular spaces.[79] The changes in morphology of the cell surface are also similar to those in toad urinary bladder epithelium.[151–153]

Several authors[154–156] have shown that microtubules and microfilaments can act as rails for intracellular motion of organelles by ATP-dependent processes. Microtubules and microfilaments are present in the terminal web of toad bladder granular cells,[117,146] but no direct evidence for a role of this mechanism in insertion or removal of aggregates is available in ADH-sensitive preparations.

Finally, there is good evidence that the fall of the hydrosmotic response to ADH is mediated at least in part by removal of the aggregates by endocytosis, which is also a process mediated by cytoskeletal elements. The rate of dissipation of the ADH-induced increase in water permeability is faster in tissues subjected to a transepithelial osmotic gradient than in tissues in which the solutions on both sides of the epithelium are of equal osmolality. Masur *et al.*[127] demonstrated with a double-label technique (HRP and ruthenium red) that endocytosis was ~6-fold greater in tissues exposed to such osmotic gradient. Exposure of the apical membrane of toad urinary bladder to cationized ferritin (but not to neutral ferritin) significantly attenuated the ADH-induced osmotic water flow and stimulated endocytosis. Furthermore, maneuvers that inhibit endocytosis (low temperature, fixation with glutaraldehyde, and treatment with metabolic inhibitors) prevented inhibition of the ADH-induced hydrosmotic response by cationized ferritin.[157] In a recent report, a method for the selective isolation of endocytic vesicles after ADH stimulation was described.[158] This approach offers great promise toward the goal of isolation of the membranes that may contain the ADH-responsive water permeability pathway. Verkman *et al.*[159] injected the volume-marker 6-carboxy-fluorescein (6CF) in rats with genetic diabetes insipidus. The 6CF was taken up by apical endocytosis in the collecting duct, the endocytic vesicles were separated by differential centrifugation, and the fluorescence quenching could be used to measure changes in vesicle volume upon imposition of osmotic gradients. In vesicles obtained from renal papilla, ADH caused a distinct change in the kinetics of osmotic shrinkage. A fast component was found only in vesicles obtained from ADH-treated animals, which on the bases of its temperature dependence and the value of P_{os} could be ascribed to the presence of water pores. In renal cortex, no measurable effect of ADH was found, as expected from the predominant content of ADH-insensitive proximal tubules in this region.

7.　Other Barriers to Osmotic Water Flow

In the toad urinary bladder, the surface density of luminal membrane aggregates correlates well with the hydrosmotic response to ADH. However, the relationship is curvilinear, i.e., saturating, suggesting a resistance to water flow in series with the apical membrane. This series resistance can become rate limiting during ADH action.[160] As summarized by Kachadorian,[161] the major arguments are the following: First, within 30 min of exposure to ADH, the osmotic water flow falls, but the number of aggregates is unchanged. Second, when naproxen, an inhibitor of prostaglandin synthesis, is employed, osmotic water flow (control or ADH-induced) is less than expected for the measured number of aggregates. By itself, naproxen caused increases in both transepithelial P_{os} and number of apical membrane aggregates.[98] Third, the increase in apical membrane P_{os} caused by treatment with both naproxen and ADH, and measured with an optical-sectioning technique, is not different from that with ADH alone.[98] Kachadorian has interpreted these discrepancies between apical membrane and transepithelial permeabilities to be due to the presence of a series barrier to water permeation, which would become apparent when apical P_{os} is massively increased by ADH. Reducing the osmolality of the serosal solution bathing toad urinary bladders fixed with glutaraldehyde results in a reversible decrease in the hydraulic resistance in series with the apical membrane. This technique seems to be excellent to assess sites of action of drugs and modulators of osmotic water flow.[162] Similar conclusions have been made for mammalian cortical collecting duct.[76,82,163] These authors have expressed this factor as a diffusion constraint factor. Finally, Levine et al.,[80] comparing P_{dw} and hexanol permeability in ADH-treated toad urinary bladder, have suggested an intracellular restriction to water diffusion, perhaps due to close packing of intracellular organelles.

8.　Remaining Questions and Future Directions

In spite of the significant recent progress in understanding the mechanisms of transepithelial osmotic water flow and of the hydrosmotic effect of ADH, it is clear that many questions remain unanswered. We wish to end this review by pointing out areas in which concentrated research efforts would be fruitful. One such area pertains to the biochemistry and cell biology of the action of ADH. It is essential to study further the regulation of the number and properties of ADH receptors, to ascertain the biochemical steps distal to the activation of cAMP-dependent protein kinases, and to elucidate the roles of endogenous modulators of ADH actions, such as Ca^{2+}, calmodulin, protein kinase C, and others. The role of the cytoskeleton in regulation of transepithelial water flow also needs further study. Understanding the processes of membrane fusion, membrane retrieval, and intracellular motility seems necessary in order to understand the mechanism of action of ADH. As pointed out earlier, such problems are at the cutting edge of our knowledge of cell function. Finally, it is clear that a complete reduction of the problem of epithelial water transport to chemical and physical concepts will ultimately require a molecular approach. Further biophysical characterization of the water transport pathway is necessary to gain insight into its mode of operation. Electrophysiologic techniques should help in this regard, and the use of fixatives such as glutaraldehyde is also a powerful tool to dissect out mechanistic events in the action of ADH. In addition, efforts at purifying the transport pathway are necessary to understand its function at a molecular level. To this end, isolation, sequencing, and reconstitution of the putative pores must eventually be accomplished. Current efforts in their purification[158] and in attempting to raise specific antibodies[164] are highly promising.

ACKNOWLEDGMENTS. We thank Guillermo A. Altenberg, Yoav Segal, and James S. Stoddard for their suggestions on a preliminary version of this chapter and Ann L. Pearce and Olwen H. Hooks for secretarial help. Studies from the authors' laboratory were supported by NIH grant DK38588.

References

1. Reuss, L. and Cotton, C. U., 1987, Isosmotic fluid transport across epithelia, in: *Contemporary Nephrology*, Volume 4 (S. Klahr and S. G. Massry, eds.), Plenum, New York, pp. 1–37.
2. Sawyer, W. H. and Manning, M., 1973, Synthetic analogs of oxytocin and the vasopressins, *Annu. Rev. Pharmacol.* **13**:5–17.
3. Sawyer, W. H. and Manning, M., 1985, The use of antagonists of vasopressin in studies of its physiological functions, *Fed. Proc.* **44**:78–80.
4. Mann, W. A., Stassen, F., Huffman, W., and Kinter, L. B., 1986, Mechanism of action and structural requirements of vasopressin analog inhibition of transepithelial water flux in toad urinary bladder, *J. Pharmacol. Exp. Ther.* **238**:401–406.
5. Eggena, P., Ma, C. L., Fahrenholz, F., Buku, A., and Schwartz, I. L., 1985, Action of photoreactive analogs of vasopressin in toad bladder, *Biol. Cell* **55**:231–238.
6. Kirk, K. L., Buku, A., and Eggena, P., 1987, Cell specificity of vasopressin binding in renal collecting duct: Computer-enhanced imaging of a fluorescent hormone analog, *Proc. Natl. Acad. Sci. USA* **84**:6000–6004.
7. Orloff, J. and Handler, J. S., 1962, The similarity of effects of vasopressin, adenosine-3′,5′-phosphate (cyclic AMP) and theophylline on the toad bladder, *J. Clin. Invest.* **41**:702–709.
8. Handler, J. S., Butcher, R. W., Sutherland, E. W., and Orloff, J., 1965, The effect of vasopressin

and of theophylline on the concentration of adenosine 3′,5′-phosphate in the urinary bladder of the toad, *J. Biol. Chem.* **240**:4524–4526.

9. Grantham, J. J. and Burg, M. B., 1966, Effect of vasopressin and cyclic AMP on permeability of isolated collecting tubules, *Am. J. Physiol.* **211**:255–259.

10. Imbert, M., Chabardes, D., Montegut, M., Clique, A., and Morel, F., 1975, Vasopressin dependent adenylate cyclase in single segments of rabbit kidney tubule, *Pflügers Arch. Eur. J. Physiol.* **357**:173–186.

11. Hall, D. A. and Varney, D. M., 1980, Effect of vasopressin on electrical potential difference and chloride transport in mouse medullary thick ascending limb of Henle's loop, *J. Clin. Invest.* **66**:792–802.

12. Hebert, S. C., Culpepper, R. M., and Andreoli, T. E., 1981, NaCl transport in mouse medullary thick ascending limbs. I. Functional nephron heterogeneity and ADH-stimulated NaCl cotransport, *Am. J. Physiol.* **241**:F412–F431.

13. DeSousa, R. C. and Grosso, A., 1985, Forskolin mimics the hydrosmotic action of vasopressin in the urinary bladder of toads *Bufo marinus, J. Physiol. (London)* **365**:307–318.

14. Dousa, T. P. and Barnes, L. D., 1977, Regulation of protein kinase by vasopressin in renal medulla in situ, *Am. J. Physiol.* **232**:F50–F57.

15. Schlondorff, D. and Franki, N., 1980, Effect of vasopressin on cyclic AMP-dependent protein kinase in toad urinary bladder, *Biochim. Biophys. Acta* **628**:1–12.

16. DeLorenzo, R. J., Walton, K. G., Curran, P. F., and Greengard, P., 1973, Regulation of phosphorylation of a specific protein in toad-bladder membrane by antidiuretic hormone and cyclic AMP, and its possible relationship to membrane permeability changes, *Proc. Natl. Acad. Sci. USA* **70**:880–884.

17. Ferguson, D. R. and Twite, B. R., 1974, Effects of vasopressin on toad bladder membrane proteins: Relationship to transport of sodium and water, *J. Endocr.* **64**:501–507.

18. Shimada, H., Mishina, T., and Marumo, F., 1983, Effects of guanine nucleotides on vasopressin-induced water flow and sodium transport of the frog bladder, *Pflügers Arch. Eur. J. Physiol.* **397**:169–175.

19. Pearl, M. and Taylor, A., 1985, Role of the cytoskeleton in the control of transcellular water flow by vasopressin in amphibian urinary bladder, *Biol. Cell* **55**:163–172.

20. Bentley, P. J., 1959, The effects of ionic changes on water transfer across the isolated urinary bladder of the toad *Bufo marinus, J. Endocr.* **18**:327–333.

21. Lorenzen, M., Frindt, G., Taylor, A., and Windhager, E. E., 1987, Quinidine effect on hydrosmotic response of collecting tubules to vasopressin and cAMP, *Am. J. Physiol.* **252**:F1103–F1111.

22. Taylor, A., Eich, E., Pearl, M., Brem, A. S., and Peeper, E. Q., 1987, Cytosolic calcium and the action of vasopressin in toad urinary bladder, *Am. J. Physiol.* **252**:F1028–F1041.

23. Taylor, A., Pearl, M., and Crutch, B., 1985, Role of cytosolic free calcium and its measurement in a vasopressin-sensitive epithelium, *Mol. Physiol.* **8**:43–58.

24. Ausiello, D. A. and Hall, D., 1981, Regulation of vasopressin-sensitive adenylate cyclase by calmodulin, *J. Biol. Chem.* **256**:9796–9798.

25. Tsien, R. Y., 1983, Intracellular measurements of ion activities, *Annu. Rev. Biophys. Bioeng.* **12**:91–116.

26. Grosso, A., Cox, J. A., Malnoe, A., and DeSousa, R. C., 1982, Evidence for a role of calmodulin in the hydrosmotic action of vasopressin in toad bladder, *J. Physiol. (Paris)* **78**:270–278.

27. Dillingham, M. A., Dixon, B. S., Kim, J. K., and Wilson, P. D., 1986, Effect of trifluoperazine on rabbit cortical collecting tubular response to vasopressin, *J. Physiol. (London)* **372**:41–50.

28. Roufogalis, B. D., 1986, Calmodulin antagonism, in: *Calcium and Cell Physiology* (D. Marme, ed.), Springer-Verlag, Berlin, pp. 148–169.

29. Masur, S. K., Sapirstein, V., and Rivero, D., 1985, Phorbol myristate acetate induces endocytosis as well as exocytosis and hydrosmosis in toad urinary bladder, *Biochim. Biophys. Acta* **821**:286–296.

30. Schlondorff, D. and Levine, S. D., 1985, Inhibition of vasopressin-stimulated water flow in toad bladder by phorbol myristate acetate, dioctanoylglycerol, and RHC-80267, *J. Clin. Invest.* **76**:1071–1078.

31. Grantham, J. and Orloff, J., 1968, Effect of prostaglandin E_1 on the permeability response of the isolated collecting tubule to vasopressin, adenosine 3',5'-monophosphate, and theophylline, *J. Clin. Invest.* **47**:1154–1161.

32. Orloff, J., Handler, J. S., and Bergstrom, S., 1965, Effects of prostaglandin (PGE_1) on the permeability response of toad bladder to vasopressin, theophylline and adenosine 3',5'-monophosphate, *Nature* **205**:397–398.

33. Lipson, L. C. and Sharp, G. W. G., 1971, Effect of prostaglandin E_1 on sodium transport and osmotic water flow in the toad bladder, *Am. J. Physiol.* **220**:1046–1052.

34. Flores, A. G. A. and Sharp, G. W. G., 1972, Endogenous prostaglandins and osmotic water flow in the toad bladder, *Am. J. Physiol.* **223**:1392–1397.

35. Omachi, R. S., Robbie, D. E., Handler, J. S., and Orloff, J., 1974, Effects of ADH and other agents on cyclic AMP accumulation in toad bladder epithelium, *Am. J. Physiol.* **226**:1152–1157.

36. Janszen, F. H. A. and Nugteren, D. H., 1971, Histochemical localisation of prostaglandin synthetase, *Histochemie* **27**:159–164.

37. Muirhead, E. E., Germain, G., Leach, B. E., Pitcock, J. A., Stephenson, P., Brooks, B., Brosius, W. L., Daniels, E. G., and Hinman, J. W., 1972, Production of renomedullary prostaglandins by renomedullary interstitial cells in tissue culture, *Circ. Res.* **30/31** (Suppl. II):161–172.

38. Zusman, R. M. and Keiser, H. R., 1977, Prostaglandin biosynthesis by rabbit renomedullary interstitial cells in tissue culture: Stimulation by angiotension II, bradykinin, and arginine vasopressin, *J. Clin. Invest.* **60**:215–223.

39. Zusman, R. M., Keiser, H. R., and Handler, J. S., 1977, Vasopressin-stimulated water permeability in the toad urinary bladder: Role of endogenous prostaglandin E biosynthesis, *Fed. Proc.* **36**:631.

40. Anderson, R. S., Berl, T., McDonald, K. M., and Schrier, R. S., 1975, Evidence for an in vivo antagonism between vasopressin and prostaglandin in the mammalian kidney. *J. Clin. Invest.* **56**:420–426.

41. Lum, G. M., Aisenbrey, G. A., Dunn, M. J., Berl, T., Schrier, R. S., and McDonald, K. M., 1977, *In vivo* effect of indomethacin to potentiate the renal medullary cyclic AMP response to vasopressin. *J. Clin. Invest.* **59**:8.

42. Berl, T., Raz, A., Wald, H., Horowitz, J., and Czaczkes, A., 1977, Prostaglandin synthesis inhibition and the action of vasopressin: Studies in man and rat, *Am. J. Physiol.* **232**:F529–F537.

43. Levine, S. D., Levine, R. D., Worthington, R. E., and Hays, R. M., 1976, Selective inhibition of osmotic water flow by general anesthetics in toad urinary bladder, *J. Clin. Invest.* **58**:980–988.

44. Hays, R. M., Franki, N., and Ross, L. S., 1979, Effect of metabolic inhibitors on vasopressin-stimulated transport systems in the toad bladder, *J. Supramol. Struct.* **10**:175–184.

45. Orloff, J. and Zusman, R., 1978, Role of prostaglandin E (PGE) in the modulation of the action of vasopressin in water flow in the urinary bladder of the toad and mammalian kidney, *J. Membr. Biol.* **40**:297–304.

46. Dillingham, M. A. and Anderson, R. J., 1986, Inhibition of vasopressin action by atrial natriuretic factor, *Science* **231**:1572–1573.

47. Svelto, M. and Lippe, C., 1978, Colchicine inhibition of ADH effect on frog skin permeability, *Experientia* **34**:360–361.

48. DeSousa, R. C., Grosso, A., and Rufener, C., 1974, Blockade of the hydrosmotic effect of vasopressin by cytochalasin B, *Experientia* **30**:175–177.

49. Eggena, P., 1983, Effect of glutaraldehyde on hydrosmotic response of toad bladder to vasopressin, *Am. J. Physiol.* **244**:C37–C43.

50. Mendoza, S. and Thomas, M. W., 1982, Effect of monensin on osmotic water flow across the toad bladder and its stimulation by vasopressin and cyclic AMP, *J. Membr. Biol.* **67**:99–102.

51. Hoch, B. S., Ast, M. B., Fusco, M. J., Jacoby, M., and Levine, S. D., 1988, Protein synthesis inhibitors attenuate water flow in vasopressin-stimulated toad urinary bladder, *Am. J. Physiol.* **254**:F139–F144.

52. DeSousa, R. C. and Grosso, A., 1979, Vanadate blocks cyclic AMP-induced stimulation of sodium and water transport in amphibian epithelia, *Nature (London)* **279**:803–804.

53. Finkelstein, A., 1986, *Water Movements through Lipid Bilayers, Pores and Plasma Membranes: Theory and Reality,* Wiley, New York.

54. Bean, C. P., 1972, The physics of porous membranes-Neutral pores, in: *Membranes I. Macroscopic Systems and Models* (G. Eisenman, ed.), Dekker, New York, pp. 1–54.

55. Levitt, D. G., 1973, Kinetics of diffusion and convection in 3-Å pores. Exact solution by computer simulation, *Biophys. J.* **13:**186–206.

56. Cotton, C. U. and Reuss, L., 1989, Measurement of the effective thickness of the mucosal unstirred layer in *Necturus* gallbladder epithelium, *J. Gen. Physiol.* **93:** 631–647.

57. Barry, P. H. and Diamond, J. M., 1984, Effects of unstirred layers on membrane phenomena, *Physiol. Rev.* **64:**763–873.

58. Diamond, J. M., 1979, Osmotic water flow in leaky epithelia, *J. Membr. Biol.* **51:**195–216.

59. Koefoed-Johnson, V. and Ussing, H. H., 1953, The contributions of diffusion and flow to the passage of D_2O through living membranes. Effects of neurohypophyseal hormone on isolated anuran skin, *Acta Physiol. Scand.* **28:**60–76.

60. Hays, R. M. and Leaf, A., 1962, Studies on the movement of water through the isolated toad bladder and its modification by vasopressin, *J. Gen. Physiol.* **45:**905–919.

61. Andersen, B. and Ussing, H. H., 1957, Solvent drag on non-electrolytes during osmotic flow through isolated toad skin and its response to antidiuretic hormone, *Acta Physiol. Scand.* **39:**228–239.

62. Dainty, J., 1963, Water relations of plant cells, *Adv. Botan. Res.* **1:**279–326.

63. Dainty, J. and House, C. R., 1966, An examination of the evidence for membrane pores in frog skin, *J. Physiol.* **185:**172–184.

64. Hays, R. M. and Franki, N., 1970, The role of water diffusion in the action of vasopressin, *J. Membr. Biol.* **2:**263–276.

65. Schafer, J. A., Troutman, S. L., and Andreoli, T. E., 1974, Osmosis in cortical collecting tubules, ADH-independent osmotic flow rectification, *J. Gen. Physiol.* **64:**228–240.

66. Pietras, R. J. and Wright, E. M., 1975, The membrane action of antidiuretic hormone (ADH) on toad urinary bladder, *J. Membr. Biol.* **22:**107–123.

67. Finkelstein, A., 1976, Water and nonelectrolyte permeability of lipid bilayer membranes, *J. Gen. Physiol.* **68:**127–135.

68. Finkelstein, A., 1976, Nature of the water permeability increase induced by antidiuretic hormone (ADH) in toad urinary bladder and related tissues, *J. Gen. Physiol.* **68:**137–143.

69. Leaf, A. and Hays, R. M., 1962, Permeability of the isolated toad bladder to solutes and its modification by vasopressin, *J. Gen. Physiol.* **45:**921–932.

70. Levine, S., Franki, N., and Hays, R. M., 1973, Effect of phloretin on water and solute movement in the toad bladder, *J. Clin. Invest.* **52:**1435–1442.

71. Grantham, J. J. and Burg, M. B., 1966, Effect of vasopressin and cyclic AMP on permeability of isolated collecting tubules, *Am. J. Physiol.* **211:**255–259.

72. Hebert, S. C. and Andreoli, T. E., 1985, Water transport and osmoregulation by terminal nephron segments, in: *The Kidney: Physiology and Pathophysiology,* (G. Giebisch, ed.), Raven, New York, pp. 933–949.

73. Finkelstein, A. and Rosenberg, P. A., 1979, Single-file transport: Implications for ion and water movement through gramidicin A channels, in: *Membrane Transport Processes,* Volume 3 (C. F. Stevens and R. W. Tsien, eds.), Raven Press, New York, pp. 73–88.

74. Gluck, S. and Al-Awqati, Q., 1980, Vasopressin increases water permeability by inducing pores, *Nature (London)* **284:**631–632.

75. Parisi, M., Wietzerbin, J., and Bourguet, J., 1983, Intracellular pH, transepithelial pH gradients and ADH-induced water channels, *Am. J. Physiol.* **244:**F712–F718.

76. Schafer, J. A. and Andreoli, T. E., 1972, Cellular constraints to diffusion. The effect of antidiuretic hormone on water flows in isolated mammalian collecting ducts, *J. Clin. Invest.* **51:**1264–1278.

77. Parisi, M. and Bourguet, J., 1983, The single file hypothesis and the water channels induced by antidiuretic hormone, *J. Membr. Biol.* **71:**189–193.

78. Levine, S. D., Jacoby, M., and Finkelstein, A., 1984, The water permeability of toad urinary bladder. II. The value of $P_f/P_{d(w)}$ for the antidiuretic hormone-induced water permeation pathway, *J. Gen. Physiol.* **83:**543–562.

79. Kirk, K. L., Schafer, J. A., and DiBona, D. R., 1984, Quantitative analysis of the structural events associated with antidiuretic hormone-induced volume reabsorption in the rabbit cortical collecting tubule, *J. Membr. Biol.* **79:**65–74.

80. Levine, S. D., Jacoby, M., and Finkelstein, A., 1984, The water permeability of toad urinary bladder. I. Permeability of barriers in series with the luminal membrane, *J. Gen. Physiol.* **83:**529–542.

81. Parisi, M., Merot, J., and Bourguet, J., 1985, Glutaraldehyde fixation preserves the permeability properties of the ADH-induced water channels, *J. Membr. Biol.* **86:**239–245.

82. Hebert, S. C. and Andreoli, T. E., 1980, Interactions of temperature and ADH on transport in cortical collecting tubules, *Am. J. Physiol.* **238:**F470–F480.

83. DiBona, D. R., Kirk, K. L., and Johnson, R. D., 1985, Microscopic investigation of structure and function in living epithelial tissues, *Fed. Proc.* **44:**2693–2703.

84. Spring, K. R., 1985, The study of epithelial function by quantitative light microscopy, *Pflügers Arch. Eur. J. Physiol.* **405:**S23–S27.

85. Welling, L. W., Welling, D. J., and Ochs, T. J., 1983, Video measurement of basolateral membrane hydraulic conductivity in the proximal tubule, *Am. J. Physiol.* **245:**F123–F129.

86. Whittembury, G., Lindemann, B., Carpi-Medina, P., González, E., and Linares, H., 1986, Continuous measurements of cell volume changes in single kidney tubules, *Kidney Int.* **30:**187–191.

87. Strange, K. and Spring, K. R., 1986, Methods for imaging renal tubule cells, *Kidney Int.* **30:**192–200.

88. Zeuthen, T., 1982, Relations between intracellular ion activities and extracellular osmolarity in *Necturus* gallbladder epithelium, *J. Membr. Biol.* **66:**109–121.

89. Reuss, L., 1985, Changes in cell volume measured with an electrophysiologic technique, *Proc. Natl. Acad. Sci. USA* **82:**6014–6018.

90. Ganote, C. E., Grantham, J. J., Mores, H. L., Burg, M. B., and Orloff, J., 1968, Ultrastructural studies of vasopressin effect on isolated perfused renal collecting tubules of the rabbit, *J. Cell Biol.* **36:**355–367.

91. Grantham, J. J., Ganote, C. E., Burg, M. B., and Orloff, J., 1968, Paths of transtubular water flow in isolated renal collecting tubules, *J. Cell Biol.* **41:**562–576.

92. Schafer, J. A., Troutman, S. L., and Andreoli, T. E., 1974, Osmosis in cortical collecting tubules. ADH-independent osmotic flow rectification, *J. Gen. Physiol.* **64:**228–240.

93. Kirk, K. L., DiBona, D. R., and Schafer, J. A., 1984, Morphologic response of the rabbit cortical collecting tubule to peritubular hypotonicity: Quantitative examination with differential interference contrast microscopy, *J. Membr. Biol.* **79:**53–64.

94. Tisher, C. C., Bulger, R. E., and Valtin, H., 1971, Morphology of renal medulla in water diuresis and vasopressin-induced antidiuresis, *Am. J. Physiol.* **220:**87–94.

95. Rick, R. and DiBona, D. R., 1987, Intracellular solute gradients during osmotic water flow: An electron-microprobe analysis, *J. Membr. Biol.* **96:**85–94.

96. Eggena, P., Christakis, J., and Deppisch, L., 1975, Effect of hypotonicity on cyclic adenosine monophosphate formation and action in vasopressin target cells, *Kidney Int.* **7:**161–169.

97. Parisi, M., Ripoche, P., Pervost, G., and Bourguet, J., 1981, Regulation by ADH and cellular osmolarity of water permeability in frog urinary bladder: A time course study, *Ann. NY Acad. Sci.* **372:**144–161.

98. Kachadorian, W. A., Sariban-Sohraby, S., and Spring, K. R., 1985, Regulation of water permeability in toad bladder at two barriers, *Am. J. Physiol.* **248:**F260–F265.

99. Cotton, C. U., Weinstein, A. M., and Reuss, L., 1989, Osmotic water permeability of *Necturus* gallbladder epithelium, *J. Gen. Physiol.* **93:** 649–679.

100. Strange, K. and Spring, K. R., 1987, Cell membrane water permeability of rabbit cortical collecting duct, *J. Membr. Biol.* **96:**27–43.

101. Strange, K. and Spring, K. R., 1987, Absence of significant cellular dilution during ADH-stimulated water reabsorption, *Science* 235:1068–1070.

102. Kirk, K. L., 1988, Origin of ADH-induced vacuoles in rabbit cortical collecting tubule, *Am. J. Physiol.* 254:F719–F733.

103. González, E., Carpi-Medina, P., and Whittembury, G., 1982, Cell osmotic water permeability of isolated rabbit proximal straight tubules, *Am. J. Physiol.* 242:F321–F330.

104. González, E., Carpi-Medina, Linares, H., and Whittembury, G., 1984, Osmotic water permeability of the apical membrane of proximal straight tubular (PST) cells, *Pflügers Arch. Eur. J. Physiol.* 402:337–339.

105. Carpi-Medina, P., González, E., and Whittembury, G., 1983, Cell osmotic water permeability of isolated rabbit proximal convoluted tubules, *Am. J. Physiol.* 244:F554–F563.

106. Carpi-Medina, P., Lindemann, B., González, E., and Whittembury, G., 1984, The continuous measurement of tubular volume changes in response to step changes in contraluminal osmolality, *Pflügers Arch. Eur. J. Physiol.* 400:343–348.

107. Persson, B-E., and Spring, K. R., 1982, Gallbladder epithelial cell hydraulic water permeability and volume regulation, *J. Gen. Physiol.* 79:481–505.

108. Chevalier, J., Bourguet, J., and Hugon, J. S., 1974, Membrane associated particles: Distribution in frog urinary bladder epithelium at rest and after oxytocin treatment, *Cell Tissue Res.* 152:129–140.

109. Kachadorian, W. A., Wade, J. B., and DiScala, V. A., 1975, Vasopressin: Induced structural change in toad bladder luminal membrane, *Science* 190:67–69.

110. Kachadorian, W. A., Levine, S. D., Wade, J. B., DiScala, V. A., and Hays, R. M., 1977, Relationship of aggregated intramembranous particles to water permeability in vasopressin-treated toad urinary bladder, *J. Clin. Invest.* 59:576–581.

111. Wade, J. B., 1985, Membrane structural studies of the action of vasopressin, *Fed. Proc.* 44:2687–2692.

112. Brown, D., Grosso, A., and DeSousa, R. C., 1983, Correlation between water flow and intramembrane particle aggregates in toad epidermis, *Am. J. Physiol.* 245:C334–C342.

113. Harmanci, M. C., Kachadorian, W. A., Valtin, H., and DiScala, V. A., 1978, Antidiuretic hormone-induced intramembranous alterations in mammalian collecting ducts, *Am. J. Physiol.* 235:F440–F443.

114. Chevalier, J., Pinto da Silva, P., Ripoche, P., Gobin, R., Wang, W-Y., Grossetete, J., and Bourguet, J., 1985, Structural and cytochemical differentiation of membrane elements of the apical membrane of amphibian urinary bladder epithelial cells. A label fracture study, *Biol. Cell* 55:181–190.

115. Humbert, F., Montesano, R., Grosso, A., DeSousa, R. C., and Orci, L., 1977, Particle aggregates in plasma and intracellular membranes of toad bladder (granular cell), *Experientia* 33:1364–1367.

116. Wade, J. B., 1978, Membrane structural specialization of the toad urinary bladder revealed by the freeze-fracture technique. III. Location, structure and vasopressin dependence of intramembrane particle arrays, *J. Membr. Biol.* 40:281–296.

117. Muller, J., Kachadorian, W. A., and DiScala, V. A., 1980, Evidence that ADH-stimulated intramembrane particle aggregates are transferred from cytoplasmic to luminal membranes in toad bladder epithelial cells, *J. Cell Biol.* 85:83–95.

118. Warncke, J. and Lindemann, B., 1981, Effect of ADH on the capacitance of apical epithelial membranes, in: *Advances in Physiological Sciences*, Volume 3, *Physiology of Non-excitable Cells*, Pergamon, New York, pp. 129–133.

119. Stetson, D. L., Lewis, S. A., Alles, W., and Wade, J. B., 1982, Evaluation by capacitance measurements of antidiuretic hormone induced membrane area changes in toad bladder, *Biochim. Biophys. Acta* 689:267–274.

120. Palmer, L. G. and Lorenzen, M., 1983, Antidiuretic hormone-dependent membrane capacitance and water permeability in the toad urinary bladder, *Am. J. Physiol.* 244:F195–F204.

121. Palmer, L. G. and Speez, N., 1984, Modulation of antidiuretic hormone-dependent capacitance and water flow in toad urinary bladder, *Am. J. Physiol.* 246:F501–F508.

122. Hays, R. M., Franki, N., and Ding, G., 1987, Effects of antidiuretic hormone on the collecting duct, *Kidney Int.* **31:**530–537.

123. Sasaki, J., Tilles, S., Condeelis, J., Carbone, J., Meiteles, L., Franki, N., Bolon, R., Robertson, C., and Hays, R. M., 1984, Electronmicroscopic study of the apical region of the toad bladder epithelial cells, *Am. J. Physiol.* **247:**C268–C281.

124. Kachadorian, W. A., Casey, C., and DiScala, V. A., 1978, Time course of ADH-induced intramembranous particle aggregation in toad urinary bladder, *Am. J. Physiol.* **234:**F461–F465.

125. Gronowicz, G., Masur, S. K., and Holtzman, E., 1980, Quantitative analysis of exocytosis and endocytosis in the hydroosmotic response of the toad bladder, *J. Membr. Biol.* **52:**221–235.

126. Wade, J. B., Stetson, D. L., and Lewis, S. A., 1981, ADH action: Evidence for a membrane shuttle mechanism, *Ann. NY Acad. Sci.* **372:**106–117.

127. Masur, S. K., Cooper, S., and Rubin, M. S., 1984, Effect of an osmotic gradient on antidiuretic hormone-induced endocytosis and hydroosmosis in the toad urinary bladder, *Am. J. Physiol.* **247:** F370–F379.

128. Ding, G., Franki, N., and Hays, R. M., 1985, Evidence for cycling of aggregate-containing tubules in toad urinary bladder, *Biol. Cell* **55:**213–218.

129. Harris, H. W., Jr., Wade, J. B., and Handler, J. S., 1986, Transepithelial water flow regulates apical membrane retrieval in antidiuretic hormone-stimulated toad urinary bladder, *J. Clin. Invest.* **78:**703–712.

130. Wade, J. B., 1980, Hormonal modulation of epithelial structures, in: *Current Topics in Membranes and Transport, Cellular Mechanisms of Renal Tubular Ion Transport* (E. L. Boulpaep, ed.), Academic Press, New York, pp. 124–147.

131. Kachadorian, W. A., Wade, J. B., Uiterwyk, C. C., and DiScala, V. A., 1977, Membrane structure and functional responses to vasopressin in toad bladder, *J. Membr. Biol.* **30:**381–401.

132. Lichtenstein, N. S. and Leaf, A., 1965, Effect of amphotericin B on the permeability of the toad bladder, *J. Clin. Invest.* **44:**1328–1342.

133. Hays, R. M., Chevalier, J., Gobin, R., and Bourguet, J., 1985, Fusion images and intramembrane particle aggregates during the action of antidiuretic hormone: A rapid freeze study, *Cell Tissue Res.* **240:**433–439.

134. DeSousa, R. C., 1985, From stimulus-secretion coupling to stimulus-hydrosmotic response, *Biol. Cell* **55:**159–162.

135. Masur, S. K., Holtzman, E., Schwartz, I. L., and Walter, R., 1971, Correlation between pinocytosis and hydroosmosis induced by neurohypophyseal hormones and mediated by adenosine 3′,5′-cyclic monophosphate, *J. Cell Biol.* **49:**582–589.

136. Masur, S. K., Holtzman, E., and Walter, R., 1972, Hormone stimulated exocytosis in the toad urinary bladder, *J. Cell Biol.* **52:**211–219.

137. Taylor, A., Mamelak, M., Reaven, E., and Maffly, R., 1973, Vasopressin: Possible role of microtubules and microfilaments in its action, *Science* **181:**347–350.

138. Burch, R. M. and Halushka, P. V., 1982, Inhibition of prostaglandin synthesis antagonizes the colchicine-induced reduction of vasopressin-stimulated water flow in the toad urinary bladder, *Mol. Pharmacol.* **21:**142–149.

139. Ausiello, D. A. and Hartwig, J. H., 1985, Microfilament organization and vasopressin action, in: *Vasopressin* (R. W. Schrier, ed.), Raven Press, New York, pp. 89–96.

140. Ausiello, D. A., Hartwig, J., and Brown, D., 1987, Membrane and microfilament organization and vasopressin action in transporting epithelia, Chapt. 17, in: *Cell Calcium and the Control of Membrane Transport*, Volume 42, (L. J. Mandel, D. C. Eaton, eds.), Rockefeller University Press, New York, pp. 259–275.

141. Ausiello, D. A., Corwin, H. L., and Hartwig, J. H., 1984, Identification of actin-binding protein and villin in toad bladder epithelia, *Am. J. Physiol.* **246:**F101–F104.

142. DiBona, D. R., 1983, Cytoplasmic involvement in ADH-mediated osmosis across toad urinary bladder, *Am. J. Physiol.* **245:**C297–C307.

143. DiBona, D. R., Civan, M. M., and Leaf, A., 1969, The cellular specificity of the effect of vasopressin on toad urinary bladder, *J. Membr. Biol.* **1:**79–91.

144. DiBona, D. R., 1981, Vasopressin action on the conformational state of the granular cell in the amphibian bladder, in: *Epithelial Ion and Water Transport* (A. D. C. Macknight, J. P. Leader, eds.), Raven Press, New York, pp. 241–256.

145. Davis, W. L., Goodman, D. B. P., Schuster, R. J., Rasmussen, H., and Martin, J. H., 1974, Effects of cytochalasin B on the response of toad urinary bladder to vasopressin, *J. Cell Biol.* **63:** 986–997.

146. Pearl, M. and Taylor, A., 1983, Actin filaments and vasopressin-stimulated water flow in toad urinary bladder, *Am. J. Physiol.* **245:**C28–C39.

147. Eggena, P., 1972, Glutaraldehyde-fixation method for determining the permeability to water of the toad urinary bladder, *Endocrinology* **91:**240–246.

148. Kachadorian, W. A., Ellis, S. J., and Muller, J., 1979, Possible roles of microtubules and microfilaments in ADH action on toad urinary bladder, *Am. J. Physiol.* **236:**F14–F20.

149. DiBona, D. R., 1978, Direct visualization of epithelial morphology in the living amphibian urinary bladder, *J. Membr. Biol.* **40:**45–70.

150. DiBona, D. R., 1979, Direct visualization of ADH-mediated transepithelial osmotic flow, in: *Hormonal Control of Epithelial Transport* (J. Bourguet, ed.), INSERM, Paris, pp. 195–208.

151. Spinelli, F., Grosso, A., and DeSousa, R. C., 1975, The hydroosmotic effect of vasopressin: A scanning electron-microscope study, *J. Membr. Biol.* **23:**139–156.

152. Mills, J. W. and Malick, L. E., 1978, Mucosal surface morphology of the toad urinary bladder. Scanning electron microscope study of the natriferic and hydro-osmotic response to vasopressin, *J. Cell Biol.* **77:**598–610.

153. LeFurgey, A. and Tisher, C. C., 1981, Time course of vasopressin-induced formation of microvilli in granular cells of toad urinary bladder, *J. Membr. Biol.* **61:**13–19.

154. Allen, R. D., Weiss, D. G., Hayden, J. H., Brown, D. T., Fujiwake, H., and Simpson, M., 1985, Gliding movement of and bidirectional transport along single native microtubules from squid axoplasm: Evidence for an active role of microtubules in cytoplasmic transport, *J. Cell Biol.* **100:** 1736–1752.

155. Hirokawa, N., Bloom, G. S., and Vallee, R. B., 1985, Cytoskeletal architecture and immunocytochemical localization of microtubule-associated proteins in regions of axons associated with rapid axonal transport: The β,β' in iminodipropionitrile-intoxicated axon as a model system, *J. Cell Biol.* **101:**227–239.

156. Spudich, J. A., Kron, S. J., and Sheetz, M. P., 1985, Movement of myosin-coated beads on oriented filaments reconstituted from purified actin, *Nature (London)* **315:**584–586.

157. Beauwens, R., Kronnie, G. T., Snauwaert, J., and Veld, P. A. I., 1986, Polycations reduce vasopressin-induced water flow by endocytic removal of water channels, *Am. J. Physiol.* **250:** C729–C737.

158. Masur, S. K., Gruenberg, J., and Howell, K. E., 1987, Endosomal compartment of toad bladder epithelium, *Am. J. Physiol.* **252:**C115–C120.

159. Verkman, A. S., Lencer, W. I., Brown, D., and Ausiello, D. A., 1988, Endosomes from kidney collecting tubule cells contain the vasopressin-sensitive water channel, *Nature* **333:**268–269.

160. Levine, S. D. and Kachadorian, W. A., 1981, Barriers to water flow in vasopressin-treated toad urinary bladder, *J. Membr. Biol.* **61:**135–139.

161. Kachadorian, W. A., 1985, Regulation of ADH-stimulated water flow at a postluminal barrier in toad bladder, *Biol. Cell* **55:**225–230.

162. Carvounis, C. P., 1985, Cell determinants of vasopressin-stimulated water flow, *Biol. Cell* **55:** 207–212.

163. Schafer, J. A. and Andreoli, T. E., 1972, The effect of antidiuretic hormone on solute flows in mammalian collecting tubules, *J. Clin. Invest.* **51:**1279–1286.

164. Wade, J. B., Guckian, V., and Koeppen, I., 1984, Development of antibodies to apical membrane constituents associated with the action of vasopressin, in: *Current Topics in Membranes and Transport*, Volume 20, *Molecular Approaches to Epithelial Transport* (A. Kleinzeller, F. Bronner, J. Wade, and S. Lewis, eds.), Academic Press, New York, pp. 217–234.

2

Renal Hemodynamics and Sodium Chloride Excretion

Ali A. Khraibi and Franklyn G. Knox

1. Renal Hemodynamics

The regulation of renal hemodynamics involves a number of integrated intrinsic and extrinsic control mechanisms. The extrinsic control mechanisms can have an important influence under many physiologic circumstances; however, much attention has been focused on intrinsic controls that are involved in the autoregulation of renal blood flow (RBF) and glomerular filtration rate (GFR).

Autoregulation of RBF and GFR may be defined as the intrinsic capability of the kidney to maintain a constant level of blood flow and glomerular filtration regardless of considerable variations in renal perfusion pressure. The actual pressure range of autoregulation may vary from one species to another, but is usually between 70 and 180 mm Hg in mammals. It is uncertain whether distinct mechanisms regulate RBF and GFR; however, the two can be dissociated under certain conditions.[1-4]

Two primary mechanisms exist to explain the phenomenon of renal autoregulation. One mechanism, called the myogenic mechanism, is mainly a phenomenon manifested by the response of renal vasculature to changes in wall tension. A second mechanism is tubuloglomerular feedback. This a complex mechanism that requires the participation of a detector, a transmitter, and an effector component.

ALI A. KHRAIBI and FRANKLYN G. KNOX • Departments of Physiology and Biophysics, and Medicine, Mayo Medical School, Mayo Foundation, Rochester, Minnesota 55905.

1.1. Myogenic Mechanism

This mechanism is thought to respond to instantaneous changes in vascular wall tension. The explanation of this phenomenon is based on Laplace's law, which states that the wall tension in a vessel is equal to the product of transmural hydrostatic pressure difference and radius of the vessel. According to this theory, the wall tension of a vessel is held constant. An increase in the transmural pressure (for example, due to an increase in renal perfusion pressure) results in a transient increase in wall tension. Under these circumstances, the radius of this vessel decreases instantaneously to maintain a constant wall tension. The reduction in vessel radius results from vasoconstriction, which leads to an increase in vascular resistance. Therefore, the controlled variable in the myogenic mechanism is wall tension. Blood flow is regulated as a secondary event by changes in vascular resistance.

Most studies that support the myogenic mechanism have been through exclusion of various other mechanisms rather than through direct evidence. Studies by Gilmore et al.[5] and Källskog et al.,[6] however, demonstrated direct evidence for the myogenic phenomenon in regulating renal hemodynamics in the renal vasculature of hamsters and rats. The observation by Gilmore et al.[5] that the radius of transplanted hamster renal afferent arterioles is very responsive to extravascular pressure supports the proposal that some purely physical parameter that depends on transmural pressure is responsible for the alteration of smooth muscle contractile activity. Edwards[7] investigated the interaction between lumen diameter and intraluminal pressures of interlobular arteries and superficial afferent and efferent arterioles isolated from rabbit kidneys. In these isolated microvessels it was found that increasing intraluminal pressure from 70 to 180 mm Hg resulted in decreases in lumen diameters of interlobular arteries and afferent arterioles. In contrast, the efferent arterioles responded in a passive manner to increases in intraluminal pressure by dilation. Thus, the results of this study provide some evidence for the involvement of the myogenic mechanism in regulating renal blood flow by the preglomerular vessels.

Mathematical analyses of the myogenic hypothesis with particular reference to autoregulation of renal blood flow have been developed by Oien and Aukland[8] and Lush and Fray.[9] In this latter myogenic model it is argued that the vascular smooth muscle contraction is initiated by stretch-induced changes in calcium permeability. The model predicts an upward and rightward shift of the autoregulatory pressure flow curve in response to increased tissue hydrostatic pressure. In this model, the autoregulatory mechanism senses stretch but simply responds to it rather than attempting to regulate it. Most of the constituent parts of the model have experimental support, except the hypothesis that stretch controls intracellular calcium. In a recent study, Aukland and Oien[10] used models to evaluate the extent of the involvement of tubuloglomerular feedback and myogenic vascular response, alone or together, in explaining the available experimental observations on renal autoregulation. It was concluded that good autoregulation of RBF and GFR may result from a myogenic mechanism alone, or in combination with tubuloglomerular feedback. The regulation of preglomerular vascular resistance predicted from the experimental feedback response to varying single nephron distal tubular flow rate is insufficient to account for renal autoregulation observed in rats and dogs. Addition of a preglomerular myogenic response to tubuloglomerular feedback may provide excellent RBF and GFR autoregulation and attenuate the distal flow response.

Moore[11] measured and analyzed the change in glomerular capillary pressure produced by elevation of arterial pressure during tubuloglomerular feedback inhibition in Sprague–Dawley rats. The data indicated that intrinsic adjustments in renal vascular resistance could provide about 50% compensation for a rise in arterial pressure. The author suggested that this mechanism is probably an intrinsic myogenic reflex of the afferent vessels stimulated by changes in intravascular pressure. In a study by Casellas and Navar[12] of *in vitro* perfusion of juxtamedullary nephrons in rats, spontaneous cyclic vasomotion in the face of a constant perfusion pressure was observed. This was first detected visually as cyclic variations of glomerular tuft perfusion and could be quantitated as cyclic alterations in glomerular capillary and tubular pressure. Kreisberg *et al.*[13] demonstrated that the smooth muscle–like cells in the cultured glomerular mesangium appear to be contractile and may play a role in regulating the surface area for ultrafiltration.

In two studies by Young and Marsh[14] and Sakai and Marsh,[15] the transient and frequency responses of RBF autoregulation and hydrostatic pressure wave propagation along the rat nephron were analyzed. The fast-acting component in renal autoregulation was attributed to an intrinsic myogenic response of the renal vessels. However, in a later study,[16] the existence of a high-frequency response could not be shown except under circumstances whereby the fast component of the response to step forcing could have been an artifact. The authors stated that their earlier results were in error, and frequency response methods detect only one regulator of RBF. They concluded that the macula densa feedback was the only flow-regulating mechanisms detected. Further, it was suggested that the available evidence indicates that renal autoregulatory mechanisms originate entirely within tubular responses. In the last 2 years, experimental studies on the myogenic mechanism in relation to the regulation of RBF have been rare, and more work needs to be done to further investigate and clarify the possible importance of this phenomenon in autoregulation of renal hemodynamics.

1.2. Tubuloglomerular Feedback Mechanism

Tubuloglomerular feedback is a well-established mechanism and is thought to be of great importance in renal autoregulation. Many studies have demonstrated the existence of a distal tubule–glomerular mechanism that is responsive to changes in flow rate in distal tubules and serves as a regulator of GFR.[17–20] This feedback mechanism may be divided into three components that take place sequentially in a series of events in response to flow-related alterations in the concentration of electrolytes and other osmolar components in the tubular fluid. First, changes in the tubular fluid concentration of one or more components are detected as the flow is exposed to the macula densa cells of the distal tubule (detector component); second, the signal is transmitted from the macula densa cells to renal vascular elements (transmitter component); and third, the elicited response is manifested by vascular smooth muscle contraction or relaxation (effector component).

1.2.1. Detector Component

The interaction between the distal tubule and glomerular vascular structures during changes in flow rates may be triggered by flow-dependent alterations in the concentration of sodium and chloride at the macula densa cells,[21-23] or by changes in distal tubular fluid osmolality.[24-26] Studies by Briggs et al.[21] and Schnermann et al.[22] have shown that increases in sodium chloride concentration—perfused retrograde in the loop of Henle—of between 15 and 60 mEq result in proportionate decreases in filtration rate. These observations support the theory that transport, especially of sodium chloride by the macula densa cells, plays an important role in the detector component of the feedback mechanism. This hypothesis has been challenged by Bell and co-workers,[24,25] who proposed that alterations in osmolality act as the luminal signal triggering feedback responses. This proposal is based on demonstration that solutions containing low concentrations of chloride and other electrolytes (for example, sodium iothionate) produce changes in filtration rate when perfused retrograde through the loop of Henle.[26] Thus, the detector component of the tubuloglomerular feedback mechanism remains controversial.

1.2.2. Transmitter Component

The mode of transmission of the signal of tubuloglomerular feedback has been studied by Bell,[27] who proposed that a cytosolic calcium system, probably in the cells of the macula densa, participates in the transmission of the luminal signals to the glomerular vasculature. According to this theory, there is a mobilization of calcium from intracellular stores as the concentration of the distal tubular fluid increases from hyposmotic toward isosmotic values. This increase in cytosolic calcium concentration may help in the transmission of the signal to glomerular vascular elements, resulting in vasoconstriction and a reduction in filtration rate. A series of micropuncture experiments utilizing agents that have been reported to increase intracellular cyclic AMP (cAMP), which in turn can modify calcium-mediated events, were performed by Bell.[27] Retrograde microperfusion with isotonic Ringer's solution decreased stop-flow pressure (SFP) from an average of 37 mm Hg to 25 mm Hg. Addition of 3-isobutyl-1-methylxanthine (IBMX), a phosphodiesterase inhibitor, to the isotonic Ringer's solution, produced a dose-dependent decrease in the magnitude of SFP feedback responses. This inhibition was abolished and tubuloglomerular feedback responses were restored to near control levels when calcium ionophore (A23187) was added to the isotonic Ringer's solution containing IBMX. Inhibitions in tubuloglomerular feedback responses were obtained when forskolin, an agent that stimulates adenylate cyclase activity, or the dibutyryl form of cAMP was administered. The author postulated that an adenylate cyclase–activated cAMP system may exist and that this mechanism can influence the transmission of tubuloglomerular feedback signals by stimulation of calcium transport across the plasma membrane or endoplasmic reticulum. Hence, elevated intracellular cAMP may prevent the mobilization of intracellular calcium, thus directly lowering cytosolic calcium concentration and impairing the feedback responses.

1.2.3. Effector Component

The controversy that exists in explaining the detector and transmitter components also extends to the explanation of the effector side of tubuloglomerular feedback mechanism. The major thrust of this controversy is centered on whether the primary segment of resistance responsible for hemodynamic autoregulation is preglomerular or located at other sites. Bell et al.[28] have shown that increases in flow rate out of the late proximal tubule lead to decreases in glomerular capillary pressure and single nephron glomerular filtration rate (SNGFR). It was also demonstrated that significant decreases in glomerular capillary pressure were obtained at rates of infusion into the late proximal tubule as low as 10 nl/min. The authors suggested that glomerular capillary pressure is responsive to changes in late proximal flow rates that are within the normal range. The results of these experiments supported the hypothesis that increases in afferent arteriolar resistance are mainly responsible for feedback-mediated decreases in glomerular filtration rate. Even though it is generally accepted that glomerular pressure exhibits an autoregulatory behavior, still other studies suggested that other sites may be involved in the effector site of tubuloglomerular feedback mechanism.[29,30] In studies performed by Tucker et al.,[29] a carbonic anhydrase inhibitor, when administered systemically, produced decreases in SNGFR, but no significant decrease in glomerular pressure. Also, Ichikawa[30] showed that tubuloglomerular feedback-induced changes in SNGFR were not coupled with alterations in glomerular hydrostatic pressure, and that the feedback regulation of glomerular filtration rate is mediated by changes in vasomotor tone of preglomerular, glomerular, and postglomerular vessel sites. It was suggested that these alterations in vasomotor tone may be mediated through mesangial cell contractility. In a study by Persson et al.[31] in angiotensin II–prostaglandin-blocked rats, glomerular capillary hydrostatic pressure and SFP feedback responses were completely eliminated, while SNGFR response persisted but to a lesser extent. The authors suggested that in angiotensin II–prostaglandin-blocked rats, tubuloglomerular feedback SNGFR responses can occur without changes in glomerular capillary pressure, possibly by parallel alterations in afferent and efferent arteriolar resistances. It remains to be seen whether there are other physiologic states where SNGFR and glomerular capillary pressure feedback responses can be dissociated.

1.3. Sensitivity of Tubuloglomerular Feedback Mechanism

The sensitivity or feedback gain of the tubuloglomerular feedback mechanism has been measured under different physiologic and experimental conditions and has been found to be variable. In two recent studies by Seney *et al.*,[32,33] the possibility that increases in GFR associated with high-protein diet are accompanied by alterations in the sensitivity of the tubuloglomerular feedback mechanism was investigated. Loop of Henle perfusion experiments showed that in male Sprague–Dawley rats fed a high-protein diet (40% casein), the tubuloglomerular feedback mechanism is less sensitive than in rats fed the low-protein diet (6% casein). It was concluded that the sensing mechanism of the tubuloglomerular feedback system becomes less responsive on a high-protein-diet intake leading to an elevated GFR.[32] In a later study,[33] micropuncture and microperfusion methods were utilized to determine whether the protein-dependent shift in the activity of tubuloglomerular feedback is a result of changes in either the signal or the sensing mechanism in the feedback pathway. In rats fed the high-protein diet, single-nephron GFR was significantly higher, sodium and chloride concentrations in the early distal tubule fluid were significantly lower, while early distal osmolality was not different in comparison with rats fed the low-protein diet. Tubuloglomerular feedback responses were not different in the two diet groups of rats when assessed by changes in SFP during perfusion of the distal nephron with sodium chloride solutions (Fig. 1). It was

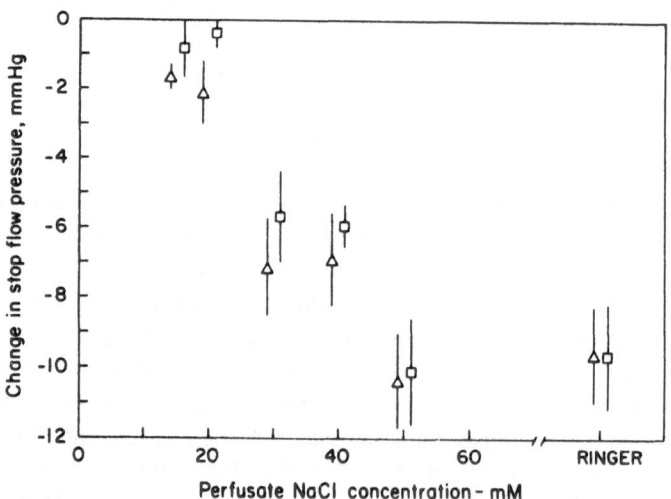

Fig. 1. Relations between concentration of NaCl in fluid perfused backward into early distal tubules and tubuloglomerular feedback response. Symbols indicate means ± SE. □, 6% protein diet; number of nephrons from lowest to highest concentrations: 5, 7, 9, 7, 7, 8. △, 40% protein diet; number of nephrons from lowest to highest concentrations: 7, 6, 10, 7, 9, 10. Osmolalities for solutions containing 15, 20, 30, 40, and 50 mM NaCl and dye were 37, 46, 65, 84, and 102 mosmol/kg, respectively. Osmolality for the Ringer's-like solution was 290 mosmol/kg.[33]

concluded that changes in dietary protein do not alter the sensing mechanism of the tubuloglomerular feedback system, but affect the signal eliciting the tubuloglomerular feedback response. The authors offered a hypothesis that may explain the steps that are involved in producing an elevated GFR during a high-protein diet. The high-protein intake initially stimulates absorption of sodium and chloride somewhere between the late proximal and early distal tubules. The low concentrations of sodium and chloride in the tubular fluid entering the macula densa weaken the signal responsible for initiating tubuloglomerular feedback. Thus, the negative feedback effect on glomerular function is suppressed and GFR increases.[33] Low-protein diet has been shown to prevent the elevation of GFR and the impairment of feedback regulation observed in the nonclipped kidneys of Goldblatt hypertensive rats.[34] The low-protein diet prevents glomerular injury in the nonclipped kidney despite the presence of hypertension, probably by maintaining an intact tubuloglomerular feedback mechanism. Also, in the remnant kidney model of hypertension, low-protein diet attenuates the proteinuria and the progressive glomerular scarring observed when rats are fed a normal-protein diet.[35] Poor renal autoregulation is demonstrated in this model when rats are given normal but not low-protein intake.

In a recent study by Moore and Mason,[36] the effect of extracellular fluid volume on tubuloglomerular feedback control of distal fluid delivery was determined in hydropenic, moderately hemorrhaged, and volume-expanded rats. In the volume-expanded rats, a rightward shift in the tubuloglomerular feedback onset threshold and operating point was demonstrated. This shift allows more tubular fluid to pass the macula densa before a compensatory reduction response in SNGFR is elicited. The reduced SNGFR observed following hemorrhage may be partly due to a modest degree of tonic suppression by tubuloglomerular feedback. The results of this study show that when extracellular fluid volume is changed, the level at which tubuloglomerular feedback stabilized distal fluid delivery is reset. Increases in SNGFR, similar to those observed during volume expansion, have been seen during atrial natriuretic factor infusion. The elevation in SNGFR caused by atrial natriuretic factor is associated with an increase in glomerular capillary pressure and with a blunted maximal tubuloglomerular feedback response.[37] Also, hyperglycemia causes a significant rise in RBF and GFR in anesthetized dogs.[38] These increases are abolished in the nonfiltering kidney in which glomerular feedback responses are blocked. Thus, it was suggested that hyperglycemia impairs renal autoregulation and the increase in RBF and GFR may be caused by a tubuloglomerular feedback mechanism.

Renal interstitial hydrostatic and oncotic pressure have been shown to have an effect on the sensitivity of tubuloglomerular feedback control. During volume expansion in rats, the net renal interstitial pressure (subcapsular interstitial hydrostatic pressure minus interstitial oncotic pressure) increased and the sensitivity of the feedback mechanism, as measured by SFP, declined.[39] In the partially obstructed kidney there is an increase in tubuloglomerular feedback sensitivity during saline volume expansion.[40] This elevation in sensitivity leads to activation of the tubuloglomerular feedback mechanism to reduce and maintain GFR at a low level.

Dilley and Arendshorst[41] demonstrated that the 6-week-old Okamoto spontaneously hypertensive rat (SHR) exhibits a more sensitive and reactive tubuloglomerular feedback than the age-matched Wistar–Kyoto rat. This hyperactivity of the feedback system seen in a young SHR is less marked with normalization of GFR and filtration dynamics in the adult SHR with established hypertension. Young prehypertensive rats of the spontaneously hypertensive Milan strain exhibit essentially no tubuloglomerular feedback response.[42] During the developmental stage of hypertension, the sensitivity of tubuloglomerular feedback, as measured by SFP, is significantly higher than in the prehypertensive stage and than in the Milan normotensive rats. The results of this study indicated that during the prehypertensive stage in Milan spontaneously hypertensive rats there is essentially no tubuloglomerular feedback activity, but during the development of hypertension the tubuloglomerular feedback system becomes highly activated to reduce glomerular filtration.

Other factors that have previously been shown to affect the sensitivity or modulate the response of the tubuloglomerular feedback mechanism include angiotensin II,[43,44] captopril,[45] a converting enzyme inhibitor, aprotinin, a kallikrein inhibitor, and prostaglandin[46]; single nephron obstruction[47] and release of 24-hr unilateral ureteral obstruction[47,48]; pregnancy[49]; growth[50]; and nephron heterogeneity.[51]

1.4. Other Factors Controlling Renal Hemodynamics

1.4.1. Angiotensin II

The renin–angiotensin system plays an important role in restoring fluid volumes and maintaining arterial pressure at normal levels.[52] The renal hemodynamic effects of angiotensin II stabilize GFR and contribute to the maintenance of sodium homeostasis.[53] There is evidence to indicate that angiotensin II has multiple effects on renal function exerted by its influence on vascular, glomerular, and tubular structures. Infusion of angiotensin II produces a reduction in nephron plasma flow, an increase in glomerular capillary hydrostatic pressure, an increase in afferent and efferent arteriolar resistances, and a reduction in the glomerular ultrafiltration coefficient.[54] The renin–angiotensin system is critically important in controlling GFR during decreases in sodium intake or renal perfusion pressure or increases in renal venous pressure.[55,56] The renal vascular site of action of angiotensin II, which is most physiologically relevant, and the resulting alterations in renal resistance have been widely studied but remain controversial.

There is strong evidence to indicate that the intrarenally formed angiotensin II controls GFR during reductions in renal perfusion pressure by a dominant effect on the efferent arteriolar resistance.[2,54] In dogs with blocked intrarenal angiotensin II formation, GFR fell by 24% RBF, increased by 29%, and calculated afferent and efferent arteriolar resistances decreased to 32% and 80% of control, respectively, as a result of reduction of renal arterial pressure to 70 mm Hg. These calculations suggested that the intrarenal renin–angiotensin system controls GFR primarily by maintaining efferent arteriolar resistance, with little effect on the tone of afferent vessels.[2] In normal kidneys, angiotensin II infusion decreased RBF to 61% of control and did not change GFR significantly, suggesting a primarily efferent arteriolar effect[57] (Fig. 2). Similar results were reported by Textor *et al.*[3] in dogs with induced renal artery stenosis. In these dogs, intrarenal infusion of the angiotensin antagonist Sar-1-Ala-8-AII produced an abrupt decrease in GFR despite maintained renal blood flow. In the same study, the converting enzyme inhibitor captopril was administered orally to 14 patients with unilateral renovascular hypertension. Over a period of 1 hr blood pressure and GFR fell significantly with no significant decrease in renal plasma flow. The differing effect on GFR and renal plasma flow reflected a significant reduction in filtration fraction. By contrast, similar blood pressure reduction with sodium nitroprusside in these patients produced no significant changes in GFR and renal plasma flow. Since GFR, following captopril administration, fell significantly below that during sodium nitroprusside infusion, the authors concluded that administration of converting enzyme inhibitor in subjects with reno-

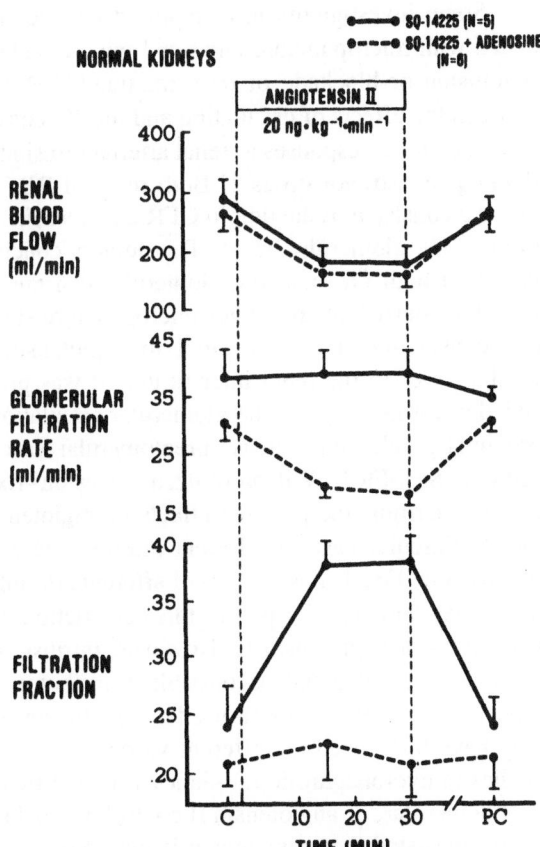

Fig. 2. Effects of intravenous infusion of angiotensin II (20 ng·kg·$^{-1}$min^{-1}) after infusion of converting enzyme inhibitor SQ 14225 (captopril) or after infusion of SQ 14225 plus adenosine (1 μmol/min into renal artery) on renal blood flow, glomerular filtration rate, and filtration fraction in normal kidneys. Values are means ±SE.[57]

vascular hypertension produced selective reduction in the efferent arteriolar resistance.

Micropuncture studies have shown that pressor and nonpressor doses of angiotensin II influence glomerular ultrafiltration.[54] The reduction in nephron plasma flow may result from increases in both afferent and efferent arteriolar resistance; however, the proportional elevation in efferent arteriolar vascular resistance is greater. The increase in preglomerular resistance with pressor doses of angiotensin II may be a secondary result of an autoregulatory response to the increase in renal perfusion pressure.[54] This proposal is supported by evidence indicating no change in preglomerular resistance when renal perfusion pressure is held constant,[58] when changes in tubuloglomerular feedback are prevented,[59] or in isolated perfused afferent arterioles.[7] Thus, in most conditions that require the renin–angiotensin system to be activated to restore fluid volume and arterial pressure toward normal, the renal vascular effects of angiotensin II stabilize GFR by maintaining blood pressure and increasing the resistance of the efferent arterioles.[52] Schnermann et al.[60] suggested that saralasin influences autoregulation through a mechanism independent of tubuloglomerular feedback and that the effect of saralasin is more likely due to its blockade of the effects of angiotensin II on the efferent arteriole.

Some investigators have reported changes in preglomerular resistance, estimated with micropuncture and renal microcirculation methods, during angiotensin II infusion or blockade of its formation.[61–65] To determine possible differences between the effects of circulating and locally converted angiotensin II, Navar et al. compared renal responses to renal arterial infusions of angiotensin I and angiotensin II in equiconstrictor doses.[62] Both reduced RBF and angiotensin I infusions produced a consistent reduction in GFR and SNGFR, which indicated effects proximal to or at the glomerulus level. The authors concluded that angiotensin I infusions increased both pre- and postglomerular resistances and decreased the glomerular filtration coefficient. In a later micropuncture study, Mitchell and Navar indicated that conversion of angiotensin I to angiotensin II can occur in the peritubular capillaries or in the renal interstitium. It was proposed that angiotensin II, either added or formed beyond the glomerular circulation, can elevate reabsorption in the proximal tubule and increase preglomerular vascular resistance and consequently decrease SNGFR.[63] Wilson utilized perfusion–fixation and vascular casting methods to determine the possible effects of angiotensin II on the afferent arterioles in rats.[64] Vascular casts of afferent arterioles were examined by scanning electron microscopy. Focal constrictions of afferent arterioles were observed in all regions of the kidney, and a major part of this constriction was attributed to a direct constrictive action of angiotensin II. However, intrinsic renal autoregulatory mechanisms could not be ruled out as possible contributors to the afferent vasoconstriction especially since this study showed that perfusion–fixation at elevated pressure alone may have influenced the afferent vasoconstriction.[64] Other renal microcirculation studies in hydronephrotic rat kidney revealed two foci, one preglomerular and one postglomerular, of angiotensin II control of renal hemodynamics.[65] The data in this study suggested that angiotensin II may produce a significant increase in vascular resistance near the glomerulus, especially in the efferent arterioles. There seems to be little doubt that angiotensin II produces efferent arteriolar constriction. This postglomerular manipulation of renal resistance might even be the principal action of angiotensin II, while its effect on afferent arterioles remains less certain.[64]

Angiotensin II may be involved in the regulation of regional medullary blood flow. Exogenous intrarenal administration of angiotensin II, at a does that did not affect GFR and RBF, induced papillary ischemia and preserved medullary hypertonicity. The prevention of the increase in papillary plasma flow may contribute to the diminished natriuretic response and sodium retention during chronic salt-retaining states.[66,67] The proposal that angiotensin II may have possible actions in the renal medulla where it could regulate medullary blood flow and modify the function of the countercurrent concentrating system is supported by receptor density studies. Angiotensin II receptors have been identified in many renal sites, and a high density of these receptors occur in longitudinal bands in the inner zone of the outer medulla in association with vasa recta bundles.[68] It is also possible that angiotensin II in the renal interstitial fluid may play a role in the regulation of renal functions.[69] It has been demonstrated that *de novo* angiotensin II is formed within the kidney in response to enhanced renin secretion rate.[70] The density of angiotensin II receptors in the glomeruli may play a role in producing glomerular hemodynamic alteration. A strong negative correlation between plasma angiotensin II and glomerular angiotensin receptor density has been shown.[71] Thus, sodium intake may regulate glomerular angiotensin receptor density by the changes it produces on plasma angiotensin levels.

The renin–angiotensin system may interact with other factors and play an important role in their renal hemodynamic responses. Such factors may include adenosine, prostaglandins, and renal nerves. Intrarenal infusion of adenosine leads to a decrease in renin release which can be dissociated from its hemodynamic effect.[72] This adenosine-induced decrease in renin release can be antagonized by theophylline.[73] Hall *et al.*[4] demonstrated that the renin–angiotensin system plays an important, time-dependent role in the renal hemodynamic responses to adenosine. Inhibition of angiotensin II formation by captopril almost totally blocks the transient renal vasoconstriction normally observed with intrarenal adenosine infusions. In a recent study by Hall and Granger,[57] the hypothesis that high renal levels of adenosine may alter GFR control by angiotensin II was tested. Endogenous formation of angiotensin II was blocked by captopril so that changes in its intrarenal formation would not affect adenosine–angiotensin II interactions. Comparisons were then made between RBF and GFR effects of angiotensin II in dogs with and without increased intrarenal levels of adenosine (Fig. 2). The results of this study suggest that adenosine markedly alters GFR control by angiotensin II, probably by causing angiotensin II to constrict preglomerular vessels. This effect is not apparent in most physiologic conditions; however, it could play a role in lowering GFR under certain pathophysiologic states when renal adenosine and angiotensin II levels are simultaneously elevated, as in severe renal ischemia. This interaction occurs in normal as well as nonfiltering kidneys, suggesting that it may be independent of changes in tubuloglomerular feedback.[57]

Interaction between angiotensin II and prostaglandins has been shown to occur in isolated human glomeruli[74] and perfused rat kidney.[75] In both studies, administration of angiotensin II enhanced the formation of prostaglandin E_2 and 6-keto-$F_{1\alpha}$. Angiotensin II also stimulated prostaglandin synthesis in mesangial cells.[76] Sar-1-Thr-8-AII, an antagonist of angiotensin II receptors, blocks stimulation of prostaglandin E_2 synthesis induced by angiotensin II in cultured rat glomerular epithelial cells.[77] Renal synthesis of prostaglandin E_2 appears to be dependent on the activity of angiotensin II, thus suggesting that angiotensin II is a physiologic modulator of renal prostaglandin E_2 synthesis.[78] This interrelationship might have a physiologic importance in the regulation of glomerular hemodynamics.[74]

Angiotensin II appears to be a critical factor for the full functional expression of renal nerve stimulation at the glomerulus.[79] This study demonstrated that generally the effects of renal nerve stimulation on glomerular hemodynamics during angiotensin II inhibition were of much less magnitude than those observed during renal nerve stimulation with the angiotensin II system intact. It has been suggested that during low sodium intake, activation of sympathetic nerve activity elicits an enhanced renin release response.[80] The renin response to continuous renal nerve stimulation is enhanced by concomitantly generated prostaglandin E_2.[81] Intact renal nerves are necessary for the development and maintenance of the mild hypertension that results from sodium restriction in uninephrectomized rats. The pressor contribution of the renal nerves to this form of hypertension appears to be related, at least in part, to the activation of the renin–angiotensin system pressor mechanism.[82] Chronic studies in conscious dogs have indicated that the renal nerves may play a role in the chronic regulation of renin release during both normal and low-sodium diet.[83]

1.4.2. Adenosine

Intrarenal adenosine may play a role in the intrinsic regulation of GFR and RBF; however, the quantitative importance of adenosine in mediating renal hemodynamics is still unclear. Studies by Premen *et al.*[84] in anesthetized dogs failed to provide evidence that adenosine plays an important role in autoregulation of GFR and RBF during acute reduction in renal artery pressure within the autoregulatory range. GFR and RBF were well autoregulated (>90%) at renal perfusion pressure equal to or greater than 85 mm Hg before and after either aminophylline, an adenosine receptor blocker, or intrarenal infusion of adenosine in two separate groups of dogs. Other studies have shown that intrarenal infusion of adenosine causes a significant reduction in baseline GFR, sodium excretion, and filtration fraction in anesthetized dogs.[85] In anesthetized rats, intravenous infusions of 5'-N-ethylcarboxamide adenosine, an A_2-selective agonist, 2-chloroadenosine, a nonselective agonist, and N^6-cyclohexyladenosine, an A_1-selective agonist, produced significant reductions in GFR.[86] Pawlowska *et al.*[87] utilized a chronically implanted polyethylene capsule to infuse adenosine or its analogs into the renal interstitium. Bolus injection followed by continuous infusion of adenosine or its metabolically stable analog 2-chloradenosine produced significant reductions in GFR while having no significant effect on RBF. Interstitial infusion of theophylline, an adenosine receptor antagonist, completely abolished the effects of both adenosine and 2-chloradenosine on GFR, suggesting an extracellular action of adenosine. Intrarenal infusion of adenosine may have an effect on vasa recta blood flow.[88]

Renal adenosine levels appear to increase under certain specific experimental conditions. Urinary excretion of endogenous adenosine increases after the intrarenal injection of contrast media in sodium-depleted anesthetized dogs.[89] This change in adenosine level was associated with a significant reduction in RBF and GFR. These results support the hypothesis that endogenous adenosine is involved in the renal hemodynamic response to contrast media. In two-kidney, one-clip Goldblatt hypertensive rats, renal venous plasma levels of adenosine were found to be elevated sixfold in comparison with sham-operated controls.[90] These data support a role for endogenous adenosine as a regulator of renin release in this renin-dependent form of renovascular hypertension.

1.4.3. Prostaglandins

Prolonged treatment (6 weeks) with indomethacin, an inhibitor of prostaglandin synthesis, does not affect basic renal hemodynamics or renal excretory function in humans with normal renal function.[91] However, such treatment significantly impairs the adaptive responses of both renal excretory function and the renin–angiotensin–aldosterone axis to sodium restriction. In anesthetized dogs, blockade of prostaglandin synthesis by ibuprofen treatment produces no significant changes in GFR and blood flow in outer cortex, inner cortex, or outer medulla, as compared with untreated dogs.[92] Also, intrarenal infusion of prostaglandin E_2 does not have a significant effect on GFR or RBF in anesthetized dogs[93] or rats.[94] Thus, renal function is not dependent on the integrity of prostaglandin synthesis, at least under ordinary circumstances. Inhibition of prostaglandin synthesis in normal animals and humans does not induce a significant decline in renal function.[94,95] Prostaglandins, however, appear to be necessary for the maintenance of glomerular filtration, especially at the lower end of the autoregulatory range. Indomethacin administration increases the pressure dependency of the filtration rate in Sprague–Dawley rats.[60] Both GFR and SNGFR fell significantly in response to reductions in arterial pressure from a normal value of 119 mm Hg to 78 mm Hg. The authors suggested that the existence of an intact prostaglandin system is critical in maintaining GFR at low pressures.[60] In anesthetized dogs, decreases in renal arterial pressure within the autoregulatory range reduce prostaglandin E_2 excretion, whereas GFR and RBF are not affected.[96] Data from isolated rat kidneys suggest that prostaglandins promote pressure natriuresis by maintaining afferent arteriolar dilation. Their inhibition leads to afferent constriction which lowers GFR and reduces sodium excretion.[97]

Prostaglandins may interact with the angiotensin II system to produce renal hemodynamic effects. Renal synthesis of prostaglandin E_2 appears to be dependent on the activity of angiotensin II.[78] In salt-loaded rats, infusion of angiotensin II stimulates glomerular prostaglandin E_2 synthesis, as assessed by tubular fluid measurements.[98] Excretory rates of prostaglandin E_2 increase significantly in association with elevated GFR and RBF during amino acid infusion in normal subjects.[99] A decrease in prostaglandin synthesis could significantly reduce the amino acid–induced hemodynamic effects by removing their permissive effects. In nephrotic animals, an enhanced renal synthesis of prostaglandin I_2 appears to play a critical role in the adaptive changes responsible for the hyperfiltration that results from high-protein diet.[100]

Other widely varied factors have been reported to cause changes in renal hemodynamics. Among these factors are protein loading[101−103] or restriction,[104] amino acid infusion,[105−107] hypoproteinemia[108] and hyperproteinemia,[109] methoxamine and norepinephrine,[110] glucagon,[111] growth hormone,[112] aging,[113] pregnancy,[114,115] thromboxane A_2,[116] leukotriene D_4,[117] renal mass reduction,[118] and spontaneous hypertension.[119]

2. Sodium Chloride Excretion and Regulation

2.1. Sodium Balance and Its Regulation

It is well established that the normal kidney alters sodium excretion in response to vast changes in sodium intake. However, the renal adaptive alterations in response to such widely varying quantities of salt intake remain unclear, particularly in humans. In a study by Roos et al.,[120] changes in extracellular fluid volume (ECFV), humoral factors, and blood pressure were measured after equilibration at three levels of sodium intake (20, 200, and 1128 mEq/day) in normal humans. Significant reductions in plasma renin activity and aldosterone were observed between successive levels of sodium intake, while blood pressure remained similar. ECFV increased significantly as the level of sodium intake was elevated, and this increase in ECFV was strongly correlated with fractional and absolute sodium excretion. Serum chloride increased significantly, but serum sodium was significantly increased only when comparison was made between the high and low sodium intake. GFR increased as the level of sodium intake was elevated. The results of this study demonstrate that in normal humans the maintenance of sodium balance during significant increases in sodium intake depends on renal adaptation of GFR, as well as proximal and distal tubular reabsorption. These changes in kidney function are associated with marked changes in neurohormonal factors and ECFV, whereas changes in blood pressure and serum sodium are only modest. The kidneys' precision in regulating sodium has been reaffirmed in Sprague–Dawley rats by Brensilver et al.[121] When sodium intake was less than the minimum daily requirement of 247 μEq/day, urinary sodium excretion was reduced to a minimum. When more than 247 μEq/day of sodium was ingested, the excess was excreted quantitatively.

The phenomenon of pressure natriuresis and diuresis has been recognized for many decades. Increases in renal perfusion pressure produce a significant increase in sodium and water excretion. Pressure natriuresis results from decreased tubular sodium reabsorption rather than increased filtered load since GFR remains well autoregulated in the face of acute changes in renal perfusion pressure.[122-124] The nephron site of changes in sodium reabsorption that occurs when renal perfusion pressure is altered remains controversial. In a recent micropuncture study by Haas *et al.*[124] it was demonstrated that increases in renal perfusion pressure have no effect on sodium reabsorption by the proximal tubule of superficial nephrons. Sodium delivery to the point of micropuncture in the descending limb of Henle's loop of deep nephrons was increased, suggesting inhibition of sodium reabsorption by proximal tubules of deep nephrons in response to elevations in renal perfusion pressure.

Activation of the renal sympathetic nerves can lead to an increase in sodium reabsorption and a decrease in sodium excretion.[125] The renal nerves act directly on the tubules to increase sodium reabsorption. In addition, activation of the renal sympathetic nervous system increases the release of renin and the formation of angiotensin II.[80-82] Under conditions of marked renal sympathetic nerve activity, renal resistance increases in a way that alters Starling physical forces in favor of increased sodium reabsorption. The importance of the renal sympathetic nerves as sodium regulator diminishes under normal or volume-expanded states.[125]

Sodium excretion and the regulation of sodium balance are influenced and controlled by many factors that often respond in an integrative manner to maintain a near-constant plasma and extracellular fluid sodium concentration.

2.2. Renin–Angiotensin–Aldosterone System

In addition to its hemodynamic effects, angiotensin II is one of the most powerful regulators of extracellular volume and renal sodium excretion.[52,126] A decrease in extracellular fluid volume leads to an increase in angiotensin II formation. Angiotensin II causes the release of aldosterone, which acts on the cortical collecting tubules to enhance sodium reabsorption. Considerable evidence suggests that the intrarenal actions of angiotensin II are quantitatively more important than its extrarenal effect on aldosterone secretion in the normal day-to-day regulation of sodium balance.[52] Angiotensin II markedly constricts efferent arterioles and causes a significant increase in renal vascular resistance. These renal vascular actions tend to increase sodium reabsorption by altering peritubular capillary physical forces. Angiotensin II may also increase sodium reabsorption and enhance urine concentrating ability by reducing renal medullary blood flow (Fig. 3).

For many years, the most widely recognized mechanism by which angiotensin II decreases sodium excretion was its stimulation of aldosterone secretion. However, more recent studies have suggested that angiotensin II has intrarenal actions that may be more important quantitatively in increasing sodium reabsorption than its indirect aldosterone-mediated effects.[125,128] Figure 4 shows results from experiments in which the acute effects of angiotensin II were blocked by infusing a converting enzyme inhibitor into the renal artery.[52,128,131] After 90 min of angiotensin II blockade, urinary sodium excretion, fractional excretion of sodium, and

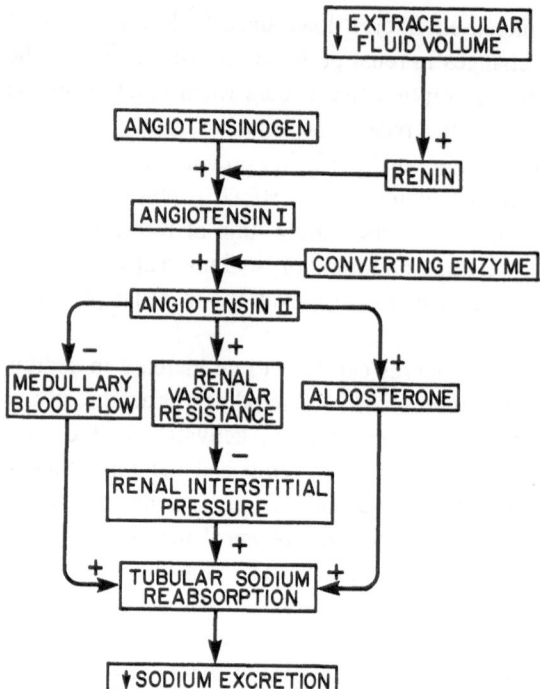

Fig. 3. Block diagram illustrating the possible mechanisms of action of the renin–angiotensin system to affect and regulate sodium excretion.[125]

urine flow rate increased significantly in the absence of a change in plasma aldosterone concentration. These observations indicated a direct intrarenal effect of angiotensin II blockade and emphasized the importance of the intrarenal effects of angiotensin II in allowing the kidney to adapt to low sodium intake.

Angiotensin II has been shown to have a direct effect on the stimulation of tubular sodium reabsorption.[52,54,126-130] Physiologic concentrations of angiotensin II (10^{-11}–10^{-9} M) increase proximal tubular reabsorption, whereas pharmacologic doses (10^{-7} M and above) inhibit reabsorption.[127] Angiotensin II may have an important effect on more distal tubular segments; however, the exact site at which angiotensin II may increase distal tubular transport is still uncertain.[52,128,130] The effects of angiotensin II on the proximal tubules are not neurally mediated since they are observed in denervated kidneys and in nerve-free isolated tubules. In addition, they appear to be mediated by receptors on the basolateral membrane of proximal tubule epithelial cells.[127]

The physiologic significance of the natriuretic and diuretic actions of extremely high levels of angiotensin II remains unclear. The mechanisms responsible for the transition from antinatriuresis to natriuresis and diuresis during progressively higher rates of infusion of angiotensin II appear to be partly related to the hemodynamic changes associated with increased arterial pressure.[52,130] Figure 5 shows the renal excretory responses to various rates of intravenous infusion of angiotensin II in dogs in which renal perfusion pressure was allowed to increase and in the same dogs when renal perfusion pressure was servo-controlled. When renal perfusion pressure was servo-controlled at the same level measured before starting angiotensin II infusion, the natriuretic and diuretic actions of angiotensin II were totally abolished even at extremely high rates of infusion (Fig. 5). These results suggest that natriuresis and diuresis associated with high infusion rates of angiotensin II result from increased renal perfusion pressure, rather than being a direct tubular effect of angiotensin II.[52] The mechanism responsible for the pressure natriuresis and diuresis observed during high rates of angiotensin II infusion appears to be partly due to the decreased fractional reabsorption of sodium in proximal and distal tubules (Fig. 5). Studies in isolated, perfused rabbit proximal tubules have

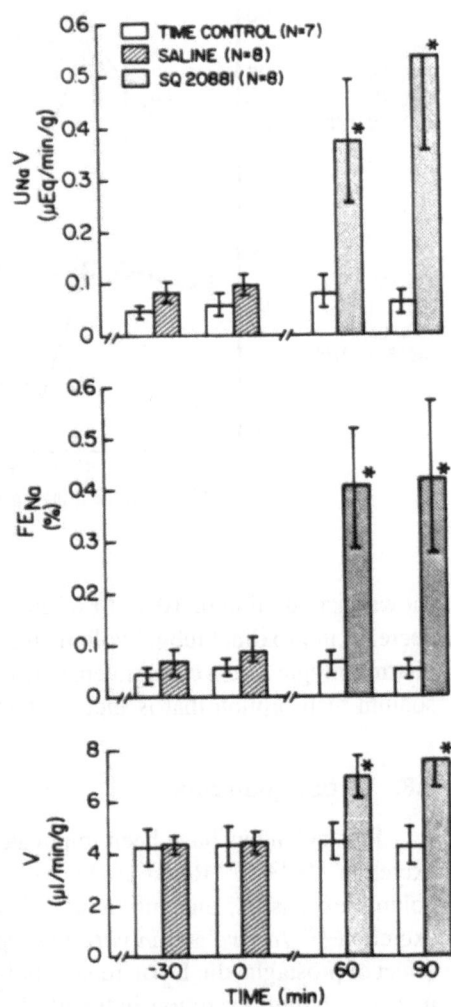

Fig. 4. Changes in urinary sodium excretion ($U_{Na}V$), fractional sodium excretion (FE_{Na}), and urine flow (V) in sodium-depleted dogs during intrarenal infusion of isotonic saline (time control) or the converting enzyme inhibitor SQ-20881.[128]

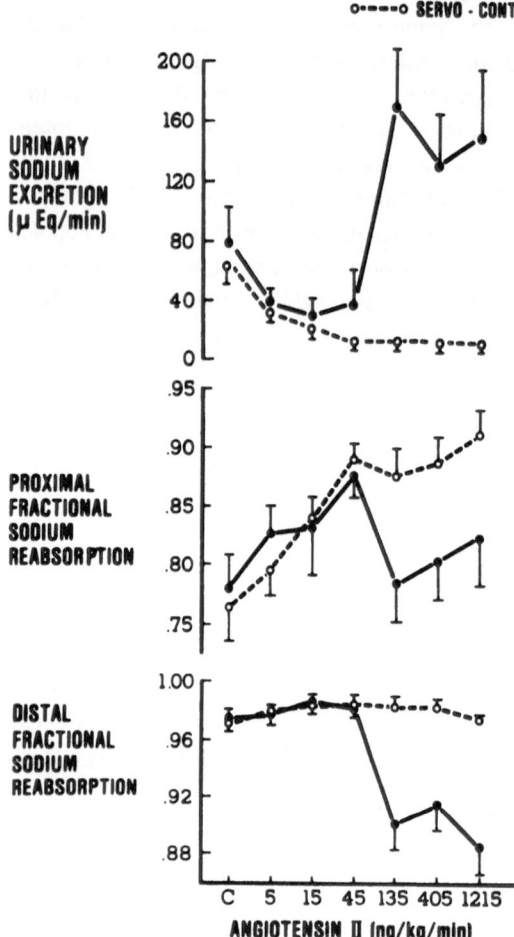

Fig. 5. Changes in urinary sodium excretion, proximal fractional sodium reabsorption (estimated from fractional lithium reabsorption), and distal fractional sodium reabsorption during increasing rates of angiotensin II infusion with renal arterial pressure either maintained at control level (servo-control) or permitted to increase (normal). Distal tubule refers to all parts of renal tubule beyond proximal tubule.[52]

shown that addition of 10^{-7} M of angiotensin II to the bath produced a significant decrease in proximal tubule volume reabsorption.[127,132] These studies indicate that pharmacologic levels of angiotensin II may have a direct inhibitory effect on tubular sodium reabsorption that is independent of increases in renal perfusion pressure.

2.3. Prostaglandins

Prostaglandins have been implicated as regulators of sodium reabsorption and excretion.[122,125,133] Renal production of prostaglandin E_2 is elevated during acute volume expansion, and intrarenal infusion of prostaglandin E_2 increases sodium excretion.[125] *In vivo* and *in vitro* microperfusion studies suggest a direct inhibitory effect of prostaglandin E_2 on renal tubule sodium transport. Prostaglandins may also increase sodium excretion indirectly by increasing medullary blood flow or renal interstitial hydrostatic pressure.[125]

Prostaglandins may play a role in sodium excretion by affecting the mechanism of pressure natriuresis.[96,97,122] Gleim *et al.*[97] studies the renal effects of changing perfusion pressure on control and indomethacin-treated isolated rat kidneys. In control kidneys, significant linear correlations exist between renal artery pressure and GFR, filtration fraction, fractional sodium reabsorption, and sodium excretion. In kidneys treated with indomethacin these correlations shift to the right. Therefore, prostaglandin-inhibited kidneys require higher renal perfusion pressures than control kidneys to maintain similar filtration rates and sodium excretion. It was suggested that prostaglandins promote pressure natriuresis in isolated perfused rat kidney by afferent arteriolar dilation mechanism. In prostaglandin-inhibited kidneys, afferent constriction may ensue, leading to an increase in renal vascular resistance and reductions of GFR, filtration fraction, and sodium excretion. In anesthetized sodium-replete dogs, prostaglandin synthesis inhibition dramatically impairs the pressure-natriuresis response.[96,122] In dogs treated with indomethacin, sodium excretion was reduced by 70% (Fig. 6), but GFR and autoregulatory capability were not affected. In dogs not treated with indomethacin there is a signifi-

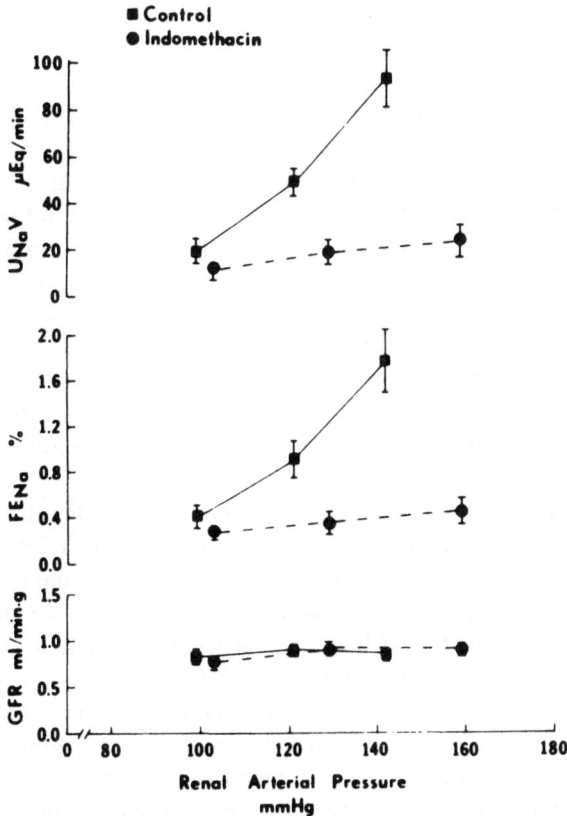

Fig. 6. Effect of prostaglandin synthesis inhibition (indomethacin) on pressure natriuresis in sodium-loaded dogs. $U_{Na}V$, urinary sodium excretion; FE_{Na}, fractional sodium excretion.[122]

cant correlation between urinary prostaglandin E_2 excretion and sodium excretion within the autoregulatory range.[122] These observations suggest that the renal prostaglandin system may have an important effect on the pressure natriuresis mechanism.

2.4. Atrial Natriuretic Factor

Atrial natriuretic factor (ANF) comprises a family of peptide hormones that was discovered in 1981 by deBold *et al.*[134] Since then, a considerable body of evidence has been accumulating on the ability of ANF to relax vascular smooth muscles[135–137] and modulate the actions of the renin–angiotensin–aldosterone system.[137,138] ANF produces a rapid and brisk natriuresis and diuresis[134,139] and may play an important role in the control of sodium balance and the regulation of ECFV.

2.4.1. Synthesis and Release of ANF

ANF is a peptide that is synthesized in atrial cardiocytes in mammals.[138,140] When released, ANF circulates and interacts with specific receptors eliciting multiple biologic actions that are mainly involved with fluid volume homeostasis and modulating the actions of the renin–angiotensin–aldosterone system.[138,140] The atrial myocytes synthesize the initial ANF precursor, process it to a 126-amino-acid polypeptide, and store this prohormone (pro-ANF: Asn 1–Tyr 126) in secretory granules.[140–143] A 28-amino-acid polypeptide identified as the C-terminal of pro-ANF (Ser 99–Tyr 126) appears to be the predominant circulating atrial peptide[142] and the major biologically active form released from isolated rat heart.[140,144] An enzyme (IRCM–SP1) has been isolated by Cantin and Genest from heart atria and ventricles.[141] This enzyme is highly specific in cleaving pro-ANF (Asn 1–Tyr 126) to yield ANF (103–126), (102–126), and (99–126). Inagami *et al.* isolated specific peptidases that are responsible for the conversion of pro-ANF to circulating ANF in rats.[143] The variety in molecular forms of rat ANF suggests that the processing system for ANF precursors differs from tissue to tissue.[145] The structure of ANF (99–126) in humans and dogs differs from that in rats, mice, and rabbits by one amino acid.[140]

Atrial distention has been consistently found to be the stimulus for the release of ANF into the circulation. In a study by Fried *et al.*[146] the relationship between right atrial pressure (RAP) and plasma ANF levels after an acute Ringer's solution volume expansion was examined in Sprague–Dawley rats. Acute volume expansion was achieved by infusing 5% of body weight Ringer's solution over a period of 5 min. RAP was manipulated by inflating or deflating a balloon catheter that was placed into the thoracic inferior vena cava through the left femoral vein. The result of this study is illustrated in Figure 7, which demonstrates a significant correlation between RAP and plasma ANF level.[146] Studies on isolated Sprague–Dawley rat hearts have shown that direct mechanical stretch of the atria results in the release of ANF.[147] This release appears to be influenced by both the extent and rate of atrial

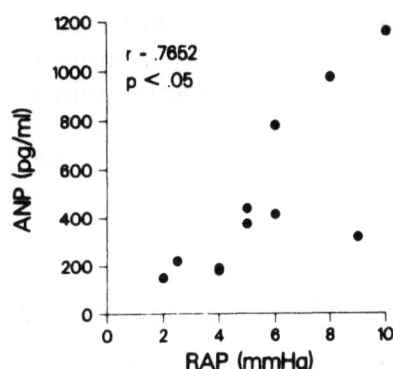

Fig. 7. Relationship between peak right atrial pressure (RAP) and plasma levels of atrial natriuretic peptide (ANP) in Sprague–Dawley rats (*n* = 10). Arterial blood was withdrawn for plasma ANP measurements after 1 min of 5% body weight volume expansion with Ringer's solution.[146]

stretch.[148] *In vivo* studies in rats[149,150] and dogs[151] have suggested that the atria detect alterations in ECFV or intravascular fluid volume and release ANF. It appears that the ANF hormonal system is functional during fetal life and that the release of ANF is stimulated, as in mature animals, by an increase in intracardiac pressure.[152] In humans, the release of ANF is at least partly regulated by right and left atrial pressures[153] and ANF is rapidly released in response to atrial volume and pressure changes.[154] It appears that atrial distention, whatever the cause, releases ANF into plasma in humans.[155] Also, head-out water immersion stimulates the release of ANF from the atria, most likely through a direct hemodynamic effect.[156] In addition, some data suggest that ANF-containing cardiocytes may respond directly to changes in systemic electrolytes such as sodium or chloride ions.[150] The release of ANF is not mediated by endogenous neurotransmitters[147] and may not be controlled by the cardiac nerves[157] since atrial distention consistently increases plasma concentrations of ANF in cardiac-denervated dogs.[158] This proposal is still controversial. Eskay *et al.*[150] have shown that complete cardiac denervation in the pithed rat preparation, which removes both humoral influences that originate in the central nervous system and direct neuronal control of the heart by the vagal and sympathetic nerves, blocks the volume loading–induced release of ANF. These results suggest that neuronal influences may be important in the release of ANF during volume expansion.

Plasma levels of ANF are elevated in patients with various heart diseases.[159] The highest plasma ANF concentrations are found in patients with the most marked impairment of ventricular function and mitral valve disease. In patients with coronary heart disease or with cardiomyopathy, a linear relationship is found between plasma ANF levels and left ventricular filling pressure or mean pulmonary artery pressure, respectively.[159] In a study by Burnett *et al.*,[160] circulating levels of ANF were measured in normal human subjects, in patients with cardiovascular disease and normal cardiac filling pressure, and in patients with cardiovascular disease and elevated cardiac filling pressure with and without congestive heart failure. The results of these studies showed that elevated cardiac filling pressure is associated with elevated circulating concentrations of ANF and that congestive heart failure is not characterized by a deficiency of, but by an increase in, ANF. Plasma levels of ANF are also elevated in patients with chronic renal failure and spontaneous tachyarrhythmias.[161] In rats with myocardial infarction induced by left coronary artery ligation, plasma ANF levels varied directly with increasing infarct and atrial sizes. However, atrial ANF concentration varied inversely with increasing infarct size.[162] These studies and others[163] suggest that chronic stimulation of ANF release from the atria is associated with turnover and depleted stores of ANF in proportion to the severity of the heart failure. In cardiomyopathic hamsters with congestive heart failure, circulating ANF is significantly higher than in control animals, indicating that secretion of ANF is stimulated and atrial storage of the peptide is reduced during congestive heart failure.[164]

Plasma levels of ANF are elevated in hypertensive human subjects with cardiac hypertrophy.[165,166] Also, studies on isolated heart–lung preparations from hypertensive inbred Dahl salt-hypertension sensitive (S) and normotensive inbred Dahl salt-hypertension resistant (R) rats revealed that at any atrial pressure, hearts of hypertensive S rats release more ANF than hearts of normotensive R rats.[167] This difference in the release of ANF between the two strains of rats is probably a consequence of hypertension. The relationships between ANF release and atrial pressure observed in this study support the proposal that atrial distention stimulates the release of ANF in normotensive and hypertensive states.[167] It appears that all of the atrial and ventricular myocardium can express the ANF gene and recruitment increases in response to passive stretch of the cardiac chambers.[168] Plasma ANF concentrations have been shown to increase during rapid atrial pacing,[169] whereas caval constriction appears to produce a significant reduction in the baseline level of plasma ANF.[170]

2.4.2. Effects of ANF on Sodium Excretion

ANF produces relaxation of aortic strips, inhibits steroidogenesis in both zona glomerulosa and zona fasciculata cells, and inhibits the release of arginine vasopressin from the isolated rat hypothalamohypophysial preparation *in vitro*, but decreases vasopressin release *in vivo* only at pharmacologic doses.[141] In mammals, ANF administration modulates renal and systemic vascular resistance and decreases mean arterial pressure, cardiac output, and plasma volume.[171] However, the most striking effect of ANF is its ability to produce enhanced sodium and water excretion and its modulatory actions on the renin–angiotensin–aldosterone system.[138] Figure 8 shows the effects of intravenous infusion of synthetic alpha-human atrial natriuretic peptide (αhANP) on renal hemodynamic and excretory function in normal human subjects.[172] In this study, the plasma concentration of αhANP averaged 58 ± 12 pg/ml under control conditions, was increased to 625 ± 87 pg/ml during αhANP infusion at a rate of 6.25 μg/min, and fell to control values during recovery. GFR, filtration fraction (FF), urine flow rate, and sodium and potassium excretions increased during αhANP infusion. In addition, systolic and diastolic

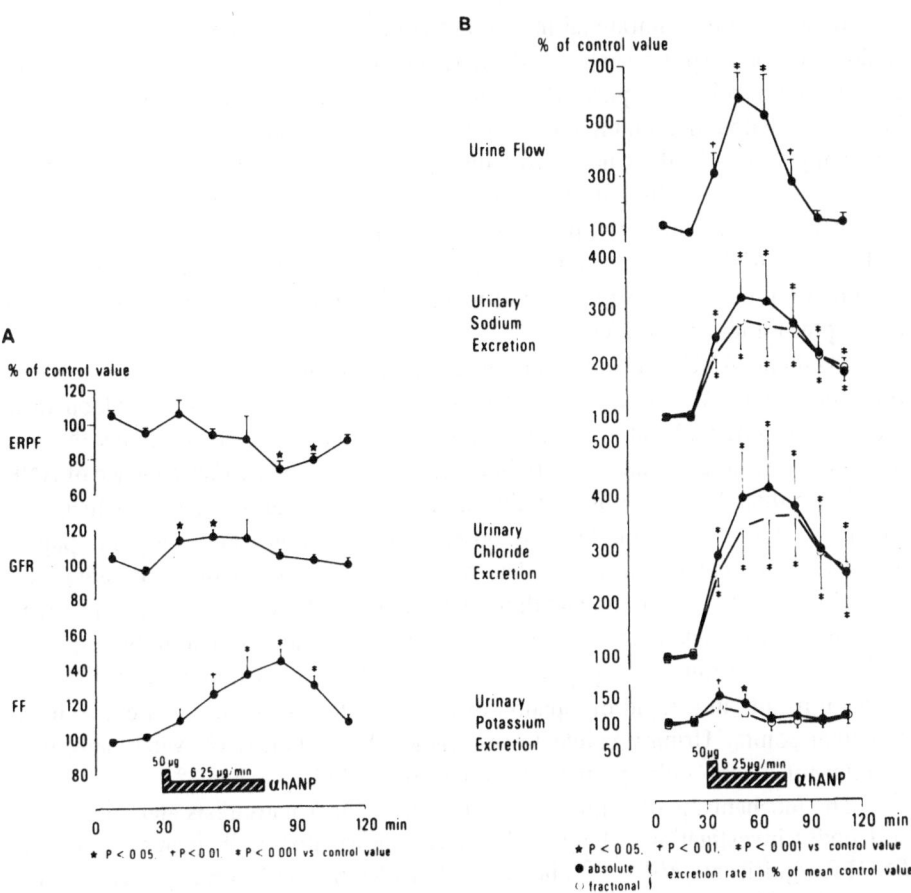

Fig. 8. Effect of synthetic alpha-human atrial natriuretic peptide (αhANP), a 50-μg bolus followed by maintenance infusion of 6.25 μg/min, on renal hemodynamics (A) and renal excretory response (B) in 10 normal human subjects (mean ± SE). The mean of two control values is taken as 100%. ERPF, effective renal plasma flow; GFR, glomerular filtration rate; FF, filtration fraction.[172]

blood pressures decreased while heart rate increased significantly.[172] Similar effects of ANF on blood pressure have been demonstrated by other investigators in humans[173] and rats.[174−176]

The natriuretic effect of ANF is not mediated by or dependent on renal prostaglandins.[177] Also, renal innervation is not necessary for natriuresis and diuresis produced by ANF.[178] However, the natriuretic responses of ANF are modulated by the prevailing levels of renal perfusion pressure.[179,180] Reductions in renal artery pressure may block the natriuretic and diuretic effects of ANF by interfering with its hemodynamic actions or by causing an increase in sodium reabsorption to limit delivery to terminal nephron segments.[181] Thus, peritubular capillary hydrostatic and oncotic pressures may modulate the natriuretic and diuretic effects of ANF.[182]

In normal dogs, intrarenal infusion of ANF results in a significant decrease in renin secretion despite a sustained decrease in mean arterial pressure. This effect of ANF on renin release requires a functional macula densa, since in the nonfiltering kidney, ANF does not inhibit renin secretion.[183] This conclusion is supported by data indicating that ANF does not have a direct action on juxtaglomerular cells.[184,185] When rabbit isolated afferent arterioles are exposed to αhANF, renin release rate does not change significantly.[184] In addition to its *in vivo* effects on renin secretion, endogenous ANF has been shown to substantially modulate the sympathetic activity by inhibiting epinephrine release and baroreceptor reflexes in conscious dogs and under physiologic conditions.[186]

Synthetic ANF infusion results in a significant increase in vasa recta blood flow that occurs 45 min after the start of ANF infusion.[187] Papillary blood flow increases significantly after 2 min of ANF infusion in anesthetized rats.[188] The increases in vasa recta and papillary blood flows appear to be a consequence of ANF infusion rather than the cause of the natriuresis and diuresis, since increases in sodium excretion and urine flow are observed before significant changes in papillary and vasa recta blood flows are detected.[187,188] The renal papilla does not play a critical role in the natriuretic and diuretic response of ANF. Anesthetized rats with papillary necrosis and control rats have a similar ANF-induced natriuretic response, indicating that a functional papilla is not required for the action of ANF.[189] ANF infusion results in a rapid dissipation of the medullary gradient for urea, sodium, and total solute. Urinary solute losses, rather than addition of water, appear to account for a substantial portion of the loss of medullary solute.[190]

The mechanisms of action by which ANF induces natriuresis and diuresis are still under investigation. Many studies have shown that ANF increases GFR or SNGFR significantly[37,191–193]; however, considerable controversy presently exists on whether ANF enhances sodium excretion primarily through an effect on increasing the filtered load of sodium by increasing filtration rate, or by inhibition of tubular reabsorption either directly or indirectly. In a study by Cogan,[191] ANF caused a significant increase in SNGFR and GFR. When these filtration rates were brought back to control levels by aortic constriction, proximal transport was reduced to normal despite continued ANF administration, and 90% of the ANF-induced natriuresis and chloruresis was abolished. The author concluded that ANF has no direct effect on reabsorption in the superficial proximal convoluted tubule independent of changes in GFR and suggested that ANF can increase renal solute excretion predominantly by increasing GFR.[191] Unfortunately, the utilization of aortic constriction to normalize GFR often results in renal perfusion pressures that are different between the two periods that are being compared. The arterial pressure was significantly reduced during the ANF plus aortic constriction period as compared with both the control period and the period of ANF infusion.[191] In a study by Haas *et al.*[124] it was demonstrated that increases in renal perfusion pressure have no effect on sodium reabsorption by the proximal tubule of superficial nephrons. Sodium delivery to the point of micropuncture in the descending limb of Henle's loop of deep nephrons was increased, suggesting inhibition of sodium reabsorption by proximal tubules of deep nephrons in response to elevation in renal perfusion pressure. Thus, it is likely that the antinatriuretic effects of the reduction in renal perfusion pressure may be counterbalancing the natriuretic effects of ANF in distal or deep nephron segments. The increase in glomerular filtration that is often observed when ANF is infused may be the result of an increase in glomerular capillary hydrostatic pressure[192] or a combined increase in both glomerular capillary hydrostatic pressure and ultrafiltration coefficient.[193] The localization of ANF glomerular receptors may explain the direct effects of ANF on glomerular capillaries and the resulting increase in the filtration rate.[194]

In a recent study by Burnett et al.,[195] controlling GFR by aortic clamping did not abolish the natriuresis of ANF in anesthetized dogs. Despite no change in GFR and thus filtered load of sodium, there was a significant increase in fractional excretion of sodium and lithium, a marker for proximal reabsorption of sodium. The contrast between this study and that of Cogan[191] is probably related to the aortic clamping. Reduction in renal perfusion pressure prevents the ANF-induced increase in GFR, but it can also have a direct effect on enhancing tubular reabsorption of sodium and water which could neutralize the proposed tubular action of ANF. Other studies have shown that ANF can cause natriuresis and diuresis without significantly altering GFR.[178,179,196-199] Data collected from uninephrectomized baboons dissociated the effects of ANF on water and solute excretion from those on GFR and filtration fraction.[200] Also, under conditions of salt loading and water diuresis, ANF induces natriuresis and diuresis in humans without altering GFR.[201] It is most likely that ANF-induced natriuresis is mediated by both an increase in GFR and a decrease in tubular reabsorption.

Several studies attempted to identify the possible nephron site at which ANF could be inhibiting sodium and water reabsorption. Some of these studies utilized whole kidney clearance[189,202-205] and in vitro microperfusion methods[204]; others used micropuncture[199,206,207] and microcatheterization procedures.[207] Burnett et al.[202] showed that intrarenal infusion of ANF in anesthetized dogs results in an increase in fractional lithium and phosphate excretion, suggesting that this factor may have an effect on proximal tubule reabsorption. Infusion of ANF in thyroparathyroidectomized rats increases fractional excretion of sodium, phosphate, and bicarbonate.[203] Luminal brush border membrane vesicles from renal cortex of these rats have significantly decreased sodium-dependent phosphate transport as measured by rapid filtration techniques. Direct addition of ANF to brush border membrane vesicles had no effect on sodium-dependent phosphate transport, and direct application of this factor to isolated proximal tubules had no effect on sodium transport. In another study by Baum and Toto,[204] in vitro microperfusion techniques were utilized to examine the effect of ANF on rabbit proximal tubule. The results of these studies showed that ANF does not have a direct inhibitory effect on transport in the proximal tubules. These results may lead to the conclusion that ANF does not directly inhibit sodium transport in the proximal tubules, but may induce changes in transport through an indirect mechanism. Physiologic concentrations of ANF act within the kidney to decrease proximal tubule reabsorption by inhibition of angiotensin-stimulated sodium and water transport.[206]

ANF may act to alter sodium transport at a nephron site distal to the proximal tubule. Infusion of synthetic ANF in Munich–Wistar rats produces a significant increase in absolute and fractional deliveries of sodium and water to the papillary end-descending limb in juxtamedullary nephrons, despite no significant changes in SNGFR.[199] The author concluded that ANF blunts sodium reabsorption in the deep nephrons presumably in the juxtamedullary proximal tubule and/or thin descending limb of Henle's loop. Results from a study by Peterson et al.[207] failed to demonstrate a significant direct peritubular effect on ANF on thick ascending limb sodium chloride permeability in outer cortical nephrons. Sonnenberg et al.[208] characterized sodium transport in the inner medullary collecting duct before and after ANF infusion in anesthetized rats. Infusion of ANF was associated with increased sodium delivery and decreased fractional sodium reabsorption in the collecting duct. Similar increase in delivery by potassium chloride had no effect on fractional sodium reabsorption. The results of this study support the proposal that ANF has a specific inhibitory effect on net sodium transport in the inner medullary collecting duct. However, other studies conflict with this proposal. Results from a study by Hildebrandt and Banks[189] indicated that the medullary collecting duct is not a major site of action of ANF and that a functional papilla is not required for its action.

There are many potential mechanisms by which ANF can have an effect on tubular sodium and water reabsorption. ANF could have a direct inhibitory effect on active tubular transport of sodium and water, or indirectly inhibit this transport via changes in medullary blood flow and intrarenal hormones. Many studies failed to provide evidence for a direct effect of ANF to inhibit sodium transport in isolated proximal tubules.[203,204] However, in a study by Cantiello and Ausiello,[209] the possible direct effect of ANF and cyclic $3',5'$-guanosine monophosphate (cGMP) on sodium transport of renal epithelial cells was investigated. Renal cell culture model, $LLC-PK_1$, which contains an amiloride-sensitive conductive sodium transport pathway and a sodium–hydrogen exchanger, was used in these experiments. ANF (10^{-7} M) or exogenous cGMP (10^{-3} M) maximally inhibited the uptake of $^{22}Na^+$ through the amiloride-sensitive conductive pathway which represented up to 60% of the total $^{22}Na^+$ uptake. It was concluded that ANF can directly inhibit sodium transport in renal epithelial cells probably through stimulation of cGMP. The biologic activity of ANF appears to be mediated by cGMP.[210,211] ANF stimulates glomerular production of cGMP[212–214] and enhances intracellular cGMP in glomerular mesangial cells.[215] cGMP mediates the transport effects of ANF in rabbit inner medullary collecting duct, indicating that cGMP may play an important role in regulation of the renal transport of sodium.[216]

ANF may decrease sodium reabsorption by dissipating the medullary tonicity via a medullary washout mechanism. Continuous intrarenal infusion of ANF in dogs caused a significant decrease in urine osmolality with maintained free-water clearance. During recovery, urine osmolality returned to control values, suggesting that medullary washout did not occur.[202] Studies on medullary hemodynamics have indicated that increases in vasa recta and papillary blood flows are a consequence rather than the cause of the natriuresis of ANF.[187,188]

Intrarenal infusion of ANF in anesthetized dogs significantly decreases renin secretion rate,[179,202] even under conditions of acute low-output heart failure, which is a state of high renin secretion.[217] Intravenous infusion of ANF has a similar effect on renin secretion.[218] The mechanism by which ANF reduces renin secretion is not completely understood. Studies by Opgenorth et al.[183] support an important role for the macula densa in ANF inhibition of renin secretion. In the nonfiltering kidney, where the macula densa is nonfunctional, ANF was found to have no inhibitory effect on renin secretion. The macula densa may have been responding to an increased delivery of sodium chloride by signaling the juxtaglomerular cells to reduce renin secretion. Although these data provide strong support for a macula densa mechanism, the possibility of ANF having a direct inhibitory effect on juxtaglomerular cells cannot be ruled out. It is possible that part of the natriuretic effect of ANF may be mediated by the ability of this factor to suppress the renin–angiotensin system.

In addition to its inhibitory effect on renin release, ANF has been shown to significantly decrease plasma aldosterone levels in anesthetized dogs[218] and rats.[219] In vitro studies have also shown that ANF directly inhibits aldosterone production by suspensions of bovine adrenal glomerulosa cells[220] as well as the angiotensin II–stimulated aldosterone release in isolated rat adrenal glomerulosa cells.[221–223] It is possible that the reduced levels of circulating angiotensin II produced by the suppressed renin secretion observed during ANF infusion could be responsible for the decrease in aldosterone release. The suppression of aldosterone secretion may not play an important role in the acute natriuretic response to ANF. However, chronic alterations in circulating levels of this hormone by ANF could mediate the long-term regulation of sodium balance.

2.4.3. ANF and Regulation of Sodium Excretion

It is universally accepted that infusion of ANF has a potent effect on sodium excretion; however, the quantitative importance of this factor in regulating sodium balance is not as clear. Plasma levels of ANF increase with increasing sodium intake in humans.[224] In conscious dogs, infusion of hypertonic saline induces an increase in plasma osmolality and a significant elevation in plasma levels of ANF.[225] Immersion to the neck in water induces central hypervolemia in normal humans that is accompanied by a prompt and marked increase in plasma ANF.[226]

In a study by Schwab et al.,[227] acute right atrial appendectomy in rats was shown to attenuate the acute volume expansion-induced increases in circulating ANF and urinary sodium excretion. The results of this study and of others[228,229] suggest that in rats the natriuresis and diuresis of acute volume expansion is mediated at least in part by an elevation in circulating ANF. These findings do not appear to be similar in dogs. Chronic bilateral atrial appendectomy failed to significantly attenuate the elevation in ANF or alter sodium excretion after dogs were volume-expanded.[230] These differences between the response of dogs and rats may suggest that in dogs the release of ANF contained in the atrial appendages is not necessary for the normal renal response to acute volume expansion. It is also possible that during the recovery period from the chronic appendectomy (10–14 days), the granules in the remaining atrial tissue proliferate and compensate for those lost by the appendectomy. This proposal may explain the increase in plasma ANF during acute volume expansion in dogs despite the chronic bilateral removal of the atrial appendages.[231]

In a recent study by Khraibi *et al.*[232] the quantitative role of ANF in mediating the natriuresis induced by acute volume loading was determined in anesthetized rats. In one group of rats, acute volume expansion was established by infusing saline (5% body weight) over a period of 30 min. A second group of rats was infused with synthetic ANF (2 μg·kg^{-1}·h^{-1}) to mimic the high plasma levels of ANF observed during acute volume loading. A third group served as control. The results of this study are shown in Figure 9. Infusion of ANF at a dose that produces a similar plasma level of ANF as does acute saline volume expansion can induce ~40% of natriuresis and diuresis of volume expansion. The fact that synthetic ANF

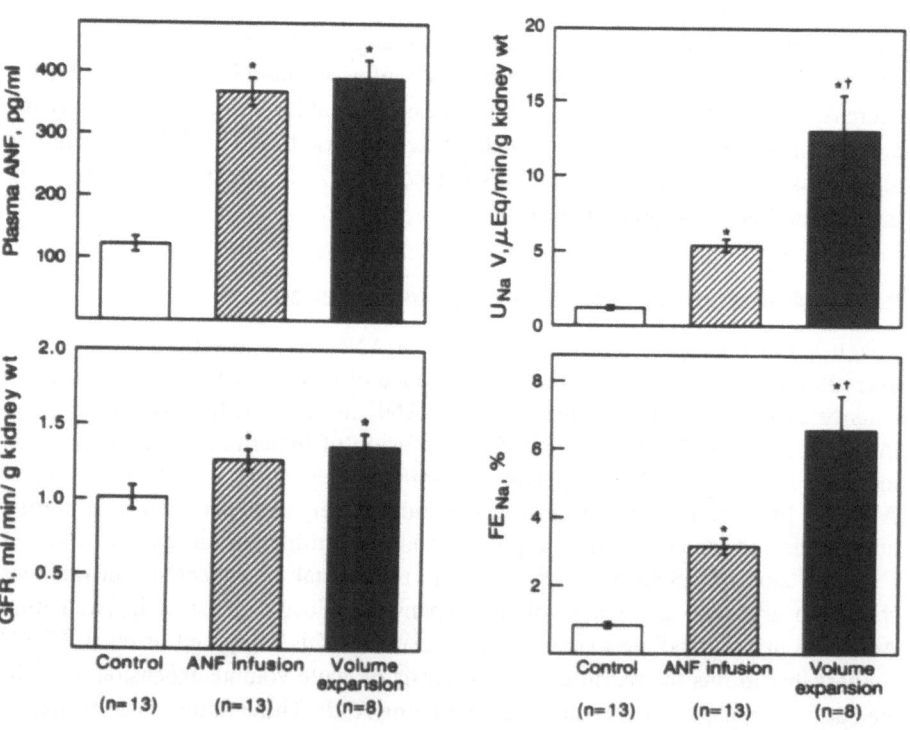

Fig. 9. Plasma circulating levels of atrial natriuretic factor (ANF) and renal responses in control rats, rats infused with ANF (2 μg·kg^{-1}h^{-1}), and saline volume-expanded rats (5% of body weight over a period of 30 min). Values are means ± SE. *$p < 0.05$ vs. control; †$p < 0.05$ vs. ANF infusion. GFR, glomerular filtration rate; $U_{Na}V$, urinary sodium excretion; FE_{Na}, fractional excretion of sodium.[232]

infusion did not totally simulate acute volume expansion indicates that factors other than circulating ANF may mediate the natriuretic and diuretic response induced by volume loading. The results of this study[232] and of others[233,234] support the proposal that circulating levels of ANF may be quantitatively important in mediating the natriuresis during acute volume expansion. In addition, ANF has been suggested by many investigators to play an important role in the regulation of sodium excretion[235] and balance,[236] blood volume[236,237] and extracellular fluid volume,[238] and blood pressure.[236,237,239]

3. Function of Discrete Nephron Segments

3.1. Proximal Tubule

The proximal convoluted tubule is responsible for the reabsorption of almost all of the filtered bicarbonate, glucose, and amino acids, as well as 40% or more of the filtered sodium, fluid, chloride, and phosphate.[240] In rats, volume absorption in this segment of the nephron occurs in two phases. In the first phase, the absorption of glucose, amino acids, organic acids, and sodium bicarbonate constitutes most of the volume absorption and is associated with an increase in luminal chloride concentration. The second phase of volume absorption occurs from a tubular fluid high in chloride and mainly involves the absorption of sodium chloride. At least 80% of sodium chloride absorption from the rat proximal convoluted tubule occurs in the second phase.[241] In the proximal tubules, several transport mechanisms are utilized to transport sodium from the lumen to the proximal tubule epithelial cells. These include sodium-dependent organic solute cotransport, sodium–hydrogen exchange, directly coupled sodium chloride transport, and rheogenic sodium entry.[242] All the forms of sodium chloride cotransport are examples of secondary active transport, and the primary active transport step is the maintenance of the sodium gradient by the basolateral Na^+,K^+-ATPase. Studies in the rabbit proximal convoluted tubule have indicated that sodium chloride transport is transcellular and electroneutral.[243] It appears that Na^+-H^+ and $Cl^--HCO^-_3(OH^-)$ antiporters mediate the neutral active sodium chloride transport in the proximal convoluted tubules.[244] In the proximal straight tubules, the active component is simple rheogenic sodium transport, with chloride absorption driven through the paracellular shunt pathway by the lumen negative potential difference.[245] In LLC-PK$_1$, a cell line derived from pig kidney epithelium, at least a fraction of the transepithelial sodium transport occurs through a simple rheogenic transport system.[246]

Harris et al.[247] studied the Na^+-H^+ exchange in 3-day primary cultures of rat proximal tubule cells which retained the functional characteristics of in vivo proximal tubules. The results of these studies demonstrate that Na^+-H^+ exchange mediates the majority of net sodium influx into these cells and that after cellular acidification, sodium content increases due to further activation of Na^+-H^+ exchange. Secondary stimulation of Na^+-K^+ pump activity is also induced by the increased intracellular sodium content, demonstrating a coupling of the Na^+-K^+ pump to Na^+-H^+ exchange in the acidification response. In posthypercapnic rabbits, there is an increase in maximum activity (V_{max}) of Na^+-H^+ antiporter mediated through the electroneutral Na^+-H^+ exchange and not through conductive hydrogen and sodium pathway.[248] Adenosine cAMP inhibits the rate of bicarbonate reabsorption and the rate of Na^+-H^+ exchange transport in the apical membrane of the proximal convoluted tubule.[249] N-ethoxycarbonyl-2-ethoxy-1,2-dihydroquino-line (EEDQ), a carboxyl-activating agent, inhibits the renal Na^+-H^+ antiporter by decreasing both the V_{max} and K_m (concentration of sodium that results in half V_{max}).[250] Several manipulations have been shown to increase the exchange rate of the renal Na^+-H^+ antiporter. These include metabolic acidosis, glucocorticoid admin-istration, chronic renal failure, and unilateral nephrectomy.[250] In isolated proximal tubule cells, acute application of glucocorticoid increases the activity of the Na^+-H^+ exchanger by increasing the V_{max} of the carrier for external Na^+ and for external H^+. The activation requires RNA and protein synthesis and is consistent with an increase in the number of carriers in the membrane.[251]

Many manipulations have been shown to affect transport in the proximal tubules. Administration of benzolamide, a carbonic anhydrase inhibitor, reduces the rate of proximal tubule fluid reabsorption and peritubular capillary water uptake forces.[252] In rabbits fed varying protein diets, a significant increase in fluid absorp-tion was observed in superficial proximal straight tubule segments obtained from remnant renal tissue harvested 3 weeks after uninephrectomy when compared with sham-operated controls. The changes in fluid absorption following uninephrectomy are attributed to elevations in the active, but not the passive, component of fluid transport in all protein-fed groups.[253] Norepinephrine stimulates solute transport in isolated rabbit proximal convoluted tubules by increasing Na^+,K^+-ATPase ac-tivity,[254] while angiotensin II decreases fluid transport in proximal convoluted and straight tubules.[255] The importance of the factors affecting proximal tubular reab-sorption may change during development. Kaskel et al.[256] suggested that during early postnatal life glomerulotubular balance is achieved by a high permeability of the proximal tubule, which compensates for the low net reabsorptive pressure. As the animal matures, proximal tubule epithelium becomes tighter; thus, in order to maintain tubuloglomerular balance, an increase in the number of intercellular chan-nels and in active transport of sodium is postulated by the authors. Nephron hetero-geneity may be a factor in determining transport in the proximal tubule. It has been demonstrated that increases in renal perfusion pressure result in decreases in sodium reabsorption by the proximal tubule of deep, but not superficial, nephrons.[124]

3.2. Loop of Henle

The medullary thick ascending limb of Henle absorbs large amounts of sodium chloride, but is impermeable to water; thus it dilutes the urine, increases medullary osmolality, and contributes to the countercurrent concentrating mechanism. In the past few years the mechanisms and factors that control sodium chloride absorption by the thick ascending limb of the loop of Henle have been substantially modified. In two reviews by Hebert and Andreoli[257] and Molony et al.,[258] evidence was presented for a model of sodium chloride absorption in the thick ascending limb. According to this model, net chloride absorption is rheogenic, involves a secondary active transport mechanism, and occurs via a furosemide-sensitive coupled electroneutral $(Na^+, K^+, 2Cl^-)$ apical chloride transport process. The apical chloride entry mechanism occurs in parallel with a large potassium conductance across the luminal membrane and a conductive chloride exit mechanism in basolateral plasma membranes. The metabolic energy needed for active transcellular sodium absorption is reduced in this model owing to the positive voltage in the lumen and the high paracellular conductance in the thick ascending limb that provides for 50% of net sodium absorption via the paracellular route. The driving force for paracellular sodium absorption is the lumen-positive potential. Molony et al.[259] proposed that in isolated segments of mouse medullary thick ascending limb, antidiuretic hormone may elevate sodium chloride absorption by increasing the functional number of apical membrane $Na^+, K^+, 2Cl^-$ transport units, enhancing the conductance of potassium across the luminal membrane, and indirectly increasing chloride conductance through the basolateral membrane. Prostaglandin E_2 inhibits antidiuretic hormone stimulation of sodium chloride transport in the isolated microperfused mouse medullary thick ascending loop of Henle.[258] In the presence of 1-desamino-8-D-arginine vasopressin, the fractional delivery of water, sodium, and chloride at the bend of the long-loop nephron decreases.[260] Elalouf et al. hypothesized that water removal along the rat descending limb of Henle increases outward sodium chloride diffusion along this segment of the nephron.[260] In addition, the descending limb of the long-loop nephron of hamsters appears to have an important role in the medullary recycling of potassium by passive diffusion mechanism.[261]

The electrically neutral Na,K,Cl cotransport in the thick ascending limb of Henle's loop is inhibited by the loop diuretics furosemide and bumetanide.[262] Elevations in tubular sodium delivery are associated with an increase in Na^+, K^+-ATPase in isolated medullary thick ascending limb of Henle's loop from sodium-loaded but not from furosemide-treated rats. The lack of inhibition of Na^+, K^+-ATPase by furosemide in the thick ascending limb of Henle may be due to elevated sodium delivery to this nephron segment, which counteracts the effect of furosemide.[263] Recently, a mathematical model has been developed by Taniguchi et al.[264] which can take species differences and internephron heterogeneity into account and illustrates the transport processes along the descending limb of Henle's loop under various physiologic and pathophysiologic conditions.

3.3. Distal Tubule

In distal tubule cells, four different pathways may mediate Na, K, and Cl transport across the luminal membrane. Two pathways permit diffusive movement of cations, one an amiloride inhibitable channel for sodium, the other a barium inhibitable channel for potassium.[265] At least two pathways mediate sodium transport across the luminal membrane of the distal tubule. One pathway is a conductive channel and the other may be a coupled Na^+-Cl^- cotransport pathway.[266] It appears that the early distal tubule has a greater capacity to transport sodium and chloride than the late distal tubule. In the early distal tubule, almost all transcellular sodium transport utilizes a Na^+-Cl^- cotransport pathway, while other pathways may mediate the majority of sodium transport by the late distal tubule.[266] Results of studies by Velazquez *et al.*[267] suggest that a mechanism that mediates K^+-Cl^- secretion is located in the luminal membrane of distal convoluted tubule and initial collecting tubule epithelium. The initial collecting tubule appears to be the major site of potassium secretion. The distal convoluted tubule secretes potassium at a low rate that is not affected by flow or high-potassium diet.[268] Thus, this segment of the distal tubule contributes to total potassium excretion.[267]

3.4. The Collecting System

The apical cell membrane ionic conductive properties of rabbit isolated perfused cortical collecting tubule have been studied using microelectrode techniques.[269] Stable cell membrane voltage recordings have been obtained by impaling cells from the bath side across the basolateral cell membrane. Amiloride addition to the luminal perfusate produces a hyperpolarization in the voltage of the apical cell membrane, a reduction in the transepithelial conductance, and an increase in the fractional resistance as estimated by the ratio of the resistance of the apical cell membrane to the sum of the apical and basolateral cell membrane resistances. Increasing potassium in the luminal perfusate indicates a high potassium conductance at the cell apical membrane. This conductive pathway can be blocked by barium or reducing luminal pH to 4.0. Addition of both amiloride and barium in the luminal perfusate results in a significant increase in fractional resistance. These results indicate that sodium and potassium conductances appear to be the dominant conductive pathways at the apical cell membrane and that this membrane contains an amiloride-sensitive sodium conductance and a barium-and-hydrogen-sensitive potassium conductance. The basolateral cell membrane appears to be predominantly chloride selective,[270] and this might be consistent with the role of this segment in electrogenic hydrogen secretion. Chloride appears to be transported by three major mechanisms in rabbit cortical and outer medullary collecting tubules (Fig. 10).[271] First, chloride can be actively reabsorbed by an electroneutral $Cl-HCO_3$ exchanger localized in the apical membrane of the HCO_3-secreting (β-type) intercalated cells. Second, chloride can diffuse passively down electrochemical gradients through the paracellular pathway. Third, chloride undergoes recycling across the basolateral membrane of the H^+-secreting (α-type) intercalated cell. These mechanisms may play an important role in regulating chloride balance.[271]

The medullary collecting duct has a high capacity for sodium chloride reabsorption and may play an important role in the final urinary salt excretion and the regulation of sodium balance.[272] Amiloride natriuresis appears to be caused pri-

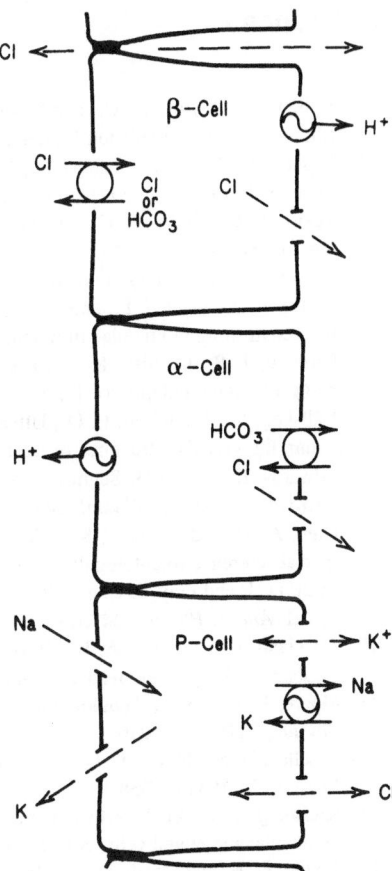

Fig. 10. Schematic representation of three cell types found in rabbit cortical collecting tubule. Apical (luminal) membrane is on left of cell. Principal cell (P-cell) and HCO_3-secreting (β) cells are found predominantly in cortical collecting tubule. Acid-secreting (α) cells are located in outer medullary collecting tubule (inner stripe) as well as in cortical collecting tubule.[271]

marily by the inhibition of sodium reabsorption in the medullary collecting duct, probably by the blockade of specific sodium channels.[273] The antikaliuresis of amiloride may be caused in part by inhibition of potassium secretion in the collecting duct. Studies by Sands *et al.*[274] on the effects of vasopressin on urea and water transport in the rat inner medullary collecting duct have shown at least two functionally distinct segments. The initial segment has low basal permeabilities to both water and urea, and vasopressin increases water but not urea transport. The terminal segment has high basal permeabilities to water and urea, and vasopressin increases both water and urea transport. The authors proposed that these functional differences may play an important role in the regulation of interstitial osmolality in the inner medulla and thus in the regulation of water excretion.

ACKNOWLEDGMENTS. The authors are grateful to June Hanke, who provided excellent editorial and secretarial assistance.

References

1. Hall, J. E., Guyton, A. C., and Cowley, A. W., Jr., 1977, Dissociation of renal blood flow and filtration rate autoregulation by renin depletion, *Am. J. Physiol.* **232:**F215–F221.
2. Kastner, P. R., Hall, J. E., and Guyton, A. C., 1984, Control of glomerular filtration rate: Role of intrarenally formed angiotensin II, *Am. J. Physiol.* **246:**F897–F906.
3. Textor, S. C., Tarazi, R. C., Novick, A. C., Bravo, E. L., and Fouad, F. M., 1984, Regulation of renal hemodynamics and glomerular filtration in patients with renovascular hypertension during converting enzyme inhibition with captorpil, *Am. J. Med.* **76:**29–37.
4. Hall, J. E., Granger, J. P., and Hester, R. L., 1985, Interaction between adenosine and angiotensin II in controlling glomerular filtration, *Am. J. Physiol.* **248:**F340–F346.
5. Gilmore, J. P., Cornish, K. G., Rogers, S. D., and Joyner, W. L., 1980, Direct evidence for myogenic autoregulation of the renal microcirculation in the hamster, *Circ. Res.* **47:**226–230.
6. Källskog, Ü., Lindblom, L. O., Ulfendahl, H. R., and Wolgast, M., 1976, Hydrostatic pressure within the vascular structures of the rat kidney, *Pflügers Arch.* **363:**205–210.
7. Edwards, R. M., 1983, Segmental effects of norepinephrine and angiotensin II on isolated renal microvessels, *Am. J. Physiol.* **244:**F526–F534.
8. Oien, A. H. and Aukland, K., 1983, A mathematical analysis of the myogenic hypothesis with special reference to autoregulation of renal blood flow, *Circ. Res.* **52:**241–252.
9. Lush, D. J. and Fray, J. C. S., 1984, Steady-state autoregulation of renal blood flow: A myogenic model, *Am. J. Physiol.* **247:**R89–R99.
10. Auckland, K. and Oien, A. H., 1987, Renal autoregulation: Models combining tubuloglomerular feedback and myogenic response, *Am. J. Physiol.* **252:**F768–F783.
11. Moore, L. C., 1984, Tubuloglomerular feedback and SNGFR autoregulation in the rat, *Am. J. Physiol.* **247:**F267–F276.
12. Casellas, D. and Navar, L. G., 1984, *In vitro* perfusion of juxtamedullary nephrons in rats, *Am. J. Physiol.* **246:**F349–F358.
13. Kreisberg, J. I., Venkatachalam, M., and Troyer, D., 1985, Contractile properties of cultured glomerular mesengial cells, *Am. J. Physiol.* **249:**F457–F463.
14. Young, D. K. and Marsh, D. J., 1981, Pulse wave propagation in rat renal tubules: implications for renal autoregulation, *Am. J. Physiol.* **240:**F466–F458.
15. Sakai, T. and Marsh, D. J., 1983, Analysis of frequency response of renal blood flow autoregulation in rats, *Fed. Proc.* **42:**1090 (Abstract).
16. Sakai, T., Hallman, E., and Marsh, D. J., 1986, Frequency domain analysis of renal autoregulation in the rat, *Am. J. Physiol.* **250:**F364–F373.
17. Wright, F. S. and Briggs, J. P., 1979, Feedback control of glomerular blood flow, pressure, and filtration rate, *Physiol. Rev.* **59:**958–1006.
18. Schnermann, J. and Briggs, J., 1985, Function of the juxtaglomerular apparatus: Local control of glomerular hemodynamics, in: *The Kidney: Physiology and Pathophysiology* (D. W. Seldin and G. Giebisch, eds.), Raven Press, New York, pp. 669–697.
19. Häberle, D. A. and Von Baeyer, H., 1983, Characteristics of glomerulotubular balance, *Am. J. Physiol.* **244:**F355–F366.
20. Häberle, D. A. and Davis, J. M., 1984, Resetting of tubuloglomerular feedback: Evidence for a humoral factor in tubular fluid, *Am. J. Physiol.* **246:**F495–F500.
21. Briggs, J. P., Steipe, B., Schubert, G., and Schnermann, J., 1982, Micropuncture studies of the renal effects of atrial natriuretic substance, *Pflügers Arch.* **395:**271–276.
22. Schnermann, J., Ploth, D. W., and Hermle, M., 1976, Activation of tubuloglomerular feedback by chloride transport, *Pflügers Arch.* **363:**229–240.
23. Wright, F. S., 1984, Intrarenal regulation of glomerular filtration rate, *J. Hypertension* **2:**105–113.
24. Bell, P. D. and Navar, L. G., 1982, Relationship between tubuloglomerular feedback responses and perfusate hypotonicity, *Kidney Int.* **22:**234–239.

25. Bell, P. D., 1982, Luminal and cellular mechanisms for the mediation of tubuloglomerular feedback responses, *Kidney Int.* **22**(12):S97–S103.

26. Bell, P. D., McLean, C. B., and Navar, L. G., 1981, Dissociation of tubuloglomerular feedback responses from distal tubular chloride concentration in the rat, *Am. J. Physiol.* **240**:F111–F119.

27. Bell, P. D., 1985, Cyclic AMP-calcium interaction in the transmission of tubuloglomerular feedback signals, *Kidney Int.* **28**:728–732.

28. Bell, P. D., Reddington, M., Ploth, D., and Navar, L. G., 1984, Tubuloglomerular feedback-mediated decreases in glomerular pressure in Munich–Wistar rats, *Am. J. Physiol.* **247**:F877–F880.

29. Tucker, B. J., Steiner, R. W., and Blantz, R. C., 1978, Studies on the tubuloglomerular feedback system in the rat. The mechanism of reduction in filtration rate with benzolamide, *J. Clin. Invest.* **62**:993–1005.

30. Ichikawa, I., 1982, Direct analysis of the effector mechanism of the tubuloglomerular feedback system, *Am. J. Physiol.* **243**:F447–F455.

31. Persson, A. E. G., Gushwa, L. C., and Blantz, R. C., 1984, Feedback pressure-flow responses in normal and angiotensin–prostaglandin-blocked rats, *Am. J. Physiol.* **247**:F925–F931.

32. Seney, F. D., Jr. and Wright, F. S., 1985, Dietary protein suppresses feedback control of glomerular filtration in rats, *J. Clin. Invest.* **75**:558–568.

33. Seney, F. D., Jr., Persson, A. E. G., and Wright, F. S., 1987, Modification of tubuloglomerular feedback signal by dietary protein, *Am. J. Physiol.* **252**:F83–F90.

34. Schnermann, J., Gokel, M., Weber, P. C., Schubert, G., and Briggs, J. P., 1986, Tubuloglomerular feedback and glomerular morphology in Goldblatt hypertensive rats on varying protein diets, *Kidney Int.* **29**:520–529.

35. Bidani, A. K., Schwartz, M. M., and Lewis, E. J., 1987, Renal autoregulation and vulnerability to hypertensive injury in remnant kidney, *Am. J. Physiol.* **252**:F1003–F1010.

36. Moore, L. C. and Mason, J., 1986, Tubuloglomerular feedback control of distal fluid delivery: effect of extracellular volume, *Am. J. Physiol.* **250**:F1024–F1032.

37. Huang, C-L. and Cogan, M. G., 1987, Atrial natriuretic factor inhibits maximal tubuloglomerular feedback response, *Am. J. Physiol.* **252**:F825–F828.

38. Woods, L. L., Mizelle, H. L., and Hall, J. E., 1987, Control of renal hemodynamics in hyperglycemia: possible role of tubuloglomerular feedback, *Am. J. Physiol.* **252**:F65–F73.

39. Boberg, U. and Persson, A. E. G., 1985, Tubuloglomerular feedback during elevated renal venous pressure, *Am. J. Physiol.* **249**:F524–F531.

40. Morsing, P., Stenbergh, A., Müller-Suur, C., and Persson, A. E. G., 1987, Tubuloglomerular feedback in animals with unilateral, partial ureteral occlusion, *Kidney Int.* **32**:212–218.

41. Dilley, J. R. and Arendshorst, W. J., 1984, Enhanced tubuloglomerular feedback activity in rats developing spontaneous hypertension, *Am. J. Physiol.* **247**:F672–F679.

42. Boberg, U. and Persson, A. E. G., 1986, Increased tubuloglomerular feedback activity in Milan hypertensive rats, *Am. J. Physiol.* **250**:F967–F974.

43. Göransson, A. and Sjöquist, M., 1984, The effect of pressor doses of angiotensin II on autoregulation and intrarenal distribution of glomerular filtration rate in the rat, *Acta Physiol. Scand.* **122**:615–620.

44. Schnermann, J. and Briggs, J., 1986, Role of the renin–angiotensin system in tubuloglomerular feedback, *Fed. Proc.* **45**:1426–1430.

45. Schnermann, J., Briggs, J. P., Schubert, G., and Marin-Grez, M., 1984, Opposing effects of captopril and aprotinin on tubuloglomerular feedback responses, *Am. J. Physiol.* **247**:F912–F918.

46. Boberg, U., Hahne, B., and Persson, A. E. G., 1984, The effect of intraarterial infusion of prostaglandin on the tubuloglomerular feedback control in the rat, *Acta Physiol. Scand.* **121**:65–72.

47. Tanner, G. A., 1985, Tubuloglomerular feedback after nephron or ureteral obstruction, *Am. J. Physiol.* **248**:F688–F697.

48. Wahlberg, J., Stenberg, A., Wilson, D. R., and Persson, A. E. G., 1984, Tubuloglomerular feedback and interstitial pressure in obstructive nephropathy, *Kidney Int.* **26**:294–302.

49. Baylis, C. and Blantz, R. C., 1985, Tubuloglomerular feedback in virgin and 12-day-pregnant rats, *Am. J. Physiol.* **249:**F169–F173.

50. Briggs, J. R., Schubert, G., and Schnermann, A. J., 1984, Quantitative characterization of the tubuloglomerular feedback response: Effect of growth, *Am. J. Physiol.* **247:**F808–F815.

51. Sjöquist, M., Göransson, A., and Källskog, Ü., 1984, The influence of tubuloglomerular feedback on the autoregulation of filtration rate in superficial and deep glomeruli, *Acta Physiol. Scand.* **122:** 235–242.

52. Hall, J. E., 1986, Control of sodium excretion by angiotensin II: Intrarenal mechanisms and blood pressure regulation, *Am. J. Physiol.* **250:**R960–R972.

53. Kotchens, T. A., Welch, W. J., Lorenz, J. N., and Ott, C. E., 1987, Renal tubular chloride and renin release, *J. Lab. Clin. Med.* **110:**533–540.

54. Blantz, R. C., 1987, The glomerular and tubular actions of angiotensin II, *Am. J. Kidney Dis.* **10:** 2–6.

55. Hall, J. E., Guyton, A. C., Jackson, T. E., Coleman, T. G., Lohmeier, T. E., and Trippodo, N. C., 1977, control of glomerular filtration rate by renin-angiotensin system, *Am. J. Physiol.* **233:**F366–F372.

56. Kastner, P. R., Hall, J. E., and Guyton, A. C., 1982, Renal hemodynamic responses to increased renal venous pressure: role of angiotensin II, *Am. J. Physiol.* **243:**F260–F264.

57. Hall, J. E. and Granger, J. P., 1986, Adenosine alters glomerular filtration control by angiotensin II, *Am. J. Physiol.* **250:**F917–F923.

58. Meyers, B. D., Deen, W. M., and Brenner, B. M., 1975, Effects of norepinephrine and angiotensin II on the determinants of glomerular ultrafiltration and proximal tubule fluid reabsorption in the rat, *Circ. Res.* **37:**101–110.

59. Hall, J. E. and Granger, J. P., 1983, Renal hemodynamic actions of angiotensin II: interaction with tubuloglomerular feedback, *Am. J. Physiol.* **245:**R166–F173.

60. Schnermann, J., Briggs, J. P., and Weber, P. C., 1984, Tubuloglomerular feedback, prostaglandins, and angiotensin in the autoregulation of glomerular filtration rate, *Kidney Int.* **25:**53–64.

61. Navar, L. G. and Rosivall, L., 1984, Contribution of the renin–angiotensin system to the control of intrarenal hemodynamics, *Kidney Int.* **25:**857–868.

62. Navar, L. G., Rosivall, L., Carmines, P. K., and Oparil, S., 1986, Effects of locally formed angiotensin II on renal hemodynamics, *Fed. Proc.* **45:**1448–1453.

63. Mitchell, K. D. and Navar, L. G., 1987, Superficial nephron responses to peritubular capillary infusions of angiotensin I and II, *Am. J. Physiol.* **252:**F818–F824.

64. Wilson, S. K., 1986, The effects of angiotensin II and norepinephrine on afferent arterioles in the rat, *Kidney Int.* **30:**895–905.

65. Steinhausen, M., Kücherer, H., Parekh, N., Weis, S., Wiegman, D. L., and Wilhelm, K., 1986, Angiotensin II control of the renal microcirculation: Effect of blockade by saralasin, *Kidney Int.* **30:**56–61.

66. Faubert, P. F., Chou, S., and Porush, J. G., 1987, Regulation of papillary plasma flow by angiotensin II, *Kidney Int.* **32:**472–478.

67. Chou, S., Faubert, P. F., and Porush, J. G., 1986, Contribution of angiotensin to the control of medullary hemodynamics, *Fed. Proc.* **45:**1438–1443.

68. Mendelsohn, F. A. O., Dunbar, M., Allen, A., Chou, S. T., Millan, M. A., and Aguilera, G., 1986, Angiotensin II receptors in the kidney, *Fed. Proc.* **45:**1420–1425.

69. Inagami, T., Kawamura, M., Naruse, K., and Okamura, T., 1986, Localization of components of the renin-angiotensin system within the kidney, *Fed. Proc.* **45:**1414–1419.

70. Rosivall, L., Narkates, A. J., Oparil, S., and Navar, L. G., 1987, De novo intrarenal formation of angiotensin II during control and enhanced renin secretion, *Am. J. Physiol.* **252:**F1118–F1123.

71. Bellucci, A. and Wilkes, B. M., 1984, Mechanism of sodium modulation of glomerular angiotensin receptors in the rat, *J. Clin. Invest.* **74:**1593–1600.

72. Arend, L. J., Haramati, A., Thompson, C. I., and Spielman, W. S., 1984, Adenosine-induced decreases in renin release: dissociation from hemodynamic effects, *Am. J. Physiol.* **247:**F447–F452.

73. Spielman, W. S., 1984, Antagonistic effect of theophylline on the adenosine-induced decrease in renin release, *Am. J. Physiol.* **247**:F246–F251.

74. Stahl, R. A. K., Paracivini, M., and Schollmeyer, P., 1984, Angiotensin II stimulation of prostaglandin E_2 and 6-keto-$F_{1\alpha}$ formation by isolated human glomeruli, *Kidney Int.* **26**:30–34.

75. Cooper, C. L., Schaffer, J. E., and Malik, K. U., 1985, Mechanism of action of angiotensin II and bradykinin on prostaglandin synthesis and vascular tone in the isolated rat kidney, *Circ. Res.* **56**: 97–108.

76. Ardaillou, R., Sraer, J., Chansel, D., Ardaillou, N., and Sraer, J. D., 1987, The effects of angiotensin II on isolated glomeruli and cultured glomerular cells, *Kidney Int.* **31**(20):S74–S80.

77. Dunn, M. J. and Scharschmidt, L. A., 1987, Prostaglandins modulate the glomerular actions of angiotensin II, *Kidney Int.* **31**(20):S95–S101.

78. Katayama, S., Attallah, A. A., Stahl, R. A., and Lee, J. B., 1987, Effect of Sar-1-Ileu-8-angiotensin on renal prostaglandin E_2 biosynthesis and excretion, *J. Lab. Clin. Med.* **109**:504–508.

79. Pelayo, J. C., Ziegler, M. G., and Blantz, R. C., 1984, Angiotensin II in adrenergic-induced alteration in glomerular hemodynamics, *Am. J. Physiol.* **247**:F799–F807.

80. Osborn, J. L. and Kinstetter, D. D., 1987, Effects of altered NaCl intake on renal hemodynamic and renin release responses to RNS, *Am. J. Physiol.* **253**:F976–F981.

81. Hayashi, Y., Hisa, H., and Satoh, S., 1987, Role of prostaglandin in norepinephrine and renin release in canine kidney, *Am. J. Physiol.* **253**:F929–F934.

82. Vari, R. C., Freeman, R. H., Davis, J. O., and Sweet, W. D., 1986, Role of renal nerves in rats with low-sodium, one-kidney hypertension, *Am. J. Physiol.* **250**:H189–H194.

83. Mizelle, H. L., Hall, J. E., Woods, L. L., Montani, J., Dzielak, D. J., and Pan, Y., 1987, Role of renal nerves in compensatory adaptation to chronic reductions in sodium intake, *Am. J. Physiol.* **252**:F291–F298.

84. Premen, A. J., Hall, J. E., and Mizelle, H. L., 1985, Maintenance of renal autoregulation during infusion of aminophylline and adenosine, *Am. J. Physiol.* **248**:F366–F373.

85. Deray, G., Branch, R. A., Herzer, W. A., Ohnishi, A., and Jackson, E. K., 1987, Adenosine inhibits β-adrenoceptor but not DBcAMP-induced renin release, *Am. J. Physiol.* **252**:F46–F52.

86. Churchill, P. G. and Bidani, A., 1987, Renal effects of selective adenosine receptor agonists in anesthetized rats, *Am. J. Physiol.* **252**:F299–F303.

87. Pawlowska, D., Granger, J. P., and Knox, F. G., 1987, Effects of adenosine infusion into renal interstitium on renal hemodynamics, *Am. J. Physiol.* **252**:F678–F682.

88. Miyamoto, M., Larson, T. S., Robertson, C. R., and Jamison, R. L., 1987, Effect of intrarenal adenosine on renal function and inner medullary vasa recta blood flow, *Clin. Res.* **35**(5):808A (Abstract).

89. Arend, L. J., Bakris, G. L., Burnett, J. C., Jr., Megerian, C., and Spielman, W. S., 1987, Role of intrarenal adenosine in the renal hemodynamic response to contrast media, *J. Lab. Clin. Med.* **110**: 406–411.

90. Jackson, E. K. and Ohnishi, A., 1987, Development and application of a simple microassay for adenosine in rat plasma, *Hypertension* **10**:189–197.

91. Ruilope, L. M., Robles, R. G., Paya, C., Alcazar, E. M., Sancho-Rof, J., Rodicio, J., Knox, F. G., and Romero, J. C., 1986, Effects of long-term treatment with indomethacin on renal function, *Hypertension* **8**:677–684.

92. Passmore, J. C., Hartupee, D. A., and Jackson, B. A., 1987, Urinary and renal papillary solutes during cyclooxygenase inhibition with ibuprofen, *J. Lab. Clin. Med.* **110**:807–812.

93. Hebert, R. L., Lamoureux, C., Sirois, P., Braquet, P., and Plante, G. E., 1985, Potentiating effects of leukotriene B_4 and prostaglandin E_2 on urinary sodium excretion by the dog kidney, *Prostaglandins Leukotrienes Med.*, **18**:69–80.

94. Kirchner, K. A., Martin, C. J., and Bower, J. D., 1986, Prostaglandin E_2 but not I_2 restores furosemide response in indomethacin-treated rats, *Am. J. Physiol.* **250**:F980–F985.

95. Patrono, C. and Dunn, M. J., 1987, The clinical significance of inhibition of renal prostaglandin synthesis, *Kidney Int.* **32**:1–12.

96. Carmines, P. K., Bell, P. D., Roman, R. J., Work, J., and Navar, L. G., 1985, Prostaglandins in the sodium excretory response to altered renal arterial pressure in dogs, *Am. J. Physiol.* **248:**F8–F14.

97. Gleim, G. W., Kao-Lo, G., and Maude, D. L., 1984, Pressure natriuresis and prostaglandin secretion by perfused rat kidney, *Kidney Int.* **26:**683–688.

98. Schlondorff, D., Aynedjian, H. S., Satriano, J. A., and Bank, N., 1987, In vivo demonstration of glomerular PGE_2 responses to physiological manipulations and experimental agents, *Am. J. Physiol.* **252:**F717–F723.

99. Ruilope, L. M., Rodicio, J., Robles, R. G., Sancho, J., Miranda, B., Granger, J. P., and Romero, J. C., 1987, Influence of a low sodium diet on the renal response to amino acid infusion in humans, *Kidney Int.* **31:**992–999.

100. Benigni, A., Zoja, C., Remuzzi, A., Orisio, S., Piccinelli, A., and Remuzzi, G., 1986, Role of renal prostaglandins in normal and nephrotic rats with diet-induced hyperfiltration, *J. Lab. Clin. Med.* **108:**230–240.

101. Rugiu, C., Oldrizzi, L., and Maschio, G., 1987, Effects of an oral protein load on glomerular filtration rate in patients with solitary kidneys, *Kidney Int.* **32(22):**S29–S31.

102. Dratwa, M., Burette, A., Van Gossum, M., Collart, F., Wens, R., Charlier, L., Tielmans, C., and Deltenre, M., 1987, No rise in glomerular filtration rate after protein loading in cirrhotics, *Kidney Int.* **32(22):**S32–S34.

103. Dhaene, M., Sabot, J., Philippart, Y., Doutrelepont, J., and Vanherweghem, J., 1987, Effects of acute protein loads of different sources on glomerular filtration rate, *Kidney Int.* **32(22):**S25–S28.

104. Viberti, G., Bognetti, E., Wiseman, M. J., Dodds, R., Gross, J. L., and Keen, H., 1987, Effect of protein-restricted diet on renal response to a meat meal in humans, *Am. J. Physiol.* **253:**F388–F393.

105. Woods, L. L., Mizelle, H. L., and Hall, J. E., 1987, Role of the liver in renal hemodynamic response to amino acid infusion, *Am. J. Physiol.* **252:**F981–F985.

106. Castellino, P., Hunt, W., and DeFronzo, R. A., 1987, Regulation of renal hemodynamics by plasma amino acid and hormone concentrations, *Kidney Int.* **32(22):**S15–S20.

107. Castellino, P., Coda, B., and DeFronzo, R. A., 1986, Effect of amino acid infusion on renal hemodynamics in humans, *Am. J. Physiol.* **251:**F132–F140.

108. Manning, R. D., Jr., 1987, Effects of hypoproteinemia on renal hemodynamics, arterial pressure, and fluid volume, *Am. J. Physiol.* **252:**F91–F98.

109. Manning, R. D., Jr., 1987, Renal hemodynamics, fluid volume, and arterial pressure changes during hyperproteinemia, *Am. J. Physiol.* **252:**F403–F411.

110. Baines, A. D., Drangova, R., and Ho, P., 1987, α_1-Adrenergic stimulation of renal Na reabsorption requires glucose metabolism, *Am. J. Physiol.* **253:**F810–F815.

111. Premen, A. J., 1987, Splanchnic and renal hemodynamic responses to intraportal infusion of glucagon, *Am. J. Physiol.* **253:**F1105–F1112.

112. Hirschberg, R. and Kopple, J. D., 1987, Effect of growth hormone on GFR and renal plasma flow in man, *Kidney Int.* **32(22):**S21–S24.

113. Corman, B. and Michel, J-B., 1987, Glomerular filtration, renal blood flow, and solute excretion in conscious aging rats, *Am. J. Physiol.* **253:**R555–R560.

114. Baylis, C., 1987, The determinants of renal hemodynamics in pregnancy, *Am. J. Kidney Dis.* **9:**260–264.

115. Barron, W. M., 1987, Volume homeostasis during pregnancy in the rat, *Am. J. Kidney Dis.* **9:**296–302.

116. Yarger, W. E., Newman, W. J., and Klotman, P. E., 1987, Renal effects of aprotinin after 24 hours of unilateral ureteral obstruction, *Am. J. Physiol.* **253:**F1006–F1014.

117. Badr, K. F., Brenner, B. M., and Ichikawa, I., 1987, Effects of leukotriene D_4 on glomerular dynamics in the rat, *Am. J. Physiol.* **253:**F239–F243, 1987.

118. Bourgoignie, J. J., Gavellas, G., Martinez, E., and Pardo, V., 1987, Glomerular function and morphology after renal mass reduction in dogs, *J. Lab. Clin. Med.* **109:**380–388.

119. Iversen, B. M., Sekse, I., and Ofstad, J., 1987, Resetting of renal blood flow autoregulation in spontaneously hypertensive rats, *Am. J. Physiol.* **252:**F480–F486.

120. Roos, J. C., Koomans, H. A., Dorhout Mees, E. J., and Delawi, I. M. K., 1985, Renal sodium handling in normal humans subjected to low, normal, and extremely high sodium supplies, *Am. J. Physiol.* **249:**F941–F947.
121. Brensilver, J. M., Daniels, F. H., Lafavour, G. S., Malseptic, R. M., Lorch, J. A., Ponte, M. L., and Cortell, S., 1985, Effect of variations in dietary sodium intake on sodium excretion in mature rats, *Kidney Int.* **27:**497–502.
122. Navar, L. G., Paul, R. V., Carmines, P. K., Chou, C., and Marsh, D. J., 1986, Intrarenal mechanisms mediating pressure natriuresis: role of angiotensin and prostaglandins, *Fed. Proc.* **45:** 2885–2891.
123. Roman, R. J., 1986, Pressure diuresis mechanism in the control of renal function and arterial pressure, *Fed. Proc.* **45:**2878–2884.
124. Haas, J. A., Granger, J. P., and Knox, F. G., 1986, Effect of renal perfusion pressure on sodium reabsorption from proximal tubules of superficial and deep nephrons, *Am. J. Physiol.* **250:**F425–F429.
125. Knox, F. G. and Granger, J. P., 1987, control of sodium excretion: the kidney produces under pressure, *NIPS* **2:**26–29.
126. Harris, P. J. and Navar, L. G., 1985, Tubular transport responses to angiotensin, *Am. J. Physiol.* **248:**F621–F630.
127. Schuster, V. L., 1986, Effects of angiotensin on proximal tubular reabsorption, *Fed. Proc.* **45:** 1444–1447.
128. Hall, J. E., 1986, Regulation of glomerular filtration rate and sodium excretion by angiotensin II, *Fed. Proc.* **45:**1431–1437.
129. Navar, L. G., Carmines, P. K., Huang, W., and Mitchell, K. D., 1987, The tubular effects of angiotensin II, *Kidney Int.* **31**(20):S81–S88.
130. Olsen, M. E., Hall, J. E., Montani, J., Guyton, A. C., Langford, H. G., and Cornell, J. E., 1985, Mechanisms of angiotensin II natriuresis and antinatriuresis, *Am. J. Physiol.* **249:**F299–F307.
131. Hall, J. E., Coleman, T. G., Guyton, A. C., Balfe, J. W., and Salgado, H. C., 1979, Intrarenal role of angiotensin II and [des-Asp¹] angiotensin II, *Am. J. Physiol.* **236:**F252–F259.
132. Schuster, V. L., Kokko, J. P., and Jacobson, H. R., 1984, Angiotensin II directly stimulates sodium transport in rabbit proximal convoluted tubules, *J. Clin. Invest.* **73:**507–515.
133. Stokes, J. B., 1981, Prostaglandins and the regulation of NaCl transport across renal epithelia, *Mineral Electrolyte Metab.* **6:**35–45.
134. deBold, A. J., Borenstein, H. B., Veress, A. T., and Sonnenberg, H., 1981, A rapid and potent natriuretic response to intravenous injection of atrial myocardial extract in rats, *Life Sci.* **28:** 89–95.
135. Frolich, E. D., 1986, "Introduction," First Intl. Symp. and Swiss Hypertension Workshop on Atrial Natriuretic Peptides, 18–19 November, 1985, Berne, Switzerland, O. Weidman, E. D. Frolich and J. H. Laragh, eds., Gower Publ. Co., London, *J. Hypertension.* **4**(2):S1–S2.
136. Knorr, M., Locher, R., Stimpel, M., Edmonds, D., and Vetter, W., 1986, Effect of atrial natriuretic polypeptide on angiotensin II–induced increase of cytosolic free calcium in cultured smooth muscle cells, *J. Hypertension* **4**(2):S67–S69.
137. Schiffrin, E. L., St-Louis, J., Garcia, R., Thibault, G., Cantin, M., and Genest, J., 1986, Vascular and adrenal binding sites for atrial natriuretic factor. Effects of sodium and hypertension, *Hypertension* **8**(I):I141–I145.
138. deBold, A. J., deBold, M. L., and Sarda, I. R., 1986, Functional-morphological studies on *in vitro* cardionatrin release, *J. Hypertension* **4**(2):S3–S7.
139. Goetz, K. L., 1986, Atrial receptors, natriuretic peptides, and the kidney: Current understanding, *Mayo Clin. Proc.* **61:**600–603.
140. Trippodo, N. C., Cole, F. E., MacPhee, A. A., and Pegram, B. L., 1987, Biological mechanisms of atrial natriuretic factor, *J. Lab. Clin. Med.* **109:**112–119.
141. Cantin, M. and Genest, J., 1987, The heart as an endocrine gland, *Hypertension* **10**(I):I118–I121.
142. Cole, B. R., Schwartz, D., Manning, P. T., Katsube, N. C., and Needleman, P., 1986, Atriopeptins: Circulating volume regulatory hormones with potential therapeutic role in chronic renal failure, *J. Hypertension* **4**(2):S13–S16.

143. Inagami, T., Misono, K. S., Fukumi, H., Maki, M., Tanaka, I., Takayanagi, R., Imada, T., Grammer, R. T., Naruse, M., Naruse, K., Pandey, K. N., Parmentier, M., Yasujima, M., and Abe, K., 1987, Structure and physiological actions of rat atrial natriuretic factor, *Hypertension* **10** (I):I113–I117.

144. Thibault, G., Garcia, R., and Gutkowska, J., 1986, Identification of the released form of atrial natriuretic factor by the perfused rat heart, *Proc. Soc. Exp. Biol. Med.* **182:**137–141.

145. Miyata, A., Kangawa, K., and Matsuo, H., 1986, Molecular forms of atrial natriuretic peptides in rat tissues and plasma, *J. Hypertension* **4**(2):S9–S11.

146. Fried, T. A., Ayon, M. A., McDonald, G., Lau, A., Inagami, T., and Stein, J. H., 1987, Atrial natriuretic peptide, right atrial pressure, and sodium excretion rate in the rat, *Am. J. Physiol.* **253:** F969–F975.

147. Schiebinger, R. J. and Linden, J., 1986, The influence of resting tension on immunoreactive atrial natriuretic peptide secretion by rat atria superfused *in vitro, Circ. Res.* **59:**105–109.

148. Bilder, G. E., Schofield, T. L., and Blaine, E. H., 1986, Release of atrial natriuretic factor. Effects of repetitive stretch and temperature, *Am. J. Physiol.* **251:**F817–F821.

149. Kohno, M., Clegg, K. B., and Sambhi, M. P., 1987, Effects of volume change on circulating immunoreactive atrial natriuretic factor in rats, *Hypertension* **10:**171–175.

150. Eskay, R., Zukowska-Grojec, Z., Haass, M., Dave, J. R., and Zamir, N., 1986, Circulating atrial natriuretic peptides in conscious rats: Regulation of release by multiple factors, *Science* **232:**636–639.

151. Verburg, K. M., Freeman, R. H., Davis, J. O., Villarreal, D., and Vari, R. C., 1986, Control of atrial natriuretic factor release in conscious dogs, *Am. J. Physiol.* **251:**R947–R956.

152. Wei, Y., Rodi, C. P., Day, M. L., Wiegand, R. C., Needleman, L. D., Cole, B. R., and Needleman, P., 1987, Developmental changes in the rat atriopeptin hormonal system, *J. Clin. Invest.* **79:**1325–1329.

153. Raine, A. E. G., Erne, P., Bürgisser, E., Müller, F. B., Bolli, P., Burkart, F., and Bühler, F. R., 1986, Atrial natriuretic peptide and atrial pressure in patients with congestive heart failure, *N. Engl. J. Med.* **315:**533–537.

154. Müller, F. B., Erne, P., Raine, A. E. G., Bolli, P., Linder, L., Resink, T. J., Cottier, C., and Bühler, F. R., 1986, Atrial antipressor natriuretic peptide: release mechanisms and vascular action in man, *J. Hypertension* **4**(2):S109–S114.

155. Anderson, J. V., Gibbs, J. S. R., Woodruff, P. W. R., Greco, C., Rowland, E., and Bloom, S. R., 1986, The plasma atrial natriuretic peptide response to treatment of acute cardiac failure, spontaneous supraventricular tachycardia and induced re-entrant tachycardia in man, *J. Hypertension* **4**(2):S137–S141.

156. Miki, K., Hajduczok, G., Klocke, M. R., Krasney, J. A., Hong, S. K., and deBold, A. J., 1986, Atrial natriuretic factor and renal function during head-out water immersion in conscious dogs, *Am. J. Physiol.* **251:**R1000–R1008.

157. Nishida, Y., Miyata, A., Morita, H., Uemura, N., Kangawa, K., Matsuo, H., and Hosomi, H., 1987, Lack of neural control of atrial natriuretic peptide release in conscious dogs, *Am. J. Physiol.* **253:**F1164–F1170.

158. Goetz, K. L., Wang, B. C., Geer, P. G., Leadley, R. J., Jr., and Reinhardt, H. W., 1986, Atrial stretch increases sodium excretion independently of release of atrial peptides, *Am. J. Physiol.* **250:** R946–R950.

159. Lang, R. E., Dietz, R., Merkel, A., Unger, T., Ruskoaho, H., and Ganten, D., 1986, Plasma atrial natriuretic peptide values in cardiac diseases, *J. Hypertension* **4**(2):S119–S123.

160. Burnett, J. C., Jr., Kao, P. C., Hu, D. C., Heser, D. W., Heublein, D., Granger, J. P., Opgenorth, T. J., and Reeder, G. S., 1986, Atrial natriuretic peptide elevation in congestive heart failure in the human, *Science* **231:**1145–1147.

161. Espiner, E. A., Nicholls, M. G., Yandle, T. G., Crozier, I. G., Cuneo, R. C., McCormick, D., and Ikram, H., 1986, Studies on the secretion, metabolism and action of atrial natriuretic peptide in man, *J. Hypertension* **4**(2):S85–S91.

162. Mendez, R. E., Pfeffer, J. M., Ortola, F. V., Bloch, K. D., Anderson, S., Seidman, J. G., and

Brenner, B. M., 1987, Atrial natriuretic peptide transcription, storage, and release in rats with myocardial infarction, *Am. J. Physiol.* **253**:H1449–H1455.

163. Tsunoda, K., Hodsman, G. P., Sumithran, E., and Johnston, C. I., 1986, Atrial natriuretic peptide in chronic heart failure in the rat: A correlation with ventricular dysfunction, *Circ. Res.* **59**:256–261.

164. Edwards, B. S., Ackermann, D. M., Schwab, T. R., Heublein, D. M., Edwards, W. D., Wold, L. E., and Burnett, J. C., Jr., 1986, The relationship between atrial granularity and circulating atrial natriuretic peptide in hamsters with congestive heart failure, *Mayo Clin. Proc.* **61**:517–521.

165. Montorsi, P., Tonolo, G., Polonia, J., Hepburn, D., and Richards, A. M., 1987, Correlates of plasma atrial natriuretic factor in health and hypertension, *Hypertension* **10**:570–576.

166. Arendt, R. M., Gerbes, A. L., Riter, D., Stangl, E., Bach, P., and Zähringer, J., 1986, Atrial natriuretic factor in plasma of patients with arterial hypertension, heart failure or cirrhosis of the liver, *J. Hypertension* **4**(2):S131–S135.

167. Onwochei, M. O., Snajdar, R. M., and Rapp, J. P., 1987, Release of atrial natriuretic factor from heart-lung preparations of inbred Dahl rats, *Am. J. Physiol.* **253**:H1044–H1052.

168. Lattion, A.-L., Michel, J.-B., Arnauld, E., Corvol, P., and Soubrier, F., 1986, Myocardial recruitment during ANF mRNA increase with volume overload in the rat, *Am. J. Physiol.* **251**:H890–H896.

169. Walsh, K. P., Williams, T. D. M., Canepa-Anson, R., Pitts, E., Lightman, S. L., and Sutton, R., 1987, Effects of endogenous atrial natriuretic peptide released by rapid atrial pacing in dogs, *Am. J. Physiol.* **253**:R599–R604.

170. Freeman, R. H., Villarreal, D., Vari, R. C., and Verburg, K. M., 1987, Endogenous atrial natriuretic factor in dogs with caval constriction, *Circ. Res.* **61**(I):I96–I99.

171. Suzuki, M., Almeida, F. A., Nussenzveig, D. R., Sawyer, D., and Maack, T., 1987, Binding and functional effects of atrial natriuretic factor in isolated rat kidney, *Am. J. Physiol.* **253**:F917–F928.

172. Weidmann, P., Hasler, L., Gnädinger, M. P., Lang, R. E., Uehlinger, D. E., Shaw, S., Rascher, W., and Reubi, F. C., 1986, Blood levels and renal effects of atrial natriuretic peptide in normal man, *J. Clin. Invest.* **77**:734–742.

173. Biollaz, J., Nussberger, J., Waeber, B., and Brunner, H. R., 1986, Clinical pharmacology of atrial natriuretic (3–28) eicosahexapeptide, *J. Hypertension* **4**(2):S101–S108.

174. Trippodo, N. C., Kardon, M. B., Pegram, B. L., Cole, F. E., and MacPhee, A. A., 1986, Acute haemodynamic effects of the atrial natriuretic hormone in rats, *J. Hypertension* **4**(2):S35–S40.

175. Garcia, R., Cantin, M., Cusson, J. R., Genest, J., Gutkowska, J., Larochelle, P., Schiffrin, E. L., and Thibault, G., 1986, Some physiopathological aspects of atrial natriuretic factor, *J. Hypertension* **4**(2):S125–S129.

176. Natsume, T., Kardon, M. B., Trippodo, N. C., Januszewicz, A., Pegram, B. L., and Frolich, E. D., 1986, Atriopeptin III does not alter cardiac performance in rats, *J. Hypertension* **4**:477–480.

177. Gaillard, C. A., Koomans, H. A., Rabelink, A. J., and Dorhout Mees, E. J., 1987, Effects of indomethacin on renal response to atrial natriuretic peptide, *Am. J. Physiol.* **253**:F868–F873.

178. Krayacich, J., Kline, R. L., Macchi, A., and Calaresu, F. R., 1986, Renal responses to atriopeptin II are not dependent on renal nerves, *Am. J. Physiol.* **251**:R187–R191.

179. Seymour, A. A., Smith, S. G., III, and Mazack, E. K., 1987, Effects of renal perfusion pressure on the natriuresis induced by atrial natriuretic factor, *Am. J. Physiol.* **253**:F234–F238.

180. Blaine, E. H., Heinel, L. A., Schorn, T. W., Marsh, E. A., and Whinnery, M. A., 1986, The character of the atrial natriuretic response: pressure and volume effects, *J. Hypertension* **4**(2):S17–S24.

181. Davis, C. L. and Briggs, J. P., 1987, Effect of reduction in renal artery pressure on atrial natriuretic peptide-induced natriuresis, *Am. J. Physiol.* **252**:F146–F153.

182. Mendez, R. E., Dunn, B. R., Troy, J. L., and Brenner, B. M., 1986, Modulation of the natriuretic response to atrial natriuretic peptide by alterations in peritubular Starling forces in the rat, *Circ. Res.* **59**:605–611.

183. Opgenorth, T. J., Burnett, J. C., Jr., Granger, J. P., and Scriven, T. A., 1986, Effects of atrial natriuretic peptide on renin secretion in nonfiltering kidney, *Am. J. Physiol.* **250:**F798–F801.

184. Itoh, S., Abe, K., Nushiro, N., Omata, K., Yasujima, M., and Yoshinaga, K., 1987, Effect of atrial natriuretic factor on renin release in isolated afferent arterioles, *Kidney Int.* **32:**493–497.

185. Deray, G., Branch, R. A., Herzer, W. A., Ohnishi, A., and Jackson, E. K., 1987, Effects of atrial natriuretic factor on hormone-induced renin release, *Hypertension* **9:**513–517.

186. Holtz, J., Sommer, O., and Bassenge, E., 1987, Inhibition of sympathoadrenal activity by atrial natriuretic factor in dogs, *Hypertension* **9:**350–354.

187. Kiberd, B. A., Larson, T. S., Robertson, C. R., and Jamison, R. L., 1987, Effect of atrial natriuretic peptide on vasa recta blood flow in the rat, *Am. J. Physiol.* **252:**F1112–F1117.

188. Takezawa, K., Cowley, A. W., Jr., Skelton, M., and Roman, R. J., 1987, Atriopeptin III alters renal medullary hemodynamics and the pressure-diuresis response in rats, *Am. J. Physiol.* **252:** F992–F1002.

189. Hildebrandt, D. A. and Banks, R. O., 1987, Effect of atrial natriuretic factor on renal function in rats with papillary necrosis, *Am. J. Physiol.* **252:**F977–F980.

190. Davis, C. L. and Briggs, J. P., 1987, Effect of atrial natriuretic peptides on renal medullary solute gradients, *Am. J. Physiol.* **253:**F679–F684.

191. Cogan, M. G., 1986, Atrial natriuretic factor can increase renal solute excretion primarily by raising glomerular filtration, *Am. J. Physiol.* **250:**F710–F714.

192. Dunn, B. R., Ichikawa, I., Pfeffer, J. M., Troy, J. L., and Brenner, B. M., 1986, Renal and systemic hemodynamic effects of synthetic atrial natriuretic peptide in the anesthetized rat, *Circ. Res.* **59:**237–246.

193. Fried, T. A., McCoy, R. N., Osgood, R. W., and Stein, J. H., 1986, Effect of atriopeptin II on determinants of glomerular filtration rate in the *in vitro* perfused dog glomerulus, *Am. J. Physiol.* **250:**F1119–F1122.

194. Shimonaka, M., Saheki, T., Hagiwara, H., Hagiwara, Y., Sono, H., and Hirose, S., 1987, Visualization of ANP receptor on glomeruli of bovine kidney by use of a specific antiserum, *Am. J. Physiol.* **253:**F1058–F1062.

195. Burnett, J. C., Jr., Opgenorth, T. J., and Granger, J. P., 1986, The renal action of atrial natriuretic peptide during control of glomerular filtration, *Kidney Int.* **30:**16–19.

196. Pollock, D. M. and Arendshorst, W. J., 1986, Effect of atrial natriuretic factor on renal hemodynamics in the rat, *Am. J. Physiol.* **251:**F795–F801.

197. Salazar, F. J., Granger, J. P., Fiksen-Olsen, M. J., Bentley, M. D., and Romero, J. C., 1987, Possible modulatory role of angiotensin II on atrial peptide-induced natriuresis, *Am. J. Physiol.* **253:**F880–F883.

198. Paul, R. V., Kirk, K. A., and Navar, L. G., 1987, Renal autoregulation and pressure natriuresis during ANF-induced diuresis, *Am. J. Physiol.* **253:**F424–F431.

199. Roy, D. R., 1986, Effect of synthetic ANP on renal and loop of Henle functions in the young rat, *Am. J. Physiol.* **251:**F220–F225.

200. Bourgoignie, J. J., Gavellas, G., and Hwang, K. H., 1986, Renal effects of atrial natriuretic factor in primate, *Am. J. Physiol.* **251:**F1049–F1054.

201. Biollaz, J., Bidiville, J., Diezi, J., Waeber, B., Nussberger, J., Brunner-Ferber, F., Gomez, H. J., and Brunner, H. R., 1987, Site of the action of a synthetic atrial natriuretic peptide evaluated in humans, *Kidney Int.* **32:**537–546.

202. Burnett, J. C., Jr., Granger, J. P., and Opgenorth, T. J., 1984, Effects of synthetic atrial natriuretic factor on renal function and renin release, *Am. J. Physiol.* **247:**F863–F866.

203. Hammond, T. G., Yusufi, A. N. K., Knox, F. G., and Dousa, T. P., 1985, Administration of atrial natriuretic factor inhibits sodium-coupled transport in proximal tubules, *J. Clin. Invest.* **75:** 1983–1989.

204. Baum, M. and Toto, R. D., 1986, Lack of a direct effect of atrial natriuretic factor in the rabbit proximal tubule, *Am. J. Physiol.* **250:**F66–F69.

205. Spinelli, F., Kamber, B., and Schnell, C., 1986, Observations on the natriuretic response to intravenous infusions of atrial natriuretic factor in water-loaded anesthetized rats, *J. Hypertension* **4**(2):S25–S29.

206. Harris, P. J., Thomas, D., and Morgan, T. O., 1987, Atrial natriuretic peptide inhibits angiotensin-stimulated proximal tubular sodium and water reabsorption, *Nature* **326**:697–698.
207. Peterson, L. N., De Rouffignac, C., Sonnenberg, H., and Levine, D. Z., 1987, Thick ascending limb response to dDAVP and atrial natriuretic factor *in vivo, Am. J. Physiol.* **252**:F374–F381.
208. Sonnenberg, H., Honrath, U., Chong, C. K., and Wilson, D. R., 1986, Atrial natriuretic factor inhibits sodium transport in medullary collecting duct, *Am. J. Physiol.* **250**:F963–F966.
209. Cantiello, H. F. and Ausiello, D. A., 1986, atrial natriuretic factor and cGMP inhibit amiloride-sensitive Na$^+$ transport in the cultured renal epithelial cell line, LLC-PK$_1$, *Biochem. Biophys. Res. Commun.* **134**:852–860.
210. Hamet, P., Tremblay, J., Pang, S. C., Skuherska, R., Schiffrin, E. L., Garcia, R., Cantin, M., Genest, J., Palmour, R., Ervin, F. R., Martin, S., and Goldwater, R., 1986, Cyclic GMP as mediator and biological marker of atrial natriuretic factor, *J. Hypertension* **4**(2):S49–S56.
211. Ballerman, B. J. and Brenner, B. M., 1986, Role of atrial peptides in body fluid homeostasis, *Circ. Res.* **58**:619–630.
212. Huang, C-L., Ives, H. E., and Cogan, M. G., 1986, In vivo evidence that cGMP is the second messenger for atrial natriuretic factor, *Proc. Natl. Acad. Sci. USA* **83**:8015–8018.
213. Zeidel, M. L. and Brenner, B. M., 1987, Actions of atrial natriuretic peptides on the kidney, *Semin. Nephrol.* **7**:91–97.
214. Edwards, R. M. and Weidley, E. F., 1987, Lack of effect of atriopeptin II on rabbit glomerular arterioles *in vitro, Am. J. Physiol.* **252**:F317–F321.
215. Appel, R. G. and Dunn, M. J., 1987, Papillary collecting tubule responsiveness to atrial natriuretic factor in Dahl rats, *Hypertension* **10**:107–114.
216. Zeidel, M. L., Silva, P., Brenner, B. M., and Seifter, J. L., 1987, cGMP mediates effects of atrial peptides on medullary collecting duct cells, *Am. J. Physiol.* **252**:F551–F559.
217. Schriven, T. A., and Burnett, J. C., Jr., 1985, Effects of synthetic atrial natriuretic peptide on renal function and renin release in acute experimental heart failure, *Circulation* **72**:892–897.
218. Laragh, J. H., 1985, Atrial natriuretic hormone, the renin-aldosterone axis, and blood pressure-electrolyte homeostasis, *N. Engl. J. Med.* **313**:1330–1340.
219. Vari, R. C., Freeman, R. H., Davis, J. O., Villarreal, D., and Verburg, K. M., 1986, Effect of synthetic atrial natriuretic factor on aldosterone secretion in the rat, *Am. J. Physiol.* **251**:R48–R52.
220. Goodfriend, T. L., Elliott, M. E., and Atlas, S. A., 1984, Actions of synthetic atrial natriuretic factor on bovine adrenal glomerulosa, *Life Sci.* **35**:1675–1682.
221. Chartier, L., Schiffrin, E., and Thibault, G., 1984, Effect of atrial natriuretic factor (ANF)-related peptides on aldosterone secretion by adrenal glomerulosa cells: Critical role of the intramolecular disulphide bond, *Biochem. Biophys. Res. Commun.* **122**:171–174.
222. Campbell, W. B., Currie, M. G., and Needleman, P., 1985, Inhibition of aldosterone biosynthesis by atriopeptins in rat adrenal cells, *Circ. Res.* **57**:113–118.
223. Chartier, L., Schiffrin, E., Thibault, G., and Garcia, R., 1984, Atrial natriuretic factor inhibits the stimulation of aldosterone secretion by angiotensin II, ACTH, and potassium in vitro and angiotensin II-induced steroidogenesis *in vivo, Endocrinology* **115**:2026–2028.
224. Sagnella, G. A., Markandu, N. D., Shore, A. C., and MacGregor, G. A., 1986, Changes in plasma immunoreactive atrial natriuretic peptide in response to saline infusion or to alterations in dietary sodium intake in normal subjects, *J. Hypertension* **4**(2):S115–S118.
225. Salazar, F. J., Granger, J. P., Joyce, M. L. M., Burnett, J. C., Jr., Bove, A. A., and Romero, J. C., 1986, Effects of hypertonic saline infusion and water drinking on atrial peptide, *Am. J. Physiol.* **251**:R1091–R1094.
226. Epstein, M., Loutzenhiser, R. D., Friedland, E., Aceto, R. M., Camargo, M. J. F., and Atlas, S. A., 1986, Increases in circulating atrial natriuretic factor during immersion-induced central hypervolaemia in normal humans, *J. Hypertension* **4**(2):S93–S99.
227. Schwab, T. R., Edwards, B. S., Heublein, D. M., and Burnett, J. C., Jr., 1986, Role of atrial natriuretic peptide in volume-expansion natriuresis, *Am. J. Physiol.* **251**:R310–R313.
228. Villarreal, D., Freeman, R. H., Davis, J. O., Verburg, K. M., and Vari, R. C., 1986, Effects of atrial appendectomy on circulating atrial natriuretic factor during volume expansion in the rat, *Proc. Soc. Exp. Biol. Med.* **183**:54–58.

229. Hirth, C., Stasch, J-P., John, A., Kazda, S., Morich, F., Neuser, D., and Wohlfeil, S., 1986, The renal response to acute hypervolemia is caused by atrial natriuretic peptides, *J. Cardiovasc. Pharm.* **8**:268–275.

230. Benjamin, B. A., Metzler, C. H., and Peterson, T. V., 1987, Renal response to volume expansion in atrial-appendectomized dogs, *Am. J. Physiol.* **253**:R786–R793.

231. Trippoda, N. C., 1987, An update on the physiology of atrial natriuretic factor, *Hypertension* **10** (I):I122–I127.

232. Khraibi, A. A., Granger, J. P., Burnett, J. C., Jr., Walker, K. R., and Knox, F. G., 1987, Role of atrial natriuretic factor in the natriuresis of acute volume expansion, *Am. J. Physiol.* **252**:R921–R924.

233. Barbee, R. W. and Trippodo, N. C., 1987, The contribution of atrial natriuretic factor to acute volume natriuresis in rats, *Am. J. Physiol.* **253**:F1129–F1135.

234. Kaneko, K., Okada, K., Ishikawa, S-E., Kuzuya, T., and Saito, T., 1987, Role of atrial natriuretic peptide in natriuresis in volume-expanded rats, *Am. J. Physiol.* **253**:R877–R882.

235. Hofbauer, K. G., Criscione, L., Sonnenburg, C., Muir, A., and Mah, S. C., 1986, Acute and chronic haemodynamic and natriuretic effects of atriopeptin II in conscious rats, *J. Hypertension* **4** (2):S41–S47.

236. Laragh, J. H., 1986, The endocrine control of blood volume, blood pressure and sodium balance: Atrial hormone and renin system interactions, *J. Hypertension* **4**(2):S143–S156.

237. Sugawara, A., Nakao, K., Morii, N., Sakamoto, M., Horii, K., Shimokura, M., Kiso, Y., Nishimura, K., Ban, T., Kihara, M., Yamori, Y., Kangawa, K., Matsuo, H., and Imura, H., 1986, Significance of α-human atrial natriuretic polypeptide as a hormone in humans, *Hypertension* **8**(I):I151–I155.

238. Ballerman, B. J. and Brenner, B. M., 1987, Atrial natriuretic peptide and the kidney, *Am. J. Kidney Dis.* **X**(1):7–12.

239. Casto, R., Hilbig, J., Schroeder, G., and Stock, G., 1987, Atrial natriuretic factor inhibits central angiotension II pressor responses, *Hypertension* **9**:473–477.

240. Maddox, D. A. and Gennari, J. F., 1987, The early proximal tubule: A high-capacity delivery-responsive reabsorptive site, *Am. J. Physiol.* **252**:F573–F584.

241. Howlin, K. J., Alpern, R. J., Berry, C. A., and Rector, F. C., Jr., 1986, Evidence for electroneutral sodium chloride transport in rat proximal convoluted tubule, *Am. J. Physiol.* **250**:F644–F648.

242. Warnock, D. G. and Eveloff, J., 1982, NaCl entry mechanisms in the luminal membrane of renal tubule, *Am. J. Physiol.* **242**:F561–F574.

243. Baum, M. and Berry, C. A., 1984, Evidence for neutral transcellular NaCl transport and neutral basolateral chloride exit in the rabbit proximal convoluted tubule, *J. Clin. Invest.* **74**:205–211.

244. Baum, M., 1987, Evidence that parallel Na^+-H^+ and Cl^--$HCO^-_3(OH^-)$ antiporters transport NaCl in the proximal tubule, *Am. J. Physiol.* **252**:F338–F345.

245. Rector, F. C., Jr., 1983, Sodium, bicarbonate, and chloride absorption by the proximal tubule, *Am. J. Physiol.* **244**:F461–F471.

246. Cantiello, H. F., Scott, J. A., and Rabito, C. A., 1987, Conductive Na^+ transport in an epithelial cell line (LLC-PK_1) with characteristics of proximal tubular cells, *Am. J. Physiol.* **252**:F590–F597.

247. Harris, R. C., Seifter, J. L., and Lechene, C., 1986, Coupling of Na-H exchange and Na-K pump activity in cultured rat proximal tubule cells, *Am. J. Physiol.* **251**:C815–C824.

248. Yang, W. C., Arruda, J. A. L., and Taylor, Z., 1987, Na^+-H^+ antiporter in posthypercapnic state, *Am. J. Physiol.* **253**:F833–F840.

249. Weinman, E. J., Shenolikar, S., and Kahn, A. M., 1987, cAMP-associated inhibition of Na^+-H^+ exchanger in rabbit kidney brush-border membranes, *Am. J. Physiol.* **252**:F19–F25.

250. Rocco, V. K., Cragoe, E. J., Jr., and Warnock, D. G., 1987, N-ethoxycarbonyl-2-ethoxy-1,2-dihydroquinoline, amiloride analogues, and renal Na^+/H^+ antiporter, *Am. J. Physiol.* **252**:F517–F524.

251. Bidet, M., Merot, J., Tauc, M., and Poujeol, P., 1987, Na^+-H^+ exchanger in proximal cells

isolated from kidney. II. Short-term regulation by glucocorticoids, *Am. J. Physiol.* **253**:F945–F951.

252. Ichikawa, I. and Kon, V., 1986, Role of peritubular capillary forces in the renal action of carbonic anhydrase inhibitor, *Kidney Int.* **30**:828–835.

253. Johnston, J. R., Brenner, B. M., and Hebert, S. C., 1987, Uninephrectomy and dietary protein affect fluid absorption in rabbit proximal straight tubules, *Am. J. Physiol.* **253**:F222–F233.

254. Beach, R. E., Schwab, S. J., Brazy, P. C., and Dennis, V. W., 1987, Norepinephrine increases Na$^+$-K$^+$-ATPase and solute transport in rabbit proximal tubules, *Am. J. Physiol.* **252**:F215–F220.

255. Dominguez, J. H., Snowdowne, K. W., Freudenrich, C. C., Brown, T., and Borle, A. B., 1987, Intracellular messenger for action of angiotensin II on fluid transport in rabbit proximal tubule, *Am. J. Physiol.* **252**:F423–F428.

256. Kaskel, F. J., Kumar, A. M., Lockhart, E. A., Evan, A., and Spitzer, A., 1987, Factors affecting proximal tubular reabsorption during development, *Am. J. Physiol.* **252**:F188–F197.

257. Hebert, S. C. and Andreoli, T. E., 1984, Control of NaCl transport in the thick ascending limb, *Am. J. Physiol.* **246**:F745–F756.

258. Molony, D. A., Reeves, W. B., and Andreoli, T. E., 1987, Some transport characteristics of mammalian renal diluting segments, *Mineral Electrolyte Metab.* **13**:442–450.

259. Molony, D. A., Reeves, W. B., Hebert, S. C., and Andreoli, T. E., 1987, ADH increases apical Na$^+$ K$^+$, 2Cl$^-$ entry in mouse medullary thick ascending limbs of Henle, *Am. J. Physiol.* **252**:F177–F187.

260. Elalouf, J-M., Sari, D. C., Roinel, N., and De Rouffignac, C., 1987, NaCl and Ca delivery at the bend of rat deep nephrons decreases during antidiuresis, *Am. J. Physiol.* **252**:F1055–F1064.

261. Tabei, K. and Imai, M., 1987, K transport in upper portion of descending limbs of long-loop nephron from hamster, *Am. J. Physiol.* **252**:F387–F392.

262. Haas, M. and Forbush, B., III., 1987, Na, K, Cl-cotransport system: Characterization by bumetanide binding and photolabelling, *Kidney Int.* **32**(23):S134–S140.

263. Scherzer, P., Wald, H., and Popovtzer, M. M., 1987, Enhanced glomerular filtration and Na$^+$-K$^+$-ATPase with furosemide administration, *Am. J. Physiol.* **252**:F910–F915.

264. Taniguchi, J., Tabei, K., and Imai, M., 1987, Profiles of water and solute transport along long-loop descending limb: analysis by mathematical model, *Am. J. Physiol.* **252**:F393–F402.

265. Ellison, D. H., Velazquez, H., and Wright, F. S., 1987, Mechanisms of sodium, potassium and chloride transport by the renal distal tubule, *Mineral Electrolyte Metab.* **13**:422–432.

266. Ellison, D. H., Velazquez, H., and Wright, F. S., 1987, Thiazide-sensitive sodium chloride cotransport in early distal tubule, *Am. J. Physiol.* **253**:F546–F554.

267. Velazquez, H., Ellison, D. H., and Wright, F. S., 1987, Chloride-dependent potassium secretion in early and late renal distal tubules, *Am. J. Physiol.* **253**:F555–F562.

268. Schnermann, J., Steipe, B., and Briggs, J. P., 1987, In situ studies of distal convoluted tubule in rat. II. K secretion, *Am. J. Physiol.* **252**:F970–F976.

269. O'Neil, R. G. and Sansom, S. C., 1984, Characterization of apical cell membrane Na$^+$ and K$^+$ conductances of cortical collecting duct using microelectrode techniques, *Am. J. Physiol.* **247**:F14–F24.

270. Koeppen, B. M., 1985, Conductive properties of the rabbit outer medullary collecting duct: Inner stripe, *Am. J. Physiol.* **248**:F500–F506.

271. Schuster, V. L. and Stokes, J. B., 1987, Chloride transport by the cortical and outer medullary collecting duct, *Am. J. Physiol.* **253**:F203–F212.

272. Cupples, W. A. and Sonnenberg, H., 1987, Load dependency of sodium chloride reabsorption by medullary collecting duct in rat, *Am. J. Physiol.* **253**:F642–F648.

273. Sonnenberg, H., Honrath, U., and Wilson, D. R., 1987, Effects of amiloride in the medullary collecting duct of rat kidney, *Kidney Int.* **31**: 1121–1125.

274. Sands, J. M., Nonoguchi, H., and Knepper, M. A., 1987, Vasopressin effects on urea and H$_2$O transport in inner medullary collecting duct subsegments, *Am. J. Physiol.* **253**:F823–F832.

3

Renal Metabolism

Anton C. Schoolwerth, Sylvia L. Betcher, and Norman P. Curthoys

1. Introduction

As in previous editions, the authors have decided to discuss selected aspects of renal metabolism rather than to attempt a survey of the literature for the past several years. Accordingly, in the present chapter, an extensive discussion on the effects of acidosis on renal gene expression is included because of the application of methods in molecular biology to the study of the kidney. Selected aspects of renal substrate metabolism will also be discussed, namely, intrarenal heterogeneity of metabolic pathways, serine metabolism, ketone body metabolism, and citrate transport and metabolism. In addition, the section on adenosine will cover new information with regard to adenosine transport across epithelial cell membranes and localization of adenosine receptors in the kidney.

2. Renal Substrate Utilization

Several excellent reviews have appeared to which the reader is referred.[1,2] It has been known for some time that the kidney utilizes significant amounts of free fatty acids, lactate, glutamine, citrate, and 3-hydroxybutyrate.[1,2] In addition, the

ANTON C. SCHOOLWERTH and SYLVIA L. BETCHER • Division of Nephrology, Department of Internal Medicine, Medical College of Virginia, Virginia Commonwealth University, Richmond, Virginia 23298-0160. NORMAN P. CURTHOYS • Department of Microbiology, Biochemistry, and Molecular Biology, University of Pittsburgh, Pittsburgh, Pennsylvania 15261.

kidney utilizes substrates present at lower arterial concentrations, such as pyruvate, α-ketoglutarate, glycerol, proline, and some other amino acids (see Section 2.2). Several recent studies have reexamined the preferred substrates for utilization by the mammalian kidney. Additional evidence indicates that substrate utilization varies along the nephron. For example, enzyme analysis has demonstrated that the gluconeogenic pathway is restricted to the proximal tubule.[3,4] In contrast, the enzymes of the glycolytic pathway are restricted to distal nephron segments, including the thick ascending limb of Henle's loop.[3] These findings are supported by recent metabolic studies in isolated nephron segments indicating that the proximal tubule does not metabolize [^{14}C]glucose to a significant extent.[5,6] Similar data indicate a geographic separation of the enzymes of glutamine metabolism in proximal and distal tubules. Although the distal convoluted tubule has higher basal activity of phosphate-dependent glutaminase, only the enzyme in proximal convoluted tubule was induced in metabolic acidosis.[7] Moreover, this activity appears to be localized to the S1 and S2 segments, with a significant activity of glutamine synthetase located only in the S3 segment of the rat, but not the dog, kidney.[8] Of particular interest are studies evaluating the metabolic contribution to transport functions of the kidney. For example, Wittner *et al.*[9] demonstrated that glucose, lactate, and pyruvate were each effective in sustaining short-circuit current in the isolated perfused thick ascending limb of the rabbit kidney.

2.1. Ketone Bodies

Based on studies originally performed in rat cortical slices, Weidemann and Krebs[10] proposed that acetoacetate was the preferred renal substrate. More recently, additional attention has been paid to the role of ketone bodies as substrates for both oxidation and esterification by kidney cortex.

Guder *et al.*[11] mapped the distribution of two of the major enzymes of ketone body metabolism along mouse and rat nephrons. They demonstrated that 3-oxoacid Co-A transferase and 3-hydroxybutyrate dehydrogenase were present throughout the nephron of these two species. In general, the activities paralleled that of mitochondrial densities and, in terms of tubular protein, were highest in activity in thick ascending limb and distal convoluted tubule. However, the activity, particularly of 3-oxoacid Co-A transferase, was also high in proximal convoluted and proximal straight tubule. The activity of 3-hydroxybutyrate dehydrogenase was similar, although in mouse, but not rat, the activity was fivefold higher in the pars recta compared to the proximal convoluted tubule. Similar results have been obtained in rabbit and human kidney, although activity of 3-oxoacid-Co-A transferase was very low in the rabbit, despite the fact that similar distributions of 3-hydroxybutyrate dehydrogenase were found in rabbit, human, and rat kidney.[12] Evidence points to the fact that, as in the liver, ketone body metabolism is directly coupled to the citric acid cycle by the Co-A transferase reaction.[1,2] All of the major reactions leading to the metabolism of ketone bodies are located in the mitochondrial matrix.

Utilizing different mixes of substrates and inhibitors, Guder *et al.* obtained further evidence *in vitro* that acetoacetate is the preferred renal substrate for oxidative purposes. This conclusion is based on the findings that uptake rates of ketone bodies were increased by addition of substrates that enhance ATP turnover (such as pyruvate, lactate, and other gluconeogenic and triacylglycerol precursors).[1,13,14] In contrast, ketone bodies decreased the oxidation of glucose, lactate, pyruvate, amino acids, and fatty acids.[2] Further studies are clearly necessary to define the role for ketone body utilization. These data do indicate that under conditions in which ketone bodies are formed in increasing amounts, the kidney has the capacity to extract ketone bodies, and to oxidize, esterify, and excrete them in increasing amounts.[2]

Additional evidence that acetoacetate may be the preferred renal substrate for oxidative purposes is the finding that when endogenous lipid oxidation was inhibited by tetradecylglycidic acid,[14] oxygen consumption was restored to normal by addition of acetoacetate. Data also indicate a tight linkage between ketone body oxidation and coupling to coenzyme A, succinate oxidation, GTP, and FAD metabolism via intermediates of the citric acid cycle. Moreover, at least in proximal tubules, ketone bodies may result in conversion of other substrates to glucose and triacylglycerol.[14] *In vivo,* renal ketone body uptake is related linearly to arterial ketone body concentration.[15] Oxygen uptake measurements *in vitro* indicated that tubule suspensions of rat kidney were saturated at ketone body concentrations of 1 mM; the exact interplay affecting the maximum rate of oxidation *in vitro* vs. *in vivo* has not been clarified. Possibly this is explained by the complex interplay between ketone body utilization, succinate oxidation, and intermediates of the citric acid cycle.[14]

In addition, other fates of ketone bodies may pertain, including enhanced excretion. This is supported by studies in rat which show ketone body transport by renal tubule membranes.[16,17] More recently, Barac-Nieto has evaluated the transport of one ketone body, D($-$)-3-hydroxybutyrate, in rat renal brush border membrane vesicles.[18] These data provide new information supporting a direct coupling of hydroxybutyrate and sodium influx into brush border membrane vesicles. This does not appear to involve the net transfer of electrical charge or proton influx.

All of these data are interesting in light of an attempted analysis of preferred substrates by the kidney. Recently, Goldstein[19] has reevaluated renal arteriovenous concentration differences of major potential respiratory substrates in the rat. The data indicate significant net uptake of both acetoacetate and 3-hydroxybutyrate under control conditions and of total ketones in both ammonium chloride metabolic acidosis and diabetic ketoacidosis. These findings were correlated with $^{14}CO_2$ production from labeled substrates by cortical slices obtained from animals under the same conditions. Substantial CO_2 production was obtained from 3-hydroxybutyrate under control conditions, particularly on slices obtained from rats with diabetic ketoacidosis. Unfortunately, total CO_2 production was not measured under these conditions, and acetoacetate was not similarly tested in this study.

2.2. Serine Production

As mentioned earlier, arteriovenous differences for amino acids have been measured across the kidney from numerous mammalian species. It has been known for many years that glutamine accounts for substantial amino acid uptake in humans and dog, particularly in metabolic acidosis.[20,21] These and other data were the basis for the conclusion that glutamine was the primary substrate for renal ammonia synthesis. However, additional data have indicated that the situation may be more complex. For example, Squires *et al.*[22] demonstrated no significant uptake of glutamine by kidneys from nonacidotic rats. A similar finding was obtained by Hughey *et al.*[23] In human studies, Tizianello *et al.*[24] demonstrated net extraction by the kidney of glutamine under control circumstances. However, following 24 hr of acute ammonium chloride metabolic acidosis, no measurable increase in glutamine extraction was observed despite the fact that ammonium production increased two-fold. These studies led to a reexamination of several metabolic pathways in kidney. Of particular interest were studies focusing on the net renal production of serine, which was consistently observed. This had also been demonstrated by Pitts and associates *in vivo* in dog and rat[25,26] and in the isolated perfused rat kidney.[27]

More recently, Scaduto and Davis demonstrated serine synthesis from two gluconeogenic substrates, aspartate and glutamate, in the isolated perfused rat kidney.[28] Inhibition of serine production from aspartate was noted in the presence of the transaminase inhibitor aminooxyacetate and in the presence of 3-mercaptopicolinic acid, an inhibitor of gluconeogenesis. The data were taken to indicate that serine synthesis in rat kidney occurred via both the so-called phosphorylated and/or nonphosphorylated pathways.

Additional studies from Brosnan's laboratory evaluated serine synthesis in greater detail.[29–32] As suggested earlier, serine can be produced via several pathways; from 3-phosphoglycerate via a phosphorylated intermediate pathway, from 2-phosphoglycerate via a so-called nonphosphorylated pathway, and from glycine involving the coupling between the glycine cleavage enzyme and serine hydroxymethyl transferase (Fig. 1). The first two pathways are cytosolic, whereas the latter pathway is mitochondrial. Measurement of serine synthesis from various precursors and enzyme activity analysis of tubules fractionated on Percoll gradients indicated that serine synthesis occurred predominantly in proximal tubule.[31] The quantitative significance of these pathways has not been fully elucidated, but it is suggested that the nonphosphorylated pathway is not of primary importance and functions principally as a catabolic pathway.

Whether the phosphorylated pathway is primary or whether other pathways yet to be discovered are involved is not yet clear. However, considerable attention has been directed at the glycine cleavage enzyme complex. This is of particular interest since net renal extraction of glycine has been demonstrated in several species. Glycine can yield serine in a stoichiometry of 2 : 1 by the combined actions of the glycine–cleavage–enzyme complex and serine hydroxymethyl transferase. In renal tubules from acidotic rats, Lowry *et al.*[32] demonstrated increased glycine metabo-

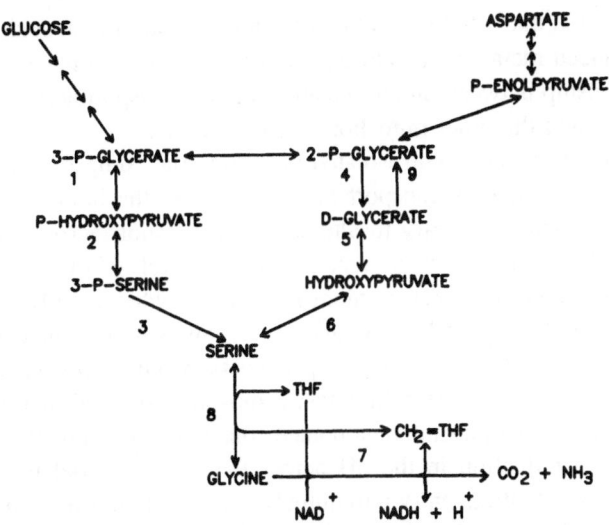

Fig. 1. Possible pathways of serine synthesis by kidney. The enzymes of the phosphorylated intermediate pathway are 3-phosphoglycerate dehydrogenase (1), phosphoserine aminotransferase (2), and phosphoserine phosphatase (3). The enzymes of the nonphosphorylated pathway are 2-phosphoglycerate phosphatase (4), D-glycerate dehydrogenase (5), and alanine-hydroxypyruvate aminotransferase (6). Serine synthesis from glycine is catalyzed by the glycine cleavage complex (7) and serine hydroxymethyltransferase (8). D-glycerate kinase (9) is also shown. (From Lowry et al.,[31] with permission, The American Physiological Society.)

lism which correlated with an increase in activity of the glycine–cleavage–enzyme complex[30]; no change in serine hydroxymethyl transferase activity was observed. These findings are of interest since by-products of these reactions are ammonium and CO_2 (potential bicarbonate); these workers postulated that glycine could supply 10–15% of the ammonium produced by the rat kidney in metabolic acidosis.[27,33] However, despite an increase in glycine extraction by rat kidney in metabolic acidosis, these workers were unable to demonstrate a significant increase in serine release.[32] Moreover, administration to control rats of cysteamine, an inhibitor of the glycine–cleavage–enzyme complex, did not alter serine release despite an inhibition of net glycine extraction. However, cysteamine administration to acidotic rats reduced serine release. These data suggest a contribution of glycine to renal ammoniagenesis in rat kidney in metabolic acidosis. Further studies should clarify substrate metabolism and metabolic pathways of renal ammoniagenesis in metabolic acidosis.

2.3. Citrate Transport in Metabolism

Considerable attention has been given to the renal excretion of citrate for several reasons: (1) Urinary citrate, by virtue of its complexation of calcium, is thought to be an endogenous inhibitor of nephrolithiasis; (2) systemic acid–base changes result in marked alterations in citrate clearance and metabolism; and (3) it has been suggested that citrate excretion has an important role in acid–base balance in diuretic-induced metabolic alkalosis.[34] Recently, attention has been focused on the interrelationship between citrate metabolism and transport across both the plasma membranes and the inner mitochondrial membrane.

Based on experiments with isolated mitochondria, Simpson[35] postulated that systemic acidosis increased transport of citrate across the luminal membranes of proximal renal tubule secondary to alterations in transport across the inner mitochondrial membrane. It had been demonstrated (see Ref. 35) that the steady-state uptake of citrate and other organic anions is increased when the pH gradient (ΔpH) across the inner mitochondrial membrane rises. This would occur when the pH of extramitochondrial medium is reduced; the converse would apply when the medium pH is increased. Based on these findings, Simpson postulated that an increase in intracellular pH and cytoplasmic bicarbonate content occurs in metabolic alkalosis, which leads to a reduction in the pH across the mitochondrial membrane. This change decreases net citrate entry into mitochondria by inhibition of the tricarboxylate carrier brought about by a reduction in the ΔpH. This inhibition of citrate transport then causes a rise in cytosolic citrate and a reduction in cell citrate uptake, with a resultant increase in renal citrate clearance. The opposite changes are postulated to occur in metabolic acidosis. Thus, citrate excretion is markedly increased in metabolic alkalosis whereas it is reduced in metabolic acidosis.

An important feature of this scheme is that it places an important role for intracellular citrate in the control of citrate transport across the plasma cell membranes of the proximal renal tubule. Support for such a statement derives from experiments performed with acetazolamide.[36] However, as noted by Hamm and Simon,[37] "the theory that the decreased reabsorption of citrate with alkalosis is due to increased intracellular citrate content has not been proven." More recent data have, in fact, indicated that the situation is more complicated and that other factors may regulate citrate transport and possibly metabolism.

In a series of experiments performed in the isolated perfused rat kidney, Anaizi et al.[38] were able to dissociate changes in intracellular citrate content from citrate reabsorption. These studies were performed in the substrate-limited kidney perfused only with citrate at different buffer pH values but with constant ionized calcium content. Although citrate transport was reduced at pH 7.6 compared to pH 7.2 or 7.4, renal tissue citrate content was not significantly increased. These workers were able to demonstrate an increase in tissue citrate content at alkaline pH only when the perfusate contained precursors of citrate, such as glucose + lactate + malate. The findings suggested that increased tissue citrate concentrations were derived by synthesis from its precursors rather than from increased uptake of extracellular fluid citrate and argued against the regulation of cellular uptake of citrate by changes in tissue citrate content secondary to alterations in mitochondrial citrate transport.

Additional evidence to support a role for extracellular, rather than intracellular, pH in the transport of citrate is found in studies by Brennan et al.,[39,40] who characterized citrate reabsorption in the rabbit nephron. In perfused nephron segments, they demonstrated that citrate reabsorption, as measured by the luminal disappearance of [^{14}C]citrate, occurred only in the proximal tubule; no significant transport occurred in cortical thick ascending limb or the cortical collecting tubule. Proximal tubule citrate transport was increased by lowering the pH in the perfusate. These findings are consistent with observations made in isolated brush border membrane vesicles[41-45] which indicated that citrate uptake occurs by a sodium-coupled electrogenic transport process with an initial rate inversely proportional to extravesicular pH. These findings have been interpreted to indicate that the protonated dicarboxylate species (citrate^{2-} or cit^{1-}) are transported in preference to the tricarboxylate, with a stoichiometry of three sodiums per one dicarboxylate citrate molecule. Moreover, the data suggested that citrate^{3-} competitively inhibits citrate^{2-} uptake (see Hamm and Simon[37] for review).

More recently, Wright and Wunz[45] compared citrate transport in renal brush border (BBMV) and basolateral membrane vesicles (BLMV). BLMV citrate uptake was stimulated to a much smaller degree by imposition of a sodium gradient. Stimulation in citrate uptake, observed on reduction of external pH, was also observed with BBMV. However, when pH was decreased from 8.0 to 5.5, citrate uptake increased only threefold in BLMV compared to 10-fold in BBMV. Jenkins et al.[47] have demonstrated an increased capacity of renal BBMV from acidotic rats to transport citrate. Although citrate clearance was enhanced in animals fed sodium bicarbonate, no significant difference compared to controls was observed in citrate transport in vesicles obtained from these animals. Additional studies have also demonstrated an increase in BBMV citrate transport in fasted rats,[48] consistent with the observation that fasting leads to a reduction in plasma citrate concentration and excretion which cannot be explained by systemic acid–base alterations.

Further studies are required to unravel the quantitative importance of citrate transport across the inner mitochondrial membrane compared to the luminal and basolateral membranes of the proximal tubule cell in the overall regulation of renal citrate clearance and metabolism.

2.4. Kinins and Kallikrein

Recent studies have provided additional information to clarify the intrarenal localization of enzymes degrading and forming kinins. Several reviews have appeared.[49,50] Immunocytochemical studies[51] and radioimmunoassay determinations[52] have provided convincing evidence that both kininase I and kininase II activity are localized primarily to the proximal convoluted tubule and the pars recta of the proximal tubule of the rabbit kidney.[53] Some discrepancy exists with regard to possible kininase II activity in other segments.[52,54] Nevertheless, the data suggest that filtered kinins are largely degraded in the proximal nephron.

In contrast to kininase localization, kallikrein (kininogenase) activity is localized to distal nephron segments.[49,55,56] In fact, in both the rat and mouse nephron, kallikrein activity is localized to connecting tubule cells of the distal nephron. Kallikrein activity was not affected by dietary sodium content in the mouse but was observed to increase fivefold in animals fed a diet of high, compared to low, potassium content.[55] Additional studies[57] have demonstrated kininogen in human medullary tissue and medullary tubule suspensions. These findings indicate that kinins are formed from kininogen by kallikrein in the distal tubule, most likely in connecting tubule cells, consistent with micropuncture localization studies in the rat nephron.[58] The exact physiologic significance of these observations remains to be determined.[56]

3. Effects of Acidosis on Renal Gene Expression

3.1. Introduction

The renal extraction and catabolism of glutamine is initiated in response to metabolic acidosis.[59-61] The extracted glutamine is both deaminated and deamidated to yield two ammonium ions. The increased renal ammoniagenesis provides an expendable cation which facilitates the excretion of titrable acids while conserving sodium and potassium ions. In the rat, the resulting α-ketoglutarate is primarily converted to glucose.[62] This process also generates bicarbonate ions which partially compensate the systemic acidosis.

During normal acid–base balance the rat kidney extracts and metabolizes very little, if any, of the plasma glutamine[22] (see Section 2.1). Within 1–3 hr following onset of acute acidosis, the arterial plasma concentration of glutamine is increased twofold due to an increased release from muscle tissue.[63] Significant renal extraction of glutamine becomes evident as the arterial plasma concentration is increased.[23] Additional responses include a prompt acidification of the urine[64] and activation of α-ketoglutarate dehydrogenase[65] due to a decreased availability of substrate and the rapid removal of the products of the mitochondrial glutaminase and glutamate dehydrogenase reactions.

During chronic metabolic acidosis many of the acute adaptations are partially compensated. In addition, the arterial plasma glutamine concentration is decreased to 65% of the normal level.[22,23] However, gradual increases in the levels of the mitochondrial glutaminase[33] and cytoplasmic phosphoenolpyruvate carboxykinase[66] make possible the continued extraction and metabolism of glutamine. The increase in the two activities occurs only within the proximal convoluted tubule,[7,67] which is the primary site of increased renal ammoniagenesis. Under these conditions, increased renal utilization of glutamine is partially compensated by a net hepatic synthesis.[68]

The mechanism by which onset of acidosis initiates the increased expression of specific genes within the renal proximal tubular epithelial cell is unknown. Increased transcription of eucaryotic genes usually occurs through the specific interaction of regulatory proteins with unique sequences of nucleotides that are contained within the promoter, the region of the gene that immediately precedes the site of initiation of transcription. The specific sequences of nucleotides are termed *cis*-acting regulatory elements, whereas the binding proteins which alter the rate of transcription are referred to as *trans*-acting factors. The coordinate expressions of the renal glutaminase and phosphoenolpyruvate carboxykinase genes are likely to utilize a common *trans*-acting factor. This factor could be a nuclear or cytoplasmic protein that undergoes significant change in conformation in response to a slight decrease in intracellular pH. In one conformation, the protein could act to stimulate transcription or stabilize the mRNA. However, the associated alterations in the interorgan metabolism of glutamine and the cell specificity of induction suggest that renal ammoniagenesis and gluconeogenesis are regulated by a specific hormone or a circulating factor. Acidosis could stimulate either the synthesis or the release of a humoral factor which leads to altered gene expression. The factor could interact directly with a nuclear receptor, which then binds to a specific *cis*-regulatory element. Alternatively, the humoral factor could cause the cell-specific increase in the concentration of a second messenger, which then activates a specific *trans*-acting factor. Recent developments in renal cell biology and in the techniques of molecular biology provide an experimental approach that can be used to investigate the mechanism by which this response is regulated.

3.2. Cellular Distribution of Adaptive Response

In normal rat kidney, the mitochondrial glutaminase is greatest in the distal portions of the nephron, intermediate in the proximal convoluted tubule, and very low in glomeruli and proximal straight tubules.[7] Within 24 hr following the onset of acidosis, the glutaminase activity is increased twofold within the proximal convoluted tubule. However, owing to the cell specificity of the increase and the greater level of activity associated with distal tubules, it requires 2–3 days to observe a significant increase in the glutaminase activity measured in a crude homogenate of whole kidney. The maximal induction is due to a 20- to 30-fold increase within the proximal convoluted tubule.

The onset of acidosis causes a more rapid induction of the renal phosphoenolpyruvate carboxykinase.[66] A significant increase in activity is detectable within 5 hr and the enzyme is maximally induced (three fold) within 13 hr. The tubular distribution of phosphoenolpyruvate carboxykinase, fructose 1,6-bisphosphatase, and glucose 6-phosphatase has been determined in microdissected segments of the rat nephron.[69] All three activities, and thus the pathway of gluconeogenesis, are localized uniquely to the entire proximal tubule. However, following onset of acidosis, the increase in phosphoenolpyruvate carboxykinase occurs only within the S1 and S2 segments of the proximal convoluted tubule.[67]

Various segments of the rat nephron have been microdissected from the kidneys of normal and chronic acidotic rats and incubated *in vitro* with 2 mM glutamine.[70] All of the segments isolated from a normal rat produce ammonia. However, the catabolism of glutamine is greatest in the distal convoluted and proximal tubules. During acidosis, increased ammonia production is observed only in the S1 and S2 segments of the proximal tubule, consistent with the cell-specific increase in glutaminase activity. From the observed rates of ammonia production and the relative abundance of the various nephron segments, it appears that the bulk of the ammonia production in a normal and acidotic rat occurs in the proximal tubule. This conclusion is also supported by previous micropuncture studies which demonstrate that at least 80% of the urinary ammonia excretion observed in normal and acidotic rats can be accounted for by ammonia contained in the fluid removed from the lumen of the proximal convoluted tubule.[71]

3.3. Altered Rates of Synthesis

In vivo pulse labeling experiments have established that the primary mechanism for the increase in the level of phosphoenolpyruvate carboxykinase is a stimulation of its synthesis.[72] During normal acid–base balance the synthesis of the carboxykinase accounts for 2% of the synthesis of the soluble proteins in rat kidney cortex. A significant increase in the relative rate of synthesis of phosphoenolpyruvate carboxykinase is observed within 2 hr after administration of an acute acid load. The relative rate of its synthesis is increased threefold within 8 hr after onset of acidosis. The increased rate of synthesis is sufficient to account for the induction of the carboxykinase. The *in vivo* degradation of the carboxykinase is not altered by acidosis and the apparent $t_{1/2}$ for the enzyme is approximately 6 hr. The administration of triamcinolone, a glucocorticoid, increases the carboxykinase activity and its relative rate of synthesis to levels similar to those observed during acidosis.

In vitro translation analysis has established that an increase in functional phosphoenolpyruvate carboxykinase mRNA occurs concomitant with the stimulation of enzyme synthesis.[73] The relative level of translatable carboxykinase mRNA is increased threefold within 6 hr after onset of acidosis or treatment with glucocorticoids. However, the inductive effect of acidosis is preserved in animals that are adrenalectomized, thyroparathyroidectomized, or hypophysectomized. Thus, acidosis and glucocorticoids apparently act independently to stimulate the renal synthesis of phosphoenolpyruvate carboxykinase.

In a normal rat the rate of glutaminase synthesis constitutes only 0.04% of the total protein synthesis.[74] During onset of acidosis, its relative rate of synthesis is increased more rapidly than the appearance of increased glutaminase activity. The increased rate of synthesis plateaus within 5 days at a value that is fivefold greater than normal. The apparent $t_{1/2}$ for glutaminase degradation is unaltered in normal and acidotic rats (5.1 days and 4.7 days, respectively). Similarly, the relative levels of translatable glutaminase mRNA are also increased gradually.[75] At various times following onset of acidosis, the change in the relative level of translatable glutaminase mRNA is very similar to the change in the relative rate of glutaminase synthesis. Therefore, induction of the mitochondrial glutaminase is not due to stimulation of the translocation and processing of its precursor or to the regulation of a required posttranslational modification.

These results indicate that induction of both glutaminase and phosphoenolpyruvate carboxykinase is due to an increase in the level of their functional mRNA. The adaptive increase in the two activities could result from the increased transcription of their respective genes. The more rapid increase in phosphoenolpyruvate carboxykinase activity may be due to a differential effect of acidosis on transcription of the two genes. Alternatively, the observed difference may reflect merely the difference in the half-lives of the two mRNAs. The half-life estimated from the increase in translatable glutaminase mRNA during onset of acidosis was approximately 3 days,[75] whereas the half-life of the renal carboxykinase mRNA is apparently 2 hr.[76] The approach of the rate of enzyme to a new steady-state level is largely a function of the degradation constant of the mRNA. Thus, the same increase in the rate of synthesis of the two mRNAs would result in a much more rapid approach of the rate of synthesis of the carboxykinase to a new steady-state level.

Alterations in the levels of functional mRNA could result from control of processes other than transcription. An altered mechanism of processing of the initial nuclear transcript, an increased rate of transport of an mRNA to the cytoplasm, a decreased rate of mRNA inactivation or degradation, or selective activation of a preexisting pool of cytoplasmic mRNA could cause an increase in the relative level of a functional mRNA. Experiments in which the decrease in glutaminase synthesis during recovery from acidosis was characterized indicate that the adaptive change in this enzyme is not regulated solely by control of transcription.

Recovery from chronic acidosis results in a rapid decrease in renal ammoniagenesis, but it causes only a very gradual decrease in glutaminase activity.[77] It requires 11 days for the induced level of the glutaminase to return to normal. In contrast, the increased rate of glutaminase synthesis[74] and the increased level of translatable glutaminase mRNA[75] return to normal within 1–2 days. The rapid decrease in functional glutaminase mRNA is inconsistent with the half-life (3 days) which was estimated from the rate of increase of translatable mRNA that occurs during onset acidosis. Thus, the rate of glutaminase mRNA inactivation or degradation must be significantly increased during recovery. Stabilization of the glutaminase mRNA could also be an important factor in its induction. The further characterization of this adaptation required the isolation of specific cDNAs that could be used to quantitate the levels of total mRNA and the rates of mRNA transcription and degradation.

3.4. Isolation of Specific cDNA

A complementary DNA for phosphoenolpyruvate carboxykinase was initially cloned from a rabbit renal pBR322 library.[78] The plasmid library was prepared using size-selected poly(A^+) RNA isolated from the kidneys of a glucocorticoid-treated, acidotic rat. Each colony was screened using four different cDNA preparations which were transcribed from poly(A^+) RNA that contained either high or low levels of translatable carboxykinase mRNA. Plasmid DNA isolated from clones selected by this procedure was rescreened by Northern blotting in order to identify a DNA that specifically hybridized to an mRNA of the appropriate size. The isolated cDNA was then confirmed by positive-hydrid selection of an mRNA which yielded immunoprecipitable phosphoenolpyruvate carboxykinase when translated. This arduous procedure yielded a recombinant plasmid that contained a 220-bp insert which encodes only a small portion of the phosphoenolpyruvate carboxykinase. However, the initial clone was used to isolate a nearly full-length cDNA (pPCK-10) which lacks only a small 5' segment of the phosphoenolpyruvate carboxykinase mRNA.[79]

A similar protocol was used to isolate cDNAs that encode the cytosolic form of rat liver phosphoenolpyruvate carboxykinase. This isoenzyme is identical to the renal phosphoenolpyruvate carboxykinase.[80] The primary structure of this mRNA was determined by sequencing the cloned DNA and by primer extension of mRNA.[81] The molecule contains 2624 nucleotides, including 143 and 615 nucleotides of 5' and 3' nontranslated segments, respectively. The 3' nontranslated sequence contains 102 alternating purine and pyrimidine nucleotides, several direct repeats, and palindromic sequences. The amino acid sequence of the carboxykinase was deduced from the mRNA sequence and confirmed by limited peptide sequencing. The protein contains 621 amino acids and has a molecular weight of 69,300.

Genomic DNA coding for phosphoenolpyruvate carboxykinase has been isolated and characterized.[79,81] The gene is composed of 10 exons and nine introns and is approximately 6 kb in length. The transcription initiation site has been identified by primer extension and S_1 nuclease mapping. The 120-bp segment of DNA that is immediately 5' to the transcription initiation site contains the typical TATA element and unique sequences that bind glucocorticoid receptors and mediate the glucagon/cAMP-dependent stimulation of the hepatic gene.[82–84] A chimeric construct containing the 600-bp segment of the phosphoenolpyruvate carboxykinase promoter fused to the chloramphenicol acetyltransferase gene was used to demonstrate that the longer segment also contains an insulin-responsive *cis*-regulatory element.[85] However, various metabolic studies indicate that the renal carboxykinase gene is not responsive to insulin or glucagon.[86]

Pulse-chase experiments carried out with primary cultures of rat renal proximal tubular epithelial cells indicate that the mitochondrial glutaminase is synthesized on cytoplasmic ribosomes as a 72-kDa precursor.[87] The precursor is rapidly translocated into the mitochondria and is processed to yield both the 68- and 65-kDa proteins that are characteristic of the mitochondrial glutaminase. Approximately 2 kb of translated nucleotides is required to encode a 72-kDa protein. Isolated rat renal poly(A$^+$) RNA was fractionated by electrophoresis on a low-melting temperature agarose gel.[75] From its relative mobility, the size of the glutaminase mRNA was estimated to be approximately 6.5 kb. Thus the glutaminase mRNA contains approximately 4.5 kb of nontranslated RNA.

A glutaminase cDNA was isolated by screening a rat renal λgtll expression library.[88] The approach used to isolate the phosphoenolpyruvate carboxykinase cDNA was not practical owing to the lower abundance and the larger size of the glutaminase mRNA. The λgtll is a phage vector that carries the structural gene for *E. coli* β-galactosidase (lac Z).[89] The λgtll DNA contains a single EcoR I restriction site that is located near the 3' end of the coding sequence of the lac Z gene. A cDNA of up to 7 kb in length can be inserted into the unique restriction site to yield a chimeric gene. When the cDNA is inserted in the same reading frame and orientation as the lac Z coding sequence, the resulting chimeric gene encodes a fusion protein that contains a segment of the β-galactosidase (110 kDa) and the sequence normally encoded by the cDNA insert (up to 250 kDa). The fusion protein is expressed in large amounts when the phages are grown in the presence of IPTG, an inducer of the lac Z gene. Thus, clonal plaques of the phage library can be transferred to nylon membranes and effectively screened with specific antibodies.

A single recombinant phage was isolated by screening a rat brain λgtll cDNA library with antibodies prepared against rat renal glutaminase.[88] A lysogen of the isolated phage produces a 145-kDa fusion protein. Partial proteolysis of the fusion protein yields a series of immunoreactive peptides that comigrate with those derived from the purified brain glutaminase. Antibodies that were affinity purified vs. the fusion protein react specifically with both the 68- and 65-kDa proteins that constitute the mitochondrial glutaminase.[90] Therefore, the two glutaminase proteins contain the same immunologic determinant as the peptide sequence that is encoded by the cloned cDNA. This result is consistent with the conclusion that the two peptides of the glutaminase are derived from a common precursor.

The two EcoR I restriction fragments of the cDNA insert were then subcloned into pGEM to yield the plasmids pGA-1 and pGA-2.[88] The former plasmid specifically hybridized an mRNA which, when translated, yields a 72-kDa protein that can be immunoprecipitated with specific glutaminase antibodies. An RNA probe transcribed from the plasmid cDNA hybridizes to an mRNA that is about 6 kb in length. This mRNA is present in rat brain and normal kidney RNA, increases sixfold in acidotic kidney RNA, but is not detectable in liver RNA. In the absence of amino acid sequence data, absolute identification of this cDNA cannot be made. However, if the isolated DNA is not a glutaminase cDNA, it is complementary to an mRNA of similar size, which has the same tissue distribution, exhibits the same level of induction in the kidney during acidosis, and encodes a protein of identical size as the initial translate of the glutaminase mRNA.

The cloned cDNA contains 1040 base pairs that apparently encode 326 amino acids from the C-terminus of the glutaminase and a short segment of 3′ untranslated nucleotides.[88] The pGA-1 and pGA-2 inserts have been used to screen a rat kidney λgt10 library. Putative clones have subsequently been isolated which apparently contain an additional 0.8 kb of coding sequence and up to 2.5 kb of 3′ nontranslated sequence. At least one additional rescreening will be required to isolate the remainder of the glutaminase cDNA.

3.5. Quantitation of mRNA Levels

Various experiments have established that glucocorticoids and cAMP act through independent mechanisms to increase transcription of the hepatic phosphoenolpyruvate carboxykinase gene.[82−84] Insulin acts as a dominant antagonist of the inductive effects of glucocorticoids and of glucagon.[91] Thus, the primary effect of all three hormones occurs at the level of transcription. However, cAMP may also act to stabilize the phosphoenolpyruvate carboxykinase mRNA.[92]

Hybridization analysis indicates that total renal phosphoenolpyruvate carboxykinase mRNA is increased in a glucocorticoid-treated, acidotic rat to the same extent as that previously observed for translatable carboxykinase mRNA.[93] Thus, activation of preexisting mRNA is not likely to contribute to the induction of the renal phosphoenolpyruvate carboxykinase. Experiments with isolated nuclei indicate that glucocorticoids and cAMP also increase expression of the renal phosphoenolpyruvate carboxykinase gene through transcriptional regulation.[94] In these experiments isolated nuclei are incubated with [^{32}P]nucleotides, and the label incorporated into a specific mRNA during transcription runoff is used as a measure of the relative rate of transcription. Dexamethasone treatment of adrenalectomized rats increases transcription of the carboxykinase gene three- to fourfold within 4 hr. Treatment with dibutyryl- or 8-bromo-cAMP causes a two to 2.5-fold increase within 15 min. In both cases, the increased rate of transcription can account for the associated increase in the level of cytosolic carboxykinase mRNA and its rate of translation.

Rats that are fasted for 24 hr exhibit a twofold increase in renal phosphoenolpyruvate carboxykinase and its mRNA (M. Gallo and N. P. Curthoys, unpublished observation). Renal nuclei isolated from 24-hr-starved rats exhibit a twofold increase in the rate of transcription of the phosphoenolpyruvate carboxykinase gene.[94] This increase is not affected by refeeding glucose, but it is partially reversed within 2 hr of administration of bicarbonate. This observation suggests that acidosis may also stimulate transcription. However, fasting a rat for 24 hr does not induce a significant metabolic acidosis (M. Gallo and N. P. Curthoys, unpublished observation). Therefore, it remains uncertain whether increased transcription is the primary mechanism by which onset of acidosis causes an increase in renal phosphoenolpyruvate carboxykinase.

The time course for onset of systemic acidosis and for induction of the carboxykinase mRNA were compared in order to determine whether alterations in pH or bicarbonate ion concentration are direct mediators of the induction.[76] Rats that are loaded with 20 mmoles ammonium chloride per kg body weight exhibit a slight decrease in blood pH after 1 hr and a maximal effect within 2 hr. In contrast, the initial increase in the amount of hybridizable phosphoenolpyruvate carboxykinase mRNA occurs 2 hr after stomach loading. Over the next 4 hr the relative level of carboxykinase mRNA increases fourfold. The increased level is sustained in rats that are made chronically acidotic. Thus, the apparent lag between the two processes suggests an intracellular mediator that regulates induction. This factor could act by stimulating the synthesis of cAMP within the rat renal proximal convoluted tubule, which could in turn mediate the tissue-specific induction of phosphoenolpyruvate carboxykinase.

Hybridization analysis using the isolated glutaminase cDNA indicates that the increase in total glutaminase mRNA during onset of chronic acidosis occurs more rapidly than the observed increase in the relative rate of glutaminase synthesis[90] and the increase in renal glutaminase activity (Fig. 2). Within 1 day, the level of glutaminase mRNA increases fivefold and by 3 days plateaus at a level that is eightfold greater than that observed in normal rats. This observation suggests that a

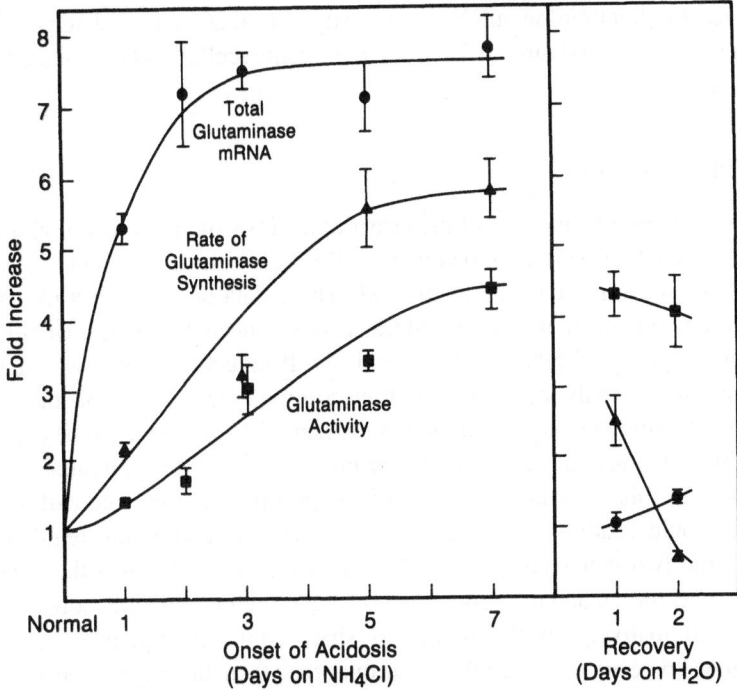

Fig. 2. Effect of chronic acidosis on rat renal levels of glutaminase mRNA and glutaminase activity. Rats were made acidotic by providing 0.28 M NH_4Cl as the sole drinking solution. The changes in glutaminase activity and in the relative rate of glutaminase synthesis were reported previously.[74] The changes in total glutaminase mRNA were measured by hybridizing rate renal RNA with a glutaminase-specific cDNA. (Unpublished data of J-J. Hwang and N. P. Curthoys.)

portion of the newly synthesized glutaminase mRNA is not translated. This could represent fully processed glutaminase mRNA that is not transported out of the nucleus. Alternatively, some of the newly synthesized cytoplasmic glutaminase may be inactive. In contrast, the decrease in total glutaminase mRNA, the level of translatable glutaminase mRNA, and the relative rate of glutaminase synthesis that occur during recovery from acidosis, all exhibit similar kinetics. Thus, the rapid reversal of the increased rate of glutaminase synthesis is probably due to both a decreased rate of synthesis and an increased rate of degradation of the glutaminase mRNA.

The effect of an acute load of NH_4Cl on the level of glutaminase mRNA was also determined (J. J. Hwang and N. P. Curthoys, unpublished observation). This protocol results in a more rapid and more pronounced acidosis than observed during development of chronic acidosis. The increase in glutaminase mRNA is initiated after a 3- to 4-hr lag. The level of glutaminase mRNA is then increased rapidly. Within 17 hr, it reaches the same level of induction as observed in a fully adapted chronic acidotic rat. The more rapid induction causes a slight (1.5-fold), but significant, increase in total renal glutaminase activity after 24 hr. The pronounced lag in appearance of glutaminase mRNA again suggests that increased renal gene expression is not mediated directly by a decrease in intracellular pH or bicarbonate ion concentration.

3.6. Future Studies

A more thorough analysis of the effect of acidosis on the levels of glutaminase and phosphoenolpyruvate carboxykinase mRNA and on the rates of transcription and mRNA turnover should be completed. These data are necessary to determine how the regulation of transcription and translation contributes to the adaptations that occur during onset and recovery from acidosis. If induction of the two enzymes is accomplished primarily by increased transcription, then it will be important to identify the required *cis*-acting regulatory element. This problem can be approached initially by isolating and sequencing the promoter region of the glutaminase gene. A comparison of this sequence with that of the phosphoenolpyruvate carboxykinase promoter would establish whether the two genes share common regulatory elements. If the two genes contain cAMP responsive elements, then this compound might serve as the second messenger that mediates their coordinate induction during acidosis. Alternatively, if the promoters share common sequences that are not homologous to recognized regulatory sequences, then the expression of the two genes may be increased by some as-yet-uncharacterized mechanism.

The rapid decrease in glutaminase mRNA during recovery from acidosis suggests that alterations in mRNA stability contribute to the adaptive changes that occur in this enzyme. Such a process might explain the presence of the large 3' nontranslated sequence that is contained in this mRNA and the low level of efficiency associated with *in vitro* translation of the glutaminase mRNA.[75] Therefore, the sequence of the 3' segment of the glutaminase mRNA should also be analyzed to determine whether it contains regulatory sequences or whether it can form unique secondary structures.

A second approach would be to characterize the regulated expression observed in transgenic mice. A strain of mice that carry the bovine growth hormone structural gene preceded by a 520-bp segment of the phosphoenolpyruvate carboxykinase promoter has been developed.[95] The growth hormone gene is expressed in liver and in kidney, but not in various tissues that lack phosphoenolpyruvate carboxykinase. Hepatic expression of the transgene is regulated by fasting and refeeding and by treatment with cAMP in a manner similar to that of the endogenous phosphoenolpyruvate carboxykinase gene. The tissue-specific expression also indicates that this segment of the carboxykinase promoter must contain sequence(s) that are required for hepatic expression. However, renal expression, although detectable, is very low relative to expression of endogenous phosphoenolpyruvate carboxykinase gene. As a result, preliminary experiments to determine whether the renal transgene could be induced by acidosis were not successful. Additional kidney-specific regulatory elements are likely to be contained further upstream within the phosphoenolpyruvate carboxykinase promoter. Transgenic constructs that contain longer segments of the promoter could be characterized in order to map the sequences that are required for renal expression or that participate in the cell-specific inductive effect of acidosis.

The development of a responsive renal cell line would greatly facilitate the mapping of the *cis*-regulatory elements. LLC-PK$_1$ cells, grown in a rocked culture, exhibit increased ammoniagenesis in response to a decrease in medium pH.[96] The increased glutamine metabolism may reflect an increased level of glutaminase. Alternatively, LLC-PK-F$^+$ cells, which can be grown in the absence of glucose, may have retained the ability to regulate expression of the phosphoenolpyruvate carboxykinase gene.[97] A cell line in which an endogenous gene responds either to decreased pH and/or bicarbonate ion concentration or to factors that are present in serum derived from acidotic animals is very likely to express the *trans*-acting factors that participate in the renal response to acidosis. Such cells could be transfected with a chimeric construct that contains the structural gene of a reporter protein (i.e., chloramphenicol acetyltransferase or neomycin phosphotransferase) and the promoter sequence of the phosphoenolpyruvate carboxykinase or glutaminase gene. If expression of the reporter protein is regulated in a manner similar to that of the endogenous gene, then constructs containing shortened segments of the promoter can be tested in order to map the *cis*-regulatory element.

Eukaryotic *trans*-acting factors bind their complementary sequence of DNA with very high affinity and specificity. Once the *cis*-regulatory element is identified, this property can be utilized to identify and to purify the regulatory proteins. Short oligonucleotides corresponding to the *cis*-regulatory elements have been used to screen expression libraries and to clone the gene for a *trans*-acting factor. Thus, this type of approach could be used to characterize the specific protein(s) that mediate the increased expression of renal genes in response to acidosis. The pH sensitivity or the ability of the regulatory protein to interact with specific second messengers or humoral factors will ultimately define the mechanism by which the adaptive changes in the interorgan metabolism of glutamine are effectively coordinated.

4. Adenosine in the Kidney

4.1. Introduction

The purine ribonucleoside adenosine is now recognized as one important mediator of physiologic events in multiple organ systems, including the kidney.[98] The primary mode of adenosine action is through binding to cell surface adenosine receptors, although an intracellular adenosine binding site also exists.[99] In addition, because adenosine is transported into most cell types and because it is an intermediary in intracellular metabolism of purines and nucleotides, perturbations of any of the components of the adenosine pathways may lead to an adenosine-related physiologic event.

The complexity of the cellular anatomy of the kidney, combined with the technical difficulties involved in dissecting the site of adenosine action for a given physiologic effect, has prevented much progress in understanding the role of adenosine in renal physiology for either normal or disease states. However, recent advances have led to more sensitive assays for adenosine, new adenosine analogs including photoaffinity labels, and new approaches to the study of renal hemodynamics.[100–103] Although this review will summarize the current state of knowledge in this area, it is assumed that application of these advances will soon lead to an even better understanding of adenosine effects in the kidney.

4.2. Adenosine Metabolic Pathways

Adenosine is produced intracellularly by enzymatic dephosphorylation of ATP to 5'AMP, which is then converted to adenosine by the enzyme 5'-nucleotidase, a process that is accelerated when the energy demands of the cell are high (Fig. 3). Adenosine is also generated as a result of methylation reactions when the product S-adenosylhomocysteine is hydrolyzed to adenosine plus homocysteine by S-adenosylhomocysteine hydrolase. Cytoplasmic adenosine is either phosphorylated by adenosine kinase to 5'-AMP or deaminated by adenosine deaminase to inosine. The former is a precursor of 5'-ATP and the latter is further catabolized to purines, like hypoxanthine, xanthine, and uric acid.[99] Adenosine is also metabolized extracellularly by adenosine deaminases associated with the external cell membrane.

Almost all cells, including those in the kidney, contain the enzymes for adenosine metabolism. However, the extent to which a particular reaction occurs

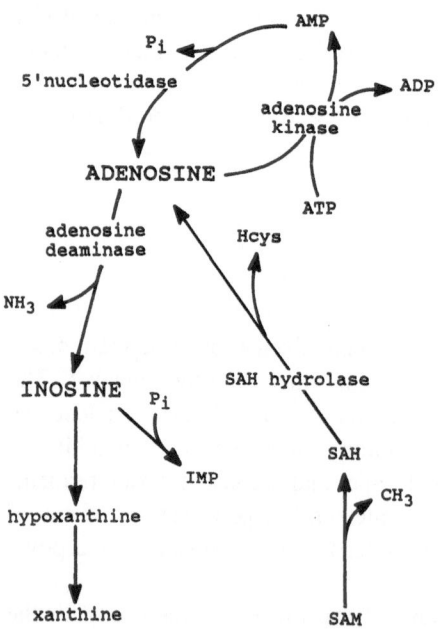

Fig. 3. Intracellular pathways of adenosine metabolism. SAM = S-adenosylmethionine, SAH = S-adenosylhomocysteine, HCys = homocysteine, P_i = phosphate.

depends on the K_m, number of molecules, and location of each enzyme, parameters that vary depending on the type of cell. The interpretation of experiments in tissues that contain the adenosine-metabolizing enzymes must take into account the action of these enzymes on added adenosine; this has not always been the case. Inhibitors of some of these pathways are available; they include adenosine deaminase inhibitors such as deoxycoformycin (DCF) and erythro-9-(2-hydroxy-3-nonyl) adenine (EHNA). The use of these inhibitors is often necessary to maintain a known experimental concentration of adenosine. An alternative approach is the use of adenosine analogs which are not metabolized by these pathways. Examples of compounds used in the studies reviewed here are listed in the next section.

4.3. Distribution of Adenosine Receptors in the Kidney

4.3.1. Background

Adenosine receptors have been identified in numerous cell types. Cell surface adenosine receptors are classified as either high-affinity A_1 receptors ($K_m \sim$ 10 nM), which lead to decreased cAMP production by adenylate cyclase when agonist binds to the receptor, or A_2 receptors ($K_m \sim 0.5-20.0$ μM), which increase intracellular levels of cAMP when stimulated by agonist binding. Both of these receptor types mediate effects on cAMP through GTP-binding proteins.[104] A third type of cell surface adenosine receptor interaction causes a physiologic effect independent of changes in cAMP levels; this is also mediated by a GTP-binding protein.[105] Both A_1 and A_2 adenosine receptors can be present simultaneously on one cell type to allow either inhibition or stimulation of a physiologic response, depending on the interstitial concentration of adenosine.

Most studies of adenosine receptors are done using synthetic analogs which interact preferentially with either A_1 or A_2 receptors. A_1 receptor–specific agonists include N^6-R-(phenylisopropyl) adenosine (L-PIA) and N^6-cyclohexyladenosine (CHA). A_2 receptor–specific agonists include adenosine 5'-ethylcarboximide (NECA) and 2-chloroadenosine. Adenosine receptor antagonists which are not receptor selective include the alkylxanthines, i.e., caffeine, theophylline, and 8-phenyltheophylline.[99,106] A recently synthesized xanthine amine congener of 1,3-dipropyl-8-phenylxanthine has been characterized as a selective inhibitor for A_1 receptors.[107]

Very little direct information is available to define the locations of adenosine receptors in the kidney, but several studies suggest that adenosine receptors are present in the glomerulus and the distal nephron.

4.3.2. Adenosine Receptors in Glomeruli

There is evidence for both A_1 and A_2 receptor sites. Rat glomeruli, isolated by the sieving method, produce cAMP in response to adenosine concentrations greater than 10^{-6} M suggestive of the presence of an A_2 receptor mechanism.[108] In rabbit glomeruli prepared by sucrose density centrifugation, an A_2 receptor agonist, NECA, stimulates adenylate cyclase activity (EC_{50} = 0.14 μM).[109] On the other hand, binding studies with the A_1 receptor agonist, [^{125}I]HPIA, identified a binding site with a K_d of 1.3 nM in this preparation.[109] The presence of A_1 receptors in glomeruli from both human and guinea pig kidneys is also suggested by specific localization of the A_1 ligand [^{3}H]CHA, using autoradiography.[110] No studies have tried to determine whether either receptor is localized to a specific glomerular cell type. Thus, it is premature to speculate about the physiologic significance of these results, although it has been suggested, based on the low binding densities of the receptors and their presence in microvascular preparations, that the measured A_1 receptors may be localized on the juxtaglomerular cells.[109]

4.3.3. Adenosine Receptors in Proximal Tubules

There is no conclusive evidence for adenosine receptors in the proximal tubule. Preparations of cortical tubules prepared by sieving techniques do not increase cAMP in response to adenosine,[108] although adenylate cyclase is stimulated about twofold by 10 μM NECA in rabbit tubules prepared by sucrose density gradient centrifugation.[111] Specific [^{125}]PIA binding in this preparation is low and its detection is complicated by the high degree of nonspecific binding (80–90%). However, studies of the perfused rat kidney have shown that PIA inhibits parathyroid hormone (PTH)-stimulated cAMP production whereas 2-chloroadenosine augments it, suggesting that both A_1 and A_2 receptors are present on proximal tubule cells that have PTH receptors.[112]

4.3.4. Adenosine Receptors in the Distal Nephron

A_6 cultured cells, a continuous cell line with characteristics of a tight distal epithelium, have basolateral membrane A_2 receptors[113] which stimulate sodium transport in an apical to basolateral direction. There is also evidence that adenosine receptors may influence water transport in the cortical collecting duct. In isolated, perfused rabbit cortical collecting tubules adenosine and the analogs NECA and 2-chloroadenosine increase hydraulic conductivity in a manner similar to arginine vasopressin (AVP).[114] In cultured cortical collecting tubule cells isolated from rabbit kidneys by immunodissection techniques, NECA, PIA, and CHA produce both inhibitory and stimulatory effects on cAMP levels at agonist concentrations consistent with the presence of both A_1 and A_2 adenosine receptors in this AVP-responsive epithelium.[98,115] The inhibitory effect of the A_1 receptor agonist CHA on AVP stimulation of cAMP is attenuated by pretreatment with pertussis toxin, evidence for the role of an inhibitory GTP-binding protein in the action of CHA.[115] Others have obtained evidence that NECA-stimulated adenylate cyclase activity in membrane preparations of rat papilla occurs by a mechanism that differs from stimulation with AVP,[116] a result consistent with the finding that an A_2 receptor effect may be localized to the luminal membrane surface in cultured rat papillary cells.[117] The presence of A_2 adenosine receptors in human renal papillae has been demonstrated.[118]

Autoradiographic localization studies have also provided evidence for the presence of adenosine receptors in the distal nephron. The A_1 receptor agonist [^{3}H]CHA labels sites in the inner and outer medulla of the guinea pig kidney.[110] Although labeling of the vasa recta could not be excluded, the authors suggested that A_1 receptors were located on the collecting duct epithelium. Similar labeling was not seen in the medulla of human kidneys. Studies in the rat kidney using [^{125}I]HPIA as an A_1 receptor ligand show the highest specific binding in the inner stripe of the outer medulla and the inner papilla, indicating that A_1 receptors could be present in the thick ascending limb and papillary collecting ducts.[119] This hypothesis is supported by the finding that PIA inhibits AVP-stimulated cAMP production in isolated preparations of both thick ascending limbs and medullary collecting ducts.[120]

4.4. Renal Handling and Production of Adenosine

Under normal circumstances, circulating plasma levels of adenosine are too low for studies of adenosine clearances. However, in situations where adenosine metabolism is prevented, e.g., in patients with adenosine deaminase deficiency or treated with DCF, circulating levels of adenosine rise to 0.4–2 µM. In a group of such patients, Kuttesch and Nelson determined that the adenosine clearance is 20–40% of the creatinine clearance, indicating that there is renal absorption of adenosine.[121] The presence of a renal absorptive pathway for adenosine was confirmed by studies in the isolated perfused rat kidney in the presence of the adenosine deaminase inhibitor EHNA.[122] The results show that adenosine is filtered and that its clearance varies with the plasma adenosine concentration; i.e., at perfusate adenosine concentrations less than 40 µM there is net absorption.

Indicator-dilution methods with radiolabeled adenosine have shown that adenosine is rapidly extracted by the kidney.[123] These studies found that glomerular filtration accounts for only 20% of the adenosine extracted, implying that most of the adenosine uptake occurs prior to reaching the tubules. The authors suggested that the nucleoside transport systems of vascular endothelial and smooth muscle cells rapidly remove adenosine from the plasma. Much of this adenosine remains in the cells, presumably because it enters various metabolic pathways (see Section 4.2). Thus, very little adenosine returns to the renal venous circulation. Of the filtered adenosine about half is excreted in the urine. The rest is probably transported into the tubular epithelial cells (see Section 4.5).

4.5. Evidence for Adenosine Transport Systems in the Kidney

Most cell types transport adenosine on membrane carrier systems operating by a facilitated diffusion mechanism.[124] Numerous investigators have provided evidence that vascular endothelial and smooth muscle cells have rapid uptake systems for nucleosides.[125]

Recently, membrane vesicles from brush borders of rat proximal tubules were shown to transport adenosine, and other purine and pyrimidine ribonucleosides, by a Na-dependent carrier.[122,126-128] There is evidence from studies of a similar transport system in rabbit ileal brush border membrane vesicles that this carrier operates by a Na–adenosine cotransport mechanism.[129] This protein carrier may be analogous to Na-dependent carriers in other epithelia, e.g., choroid plexus.[130] It is inhibited by some of the classic inhibitors of nucleoside transport (i.e., dipyridamole) but, as studied in membrane vesicle preparations, is resistant to inhibition by 6-[(4-nitrobenzyl)thio]-9-β-D-ribofuranosylpurine (NBMPR). Although its exact role in the proximal tubule has not been studied, it is reasonable to assume that this transporter reabsorbs at least part of the adenosine filtered by the glomerulus.

From studies in membrane vesicles of the rat proximal tubule and the rabbit ileum, it appears that the basolateral membrane of absorptive epithelia has a Na-independent carrier system for adenosine transport.[122,129] Thus, nucleoside transport in epithelia appears to be polarized due to a Na-dependent transport system on the luminal membrane and a Na-independent carrier on the basolateral membrane (Fig. 4). The Na-independent carrier is similar to the nucleoside transporters described in the erythrocyte, endothelium, and in nonepithelial cells in culture since it is inhibited by all of the classic nucleoside transport inhibitors including NBMPR.[124] Like the Na–adenosine cotransport system, the role of this carrier in the renal tubule is speculative, but it may be important in regulating the interstitial adenosine concentration.

Because of the rapid transport systems for adenosine in the endothelial cells lining the renal vessels, it is difficult to draw conclusions about the effects of adenosine on any of the described receptor locations in the kidney by using a perfused or whole animal experimental model, unless the experiment is done using effective concentrations of both inhibitors of adenosine uptake and extracellular adenosine catabolism. To circumvent these experimental difficulties, an ingenious approach has been used to study the role of interstitial adenosine on renal hemo-

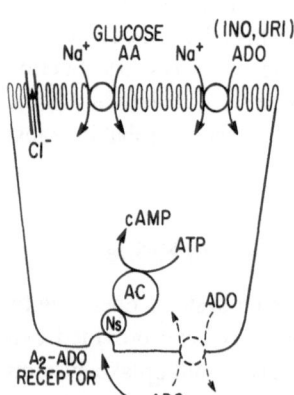

Fig. 4. Hypothetical model for polarization of adenosine transport in a single epithelial cell with a basolateral A_2–adenosine receptor. A brush border chloride channel and Na-dependent glucose or amino acid (AA) transporters are also represented. ADO = adenosine, INO = inosine, URI = uridine, AC = adenylate cyclase, N_S = stimulatory GTP-binding protein.

dynamics in Sprague–Dawley rats.[103] Micropolyethylene capsules with 50-μM pores and attached catheters were surgically placed in the interstitium of one kidney and unmetabolizable adenosine receptor analogs were infused directly into the interstitium. This method allows study of the effects of different interstitial concentrations of adenosine analogs in the absence of inhibitors of the powerful adenosine transport systems in the preglomerular vasculature (see Section 4.6.1).

4.6. Physiologic Roles for Adenosine and Adenosine Receptors

4.6.1. Renal Hemodynamics

Adenosine is a popular candidate for the role of mediator in the metabolic theory of tubuloglomerular feedback because, unlike its effects in most vasculatures, adenosine is a vasoconstrictor in the kidney.[131] Renal vasoconstriction was first reported by Szent-Györgyi in 1929 and was promoted by Thurau during the 1960s.[132,133] The reader is referred to recent reviews by prominent workers in this area for a more complete overview.[134,135] An abbreviated update is presented here.

Exogenous adenosine perfused into the renal artery causes an initial transient decrease in renal blood flow and a decrease in glomerular filtration rate (GFR) of 10–20% in the dog.[136] The vascular response of the kidney is vasoconstriction of the outer cortex accompanied by vasodilation of the deep cortex.[137] These hemodynamic effects occur only in animals that are NaCl restricted and have high plasma renin activity.[138] Antagonism by the adenosine receptor antagonist theophylline suggested that this effect might be receptor mediated. One proposed mechanism is that increased transport of NaCl by the tubules and the necessary increase in oxygen consumption lead to increased breakdown of ATP to ADP, AMP, and adenosine. Accumulated adenosine is transported out of the cell, into the interstitium, via a nucleoside transport system, where its presence can then activate cell surface receptors.

To date there is no evidence that renal cells produce interstitial increases of adenosine under normal conditions. However, studies showing that increases in interstitial adenosine concentrations can cause decreased GFR suggest that in certain situations, such as ischemia (as in acute renal failure) or in the presence of inhibitors of adenosine transport, i.e., dipyridamole, adenosine receptor–mediated control of GFR may be important. For example, infusion of dipyridamole into the sodium-depleted dog causes increased excretion of adenosine, presumably because adenosine uptake into cells is inhibited.[139] The GFR is decreased by 59%, an effect that is absent in sodium-loaded animals and completely reversed by the adenosine antagonist theophylline. Using an infusion of adenosine or an adenosine analog into the renal interstitium via a catheter connected to a surgically implanted permeable capsule, it can be demonstrated that adenosine, 2-chloroadenosine, and NECA are all effective in decreasing GFR by 54–71% in the absence of a decrease in renal blood flow.[103] The decrease in GFR is reversible when the infusion is stopped or if theophylline is present. Recent studies using perfusion of single nephrons suggest that the effect on GFR occurs by activation of A_1 adenosine receptors.[140,141]

Whether the site of this receptor effect corresponds to any of the receptor locations described in Section 4.3 remains to be established. However, studies in which a wide range of concentrations of the analogs NECA and CHA were infused into isolated rat kidneys show that afferent arteriole resistance increases with a specificity consistent with an A_1 receptor–mediated process. This is accompanied by concurrent vasodilation of the efferent arteriole, via an A_2 receptor mechanism. The data are also consistent with the presence of A_2 receptors on the afferent arteriole which mediate its vasodilation.[142]

The decrease in GFR during adenosine perfusion of the dog kidney is associated with decreases in SNGFR as measured by micropuncture studies. In these experiments, the decrease in SNGFR is due mainly to an increase in afferent arteriole resistance.[143] Previous studies showed that angiotensin II is necessary for adenosine to effectively vasoconstrict the afferent arteriole. Infusion of the angiotensin II antagonist Sar^1-Ile^8-AII attenuates adenosine-induced vasoconstriction.[144] This finding appears to explain the absence of effects of adenosine on GFR in salt-loaded animals that have suppression of the renin–angiotensin axis. In mongrel dogs, when endogenous angiotensin II concentrations were suppressed with infusions of captopril, adenosine caused small, insignificant increases in both pre- and postglomerular resistance in nonfiltering kidneys; preglomerular resistance increased markedly when exogenous angiotensin II was infused in the presence of adenosine.[145]

4.6.2. Adenosine Effects on Renin Secretion

Many studies have suggested that adenosine affects renin secretion directly. Exogenous adenosine inhibits renin secretion,[146] but interpretation of experiments using perfused kidney models to support a possible intrarenal role for endogenous adenosine modulation of juxtaglomerular apparatus activity is difficult because of the concomitant adenosine effects on hemodynamics. The use of A_1 and A_2 receptor analogs to evaluate the effect of adenosine on the secretion of renin in rat renal cortical slices has led to the conclusion that adenosine increases renin secretion via A_2 receptors and inhibits secretion via A_1 receptor effects.[142,147,149] Intracellular calcium may be an intermediary in this mechanism.[149] Since pertussis toxin is capable of blocking the inhibitory effect of the A_1 adenosine analog CHA on renin production, this receptor pathway probably requires the inhibitory GTP-binding protein and adenylate cyclase activity.[150] Perfusion studies in rats using selective A_1 and A_2 agonists confirm these effects on renal renin production.[151] The role of adenosine as a possible second messenger in the regulation of renin secretion has been discussed recently.[135,149]

Interstitial adenosine levels may be regulated by the macula densa and could provide the intercellular communication signal to control renin secretion by the juxtaglomerular cells in addition to mediating the vasoactive response needed for tubuloglomerular feedback. However, as discussed by Briggs and Schnermann, this concept is contradicted by the finding that adenosine potentiates the effect of angiotensin on the afferent arterioles; A_1 receptor activation by nanomolar concentrations of adenosine would decrease renin production, yet require angiotensin II to promote vasoconstriction.[152] An alternative theory is that vasodilation mediated by the macula densa (using some other mechanism) serves to counteract the vasoconstrictive effects of adenosine; thus, a decrease in renin secretion would attenuate the arteriolar vasoconstrictive effect of adenosine.[152] Recent evidence supports the concept that A_1 receptors and angiotensin II receptors can be activated independently to produce vasoconstriction, thus eliminating the requirement for synergistic effects of adenosine and angiotensin II to vasoconstrict the afferent arteriole. For example, when isolated rat kidneys from Na-loaded, renin-suppressed animals are perfused at constant flows, the vasoconstriction induced by the A_1 receptor agonist CHA is enhanced and is not attenuated by saralasin.[153] The independence of adenosine-mediated renal hemodynamic effects from renin concentrations has also been demonstrated in the two-kidney, one-clip Goldblatt rat.[154] These results contradict those from previous studies.[144,145]

One of the major factors leading to contradictory experimental results is likely to be the use of high concentrations of adenosine in perfused systems where it is not possible to define the site of the receptors activated by adenosine, the concentration of adenosine available at a particular receptor site, or the effects of intracellular adenosine metabolism. The actual metabolic fate of many of the adenosine analogs has not been determined in the kidney. Experiments that try to define and control these variables are needed to further dissect the role of specifically localized adenosine receptors in renal hemodynamics, as well as salt and water handling. Until these experimental difficulties are addressed, the physiologic significance of adenosine in the kidney will remain unclear.

References

1. Guder, W. G., Wagner, S., and Wirthensohn, G., 1986, Metabolic fuels along the nephron: Pathways and intracellular mechanisms of interaction, *Kidney Int.* **29**:41–45.
2. Wirthensohn, G. and Guder, W. G., 1986, Renal substrate metabolism, *Physiol. Rev.* **66**:469–497.
3. Guder, W. G. and Ross, B. D., 1984, Enzyme distribution along the nephron, *Kidney Int.* **26**:101–111.
4. Endou, H., Nonoguchi, H., Nakada, J., Takehara, Y., and Yamada, H., 1985, Glutamine metabolism in the kidney: Ammoniagenesis and gluconeogenesis in isolated segments of rats, in: *Kidney Metabolism and Function* (R. Dzurik, B. Lichardus, and W. G. Guder, eds.), Nijhoff, Boston, pp. 26–33.
5. LeBouffant, F., Hus-Citharel, A., and Morel, F., 1982, *In Vitro* $^{14}CO_2$ production by single pieces of rat cortical thick ascending limbs and its coupling to active salt transport, in: *Biochemistry of Kidney Functions* (F. Morel, ed.), Elsevier Biomedical Press, Amsterdam, pp. 363–370.
6. LeHir, M. and Dubach, U. C., 1982, Distribution of two enzymes of beta-oxidation of fatty acids along the rat nephron, in: *Biochemistry of Kidney Functions* (F. Morel, ed.), Elsevier Biomedical Press, Amsterdam, pp. 87–94.

7. Curthoys, N. and Lowry, O. H., 1973, The distribution of glutaminase isoenzymes in the various structures of the nephron in normal, acidotic and alkalotic rat kidney, *J. Biol. Chem.* **248:**162–168.
8. Lemieux, G., Baverel, G., Vinay, P., and Wadoux, P., 1976, Glutamine synthetase and glutamyltransferase in the kidney of man, dog, and rat, *Am. J. Physiol.* **231:**1068–1073.
9. Wittner, M., Weidtke, C., Schlatter, E., DiStefano, A., and Greger, R., 1984, Substrate utilization in the isolated perfused cortical thick ascending limb of rabbit nephron, *Pflügers Arch.* **402:** 52–62.
10. Weidemann, M. J. and Krebs, H. A., 1969, The fuel of respiration of rat kidney cortex, *Biochem. J.* **112:**149–166.
11. Guder, W. G., Purschel, S., and Wirthensohn, G., 1983, Renal ketone body metabolism: Distribution of 3-oxoacid Ca-Transferase and 3-hydroxybutyrate dehydrogenase along the mouse nephron, *Hoppe-Seyler's Z. Physiol. Chem.* **364:**1727–1737.
12. Guder, W. G., Purschel, S., Vandewalle, A., and Wirthensohn, G., 1984, Bioluminescence procedures for the measurement of NAD(P) dependent enzyme catalytic activities in submicrogram quantities of rabbit and human nephron structures, *J. Clin. Chem. Clin. Biochem.* **22:**129–140.
13. Baverel, G., Martin, G., Ferrier, B., and Pellet, M., 1982, Characteristics of ketone body metabolism in body renal cortex and outer medulla, in: *Biochemistry of Kidney Functions* (F. Morel, ed.), Elsevier Biomedical Press, Amsterdam, pp. 177–185.
14. Guder, W. G., Purschel, S., and Wirthensohn, G., 1985, Renal ketone body metabolism, in: *Kidney Metabolism and Function* (R. Dzurik, B. Lichardus, and W. G. Guder, eds.), Nijhoff, Boston, pp. 93–102.
15. Guder, W. G. and Wirthensohn, G., 1981, Renal turnover of substrates, in: *Renal Transport of Organic Substrates* (R. Greger, T. Lang, and S. Silbernagl, eds.), Springer-Verlag, Berlin, pp. 66–77.
16. Barac-Nieto, M., 1985, Renal hydroxybutyrate and acetoacetate reabsorption and utilization in the rat, *Am. J. Physiol.* **249:**F40–F48.
17. Barac-Nieto, M., 1986, Renal absorption and utilization of hydroxybutyrate and acetoacetate in starved rats, *Am. J. Physiol.* **251:**F257–F265.
18. Barac-Nieto, M., 1987, D(−)3-Hydroxybutyrate cotransport with Na in rat renal brush border membrane vesicles, *Pflügers Arch.* **408:**32–327.
19. Goldstein, L., 1987, Renal substrate utilization in normal and acidotic rats, *Am. J. Physiol.* **253:** F351–F357.
20. Owen, E. E., and Robinson, R. R., 1963, Amino acid extraction and ammonia metabolism by the human kidney during prolonged administration of ammonium chloride, *J. Clin. Invest.* **42:**263–276.
21. Shalhoub, R., Webber, W., Glabman, S., Canessa-Fischer, M., Klein, J., DeHaas, J., and Pitts, R. F., 1963, Extraction of amino acids from and their addition to renal blood plasma, *Am. J. Physiol.* **204:**181–186.
22. Squires, E. J., Hall, D. E., and Brosnan, J. T., 1976, Arteriovenous differences for amino acids and lactate across kidneys of normal and acidotic rats, *Biochem. J.* **160:**125–128.
23. Hughey, R. P., Rankin, B. B., and Curthoys, N. P., 1980, Acute acidosis and arteriovenous differences of glutamine in normal and adrenalectomized rats, *Am. J. Physiol.* **238:**F199–F204.
24. Tizianello, A., Deferrari, G., Garibotto, G., Robando, C., Acquarone, N., and Ghiggeri, G. M., 1982, Renal ammoniagenesis in an early stage of metabolic acidosis in man, *J. Clin. Invest.* **69:** 240–250.
25. Pitts, R. F. and MacLeod, M. B., 1972, Synthesis of serine by the dog kidney *in vivo*, *Am. J. Physiol.* **222:**394–398.
26. Pitts, R. F., Damian, A. C., and MacLeod, M. B., 1970, Synthesis of serine by rat kidney *in vivo* and *in vitro*, *Am. J. Physiol.* **219:**584–589.
27. Pitts, R. F., 1971, Metabolism of amino acids by the perfused rat kidney, *Am. J. Physiol.* **220:** 862–867.
28. Scaduto, R. C., Jr. and Davis, E. J., 1985, Serine synthesis by an isolated perfused rat kidney preparation, *Biochem. J.* **230:**303–311.

29. Lowry, M., Hall, B., Hall, D. E., and Brosnan, J. T., 1985, Pathways of serine synthesis in the rat kidney, *Contrib. Nephrol.* **47:**203–208.

30. Lowry, M., Hall, D. E., and Brosnan, J. T., 1985, Increased activity of renal glycine–cleavage–enzyme complex in metabolic acidosis, *Biochem. J.* **231:**477–480.

31. Lowry, M., Hall, D. E., and Brosnan, J. T., 1986, Serine synthesis in rat kidney: Studies with perfused rat kidney and cortical tubules, *Am. J. Physiol.* **250:**F649–F658.

32. Lowry, M., Hall, D. E., Hall, M. S., and Brosnan, J. T., 1987, Renal metabolism of amino acids *in vivo*: Studies on serine and glycine fluxes, *Am. J. Physiol.* **252:**F304–F309.

33. Davies, B. H. A. and Yudkin, J., 1952, Studies in biochemical adaptation. The origin of urinary ammonia as indicated by the effects of chronic acidosis and alkalosis on some renal enzymes in the rat, *Biochem. J.* **52:**407–412.

34. Kaufman, A. M., Brod-Miller, C., and Kahn, T., 1985, Role of citrate excretion in acid-base balance in diuretic-induced alkalosis in the rat, *Am. J. Physiol.* **248:**F796–F803.

35. Simpson, D. P., 1983, Citrate excretion: A window on renal metabolism, *Am. J. Physiol.* **244:** F223–F234.

36. Simpson, D. P., 1964, Effect of acetazolamide on citrate excretion in the dog, *Am. J. Physiol.* **206:** 883–886.

37. Hamm, L. L. and Simon, E. E., 1987, Roles and mechanisms of urinary buffer excretion, *Am. J. Physiol.* **253:**F595–F605.

38. Anaizi, N. H., Cohen, J. J., Black, A. J., and Wertheim, S. J., 1986, Renal tissue citrate: Independence from citrate utilization, reabsorption and pH, *Am. J. Physiol.* **251:**F547–F561.

39. Brennan, T. S., Klahr, S., and Hamm, L. L., 1986, Citrate transport in rabbit nephron, *Am. J. Physiol.* **251:**F683–F689.

40. Brennan, S., Klahr, S., and Hamm, L. L., 1986, Effect of luminal and peritubular pH on citrate reabsorption in the rabbit proximal convoluted tubule, *Kidney Int.* **29:**413.

41. Wright, S. H., Kippen, I., Klinenberg, J. R., and Wright, E. M., 1980, Specificity of the transport system for tricarboxylic acid cycle intermediates in renal brush borders, *J. Membr. Biol.* **57:**73–82.

42. Wright, S. H., Kippen, I., and Wright, E. M., 1982, Effect of pH on the transport of Krebs cycle intermediates in renal brush border membranes, *Biochim. Biophys. Acta* **684:**287–290.

43. Wright, S. H., Kippen, I., and Wright, E. M., 1982, Stoichiometry of Na^+-succinate cotransport in renal brush border membranes, *J. Biol. Chem.* **257:**1773–1778.

44. Jorgensen, K. E., Kragh-Hansen, U., Roigaard-Petersen, H., and Iqbal-Sheikh, M., 1983, Citrate uptake by basolateral and luminal membrane vesicles from rabbit kidney cortex, *Am. J. Physiol.* **244:**F686–F695.

45. Barac-Nieto, M., 1984, Effects of pH, calcium, and succinate on sodium citrate cotransport in renal microvilli, *Am. J. Physiol.* **247:**F282–F290.

46. Wright, S. H. and Wunz, T. M., 1987, Succinate and citrate transport in renal basolateral and brush border membranes, *Am. J. Physiol.* **253:**F432–F439.

47. Jenkins, A. D., Dousa, T. P., and Smith, L. H., 1985, Transport of citrate across renal brush border membrane: Effects of dietary acid and alkali loading, *Am. J. Physiol.* **249:**F590–F595.

48. Windus, D. W., Cohn, D. E., and Heifets, M., 1986, Effects of fasting on citrate transport by the brush border membranes of rat kidney, *Am. J. Physiol.* **251:**F678–F682.

49. Scicli, A. G. and Carretero, D. A., 1986, Renal kallikrein-kinin system, *Kidney Int.* **29:**120–130.

50. Fuller, P. J. and Funder, J. W., 1986, The cellular physiology of glomerular kallikrein, *Kidney Int.* **29:**953–964.

51. Barajas, L., Powers, K., Carretero, D., Scicli, A. G., and Inagami, T., 1986, Immunocytochemical localizations of renin and kallikrein in the rat renal cortex, *Kidney Int.* **29:**965–970.

52. Marchetti, J., Roseau, S., and Alnenc-Gelas, T., 1987, Angiotensin I converting enzyme and kinin-hydrolyzing enzymes along the rabbit nephron, *Kidney Int.* **31:**744–751.

53. Omata, K., Carretero, O. A., Scicli, A. G., and Jackson, B. A., 1982, Localization of active and inactive kallikrein (kininogenase activity) in the microdissected rabbit nephron, *Kidney Int.* **232:** 602–607.

54. Omata, K., Abe, K., Yoshinga, K., and Carretero, O., 1987, Distribution of kininase activity along the rabbit nephron, *Clin. Exp. Theory Practice* **A9**(2–3):469–472.
55. Guder, W. G., Hallback, J., Fink, E., Kaissling, B., and Wirthensohn, G., 1987, Kallikrein (Kininogenase) in the mouse nephron: Effect of dietary potassium, *Biol. Chem. Hoppe-Seyler*, **368**:637–645.
56. Guder, W. G., Hallback, J., Wirthensohn, G., Linke, R., Fink, E., and Muller-Estesl, W., 1987, Studies on the renal kallikrein system, in: *Molecular Nephrology. Biochemical Aspects of Kidney Function* (Z. Kovačevic and W. G. Guder, eds.), Walter de Gruyter, Berlin, pp. 377–384.
57. Hallback, J., Adams, G., Wirthensohn, G., and Guder, W. G., 1987, Quantification of kininogen in human renal medulla, *Biol. Chem. Hoppe-Seyler*, **368**:1151–1155.
58. Beasley, D., Oza, N. B., and Levinsky, N. G., 1987, Micropuncture localization and kallikrein secretion in the rat nephron, *Kidney Int.* **32**:26–30.
59. Kovacevic, Z. and McGivan, J. D., 1983, Mitochondrial metabolism of glutamine and glutamate and its physiological significance, *Physiol. Rev.* **63**:547–605.
60. Tannen, R. L. and Sastrasinh, S., 1984, Response of ammonia metabolism to acute acidosis, *Kidney Int.* **25**:1–10.
61. Brosnan, J. T., Vinay, P., Gougoux, A., and Halperin, M. L., 1988, Renal ammonium production and its implications for acid-base balance, in: *pH Homeostasis: Mechanisms and Control* (D. Haussinger, ed.), Academic Press, New York, pp. 281–304.
62. Vinay, P., Lemieux, G., Gougoux, A., and Halperin, M. L., 1986, Regulation of glutamine metabolism in dog kidney *in vivo*, *Kidney Int.* **29**:68–79.
63. Schrock, H., Chu, C. J., and Goldstein, L., 1980, Glutamine release from hindlimb and uptake by kidney in the acutely acidotic rat, *Biochem. J.* **188**:557–560.
64. Tannen, R. L. and Ross, B. D., 1979, Ammoniagenesis by isolated perfused rat kidney: The critical role of urinary acidification, *Clin. Sci.* **56**:353–364.
65. Lowry, M. and Ross, B. D., 1980, Activation of oxoglutarate dehydrogenase in the kidney in response to acute acidosis, *Biochem. J.* **190**:771–780.
66. Alleyne, G. A. O. and Scullard, G. A., 1969, Renal metabolic response to acid-base change. I. Enzymatic control of renal ammoniagenesis in the rat, *J. Clin. Invest.* **48**:364–370.
67. Burch, H. B., Narins, E., Chu, Fagioli, S., Choi, S., McCarthy, W., and Lowry, O. H., 1978, Distribution along the rat nephron of three enzymes of gluconeogenesis in acidosis and starvation, *Am. J. Physiol.* **235**:F246–253.
68. Welbourne, T. C., Phrompetcharat, V., Givens, G., and Joshi, S., 1986, Regulation of interorganal glutamine flow in metabolic acidosis, *Am. J. Physiol.* **250**:E457–E463.
69. Guder, W. G. and Schmidt, U., 1974, The localization of gluconeogenesis in rat nephron, *Hoppe-Seyler's Z. Physiol. Chem.* **355**:273–278.
70. Good, D. W. and Burg, M. B., 1984, Ammonia production by individual segments of the rat nephron, *J. Clin. Invest.* **73**:602–610.
71. Sajo, I. M., Goldstein, M. B., Sonnenberg, H., Stinebaugh, B. J., Wilson, D. R., and Halperin, M. L., 1981, Sites of ammonia addition to tubular fluid in rats with chronic metabolic acidosis, *Kidney Int.* **20**:353–358.
72. Iynedjian, P. B., Ballard, F. J., and Hanson, R. W., 1975, The regulation of phosphoenolpyruvate carboxykinase (GTP) synthesis in rat kidney cortex. The role of acid-base balance and glucocorticoids, *J. Biol. Chem.* **250**:5596–5603.
73. Iynedjian, P. B. and Hanson, R. W., 1977, Messenger RNA for renal phosphoenolpyruvate carboxykinase (GTP). Its translation in a heterologous cell-free system and its regulation by glucocorticoids and by changes in acid–base balance, *J. Biol. Chem.* **252**:8398–8403.
74. Tong, J., Harrison, G., and Curthoys, N. P., 1986, The effect of metabolic acidosis on the synthesis and turnover of rat renal phosphate-dependent glutaminase, *Biochem. J.* **233**:139–144.
75. Tong, J., Shapiro, R. A., and Curthoys, N. P., 1987, Changes in the levels of translatable glutaminase mRNA during onset and recovery from metabolic acidosis, *Biochemistry* **26**:2773–2777.

76. Gallo, M., Shapiro, R. A., and Curthoys, N. P., 1987, Effect of glucocorticoids and metabolic acidosis on the level of rat renal phosphoenolpyruvate carboxykinase mRNA, in: *Molecular Nephrology, Biochemical Aspects of Kidney Function* (Z. Kovacevic and W. G. Guder, eds.), Walter de Gruyter, Berlin, New York, pp. 191–197.

77. Parry, D. and Brosnan, J. T., 1978, Glutamine metabolism in the kidney during induction of, and recovery from, metabolic acidosis in the rat, *Biochem. J.* **174**:387–396.

78. Yoo-Warren, H., Cimbala, M. A., Felz, K., Monahan, J. E., Leis, J. P., and Hanson, R. W., 1981, Identification of a DNA clone to phosphoenolpyruvate carboxykinase (GTP) from rat cytosol, *J. Biol. Chem.* **256**:10224–10227.

79. Yoo-Warren, H., Monahan, J. E., Short, J., Short, H., Bruzel, A., Wynshaw-Boris, A., Meisner, H. M., Samols, D., and Hanson, R. W., 1983, Isolation and characterization of the gene coding for cytosolic phosphoenolpyruvate carboxykinase (GTP) from the rat, *Proc. Natl. Acad. Sci. USA* **80**:3656–3660.

80. Beale, E. G., Hartley, J. L., and Granner, D. K., 1982, N^6-O^2-Dibutyryl cyclic AMP and glucose regulate the amount of messenger RNA coding for hepatic phosphoenolpyruvate carboxykinase (GTP), *J. Biol. Chem.* **257**:2022–2028.

81. Beale, E. G., Chrapkiewicz, N. G., Scoble, H. A., Metz, R. J., Quick, D. P., Noble, R. L., Donelson, J. E., Biemann, K., and Granner, D. K., 1985, Rat hepatic cytosolic phosphoenolpyruvate carboxykinase (GTP). Structures of the protein, messenger RNA and gene, *J. Biol. Chem.* **260**:10748–10760.

82. Wynshaw-Borris, A., Lugo, T. G., Short, J. M., Fournier, R. E. K., and Hanson, R. W., 1984, Identification of cAMP regulatory region in the gene for rat cytosolic phosphoenolpyruvate carboxykinase (GTP), *J. Biol. Chem.* **259**:12161–12169.

83. Wynshaw-Borris, A., Short, J. M., Loose, D. S., and Hanson, R. W., 1986, Characterization of the phosphoenolpyruvate carboxykinase (GTP) promoter–regulatory region. Multiple hormone regulatory elements and the effects of enhancers, *J. Biol. Chem.* **261**:9714–9720.

84. Short, J. M., Wynshaw-Borris, A., Short, H. P., and Hanson, R. W., 1986, Characterization of the phosphoenolpyruvate carboxykinase (GTP) promoter-regulatory region. Identification of cAMP and glucocorticoid regulatory domains, *J. Biol. Chem.* **261**:9721–9726.

85. Magnuson, M. A., Quinn, P. G., and Granner, D. K., 1987, Multihormonal regulation of phosphoenolpyruvate carboxykinase–chloramphenicol acetyltransferase fusion gene, *J. Biol. Chem.* **262**:14917–14920.

86. Guder, W. G. and Rupprecht, A., 1976, Hormonal regulation of gluconeogensis in isolated rat kidney tubule fragments, in: *Use of Isolated Cells and Kidney Tubules in Metabolic Studies* (J. M. Tager, H. D. Solling, and J. R. Williamson, eds.), North Holland, Amsterdam, pp. 379–388.

87. Samaranayake, S. and Curthoys, N. P., 1987, Biosynthesis and processing of mitochondrial glutaminase, *Fed. Proc.* **46**:2109.

88. Banner, C., Hwang, J. J., Shapiro, R. A., Wenthold, R. J., Nakatani, Y., Lampel, K. A., Thomas, J. W., Huie, D., and Curthoys, N. P., 1988, Isolation of a cDNA for rat brain glutaminase, *Mol. Brain Res.* **3**:247–254.

89. Young, R. A. and Davis, R. W., 1983, Efficient isolation of genes by using antibody probes, *Proc. Natl. Acad. Sci. USA* **80**:1194–1198.

90. Shapiro, R. A., Banner, C., Hwang, J. J., Wenthold, R. J., and Curthoys, N. P., 1988, Regulation of renal glutaminase gene expression during metabolic acidosis, in: *Contributions to Nephrology* (G. Baverel, A. C. Schoolwerth, H. Endow, M. Rengel, and A. Tizianello, eds.), S. Karger, Basel **63**:141–146.

91. Sasaki, K., Cripe, T. P., Kock, S. R., Andreone, T. L., Paterson, D. D., Beale, E. G., and Granner, D. K., 1984, Multihormonal regulation of phosphoenolpyruvate carboxykinase gene transcription. Dominant role of insulin, *J. Biol. Chem.* **259**:15242–15251.

92. Hod, Y. and Hanson, R. W., 1987, Dual effect of cAMP on PEP-carboxykinase gene expression, *Fed. Proc.* **46**:2057.

93. Cimbala, M. A., Lamers, W. H., Nelson, K., Monahan, J. E., Yoo-Warren, H., and Hanson, R. W., 1982, Rapid changes in the concentration of phosphoenolpyruvate carboxykinase mRNA in rat liver and kidney, *J. Biol. Chem.* **257**:7629–7636.

94. Meisner, H., Loose, D. S., and Hanson, R. W., 1985, Effect of hormones on transcription of the gene for cytosolic phosphoenolpyruvate carboxykinase (GTP) in rat kidney, *Biochemistry*, **24:** 421–425.

95. McGrane, M. M., deVente, J., Yun, J., Bloom, J., Park, E., Wynshaw-Borris, A., Wagner, T., Rottman, F. M., and Hanson, R. W., 1988, Tissue specific expression and dietary regulation of a chimeric phosphoenolpyruvate carboxykinase/bovine growth hormone gene in transgenic mice, *J. Biol. Chem.* **263**:11443–11451.

96. Cole, L. A., Scheid, J. M., and Tannen, R. L., 1986, Induction of mitochondrial metabolism and pH-modulated ammoniagenesis by rocking LLC-PK₁ cells, *Am. J. Physiol.* **251**:C293–C298.

97. Gstraunthaler, G. and Handler, J. S., 1987, Isolation, growth and characterization of a gluconeo-genic strain of renal cells, *Am. J. Physiol.* **252**:C232–C238.

98. Spielman, W. S., Arend, L. J., and Forrest, J. N. Jr., 1987, The renal and epithelial actions of adenosine, in: *Topics and Perspectives in Adenosine Research* (F. Gerlach and B. F. Becker, eds.), Springer-Verlag, Berlin, Heidelberg, pp. 249–260.

99. Daly, J. W., 1982, Adenosine receptors: Targets for future drugs, *J. Med. Chem.* **25**:197–207.

100. Jackson, E. K. and Ohnishi, A., 1987, Development and application of a simple microassay for adenosine in rat plasma, *Hypertension* **10**:189–197.

101. Klotz, K-N., Cristalli, G., Grifantini, M., Vittori, S., and Lohse, M. J., 1985, Photoaffinity labeling of A₁-adenosine receptors, *J. Biol. Chem.* **260**:14659–14664.

102. Stiles, G. L., Daly, D. T., and Olsson, R. A., 1986, Characterization of the A₁ adenosine receptor–adenylate cyclase system of cerebral cortex using an agonist photoaffinity ligand, *J. Neurochem.* **47**:1020–1025.

103. Pawlowska, D., Granger, J. P. and Knox, F. G., 1987, Effects of adenosine infusion into renal interstitium on renal hemodynamics, *Am. J. Physiol.* **252**:F678–F682.

104. Stiles, G. L., 1986, Adenosine receptors: Structure, function and regulation, *Trends Pharmacol. Sci.* **7**:486–490.

105. Kurachi, Y., Nakajima, T., and Sugimoto, T., 1986, On the mechanism of activation of mus-carinic K⁺ channels by adenosine in isolated atrial cells: Involvement of GTP-binding proteins, *Pflügers Arch.* **407**:264–274.

106. Daly, J. W., 1985, Adenosine receptors, in: *Advances in Cyclic Nucleotide and Protein Phos-phorylation Research*, Volume 19 (D. M. F. Cooper and K. B. Seamon, eds.), Raven Press, New York, pp. 29–46.

107. Jacobson, K. A., Ukena, D., Kirk, K. L., and Daly, J. W., 1986, [³H]Xanthine amine congener of 1,3-dipropyl-8-phenylxanthine: An antagonist radioligand for adenosine receptors, *Proc. Natl. Acad. Sci. USA* **83**:4089–4093.

108. Abboud, H. E. and Dousa, T. P., 1983, Action of adenosine on cyclic 3',5'-nucleotides in glomeruli, *Am. J. Physiol.* **244**:F633–F638.

109. Freissmuth, M., Hausleithner, V., Tuisl, E., Nanoff, C., and Schuetz, W., 1987, Glomeruli and microvessels of the rabbit kidney contain both A₁- and A₂-adenosine receptors, *Naunyn-Schmiedeberg's Arch. Pharmacol.* **335**:438–444.

110. Palacios, J. M., Fastbom, J., Wiederhold, K-H., and Probst, A., 1987, Visualization of adenosine A₁ receptors in the human and the guinea-pig kidney, *Eur. J. Pharmacol.* **138**:273–276.

111. Freissmuth, M., Nanoff, C., Tuisl, E., and Schuetz, W., 1987, Stimulation of adenylate cyclase activity via A₂-adenosine receptors in isolated tubules of the rabbit renal cortex, *Eur. J. Phar-macol.* **138**:137–140.

112. Coulson, R., Wolszczak, E. A., and Scheinman, S. J., 1986, Effect of 2-chloroadenosine and R(−)phenylisopropyladenosine on the response of the isolated perfused rat kidney to parathyroid hormone. *Fed. Proc.* **45**:424 (Abstract).

113. Lang, M. A., Preston, A. S., Handler, J. S., and Forrest, J. N., Jr., 1985. Adenosine stimulates sodium transport in kidney A₆ epithelia in culture, *Am. J. Physiol.* **249**:C330–C336.

114. Dillingham, M. A. and Anderson, R. J., 1985, Purinergic regulation of basal and arginine vasopressin-stimulated hydraulic conductivity in rabbit cortical collecting tubule, *J. Membr. Biol.* **88:** 277–281.

115. Arend, L. J., Sonnenburg, W. K., Smith, W. L., and Spielman, W. S., 1987, A_1 and A_2 adenosine receptors in rabbit cortical collecting tubule cells: Modulation of hormone-stimulated cAMP, *J. Clin. Invest.* **79:**710–714.

116. Woodcock, E. A., 1986, Evidence for two different stimulatory adenylate cyclase coupling mechanisms in rat renal papilla, *J. Cyclic Nucleotide Protein Phosphor. Res.* **11:**301–316.

117. Clancy, G. P., Husted, R. F., and Stokes, J. B., 1986, Adenosine and vasopressin stimulate cyclic-AMP accumulation in rat papillary collecting duct cells (RtPC) in culture, *Fed. Proc.* **45:** 424 (Abstract).

118. Woodcock, E. A., Leung, E., and Johnston, C. I., 1986, Adenosine receptors in papilla of human kidneys, *Clin. Sci.* **70:**353–357.

119. Brines, M. L. and Forrest, J. N., Jr., 1987, Autoradiographic localization of A_1 adenosine receptors to tubules in the red medulla and papilla of the rat kidney, *Kidney Int.* **33:**256 (Abstract).

120. Torikai, S., 1987, Effect of phenylisopropyladenosine on vasopressin-dependent cyclic AMP generation in defined nephron segments from rat, *Renal Physiol.* **10:**33–39.

121. Kuttesch, J. F., Jr. and Nelson, J. A., 1982, Renal handling of 2'-deoxyadenosine and adenosine in humans and mice, *Cancer Chemother. Pharmacol.* **8:**221–229.

122. Trimble, M. E. and Coulson, R., 1984, Adenosine transport in perfused rat kidney and renal cortical membrane vesicles, *Am. J. Physiol.* **246:**F794–F803.

123. Thompson, C. I., Sparks, H. V., and Spielman, W. S., 1985, Renal handling and production of plasma and urinary adenosine, *Am. J. Physiol.* **248:**F545–F551.

124. Plagemann, P. G. W. and Wohlhueter, R. M., 1980, Permeation of nucleosides, nucleic acid bases, and nucleotides in animal cells, *Curr. Top. Membr. Transp.* **14:**225–330.

125. Pearson, J. D. and Gordon, J. L., 1985, Nucleotide metabolism by endothelium, *Annu. Rev. Physiol.* **47:**617–627.

126. Le Hir, M. and Dubach, U. C., 1984, Sodium gradient-energized concentrative transport of adenosine in renal brush border vesicles, *Pflügers Arch.* **401:**58–63.

127. Le Hir, M. and Dubach, U. C., 1985, Concentrative transport of purine nucleosides in brush border vesicles of the rat kidney, *Eur. J. Clin. Invest.* **15:**121–127.

128. Le Hir, M. and Dubach, U. C., 1985, Uphill transport of pyrimidine nucleosides in renal brush border vesicles, *Pflügers Arch.* **404:**238–243.

129. Betcher, S. L., Forrest, J. N., Jr., Knickelbein, R. G., and Dobbins, J. W., Sodium–adenosine cotransport in brush border membranes from rabbit ileum, *Am. J. Physiol.* (submitted).

130. Spector, R. and Huntoon, S., 1984, Specificity and sodium dependence of the active nucleoside transport system in choroid plexus, *J. Neurochem.* **42:**1048–1052.

131. Osswald, H., Nabakowski, G., and Hermes, H., 1980, Adenosine as a possible mediator of metabolic control of glomerular filtration rate, *Int. J. Biochem.* **12:**263–267.

132. Drury, A. N. and Szent-Györgyi, A., 1929, The physiological activity of adenine compounds with special reference to their action upon the mammalian heart, *J. Physiol. (London)* **68:**213–237.

133. Thurau, K., 1964, Renal hemodynamics, *Am. J. Med.* **36:**689–719.

134. Osswald, H., 1983, Adenosine and renal function, in *Regulatory Function of Adenosine* (R. M. Berne, T. W. Rall, and R. Rubio, eds.), Martinus Nijhoff, The Hague/Boston/London, pp. 399–415.

135. Spielman, W. S. and Thompson, C. I., 1982, A proposed role for adenosine in the regulation of renal hemodynamics and renin release, *Am. J. Physiol.* **242:**F423–F435.

136. Osswald, H., 1975, Renal effects of adenosine and their inhibition by theophylline in dogs, *Naunyn-Schmiedeberg's Arch. Pharmacol.* **288:**79–86.

137. Spielman, W. S., Britton, S. L., and Fiksen-Olsen, M. J., 1980, Effect of adenosine on the distribution of renal blood flow in dogs, *Circ. Res.* **46:**449–456.

138. Osswald, H., Hermes, H. H., and Nabokowski, G., 1982, The role of adenosine in signal transmission of tubuloglomerular feedback, *Kidney Int.* **22**(Suppl):S136–S142.

139. Arend, L. J., Thompson, C. I., and Spielman, W. S., 1985, Dipyridamole decreases glomerular filtration in the sodium-depleted dog: Evidence for mediation by intrarenal adenosine, *Circ. Res.* **56:**242–251.

140. Franco, M., Bell, P. D., and Navar, L. G., 1987, Intratubular effect of adenosine A_1 analog on tubuloglomerular feedback (TGF) mechanism, *Kidney Int.* **33:**263 (Abstract).

141. Soejima, H. and Schnermann, J., 1987, The effect of adenosine analogues on tubuloglomerular feedback responses, *Kidney Int.* **33:**413 (Abstract).

142. Murray, R. D. and Churchill, P. C., 1985, Concentration dependency of the renal vascular and renin secretory responses to adenosine receptor agonists, *J. Pharmacol. Exp. Ther.* **232:**189–193.

143. Osswald, H., Spielman, W. S., and Knox, F. G., 1978, Mechanism of adenosine-mediated decreases in glomerular filtration rate in dogs, *Circ. Res.* **43:**465–469.

144. Spielman, W. S. and Osswald, H., 1979, Blockade of post-occlusive renal vasoconstriction by an angiotensin II antagonist: Evidence for an angiotensin–adenosine interaction, *Am. J. Physiol.* **237:** F463–F467.

145. Hall, J. E. and Granger, J. P., 1986, Adenosine alters glomerular filtration control by angiotensin II, *Am. J. Physiol.* **250:**F917–F923.

146. Tagawa, H. and Vander, A. J., 1970, Effects of adenosine compounds on renal function and renin secretion in dogs, *Circ. Res.* **26:**327–338.

147. Churchill, P. C. and Churchill, M. C., 1985, A_1 and A_2 adenosine receptor activation inhibits and stimulates renin secretion of rat renal cortical slices, *J. Pharmacol. Exp. Ther.* **232:**589–594.

148. Barchowsky, A., Data, J. L., and Whorton, A. R., 1987, Inhibition of renin release by analogues of adenosine in rabbit renal cortical slices, *Hypertension* **9:**619–623.

149. Churchill, P. C., 1985, Second messengers in renin secretion, *Am. J. Physiol.* **249:**F175–F184.

150. Rossi, N. F., Churchill, P. C., and Churchill, M. C., 1987, Pertussis toxin reverses adenosine receptor-mediated inhibition of renin secretion in rat renal cortical slices, *Life Sci.* **40:**481–487.

151. Churchill, P. C. and Bidani, A., 1987, Renal effects of selective adenosine receptor agonists in anesthetized rats, *Am. J. Physiol.* **252:**F299–F303.

152. Briggs, J. P. and Schnermann, J., 1986, Macula densa control of renin secretion and glomerular vascular tone: Evidence for common cellular mechanisms, *Renal Physiol.* **9:**193–203.

153. Rossi, N. F., Churchill, P. C., Jacobson, K. A., and Leahy, A. E., 1987, Further characterization of the renovascular effects of N^6-cyclohexyladenosine in the isolated perfused rat kidney, *J. Pharmacol. Exp. Ther.* **240:**911–915.

154. Churchill, P. C., Bidani, A. K., Churchill, M. C., and Prada, J., 1984, Renal effects of 2-chloroadenosine in the two-kidney Goldblatt rat, *J. Pharmacol. Exp. Ther.* **230:**302–306.

4

Acid–Base Physiology and Pathophysiology

Melvin E. Laski and Neil A. Kurtzman

1. Introduction

In the past 2 years a considerable amount of new data has been introduced in acid–base physiology, to a large degree because of the emergence of technology for fluorometric measurement of intracellular pH. While fluorescence techniques have blossomed, the last 2 years witnessed very few studies performed with classic micropuncture, clearance, or balance techniques. Another major trend is the shift of interest to aspects of cell biology, including mechanisms of cell pH regulation and the roles of intracellular and extracellular messengers. Finally, the loudest discussions occurred regarding the role of urea metabolism in overall acid–base balance, despite the fact that few new data were produced in regard to the question.

Over 200 papers were reviewed for this discussion; rather than including all, we have chosen to present those which we felt had the greatest impact in the field. Since such choice is a matter of taste as well as quality, we acknowledge that some will disagree with our decisions, but given the increasing number of papers from which to choose, selection is unavoidable.

Because fluorescent dye techniques are a part of so many of the studies, especially of those in the proximal tubule, a short introduction seems in order for those unfamiliar with such measurement. While a variety of dyes have been used, the emerging favorite appears to be (2′,7′)-*bis*(carboxyethyl)-(5,6)-carboxyfluores-

MELVIN E. LASKI and NEIL A. KURTZMAN • Department of Internal Medicine, Texas Tech University Health Sciences Center, Lubbock, Texas 79430 cein (BCECF). This agent provides an effective pH because its fluorescent spectrum contains two regions with differing pH sensitivity. If excited in the region of 450 nm, the intensity of the fluorescence is pH independent (the isosbestic point); in contrast, the fluorescent response to excitation at 504 nm is markedly pH dependent (Fig. 1).[1] The latter quality defines the dye as a pH marker, but the former quality provides its usefulness for intracellular conditions. The lack of pH influence on the response at 450 nm removes the necessity to measure actual dye concentration. pH is related to the ratio of fluorescence at 500 nm to that at 450 nm, and this ratio is standard for any concentration. The dye does not permeate cell membranes to an appreciable extent as BCECF. Cells are loaded by application of an acetoxymethyl derivative of BCECF (BCECF-AM) which is capable of cell entry. Once in the cell the acetyxymethyl group is cleaved off by ubiquitous nonspecific esterases, trapping the dye in the cell. The dye appears to be quite nontoxic. There are some problems with photobleaching as well as photic injury when any dye technique is used, of course. The effects of cellular subcompartments and the buffering capacity of the dye remain unresolved. Given these considerations, however, the technique has proved to be extremely useful, as will be evident from the studies we will discuss.

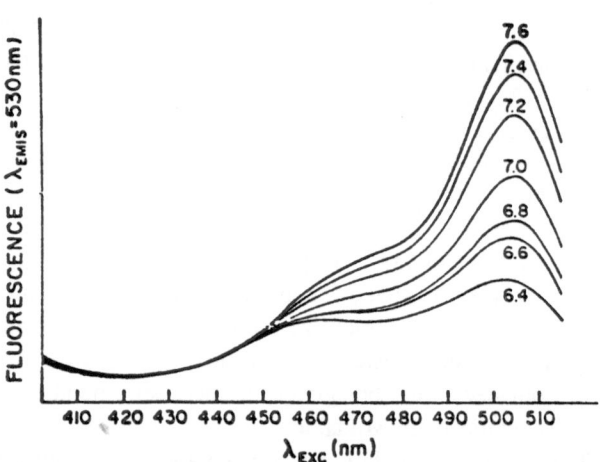

Fig. 1. The pH dependence of the fluorescence of BCECF. The effect of pH on the fluorescence of BCECF is illustrated. When the dye is excited at wavelengths of 450 nm or less, the amplitude of the emitted fluorescence, which is read through a filter allowing passage of wavelengths approximately 530 nm, is not altered by the pH of the solution in which the dye is dissolved. In contrast, if the exciting beam has a wavelength of between 500 and 510 nm, the amplitude of the emitted signal is highly pH-dependent in the physiologic range. The ratio of the signal read during excitation of the dye by 500 nm light to the signal emerging when excitation at 450 nm is performed can therefore be used to calculate the pH of the solution in which the dye is present. (Reprinted from Alpern,[1] with permission.)

2. The Proximal Tubule

2.1. Base Exit from the Proximal Tubule Cell

At the time acid–base physiology was last reviewed in this series, evidence had just become available describing the presence of a conductive, basolateral, sodium–bicarbonate cotransport mechanism which served as the major route of base exit from the proximal tubule cell.[1,2] In the past 2 years a variety of studies have served to confirm this hypothesis and to characterize the process further. A flurry of manuscripts addressed the hypothesis that this symport was electrogenic in nature, using more direct methods to examine this issue than had been present in the first descriptions. Biagi and Sohtell[3] impaled the basolateral membrane of rabbit proximal tubule cells and observed the effects of shifts in bath bicarbonate concentration on the transmembrane potential. Shifts in bicarbonate altered basolateral potential, but so did changes in pH in the absence of bicarbonate (HEPES-buffered solutions). Response to bath potassium shifts was altered by bath pH but not by bath bicarbonate *per se,* suggesting that potassium conductance was altered by pH, a suggestion supported by earlier studies showing major barium sensitivity of this membrane.[4] If a base conductance was present, it was not specifically for bicarbonate and was remarkably large. The same individuals then further examined the electrical response of the basolateral membrane to alterations of bicarbonate and sodium at constant pH.[5] In these studies they demonstrate the presence of a rapid transient in potential immediately upon lowering bath bicarbonate at constant pH. This spike was abolished by acetazolamide. In addition, the authors found a significant depolarization of the basolateral membrane after replacement of sodium with tetramethyl ammonium (TMA) or *n*-methyl *d*-glucamine (NMDG), a response which could be prevented by the presence of 4-acetamido-4′-isothiocyanostilbene-2-2′-disulfonate (SITS), thus providing evidence of a basolateral sodium conductance which is SITS inhibitable, which corresponds to the predictions of Alpern.[1] Similar studies were performed by Sasaki *et al.*,[6] with the additional observation that the effect of changing bath bicarbonate on Vbl was limited if the bicarbonate concentration was altered in the presence of nominally sodium-free bath. The effect of bath chloride on the response of basolateral membrane potential to bicarbonate shifts was minimal. These authors also noted the presence of considerably greater intracellular sodium levels than previously measured, and this value decreased when bath bicarbonate was lowered. Akiba *et al.*[7] assessed the entry of labeled sodium into basolateral membrane vesicles, evaluating the effects of a variety of anions on this entry in the presence and absence of SITS. The effect of clamping the potential across the vesicle membrane by use of valinomycin and potassium was also measured. All data supported the presence of sodium bicarbonate electrogenic cotransport. In a similar vein, Jentsch *et al.*[8] studied bicarbonate-linked conductance in cultured kidney cells (BSC 1, from African green monkey) and found sodium bicarbonate conductance and no potassium conductance, but since the cells were grown on solid support the sidedness of the processes was not known. Finally, Lopes et al.[9] demonstrated the presence of sodium bicarbonate cotransport of a conductive nature in the basolateral membrane of the *Necturus* proximal tubule, a process they had previously shown in *Ambystoma*. It would thus seem that there is uniformity of opinion that the sodium bicarbonate–linked transport step is conductive in nature.

A second question with regard to this mechanism is its specificity for bicarbonate. Two carefully performed studies approached this issue with similar, but not identical techniques. Krapf et al.[10] measured intracellular pH with BCECF in isolated, perfused rabbit proximal convoluted tubules and altered the bath pH, bicarbonate, and sodium. SITS effectively blocked cell pH regulation under the conditions of the study, and removal of bath sodium was seen to result in acidification of the cells. Removing exogenous CO_2/HCO_3 limited the effect of bath pH on pHi and also greatly lowered the effect of zero sodium bath on cell pH. The effect of nominally sodium-free bath on cell pH was abolished when acetazolamide was used in CO_2-free systems, indicating that residual effects of low sodium in CO_2-free systems were due to endogenous bicarbonate generation. Similarly, cyanide abolished pH regulation in CO_2-free systems. These data indicate that sodium bicarbonate cotransport is the dominant pH regulatory process in the basolateral membrane, and that the system is fairly tightly dependent on the CO_2/HCO_3 moiety. Burckhardt and Fromter[11] perfused rat proximal tubule *in vivo*, using peritubular capillary perfusion to create a CO_2/HCO_3-free system. The pH of the peritubular fluid was altered using a variety of nonbicarbonate buffer systems and the effects of these changes on cell pH and buffer capacity were measured. Basolateral potential was measured as changes were performed, and while some change was noted that was attributable to pH itself, changes in potential were much greater in the presence of bicarbonate than in its absence. Barium did not alter the rapid response, which shows that potassium channels are not involved. There was no effect of SITS on the potential change in response to pH shifts in bicarbonate-free solutions, suggesting that the conductive process that occurred was not mediated by the sodium base cotransporter. The bottom line from both of these studies is thus that the electrogenic sodium bicarbonate symport requires bicarbonate (or carbonate), and that other bases cannot substitute.

Yet another question about sodium bicarbonate cotransport is its stoichiometry. This seems resolved by the work of Soleimani et al.,[12] who examined the effects of varying sodium and bicarbonate gradients on transport across basolateral membrane vesicles. Studies were performed with and without valinomycin and potassium gradients. At $[K+]i = [K+]o$, the authors established the inward bicarbonate gradient which balanced an outward sodium gradient to precisely zero flux, and also defined the potassium gradient which balanced an outward sodium gradient at $[HCO_3-]i = [HCO_3-]o$. Their results fit a sodium : bicarbonate ratio of $3:1$, which agrees with a previous estimate of Yoshitomi et al.[13]

In a final study that deserves mention, Alpern[14] performed *in vivo* microperfusion studies which examined the effects of apical chloride concentration on cell pH in proximal tubules studied in the presence of low peritubular bicarbonate. Addition of chloride to perfusate in these conditions did not alter cell pH, and no effect of the addition of formate to the perfusate was noted. The latter maneuver was performed because of suggestions that formate may modulate acid–base transport at the apical membrane. When the studies were repeated with addition of basolateral SITS, luminal chloride addition acidified the cells, and the effect was enhanced by formate. Perfusate DIDS blocked the effect. These results are consistent with apical chloride bicarbonate exchange which is formate sensitive. Although this mechanism is unlikely to play a role in acid–base transport or cell pH regulation under normal conditions, these findings do support previous theories which suggest that salt reabsorption in the proximal tubule occurs in part via parallel sodium–proton and chloride–bicarbonate exchangers.

2.2. Apical Membrane Proton Transport Mechanisms

No major new discoveries appeared about the sodium–proton exchanger during the past 2 years. Rocco et al.[15] showed that amiloride analogs can protect the exchanger from the effects of an irreversible inhibitor which alters the molecule by carboxyl activation. This result suggests that amiloride and transported cations bind somewhere near a carboxyl group. This study and others like it are early steps along the road to a molecular understanding of cation exchange. Goldfarb and Nord[16] followed pH in MDCK-D-1 cell cultures to measure sodium–proton exchange rates. Cell pH was altered by combinations of bath potassium and pH in the presence of nigericin. Cell sodium was set with use of monensin and varying bath sodium, and ouabain was used to prevent the normal basolateral transport from rebalancing the system. Results were compatible with differing sensitivity to sodium at the inner to outer site of the exchanger (about three to four times greater on the external site). While clever, these are very complicated experiments with many assumptions, and the significance of the finding is unclear. This group and another[17,18] have performed studies of sodium–proton exchange in intact cell suspensions, achieving results similar to those in brush border vesicles, but except for a role in studies of acute in vitro adaptation of the exchanger, the technique does not seem to offer any significant advantages over vesicle studies.

The other mechanism for apical acid extrusion was investigated by Kinne-Saffran and Kinne,[19] who assayed brush border membrane vesicles for the presence of Mg-ATPase activity with a luciferase technique. The effect of protonophore on free ATP hydrolysis was used to determine how much of the activity present was proton ATPase. This appeared to be 35%. This ATPase was inhibited by DCCD and filipin to a greater degree than the other Mg-ATPase, while the proton ATPase was less inhibited by diethylstilbesterol and duramycin. Vanadate and NEM had no effect. These characteristics differ from other proton ATPases along the nephron, and in addition, the authors calculate that the activity could account for the levels of proton pump activity estimated in perfusion studies.

The next two studies discussed should be kept in mind when considering data acquired from biochemical studies of intact cells. Specifically, they remind us that not all proton transport mechanisms are related to transepithelial acidification. Gurich and Warnock[20] examined proton transport in endosomes defined by the presence of intravesicular horseradish peroxidase. When studied by techniques normally used with brush border vesicles, both a proton translocating ATPase and a sodium–proton exchanger were found to be present. More notably, the sodium–proton differed from the normal BBMV variety by its insensitivity to amiloride. Thus a cell may have two types of exchanger, which might explain results in tissue from hypertrophied kidneys. In a similar vein, Sabolic and Burckhardt[21] examined the proton ATPase found in endocytic vesicles. They found that this enzyme required magnesium and ATP, but that it was insensitive to ouabain, vanadate, ethoxyzolamide, and levamisole and was partially sensitive to oligomycin. Thiocyanate was the most effective anion for this pump, followed by chloride and the halides. No other cation was required beyond magnesium. Again, this enzyme is unique to endocytic vesicles, but might influence the results of studies performed in whole cell preparations.

2.3. Cell pH Regulation in the Proximal Tubule

These studies are presented together because their intent is to accurately measure baseline cell pH, examine the regulation of cell pH, or delineate whether apical acid extrusion or basolateral base exit is the main regulator of cell pH. Perhaps the most carefully performed used cultures of LLC-PK1 cells in culture, either on glass coverslips or on filterslips. Montrose et al.[22] used these cultured cells and a specially prepared chamber to evaluate the effects of changing apical and basolateral solutions on pHi, finding that basolateral sodium–proton exchange is the important regulator in these cells. Within this study are data using nigericin and potassium to set cell pH, which validate many other studies. A number of earlier studies have used valinomycin, potassium, and bath solution with a defined pH to set pHi, assuming that these conditions render pHi equal to pHo. The authors of this study specifically measured cell pH after such maneuvers by null point techniques, showing that the assumption was correct. The chamber system devised also has great value for future studies in cultured cells.

In the rat proximal tubule, Alpern and Chambers[23] used BCECF measurement of cell pH to follow the effects of changing luminal and peritubular bicarbonate concentration. Altering peritubular bicarbonate proved to be more influential. When SITS was present, varying sodium in the perfusate altered cell pH. The data support the presence of luminal sodium–proton exchange, which has been suggested by investigators using brush border vesicles and perfusion and micropuncture techniques. Overall, these data indicate that basolateral base exit is the main pH regulatory mechanism. Akiba et al.[24] also examined both sodium–proton exchange in the apical membrane and basolateral sodium–bicarbonate cotransporter, extracting both apical brush border membrane vesicles and basolateral membrane vesicles from control, acidotic, and alkalotic rabbits. Up-regulation of both mechanisms was seen in acidosis. Alkalosis decreased the V_{max} of the basolateral cotransporter, while the effect on the apical antiporter did not reach significance. Linear regression analysis showed significant relationship of both mechanisms with pH and also with each other. The authors point out the significance of the parallel nature of adaptation, but one wonders if any other result would be compatible with maintenance of reasonable cell pH. Kurtz[25] studied the nature of cell pH regulation in the S3 segment of the rabbit proximal tubule using BCECF and the isolated perfusion technique. In this segment, he found that the major response to lowering intracellular pH occurred at the apical membrane, and that this response was only partially amiloride inhibitable. The slow recovery of pHi that was present in the presence of sodium free perfusate was blocked by n-ethylmaleimide (NEM), N,N-dicyclohexylcarbodiimide (DCCD), iodoacetic acid and colchicine. An effect of prolonged chloride absence was also noted. These results seem compatible with a dual mechanism of proton extrusion here, a sodium–proton antiporter and a proton pump.

Two papers that presented studies in amphibian tubules raise important issues concerning the control of cell pH and acidification. In the first, Steels and Boulpaep[26] examined the effect of lowering peritubular pH on basolateral potential and fluid reabsorption using tris(hydroxymethyl)-aminomethane (TRIS) buffered solutions and the *Necturus* proximal tubule in isolation. Lowering pH inhibited fluid absorption, but raising pH did not have any effect. The basolateral membrane potential rose as bath pH rose and fell as bath pH was lowered. The importance here is in the linkage between volume absorption and pH, which may be related to the effects on basolateral potential. Wang et al.[27] used a unique preparation–a fused giant cell induced on the surface of the frog kidney at a site along the diluting segment–to study the linkage between membrane potential and cell pH and its regulation. The giant cell allows the investigators to impale a single cell with multiple electrodes and follow internal pH and potentials. These authors found that depolarizing the cell membrane with barium or absent potassium resulted in cell alkalinization, while furosemide hyperpolarized the cell and acidified it as well. They were able to construct a pH/V curve linking pH and potential. Their conclusion, which seemed quite justified, was that the cell membrane potential could be a signal to control intracellular pH, and also the rate of urinary acidification.

Adam et al.[28] used nuclear magnetic resonance (NMR) to arrive at a measurement of cell pH, equating this to the total renal pH estimated from ratios of phosphocreatine and ATP to free phosphate. A control value of 7.39 was arrived at, with a fall to 7.16 in acute acidosis, to 7.3 in chronic acidosis, and to 7.17 in potassium depletion. The authors argue that the pH effect of potassium depletion explains the rise in ammonia production seen in this condition, but the arguments are not totally convincing. The overall estimate of pHi seems high. In contrast to the 7.39 value of Adam et al.,[28] Henderson et al.[29] found a value of 7.1 in proximal tubule cells blindly impaled with double-barreled electrodes. Interestingly, the authors suggest that interstitial bicarbonate concentration may be as high as 40 mM. There are significant questions regarding the electrode, which uses a proton cocktail, and the data generated with it lead to calculations that permit passive bicarbonate exit from the cell, which other studies deem unlikely.

2.4. Regulation of Sodium–Proton Exchange

Change in the rate of sodium–proton exchange and subsequently cell pH is one of the earliest effects noted in many hormonally stimulated cells. The effect of hormones and other mediators on the exchanger in the proximal tubule was the subject of several investigations. Stimulation of sodium–proton exchange was noted in response to glucocorticoids, thyroid hormones, alpha$_2$-adrenergic agents, and phorbol esters.[30–33] Glucocorticoids but not mineralocorticoids were found to stimulate exchange *in vitro*, using the multiply inhibited cell preparation described previously. Cyclohexamide and actinomycin were inhibitory, suggesting that protein production was required for the response.[30] The effect of thyroid hormone was shown when membrane vesicles from hyperthyroid rats were compared to those from controls.[31] There was an increase in V_{max} but not K_m, consistent with an increase in the number of transporters or an increase in their individual rates. However, it is difficult to separate direct effects of the hormone on transport from an adaptive increase in transport secondary to increased filtered load. Alpha$_2$-adrenergic agents were also noted to be stimulatory, but whole cell suspensions were also used in this study, which used measurements of internal sodium space and DMO measurements of pHi for the assay.[32] Results are therefore somewhat indirect. The effect of phorbol esters was demonstrated in cultures of canine proximal tubule cells. Physiologically active forms were stimulatory but inert forms were not.[33]

Inhibition of sodium–proton exchange was found with parathyroid hormone (PTH) and cyclic AMP.[34,35] The study showing the effect of cAMP was the most elegant of this entire group. Weinman *et al.*[35] performed this study in proximal tubule brush border membrane vesicles which were phosphorylated by exposure to $MgCl_2$, KF, and ATP in the presence of a protein phosphorylating subunit. cAMP was added in varying concentrations with and without inhibitors of cAMP protein kinase inhibitors. After vesicles were resealed, standard vesicle studies were performed. cAMP exposure was found to inhibit total and amiloride inhibitable sodium–proton exchange. No other transport mechanism was affected and the authors showed by electrophoresis that phosphorylation did occur.

It is known that PTH inhibits proximal bicarbonate reabsorption. To assess the effect of PTH on sodium–proton exchange, the next study used cultures from the OK cell line. 5,5-Dimethyl-2,4-oxazolidinedione (DMO) was used to measure cell pH and the medium sodium was manipulated.[35] Incubation with PTH resulted in a lower equilibrium pHi, indicating inhibition of the exchanger.

The final study of the group does not show a direct effect of a hormone, but what is probably an indirect effect of the absence of another. Harris *et al.*[36] examined sodium–proton exchange in brush border membrane vesicles from the streptozotocin diabetic rat. The velocity of exchange was increased in the diabetic animal and this could be returned toward normal by treatment of the animals with insulin or with sodium bicarbonate. A sodium–glucose transport defect was also present and was reversible by insulin but not by bicarbonate. The authors interpreted their findings as indicating that the sodium–proton exchange was increased in response to the acidosis of increased ketone production even at normal pH. Their argument is that bicarbonate decreases the acidosis, thus lowering exchange. One wonders if other conclusions also follow. If there is a significant increase in exchange in the face of minor acidosis, this might result in increased proximal volume reabsorption as a direct result. This might result in significantly increased volume. Is this the link between diabetes and hypertension?

3. Bicarbonate Reabsorption in the Proximal Tubule

In addition to the studies that considered the processes of the proximal tubule at the cellular level, a fairly large body of new information was generated about the function and regulation of the proximal tubule as a unit. Perhaps the most remarkable of these was a study addressing the axial heterogeneity of transport in the proximal tubule. Liu and Cogan[37–40] published four studies which explored the segmental nature of bicarbonate reabsorption in the proximal tubule. In the first they performed millimeter-by-millimeter analysis of transport in hydropenia, euvolemia, atrial natriuretic factor (ANF) infusion, glucagon infusion, and alkalosis, using rats with surface glomeruli and classic repetitive micropuncture.[37] Bicarbonate reabsorption increased in the first millimeter in response to increased flow in a direct manner and increased in the second millimeter as well, but to a lesser degree. ANF and glucagon resulted in increases in filtrated load which overwhelmed bicarbonate reabsorption in the first millimeter. There were increases in the third through fifth millimeters. Alkalosis did not alter bicarbonate reabsorption in first 2 mm, but depressed it in the later nephron, where there was no increase in filtered load despite the increase in bicarbonate concentration. Chloride reabsorption increased with load in the first 2 mm, with little effect further along. Volume reabsorption was increased in the first millimeter in response to filtered load, but not if the cause of the increase was ANF or glucagon. Baseline rates in the first 2 mm were much greater than in the remainder of the accessible proximal tubule. Glomerular tubular balance for bicarbonate and volume absorption thus seems to occur in the first 2 mm of the tubule. The basic issue of axial heterogeneity was also examined in an *in vivo* microperfusion paper, where rates of reabsorption in the first 2 mm were compared with those in later segments.[38] Higher bicarbonate permeability was noted in the early segments but there were also markedly greater reabsorptive rates for bicarbonate. When calculated from net reabsorption and passive flux rates, the rate of proton secretion proved to be much greater in the earliest portions of the proximal tubule. In the third paper, angiotensin II was shown to be a major stimulant for bicarbonate, chloride, and volume reabsorption in the early proximal tubule.[39]

Saralasin could be shown to have the opposite effect. The effect of angiotensin II was separated from changes in filtration, demonstrating that the angiotensin II is a major regulator in the proximal tubule. To complete their investigation of axial heterogeneity, Liu and Cogan[40] also studied the effects of systemic alkalosis on segmental reabsorption of bicarbonate in the *in vivo* perfused tubule. Late proximal tubule bicarbonate reabsorption was depressed compared to controls, and this effect was present regardless of perfusate bicarbonate. The decrease was some 30% from control. It should be remembered that a majority of bicarbonate transport occurs early in the proximal tubule, so the role of this depression in the later tubule is not clear.

Other investigators also examined the axial differences along the proximal tubule. Pastoriza-Munoz *et al.*[41] used a fluorescent dye to measure intracellular pH along the proximal nephron, in this case 4-methylumbelliferone (4MU), which this group feels is superior to BCECF because of closer superimposition of extracellular and intracellular titration curves. Their data demonstrate a steady fall of pHi as measurement proceeded axially along the segment. Midpoint pH was 6.96, a value lower than most previous estimates. Lowering perfusate bicarbonate from 15 to 0 mM acidified the cells further. However, if bicarbonate backleak occurs at rates as high as previously suggested, the luminal HCO_3 at the end of the accessible tubule should be roughly five or so; given that this would not greatly lower tubular pH, it seems surprising that a major effect on pHi was noted.

The last 2 years brought still more investigations into the nature of chloride depletion alkalosis from the laboratories of Luke and Galla, who approached their goal of proving the importance of chloride repletion closer than ever. Three studies appeared, all of which used the dialysis-induced chloride depletion alkalosis model in the rat. In the first of these, the effect of a variety of infusions was tested on intact and anephric rats.[42] When volume was supplied in the form of fluid with similar electrolyte composition to the plasma of the animal, intact but not anephric animals recovered. This result supports the proposition that the kidneys are required for correction of alkalosis, but this point seemed obvious prior to the experiment. In the second study, both intact and anephric animals were again considered, and infusates included salt-free albumin and solutions containing non–sodium chloride salts.[43] Restoration of volume with albumin did not correct alkalosis, whereas provision of chloride did, even when performed without the addition of sodium. Correction occurred in some groups without return of GFR to normal levels, and the addition of salt-poor albumin increased GFR to normal without correcting the bicarbonate level. Several problems are still present, though. Serum potassium rose to normal only in the chloride-fed group, and the urine parameters reveal the presence of massive amounts of unaccounted cation. In addition, the substitute cations used are troublesome, including lithium and calcium chloride salts, which have independent effects on the kidney and acid–base balance. In the third study, a 5% glucose, choline bicarbonate, or choline bicarbonate with choline chloride solution was used after induction of alkalosis by dialysis and a maintenance period during which sodium phosphate, sulfate, and acetate with 20 meq/liter sodium chloride were administered.[44] Correction of pH and bicarbonate occurred only in the group that received the increased chloride. Again, only the group that received chloride had a return of serum potassium to normal. However, this occurred without a difference in dietary or administered potassium. It is difficult to account for the rise in potassium or the correction of the alkalosis except by a chloride effect. These studies still leave unresolved whether chloride plays a critical role in the pathogenesis of metabolic alkalosis independent of volume and/or potassium.

Metabolic alkalosis was the concern of several other studies. Borkan et al.[45] used hemofiltration combined with carefully designed replacement fluids to induce metabolic alkalosis while maintaining constant volume and sodium content. Once the system was released, there was a bicarbonate diuresis and a natriuresis. GFR was normal despite the alkalosis. Bicarbonate excretion decreased as volume began to contract. The model here has possibilities, but the data merely reassert the fact that bicarbonate can function as an osmotic diuretic when circumstances make it a nonreabsorbable anion.

Maddox and Gennari[46] attempted to determine whether metabolic alkalosis is preserved by a decrease in GFR without a change in absolute proximal reabsorption or by a direct increase in bicarbonate reabsorption. Chronic alkalosis was first induced with furosemide and a salt- and potassium-poor diet with sodium bicarbonate in the drinking water. Controls received the same diet but with sodium chloride and adequate potassium. Three weeks into the study micropuncture was performed. Chronic alkalosis animals demonstrated elevated blood bicarbonate and greater GFR and SNGFR than controls, leading the authors to the conclusion that the maintenance of alkalosis did not require a drop in GFR.

A variety of studies addressed other sundry issues related to bicarbonate reabsorption in the proximal tubule. Kurtz et al.[47] followed the intraluminal pH of S2 and S3 segments perfused in vitro, utilizing 1,4-dihydroxyphthalonitrile (1,4-DHPN), yet another fluorescing, pH-sensitive dye. In studies of the S3 segment, pHi dropped from 7.43 to 6.89 while total CO_2 concentration did not change, and only minimal fluid absorption occurred. If carbonic anhydrase B was added, neither pH nor total CO_2 content of the fluid altered along the length. In the S2 segment, no disequilibrium occurred. If perfusion rates were slowed, and 4 mM ammonia was added to the bath, then ammonia appeared in the perfusate if the disequilibrium pH was allowed to occur but not if carbonic anhydrase was present. The data thus clearly demonstrate the development of a disequilibrium pH. The rabbit S3 has no functional carbonic anhydrase and the disequilibrium pH that results increases ammonia secretion here. A similar collected fluid pH in rabbit proximal straight tubules was noted by Atkins and Burg,[48] who measured pH of fluid exiting tubules perfused in vitro at very slow rates. Steady-state pH at slow rates here was 6.85, and this value could be increased by raising bath bicarbonate or pH, but not by alteration of bath pCO_2. Chloride-free bath had no effect, in agreement with previous studies of this question.

In a very detailed and precise investigation, Preisig et al.[49] used t-butyl amiloride, which was the most specific inhibitor of sodium–proton exchange they could locate, to determine the importance of sodium–proton exchange to overall bicarbonate reabsorption. With this inhibitor, about 50% of baseline bicarbonate absorption was inhibited. The drug binds to the cells at appropriate rates, and peritubular perfusion was performed to remove effect of basolateral drug. Cell pH, measured by BCECF, did not change with the use of the inhibitor, but it did alter the ability of the cell to recover from acid pH. Thus, a maximum of two-thirds of proximal reabsorption can result from sodium–proton exchange. The careful exclusion of technical errors by tracking drug levels and drug position makes these results very solid.

Bomsztyk and associates[50] perfused proximal tubules *in vivo* with a variety of bicarbonate-free perfusates in an attempt to measure bicarbonate permeability and the generation of bicarbonate from CO_2. The various solutions had different pH values, and the authors measured steady-state total CO_2 concentration. The calculations result in a higher bicarbonate backleak than earlier estimates, with a maximum of 11.7×10^{-7} and a minimum of 2.4×10^{-7} cm/sec. The investigators conclude that continued acid secretion must occur at appreciable rates if bicarbonate concentration is to remain low. The most significant problem with the paper is the complexity of corrections for "actual" pCO_2 in situ. Bomsztyk[51] also delved into the relationship between chloride and bicarbonate reabsorption, finding that addition of bicarbonate to perfusates lowered chloride reabsorption. A puzzling finding here was the absence of any effect of cyanide on chloride flux, causing one to wonder if predominantly passive fluxes were measured. Perhaps related to these findings is Baum's study[52] of the effects of luminal SITS on volume reabsorption when high chloride solutions are perfused through proximal straight tubules. With high chloride perfusate, SITS depressed volume flux, and the residual flux was ouabain inhibitable. When ultrafiltrate-like solutions were used, SITS caused no change in volume flux, but decreased bicarbonate flux, a result consistent with the existence of parallel, apical, sodium–proton, and chloride–bicarbonate exchangers which mediate salt reabsorption. The data then, like those reviewed earlier, support the presence of tight interactions between bicarbonate, salt, and fluid fluxes.

Several studies appeared that dealt with proximal bicarbonate reabsorption in pathophysiologic states. The relationship between filtered load and bicarbonate reabsorption in remnant kidneys was examined by Maddox et al.[53] Bicarbonate reabsorption was examined in 5/6 nephrectomized rats. The SNGFR in these animals was varied by altering dietary protein.[53] SNGFR was highest for remnant kidney rats on high protein, less in remnant kidney animals on low protein, and least in controls. The absolute proximal reabsorption of bicarbonate followed the identical pattern. SNGFR and bicarbonate reabsorption were appropriately matched. Some of the increase in tubular capacity could be accounted for by increased tubular length and mass. These data thus echo some of the findings of Fine et al.[54] in isolated tubules. Cogan[55] also measured bicarbonate reabsorption in partially nephrectomized animals, comparing reabsorption in controls and uninephrectomy models in the presence and absence of prior renal denervation. Denervation was noted to decrease proximal bicarbonate reabsorption by 12%, chloride reabsorption by 18%, and volume reabsorption by 16%. Uninephrectomized animals also demonstrated decreased proximal reabsorption, but prior denervation modified this so that reabsorption was similar in denervated control and denervated uninephrectomy animals. Cogan concludes that the response to uninephrectomy may be neurally mediated, but the data seem indirect with regard to this point. The reabsorption of bicarbonate in the maleic acid model of proximal RTA was the subject of a paper by Bank *et al.*[56] No increase in bicarbonate backleak in comparison to controls was detectable when proximal tubules were perfused *in vivo* with zero bicarbonate fluids, but there was an overall decline of fluid, bicarbonate, and chloride transport. The authors conclude that there is depression of Na, K-ATPase activity or a direct effect on transcellular salt transport. One wishes that studies had also been performed utilizing a variety of peritubular protein concentrations and that the effect of perfusate amiloride had been studied.

4. Loop of Henle

In contrast to the amount of new information regarding this segment in *Contemporary Nephrology*, Volume 4, only a handful of papers appeared in the past 2 years which dealt with acid–base physiology and the loop of Henle. Two papers examined the effects of pH on chloride transport in the thick ascending limb. Wingo[57] manipulated bath pCO_2 and bicarbonate, as well as luminal bicarbonate and potassium. Increased bath pCO_2 lowered transepithelial potential and chloride reabsorption, as did lowering bath bicarbonate. In addition, low perfusate bicarbonate also lowered these parameters. The effects were magnified in the presence of low perfusate potassium, suggesting that the effect probably does not involve the NaK_2Cl cotransporter. The effect noted here may be a significant contributor to the diuresis and kaliuresis of acidosis. Kondo *et al.*[58] also examined effects of pH on chloride flux, this time in hamster thick ascending limbs. Again, lowering of pH also decreased chloride flux, but the pH range was from 7.4 to 6.2, and thus the results are difficult to relate to the physiologic range. The interesting argument, though, is that the results might be interpreted as indicating the presence of protein carrier. In the mouse, Friedman and Andreoli[59] also found a relationship of CO_2/HCO_3 to chloride transport. The presence of potassium is required for the effect. The effect of CO_2/HCO_3 seemed to be due to change in cellular potassium conductance. In nonmammalian systems, Munich *et al.*[60] studied the effects of acidosis and amiloride on transport in frog diluting segment, which may be a thick ascending limb analog. In this study, high pCO_2 was noted to increase resistance and inhibit chloride flux, and the effect was additive to that of amiloride. Intracellular acidosis was felt to alter cellular potassium conductance, as in the mammalian study.

These four papers thus assemble a compatible mass of data indicating that acidosis, whether of metabolic or respiratory origin, has direct effects on salt and potassium handling in the thick ascending limb. The effect is present in widely divergent species and thus is most likely to be present in the human as well. Another link between acid–base and potassium and volume physiology therefore seems established.

5. The Distal Nephron

5.1. Distal Convoluted Tubule

Most of the current work in distal nephron acidification and alkali secretion is concerned with the processes in the collecting tubule segments and their analog bladders. Still, several notable papers have appeared that deal with acidification in the micropuncture-accessible distal tubule of the rat. Since this segment anatomically precedes the collecting tubule, we will first discuss these, and then follow with the review of the work performed in bladders, the collecting tubule, and vesicles.

Since the last review, four studies examining acidification in the distal convoluted tubule have appeared. Iacovitti et al.[61] utilized the in vivo perfused distal tubule technique to determine the effect of flow and transtubular bicarbonate gradient on bicarbonate flux in normal, alkalotic, and amiloride- and acetazolamide-treated rats. Perfusate bicarbonate, potassium, and osmolarity were varied, and perfusion was performed at three different rates. At higher rates of flow, bicarbonate secretion could be demonstrated in the normal rat, and the presence of amiloride increased this process. Rates of entry were higher at lower intratubular bicarbonate concentration, and acetazolamide slowed the flux somewhat. Alkaline serum pH increased bicarbonate entry. In the same issue of the Journal of Clinical Investigation, Capasso et al.[62] presented data obtained with micropuncture and in vivo perfusion which illustrate the presence of bicarbonate reabsorption in the distal convoluted tubule under control conditions. Hypokalemic rats had higher proximal reabsorptive rates, but the bicarbonate flux in the distal tubule was not increased. However, it is notable that the rates remained normal despite decreased flow and increased gradient (low intratubular bicarbonate). In addition, the authors noted the presence of a pH disequilibrium and suggested that the omission of ammonia from perfusate in previous in vivo studies may have led to ammonia trapping which buffered pH change and lowered the apparent bicarbonate reabsorption. The presence of disequilibrium would also complicate interpretation of earlier microelectrode studies. Significant also was the effect of carbonic anhydrase infusion on delivery to the distal tubule. Bicarbonate flux in the loop of Henle rose with this maneuver. These data thus illustrate that significant bicarbonate reabsorption occurs in the distal tubule in control conditions.

This same group also provided a follow-up study[63] which addressed the effects of delivered load and hypokalemia on bicarbonate reabsorption. Hypokalemic animals had greater serum bicarbonate and pH and lower GFR and fraction excretion of bicarbonate. Despite these factors, bicarbonate reabsorption was greater in the hypokalemic animals than in controls. When the question of delivered load was examined, the data show that distal tubule bicarbonate reabsorption increases as load increases. Peritubular pH did not seem to play a role. Even in hypokalemia then, there is considerable bicarbonate reabsorption in the distal tubule, which is detectable with micropuncture techniques despite alkalemia. The rates of the process were impressive.

Finally, Kunau and Walker[64] performed *in vivo* microperfusion studies in normal and casein-fed rats. Bicarbonate reabsorption occurred in both groups and rose from about 15 pmol/mm per minute to more than 40 pmol/mm per minute in acidosis. Amiloride lowered transepithelial potential and reabsorption in the acidotic group. These results are closely related to the previous work, and also, in terms of rates and the effect of amiloride, to studies performed in the isolated perfused cortical collecting tubule. If one views all these studies as a group, there appears to be a simple message—the distal convoluted tubule reabsorbs bicarbonate, and this process is load and flow dependent and amiloride inhibitable. Under specific conditions bicarbonate entry can be shown as well. For those who have studied the cortical collecting tubule in the rabbit, this is a familiar pattern of behavior.

5.2. Studies in Bladder Analogs of Collecting Tubule

The studies of acidification which used urinary bladder techniques largely addressed the same recurring topics we have been discussing in tubules. Intracellular pH was measured in a number of papers. Arruda et al.[65] used 6-carboxyfluorescein to measure intracellular pH in intact bladders and in suspensions consisting of primarily mitochondrial-rich or granular cells. Overall pH was 7.02, but suspensions of mitochondrial rich cells had a mean pH of 6.43 and granular cells averaged 6.44. This seems to be considerable variation, and there seem to be problems with linearity in the range of measurement. The differences between the sum and its parts remain difficult to explain. Graber et al.[66] used 4-MU again and searched for a cell population with a relatively elevated intracellular pH. They did this because cells whose explicit function is to excrete acid might be predicted to have an intracellular pH that is alkaline relative to cells that do not perform this function. A subpopulation of cells that exhibited an elevated pH and seemed to correspond to carbonic anhydrase–rich cells was uncovered, a result which differs from the findings of Arruda et al.[65] in cell suspensions. Finally, Brem et al.[67] examined cell pH in toad bladders before and after exposure to vasopressin. In this instance, measurements were made with 5,5-dimethyl-2,4-oxaloadinedione (DMO) and NMR. These measurements are complicated by the degree of cell swelling in response to argenine vasopressin (AVP), but both techniques appeared to show a drop in pH after the hormone. There may be a later alkalinization phase as well. The significance of this finding relates to previous data which show that the response to vasopressin in toad bladders may be modified by external pH.

Other basic properties of the bladder acidification process were also elucidated in recent papers. A precise catalogue of anions that support chloride exchange was generated by the work of Husted and Fischer.[68] While this sequence may seem rather prosaic, it provides a way to determine whether or not the basolateral and apical anion exchange process occur via identical transporters. These transporters had previously been shown to be different by immunochemistry, but this theoretically could be due to the presence of subunits that function primarily to direct the protein to the proper membrane. The results of future studies on the apical transporter will therefore be quite interesting.

Perhaps the most interesting investigations in these membranes were those which addressed the adaptation of acidification. Acute lowering of pH in the mucosal chamber which is maintained for 2–6 min (acid pulse) was shown by Nero and colleagues[69] to result in an overshoot increase in acidification rate of short duration. The phenomenon could be enhanced further by the presence of a protonophore. When the results of sequential pulses performed with steadily lower pH were compared to similar pulses as pulse pH was sequentially higher in a single bladder, a hysteresis function was apparent (Fig. 2). Rebound acidification was clearly higher after the lowest pH challenge. Only the apical acidification rate overshot; the basolateral alkalinization did not exceed zero. These results were only obtained in the absence of exogenous CO_2. The effect seems to be due to cell acidification, which may be countered by an increase in apical pump sites (authors' opinion) while basolateral processes are inflexible. The hysteresis has important consequences to studies performed with voltage clamping. The speed of the up-and-down regulation of acidification raises significant questions; this phenomenon may not be responsible for chronic adaptation as seen in collecting tubules. Stetson and Steinmetz[70] presented data that support the concept that adaptation is due to inser-

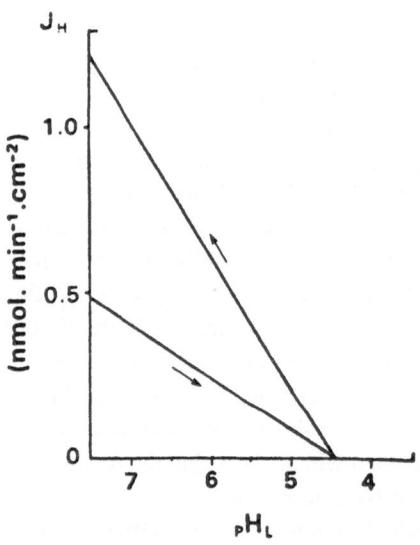

Fig. 2. The effect of increasing and decreasing luminal pH on J_H in the toad bladder. Shown is the relationship between J_H and luminal pH obtained by Nero et al.[69] as luminal pH was lowered (downward arrow) and when pH was raised (upward arrow). The regression lines summarize the results of six experiments. J_H at any luminal pH was greater if the period of measurement followed one in which the luminal pH was lower. These results were only obtained in the absence of exogenous CO_2. The results, when coupled with the finding of no effect of luminal pH on serosally directed base disposal, are consistent with the hypothesis that lowering intracellular pH in this epithelium leads to increase in J_H. (Reprinted from Nero et al.,[69] with permission.)

tion of membrane at the apical surface. Histomorphometric analysis was applied to turtle hemibladders, one member of the pair serving as control and the other exposed to elevated CO_2 tension. Data from type A and type B carbonic anhydrase–rich cells were obtained. CO_2 exposure increased the surface area of type A cells and also resulted in increased area at the basolateral surface of type B cells. In three bladders the density of rod-shaped particles in type A cell apical membrane was assessed as well, but the increase did not achieve statistical significance. If one nevertheless combines the percent increase in particle density and the amplification factor (3.8), one can estimate a fivefold increase in acidification. This number is approximately half the actual increase, a remarkable degree of agreement. The data also suggest that at least some increase in acidification may occur without membrane amplification. In the final study we will review here, Wheeler and Arruda[71] examined the effect of preloading turtles with acid on bladder structure, cell pH, and acidification. The rate of acidification was increased both *in vitro* and *in vivo*, and there was a marked increase in the number of acridine orange–positive cells, but only modest increases in the number of rhodamine- and carboxyfluorescein-positive cells. No change was noted in measurable proton ATPase. It is clear from the data that there must be an increase in acridine orange staining in granular cells, but the authors reject the possibility that these cells might be involved in acidification. This alternative is improbable, but it cannot be said to be impossible.

5.3. Mechanisms and Intracellular pH Regulation

As was true for the proximal tubule, a number of studies searched for the mechanisms that regulate intracellular pH in cells of the collecting tubule. Most studies were performed in the deep medullary collecting tubule where less cellular heterogeneity seems to be present. Zeidel and associates[72,73] published two papers examining intracellular pH regulation in rabbit renal medullary collecting duct cells. They minced medullary inner stripes, exposed the tissue to digestion, and then performed differential centrifugation to obtain a suspension composed of medullary collecting duct cells. Carboxyfluorescein was used as the pH indicator. The first study followed the rate of cell recovery from acidification with the dye and with a titrimeter in the bath as well as ATP content.[72] Recovery of pHi was measured in control conditions and in the presence of cyanide with or without glucose. pH recovery was prevented by cyanide if, in addition, glucose was removed from the media. ATP depletion prevented acidification of the media, as did exposure to digitonin. The restoration of the recovery curve when glucose was added to cyanide-containing bath proves that anaerobic metabolism can indeed drive the system. As a final point, lowering the media pH tended to preserve the ATP levels of the system. In the second study recovery from alkalinization induced by removal of CO_2 from the system was followed with the dye.[73] There was intracellular acidification which restored cell pH which was SITS and acetazolamide sensitive. Furosemide and bumetenide had no effect. An anion specificity could be shown. All of these findings suggest the presence of chloride–bicarbonate exchange as a pH regulatory process. There are difficulties here though. The suspension technique does not allow identification of sidedness, and the uniformity of the cell population in the inner stripe is not absolutely certain. The presence of proton ATPase and a basolateral anion exchanger was known previously. The major discovery is thus that acidification can apparently take place when only anaerobic metabolism is operative.

The regulation of pH was also the subject of two studies performed with cultured cells. Kleinman et al.[74] grew rat papillary tubule cells on coverslips and inserted these into cuvettes in a spectrofluorometer. BCECF was used. The rapid phase of pH recovery from an acid pulse was found to be sodium dependent, suggesting sodium–proton exchange. A second slow phase was also present, and this process was energy dependent (again glucose dependent in the presence of cyanide) and was NEM and oligomycin inhibitable. The second result is quite similar to that of Zeidel et al.[73] Once again, the sidedness of the process cannot be determined in this case because cells grown on solid surfaces lose polarity. It is doubtful that a sodium–proton exchanger could perform any function at the apical surface given pH gradients in this segment of the nephron. Wall et al.[75] grew papillary cells in culture and studied them in suspension, using BCECF to assay pH changes. These authors found a sodium-sensitive pH recovery process which was amiloride sensitive as well. DIDS had little effect. Again, the findings are similar to those just mentioned. If one accepts all the data just offered, the suggestion is that inner medullary cells have a proton ATPase pump and an anion exchanger, while papillary collecting tubule cells have a pump and a sodium–proton exchanger. Logic would put the pump at the apical surface and the antiporters at the basolateral surface, but the data do not extend that far.

The final study in this section that examined basic transport mechanisms was performed in vesicles prepared from human renal tissue. Diaz–Diaz et al.[76] produced medullary vesicles from human kidneys which became available for a variety of reasons. A number of ATPases were present, including ouabain-sensitive, NEM-sensitive, vanadate-sensitive enzymes. The vesicles could be shown to acidify their interiors, and this process was NEM sensitive and oligomycin insensitive. Preincubation with valinomycin and potassium increased the rate of acidification, suggesting that the process here is electrogenic. The most effective nucleotide was ATP, with some effect of GTP. These data show that studies performed in other mammalian systems probably yield data that apply well to human physiology.

5.4. Collecting Tubule Acidification

The investigations of the last 2 years produced, among other concepts, yet another subsegment of the collecting tubule. Koeppen[77,78] placed microelectrodes through the basolateral membranes of cells along collecting tubules from the outer stripe of the inner medulla, showing the presence of two cell types along this segment. In the first, the fractional resistance of the apical membrane was near unity, basolateral conductance was predominantly via a chloride path, amiloride had little effect, but acetazolamide and SITS hyperpolarized the basolateral membrane. These properties fit the profile of an intercalated cell. The second cell type had an apical fractional resistance of 0.8 and a predominant potassium conductance basolaterally. Amiloride was the effective agent inducing hyperpolarization here. Thus these are principal cells. There were crossover effects of each drug however, with changes in apical voltage of intercalated cells probably caused by the impact of drug-induced changes in transport in the principal cells, and vice versa. This crossover effect shows that acidification will be altered by transepithelial voltage change in this segment as it is in bladders and the cortical collecting tubule. McKinney and Davidson[79] examined total CO_2 transport in this segment, finding that total CO_2 flux is always reabsorptive and that bath chloride removal or DIDS exposure inhibits flux. Ouabain had no effect, which is difficult to reconcile with the findings of Koeppen.[78] In addition, these authors found relative acetazolamide resistance. The net sum of the data on this segment is thus unclear, and further study will be needed. It should be noted that the continuing division of the collecting tubule increases the complexity of performing studies in this area.

Laski[80] studied total CO_2 flux in collecting tubules exposed to carbonic anhydrase inhibitors and ouabain or amiloride. Ethoxyzolamide or acetazolamide decreased acidification in the cortical collecting tubule, as expected. However, although the addition of amiloride to the perfusate tended to diminish any residual bicarbonate flux present after ethoxyzolamide, the addition of ouabain to the bath of ethoxyzolamide-treated tubules resulted in the return of bicarbonate reabsorption to control levels or greater. This did not occur if amiloride was present in the lumen at the time ouabain was added to the bath. These results illustrate carbonic anhydrase–independent acidification *in vitro* and were also felt to suggest the presence of a sodium–proton exchanger in the basolateral membrane of a bicarbonate-reabsorbing cell. To test this further, the effect of bath amiloride (10^{-3} M) on acidification was measured in the absence of carbonic anhydrase inhibitors. An increase in reabsorptive total CO_2 flux was noted in cortical collecting tubules from fasted animals but not in tubules from controls. No effect was noted in the medullary collecting tubule. The absence of effect of basolateral amiloride on acidification in the medullary collecting tubule and the ability of luminal amiloride to block the ouabain effect on the ethoxyzolamide-inhibited cortical collecting tubule lead one to speculate that the cell that increases acidification in response to bath amiloride and ouabain could be a principal cell. This issue is far from proven, however.

Regulation of acidification and base secretion in the cortical collecting tubule was the subject of several papers. Hays and associates[81] first examined the effect of various autocoids on acidification in the perfused outer medullary collecting duct. PGE_2 decreased acidification slightly, and without recovery. Indomethacin had the opposite effect, and this was enhanced if the tubule was obtained from an adrenalectomized rabbit. Lysyl bradykinin had no effect, whether given alone or together with arachidonate or angiotensin II. Br-cAMP and forskolin increased reabsorption of bicarbonate. The changes observed in electrical potential were appropriate to the changes noted in bicarbonate flux. Prostaglandins and cyclic AMP (cAMP)-mediated processes therefore seem to regulate acidification here, and the prostaglandin effects resemble those seen in bladders. In a second paper, the same group noted no effect of phorbol esters on total CO_2 flux despite effects on sodium and chloride handling.[82]

Schuster[83] studied cAMP-stimulated anion transport in cortical collecting tubules using isotopic and electrode measurement of chloride fluxes. The kinetics of transport seem to demand a carrier-mediated system. Both cAMP and CO_2/HCO_3 may alter the function of a conductive chloride path parallel to an exchanger. Luminal K_m for chloride was measured at 4–11 meq/liter. The effect of chloride delivery on bicarbonate secretion is well within the physiologic range of chloride delivery to this segment.

Because of the clinical observations that serum bicarbonate does not decrease when patients develop hyposmotic states during conditions marked by excess antidiuretic hormone, and that water diuresis depresses acidification, an hypothesis has been generated which proposes that AVP serves to stimulate urinary acidification. In a study using isolated rat cortical collecting tubules, Tomita et al.[84] observed the effect of vasopressin and bradykinin on anion transport in tubules obtained from DOCA-treated subjects. AVP increased chloride and volume reabsorption and reversed bicarbonate secretion to reabsorption or lowered this flux to zero. Bradykinin reversed the effect of AVP on chloride and volume, but did not affect bicarbonate flux. These data demonstrate a bradykinin effect on this segment in the rat, in contrast to the previous results. Whether this is a species difference or whether one or the other conclusion is in error is not clear.

Bichara et al.[85] also investigated the effects of vasopressin on acidification, using micropuncture of the accessible distal convoluted tubule in endocrine-deficient rats. The data show an increase in bicarbonate reabsorption along the distal convoluted tubule after DDAVP; however, there was no increase in net acid excretion. The authors feel they have shown an effect of AVP on acidification. One must question the model, though. While the acute thyroparathyroidectomized, somatostatin-infused rat may be theoretically justified, it remains a highly complex preparation, and conclusions arising from these studies must be considered in such light.

Given the response of the kidney to respiratory acidosis in vivo and the data of Sasaki et al.[86] concerning the effects of raising bath pCO_2 on bicarbonate reabsorption in the perfused proximal tubule, one might reasonably expect that acute elevation of bath pCO_2 would increase bicarbonate reabsorption in perfused cortical collecting tubules. Surprisingly, when Breyer et al.[87] performed this maneuver, this result was not obtained. Elevation of pCO_2 did not increase acidification, although acute decrease in CO_2 tension did have an inhibitory effect. In contrast, alteration of bath pH by raising or lowering bicarbonate concentration produced significant results. Elevation of bicarbonate concentration inhibited acidification whether performed while allowing pH to rise or in an isohydric manner. The converse was also true. It made no difference whether there was an anion gap or not. The authors were forced to conclude that respiratory acidosis induced by raising pCO_2 does not alter acidification in the cortical collecting tubule, which seemed to be influenced only by "metabolic" acidosis. It is not clear why these results, which seem to contradict prior indirect studies, were obtained. On the one hand, one might recall that increasing pCO_2 above moderate levels has no effect on the turtle bladder, but two abstracts have appeared since the publication of this paper which contradict these results in collecting tubules. Both McKinney and Davidson[88] and Laski et al.[89] found significant effects of respiratory acidosis on acidification in perfused cortical collecting tubules.

The effects of mineralocorticoids on acidification were the subject of investigation in several laboratories. Abdelkhalek and associates,[90] in Doucet's laboratory, performed studies to further characterize an anion-sensitive ATPase (a non-Mg-dependent ATPase activity seen in the presence of ouabain and which is stimulated by the addition of bicarbonate to the media) and establish its cellular location. Activity was noted in both microsomal and mitochondrial fractions of centrifuged preparations, but the sensitivity to a variety of inhibitors differed significantly and the anion sensitivity also distinguished the enzymes from the two sources. Activity was highest in the proximal tubule, with appreciable activity also present in the distal convoluted tubule and the cortical and medullary collecting tubule. DOCA pretreatment resulted in increased activity in the distal nephron, with increases in terms of activity per milligram protein only in the collecting tubule. In a related study Khadouri et al.,[91] from the same laboratory, followed anion-sensitive ATPase activity in adrenalectomized rats as opposed to controls. Adrenalectomized animals were acidotic and had elevation of urine pH but normal serum pH while ingesting saline in place of water. They demonstrated less NEM-sensitive ATPase by their assay in the adrenalectomized group as compared to controls. It is not clear, though, whether it was the absence of mineralocortoid or glucocorticoid which induced this result. Otherwise the data from the two studies must be said to show that mineralocorticoids probably alter the function of this enzyme, but what this ATPase does remains unclear.

Other studies examined the interrelationship between mineralocorticoid effect and sodium delivery. Harrington and co-workers[92] remedied a long-standing deficiency by performing a neglected clearance study on the effect of dietary salt on the response to DOCA in the dog. Recent studies demonstrating the effect of mineralocorticoids on acidification in isolated tubules noted increased bicarbonate flux only in the medullary collecting tubule, which is sodium insensitive.[93] One might then argue that salt delivery is unnecessary for an increase in urinary acid excretion to occur. To readdress the issue, dogs on DOCA were fed a diet containing an acid load (7.0 mmole/kg HCl per day) with or without the addition of salt to a salt-poor basic diet. Only the salt-fed animals increased acid excretion, ammonium excretion, and potassium excretion or developed elevation of serum bicarbonate and pH. The study therefore clearly demonstrates the importance of salt delivery to the effectiveness of mineralocortoid action and suggests that the cortical collecting tubule is significant with regard to mineralocortoid-induced acidification. Mujais et al.[94] examined the converse of the question. Aldosterone-deficient animals are known to be capable of lowering urine pH normally when acidotic, if given adequate salt. To show that this is not merely an effect of metabolic acidosis, these investigators studied adrenally insufficient rats given water, sodium bicarbonate, or sodium bicarbonate and glucocorticoids, and appropriate shams. The animals were studied while acid-base parameters were normal. Despite the absence of mineralocorticoids or acidosis, the glucocorticoid-replete group which was fed bicarbonate was able to lower urine pH normally in response to acute sodium sulfate loading. Urine–blood pCO_2 values were also normal. In an interesting sidelight, it was noted that amiloride inhibited acidification in these animals as well as in normals. Both studies thus show a major link between distal acidification and salt delivery, which is seen in the presence and in the absence of mineralocorticoids.

The responses of the inner medullary collecting duct to acidosis and its release were studied by Bengele et al.,[95,96] who used the technique of retrograde collecting duct cannulation to collect tubular fluid samples. In the first paper, the effect of chronic metabolic acidosis on acidification detectable by this technique was assayed.[95] Metabolic acidosis was induced in rats studied while eucapnia was maintained by ventilator control. Samples were analyzed to determine pH in situ and carbonic anhydrase was not infused. Compared to controls, pH decreased, addition of ammonia increased, and net delivered acid increased to a greater extent in the acidotic group. The equilibrium pH measurements were very complex. In the second paper the authors studied acidification in the retrocannulated medullary collecting duct of animals which were rendered acidotic by ammonium chloride feeding and had the feeding rapidly discontinued.[96] This results in the development of a temporary metabolic alkalosis. When rats in this state were subjected to study, the authors found that acidification in the inner medullary collecting duct, though less than during the preceding acidotic state, still exceeded that in controls. From this finding the authors argue that acidification is not regulated by systemic pH. The problem with this interpretation is the same one which arises when one considers posthypercapneic metabolic alkalosis, a totally comparable situation. Although acidification is higher than in controls despite the presence of alkalosis, it decreased more than 80% in the 24 hr after the acid load was abruptly discontinued. This is not a steady-state condition from which one can draw conclusions regarding the nature of acid–base regulation. It seems more than likely that a finite time period is required to dismantle the metabolic machinery that had been marshalled to defend against the acid insult. Studies performed while this is occurring yield data that do not relate to steady-state conditions.

McKinney and Davidson[97] looked into the effects of prior potassium depletion on bicarbonate flux in cortical collecting tubules in vitro in the rabbit. A potassium-depleted diet increased bicarbonate reabsorption in the cortical collecting tubule compared to controls on normal diet, but the readdition of potassium to the diet resulted in the presence of still greater reabsorptive rates. Potassium deficiency inhibited bicarbonate flux in collecting tubules from the inner stripe of the outer medulla and this was reversible by in vivo and in vitro potassium replacement. The response to DOCA was greater than in normals though. Potassium depletion thus is an inhibitor of acidification here, in agreement with its general effect of producing acidosis in the rabbit, a result similar to that in the dog. Humans, however, behave in this instance like the rat, which becomes alkalotic when potassium deficient, so the value of the data to human physiology is questionable.

In the final study to be discussed in this section, Ribiero and Suki[98] measured total CO_2 flux in the medullary collecting tubule from postobstructed kidneys. They found inhibition of acidification to be present 24 hr after induction of ureteral obstruction. They felt this was not due to backleak or depressed proton motive force, because slow rates of perfusion produced collected fluid total CO_2 concentration equal to that in control. (However, lowering urine pH to a level at which bicarbonate concentration is still measurable is not a major test of proton motive force.) Unfortunately, no sham animals were studied; therefore no true control group is available for data comparison. Also, despite a variety of *in vivo* studies which proposed that the disorder of acidification in obstruction was a cortical collecting tubule event, no study of the cortical collecting tubule was performed. More studies are clearly needed.

6. Respiratory Acidosis

Studies of the effect of respiratory acidosis on renal function span the full extent of the nephron, and therefore this topic is considered in a separate section. Yang *et al.*[99] followed the kinetics of a proximal brush border membrane sodium–proton exchange in the posthypercapneic period. Rabbits were rendered hypercapneic in an environmental chamber. Control and 48-hr hypercapnea animals were used, as well as others which had undergone 48 hr of hypercapnea followed by 3, 24, or 48 hr of return to normal conditions. Exchanger kinetics were studied in brush border membrane vesicles. The V_{max} of exchange was found to be elevated by hypercapnea, and this increase remained for 24 hr after return of the animal to the eucapneic state. There was no alteration of amiloride sensitivity, proton permeability, or sodium–glucose cotransport. These data clearly show that increased sodium–proton exchange is induced by hypercapnea, and that there is a 24-hr lag in return of the kinetics of this transport to normal. Proximal bicarbonate handling was also the subject of a study by Winaver *et al.*[100] Micropuncture data from the proximal tubule of four groups of rats (acetazolamide-treated controls and acetazolamide-treated hypercapneic rats, both with and without prior renal denervation) were obtained. Acute hypercapnea lowered fractional bicarbonate excretion, as expected. This was accompanied by a decrease in filtered load in the intact animals, but denervated subjects had an increased filtered load. Fractional delivery to the end of the proximal tubule was diminished. This occurred in the presence of carbonic anhydrase inhibition, meaning that carbonic acid recycling or some other mechanism must be effective. Catecholamines probably exert no major effect. Finally, Trivedi and Tannen[101] estimated the effect of respiratory acidosis on proximal tubule by following the concentrations of citrate and alpha-ketoglutarate. The theory is that the levels of these metabolites will mirror intracellular pH. Malate and glutamate levels are used as controls, and the effects of metabolic and respiratory acidosis on all these concentrations are compared. In acute situations either form of acidosis had the same effect on this profile, but in the chronic state the respiratory acidosis animals demonstrated a return to a normal chemical state while the metabolic acidosis group remained abnormal. Although it is interesting that these metabolites behave differentially in the two forms of acidosis, it is questionable if cell pH changes can necessarily be inferred from this. The data remain indirect.

Three studies dealt with the effect of hypercapnea on the collecting tubule and its analogs. Verlander et al. [102] performed histomorphometric analysis in the cortical collecting tubule in respiratory acidosis, following changes in both types of intercalated cell. The type a cells increased apical membrane area, while type b cells decreased apical membrane and increased basolateral surface area. Cell numbers per se did not appear to change. While this concept no longer seems new, these data are the evidence that this happens in the mammalian collecting tubule, and they have singular importance. The alternative hypothesis, that cells transform from acidifying to base-secreting forms and back again, is gradually disappearing. A retrograde microcatheterization study of respiratory acidosis is offered by Bengele et al. [103] Because previous investigations had not shown enhancement of acidification along inner medullary collecting ducts when pCO_2 was elevated, these authors postulated that this may have happened because of a decrease in delivered buffer secondary to lowered GFR and increased proximal absorption. In these experiments carbonic anhydrase was infused to eliminate disequilibrium which might lead to acid backleak, and creatinine was infused to serve as a distal buffer. All parameters measured as assays of acidification in the collecting tubule (ammonia entry, pH drop, titratable acid delivery, and net acid delivery) were enhanced by respiratory acidosis when compared with control. The data from this technique now agree with the bulk of the data which suggest distal acidification is increased in this condition. The percent of acidification assigned to the papillary collecting tubule was impressive, but this issue is problematic because of the nature of retrograde microcatheterization techniques.

The last study we will discuss in this section raises more problems. Androgue and Madias[104] induced prolonged hypercapnea in conscious dogs and followed acidification with balance and urine minus blood pCO_2 techniques. An early rise in net acid excretion was noted, but this declined by day 10. Titratable acidity rose at first and fell by day 5. Ammonium excretion rose early and was the only parameter to remain elevated. When urine minus blood pCO_2 was measured during bicarbonate infusion, it was not increased as compared to eucapnea. The authors argue that these data show that the adaptation to chronic respiratory acidosis is a proximal event due to an increase in ammonia metabolism. The data are important because of the length of the study, but the final conclusion is not so certain. Other investigators now reject the use of urine minus blood pCO_2 in hypercapnea, preferring to use the degree of rise of pCO_2 in response to bicarbonate infusion instead.[105] While the proximal tubule is the site of ammonia generation, acid excretion in the distal tubule serves to trap ammonium and thus excrete acid.

7. Effects of Acidosis

Ignored for some time, the effects of acidosis on a variety of physiologic and biochemical processes are now of interest to a number of renal physiologists as well as other investigators. The new material is quite interesting and has the potential of having considerable clinical impact in the relatively near future. The purpose of this section is to present a smattering of the new data in this diverse area.

Perhaps the most intriguing of the material recently published are a trio of papers from a single institution which examine the impact of acidosis on muscle and protein metabolism. Data showing effects of acidosis on growth in children have been available for some time, but seem to be forgotten. The issue was reopened in 1986 by May et al.,[106] who began by studying the effects of acid loads on protein metabolism in rats. Rats were made acidotic by dietary loads, given with and without ammonium. Ammonium acetate controls for ammonium chloride loads were also studied. Urinary nitrogen was followed in balance studies, and biochemical measurements were made in isolated hindquarter preparations and muscle cell materials. Acidotic animals had lower growth rates, higher urinary nitrogen concentration, and elevation of urinary glucocorticoid excretion. Urea production did not increase. Ammonium chloride diet induced such changes, but ammonium acetate did not. Muscle preparations from acidotic animals had greater rates of proteolysis, but synthesis was normal. If acidosis was induced in adrenalectomized animals, no change in protein synthesis occurred, but repletion of glucocorticoids restored the defect in metabolism. Prostaglandin inhibitors did not affect the results, and lowering pH *in vitro* did not alter muscle catabolism in tissues from normal rats. The data therefore demonstrate that acidosis has catastrophic consequences for protein metabolism, and that these effects appear to be mediated by an increase in glucocorticoid production.

The same scientists then turned their attention to protein metabolism in uremia.[107] Uremia was induced by partial nephrectomy, and nitrogen metabolism was followed both in rats allowed to become acidotic and in pair-fed uremic rats given bicarbonate supplementation to maintain normal pH. Blood urea nitrogen was similar in the bicarbonate-fed and acidosis groups. Protein turnover was studied in isolated hindlimbs and muscle tissue from both groups. Protein turnover in hindquarters from acidotic uremics was twice control level, and correction of the acidosis resulted in a return of this parameter to normal. Not all of this effect was due to corticosteroid excess, as suggested in the previous paper, because bicarbonate was largely corrective. Not all the defects were correctable by alkali. Insulin-stimulated protein synthesis was abnormal in uremic rats and remained so despite return of pH to control levels. Again, the data support the concept that acidosis is a major factor in regulation of protein metabolism, and that its correction is quite effective in normalizing this metabolism, even in uremia.

The final study was performed by Hara and the previous three authors in uremic rats.[108] In this paper, the metabolism of branched-chain amino acids was specifically considered. Animal groups included uremic and normal controls and uremic and normal animals fed bicarbonate. Uremic acidosis was associated with detectable increases in valine and leucine catabolism, and treatment with bicarbonate reversed this. Uremic rats given bicarbonate grew normally. Again, the data show an increase in muscle catabolism in uremic acidosis which is reversed by bicarbonate. These studies make a major point which has marked clinical significance. Loss of muscle mass is a severe problem in the chronic renal failure patient, and malnutrition is common in this group. If bicarbonate addition in amounts significant to correct acidosis can prevent muscle losses, this should produce major benefits for these patients. There already are studies of acidosis and growth in children with acidosis; more attention needs to be paid to these issues in adult medicine.

Another publication with a potential for great impact was produced by Carroll et al.[109] These investigators exposed isolated adrenal tissues to solutions with a variety of pH levels. Lower pH was associated with increased angiotensin II binding, a finding that of itself might or might not be significant. Lowered pH was also associated with significant increases in aldosterone production at any level of angiotensin II stimulation (Fig. 3). This did not occur due to change in pH-dependent

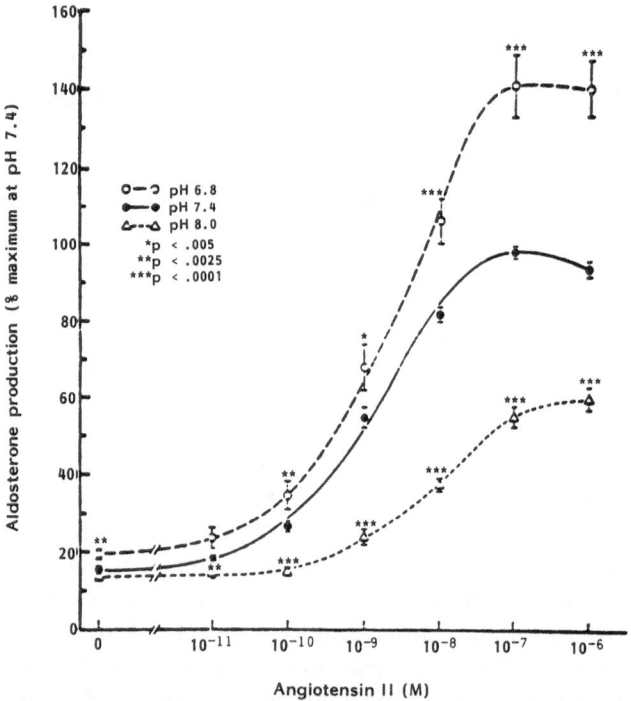

Fig. 3. The effect of pH on the angiotensin II stimulation of aldosterone secretion. The data plotted illustrate the relationship found between angiotensin II concentration and aldosterone release from isolated adrenal tissue at three pH levels. Tissues incubated in acidic media (pH 6.8) release more aldosterone in response to angiotension stimulation than tissues incubated at pH 7.4. Raising bath pH to 8.0 depressed release of aldosterone in response to angiotensin. (Reprinted from Carroll et al.,[109] with permission.)

change in calcium entry or to alteration of phosphatidyl inositol production. There was an apparent increase in binding sites for angiotensin II without increase in site affinity. These data quite clearly describe an alteration by pH of the response of aldosterone production to angiotensin II stimulation. If this is true, the study has remarkable importance. It links aldosterone production and blood pH. When combined with the known stimulation of acidification by aldosterone, the result may be a feedback loop for control of acidification.

It is well appreciated that acidosis has consequences for bone metabolism which can be severe. Several studies from the past 2 years cast new light on the processes involved. Bushinsky and Lechleider[110] used mouse calvaria exposed to acid pH solutions with variable concentrations of calcium and carbonate. The movement of calcium in terms of deposition to bone or dissolution of bone and movement into the solution was found to follow the demands of physical chemistry directly. If the free energy of the potential processes favored bone formation, this happened. If the free energy favored solubilization of bone, it occurred. Brushite and apatite were not involved. The effect of pH on calcium carbonate release is direct. These are wonderfully clear studies with a simple result.

More complex interactions in the intact animal were studied by Kraut et al.[111] The rats used were thyroparathyroidectomized prior to study, and thyroid hormone was replaced. Acidosis was induced by ammonium chloride feeding. There were pair-fed controls. Sham-operated rats were also studied on control diet. The parathyroid-deficient rats had low serum calcium to start, but developed more normal calcium and hypophosphatemia with time. Parathyroid hormone deficiency decreased bone formation and mineralization, which were worsened by acidosis. Acidosis increased bone reabsorption, which rose to levels similar to those of controls. The results are consistent with an effect of acidosis to induce osteopenia, but not osteomalacia: here, again, a direct effect of pH on mineralization. Clinically the relationship of acidosis and osteopenia is more complex than in these rats, but these findings are probably clinically relevant.

Two broad studies on the effects of acidosis on myocardial performance and metabolism appeared. Orchard et al.[112] used a fluorescing calcium-binding protein to observe the effects of pH on intracellular calcium while also measuring membrane potential and contractility. Acidifying the medium depressed contraction, and this was associated with a rise in cytosolic calcium and an increase in calcium release from sarcoplasmic reticulum following stimulation. Acid media also depolarized the cells slightly and increased the occurrence of spontaneous depolarization. Rest tension of the muscle increased, but twitch tension was impaired. A study of myocardial metabolism performed with nuclear magnetic resonance spectroscopy showed that energy metabolism was significantly inhibited by perfusion of the heart with acid media.[113] This was again associated with decreased muscle function. Thus, new data are emerging that explain the clinical observation that myocardial performance declines at low pH.

Unique interrelationships exist between acid–base balance and the renal and gastrointestinal tract transport of phosphate. Both direct effects and effects modulated by alterations in vitamin D and parathyroid hormones occur. Respiratory alkalosis is, along with phosphate deprivation, a model of a phosphate conservation state. Earlier studies show that tubular reabsorption maximum per unit glomerular filtration rate (GFR) is increased in phosphate deprivation but not respiratory alkalosis. Awazu et al.[114] examined phosphate handling in the proximal tubule with micropuncture in each of these models while blood phosphate concentration was held normal by infusion of phosphate. This infusion increased GFR in phosphate-depleted rats, but not in rats with respiratory alkalosis. The excretion of phosphate increased to a much greater extent in the respiratory acidosis rats despite the greater rise in filtered load in the phosphate depletion group. The site of much of this change appeared to be the proximal tubule. Respiratory alkalosis is thus considerably less powerful than phosphate depletion in inducing phosphate retention.

Levine et al.[115] performed clearance studies which reaffirmed that respiratory acidosis, but not metabolic acidosis, increases phosphate excretion, controlling for change in serum phosphate. They then examined phosphate uptake in cortical slices from thyroparathyoidectomized animals during control conditions and elevation of pCO_2 and found no differences. Similarly, no effect was noted in uptake by proximal tubule brush border membrane vesicles studied in this way. Brush border vesicle transport was also examined, using vesicles obtained from animals with respiratory or metabolic acidosis. Prior respiratory acidosis was found to modify transport somewhat, but metabolic acidosis did not. Vesicles from normal animals that had had serum phosphate raised to levels equal to those seen in respiratory acidosis had similar decreases in transport measured in vesicle preparations. These data suggest that the effect of respiratory acidosis on transport is due to its effect on serum phosphate level. However, an effect of intracellular pH was not ruled out.

Finally, a number of articles reported effects of acidosis on renal tubular handling of a variety of substances. In vivo microperfusion and micropuncture were used to show that metabolic acidosis increased magnesium loss. The effect of pH seemed to be located in the loop and along the distal nephron.[116] The leak could be corrected by bicarbonate infusion. Lau et al.[117] also looked at effects of acidosis on renal calcium, magnesium, and phosphate reabsorption, using balance techniques during metabolic and respiratory acidosis. Only metabolic acidosis caused urinary losses of these ions. The authors argued that these findings show that pH itself is not the cause of the transport changes. Since the effects of respiratory acidosis and metabolic acidosis on bone have long been known to differ, this is not surprising.

Boross et al.[118] studied the effects of acidosis on the handling of phosphate, calcium, and ammonium in brush border membrane vesicles. Prior acidosis inhibited phosphate uptake in normals, but not in vesicles from adrenalectomized rats. Dexamethasone replacement restored sensitivity. The response of brush border phosphate handling to acidosis seems to be steroid dependent in a manner similar to the effect of acidosis on muscle metabolism. Rising aldosterone levels were held responsible for the increase in potassium excretion noted in chronic metabolic acidosis by Scandling and Ornt.[119] Adrenalectomized animals not given high-dose aldosterone replacement did not develop potassium losses. Finally, in an unrelated study, sulfate excretion was noted to decrease in acidosis in a clearance experiment.[120]

8. Ammonia and Urea

Data relevant to ammonia metabolism have been overshadowed to some degree by arguments about the relative roles of the liver and kidney in acid–base balance. These are based on, among other issues, a basic disagreement over whether or not excretion of ammonium ion represents excretion of acid from the body. The answer classically given by renal physiologists is that it does, and that excretion of ammonium chloride is equivalent to excretion of ammonia plus hydrochloric acid. Because the addition of ammonium chloride serves to raise pH of some solutions, Atkinson and Bourke[121] have disagreed, but argue that ammonium serves as a proton donor in ureagenesis. In addition, these authors believe that the predominant factor regulating the acid–base balance of the body is the consumption of bicarbonate generated from metabolism by its incorporation into urea. Although these individuals have performed a service to the nephrologic community by pointing out that the equations of ureagenesis have long been written incorrectly and that bicarbonate is consumed rather than acid generated in the equation, the expansion of this truth to the elevation of ureagenesis as the only defense against inexorable alkalosis has no defense. Atkinson and Bourke[121,122] consider the processes of urea generation, glutamine and glutamate metabolism, and ammoniagenesis to be a single cycle and feel this is ultimately controlled by hepatic pathways through control of ureagenesis. Finally, they argue, it is urea production which is altered by serum pH. A flurry of editorials with letters in reply have appeared debating the issue.[123–126]

It is our opinion that the classical view is largely correct. The argument that ammonium excretion does not constitute acid removal from the body is specious. Ammonium indeed functions as a urinary buffer, the pH of the urine trapping ammonia and permitting increased proton excretion. That there is a link between kidney and liver in the realm of ammonia, glutamine, and urea is undoubtedly true, but it is also true that elimination of exogenous acid requires that excretion occurs to the external milieu. This function rests with the lungs and kidneys. The gastrointestinal tract plays little role. Still, though, the most significant issue is whether or not urea synthesis can be shown to be sensitive to pH variation, a necessary fact if an acid–base regulatory role is assumed to exist.

Halperin and co-workers[127] addressed this question by studying urea production during hydrochloric acid and ammonium chloride infusion, following serum glutamine, and urea production. A bicarbonate infusion group was also studied. Urea production in this study responded to nitrogen load, but had no relationship with pH. On the other hand, glutamine metabolism did relate to pH status. At least in the acute state, then, the kidneys seem to regulate pH rather than the liver. A second study from the same laboratory[128] used infusion of ammonium chloride, ammonium bicarbonate, hydrochloric acid, and hydrochloric acid plus ammonium chloride to dissect the roles of ammonium and pH on glutamine, glutamate, ammonia, and urea. Although ammonium bicarbonate rats maintained pH and bicarbonate at normal levels and ammonium chloride rats became acidotic, urea generation remained constant. At normal pH, ammonium excretion was 3% of the urea generation rate; in acidosis, it was 7% of the urea generation rate. While calculated urea generation rates did not relate to pH, they did relate to ammonia concentration, showing that ammonia and not ammonium regulates urea production. The data show that acid–base status regulates urea production only to the degree that ammonia concentration is affected. In addition, the key to ammonia excretion rates may be glutamine release from the liver, but this would be futile in the absence of increased renal glutamine uptake and ammonia synthesis.

In contrast to the lack of effect of pH on ureagenesis, the effects of acidosis on glutamine synthesis and ammoniagenesis were apparent in a variety of studies. In addition to the aforementioned studies on ureagenesis, Halperin and Bun-Chen[129] also evaluated the effect of varying blood glutamine levels on renal ammoniagenesis. Infusion of glutamine resulted in increased urinary ammonium excretion without change in other parameters. There was close correlation between delivery of glutamine and ammonium synthesis, suggesting that glutamine production might regulate ammonium production and excretion. In contrast, in the isolated tubule, Kuwuhara et al.[130] found changes in glutamine transport with bath pH alterations, with increased uptake from the bath when pH was lowered. The pH did not alter uptake of glutamine from the lumen. These findings suggest that glutamine uptake, and thus ammoniagenesis, may respond to acidosis itself. Perfused mouse tubules removed from acidotic mice were found to have increased ammoniagenesis from glutamine compared to control.[131] When control tubules were acutely exposed to lowered pH in the bath, the rate of ammoniagenesis increased, but this response was not apparent in the tubules from acidotic mice. Production of ammonia was also increased by preincubation of control tubules for 10 or more minutes in a bath of pH 7.0. If bicarbonate in the bath was lowered without change in pH, the low bath bicarbonate had no effect on ammoniagenesis, in contrast to earlier findings of Scaduto and Schoolwerth.[132] The data of Nagami and co-workers,[131] which were obtained in single tubules using ultramicroanalytic techniques, support the contention that ammoniagenesis is regulated by acid–base status, in contrast to findings with regard to ureagenesis.

In addition to acid–base status, there are other regulators of ammoniagenesis. Chobanian and Hammerman[133,134] measured ammonia production and gluconeogenesis in canine proximal tubule segments with a fluorimetric assay for glucose and a flow-through ammonium electrode. Phorbol 12,13-dibutyrate and 4-alpha-phorbol inhibited both ammonia and glucose production. The action of these agents appeared to be mediated by an effect on sodium–proton exchange because low bath sodium or high bathing solution pH prevented the effects of the phorbol esters. These data thus suggest that ammoniagenesis and gluconeogenesis are regulated by processes mediated by protein kinase C and sodium–proton exchange. The second paper reported the effect of insulin on both processes. Insulin increased ammoniagenesis from glutamine and led to decreased gluconeogenesis. Alteration of sodium–proton exchange again appeared to be involved.

In all the preceding studies, the source of nitrogen for ammoniagenesis was the glutamine that was provided to the media. Is this the only source of ammonia nitrogen? Nissim and associates[135] tested the metabolism of a wide display of amino acids in complex media on ammoniagenesis. Glutamine could be shown to be the preferred nitrogen source, although small amounts of synthesis were supported by the other compounds. Studies that purport to demonstrate that another source is significant cannot be taken as appropriate if the secondary source is provided as a single possibility; testing in complex solutions will be necessary to make such a point.

Several studies performed experiments which included the use of acidivin, which was felt to be an inhibitor specific for phosphate-independent, but not phosphate-dependent, glutamine transferase. Most were rendered questionable by the work of Sastrasinh and Sastrasinh,[136] who demonstrated that this agent inhibits glutamine uptake at the cell membrane. This finding casts doubt on a number of prior studies.

Another issue with regard to ammoniagenesis that was investigated in 1986 was the tubular heterogeneity of this process. The painstaking work of Nonoguchi et al. [137] shows that the S1 and S2 segments of the proximal tubule had high rates of ammonia generation in control and also responded to acidosis and potassium depletion. S3 segments produced ammonia well in control but did not increase after such perturbations. Juxtamedullary and superficial tubules performed equally under control conditions, but only the superficial tubules showed adaptability. These findings demand that future studies provide careful identification of the tubule segments used.

Tannen and Goyal[138] investigated the factors responsible for the depression of the normal ammoniagenic response to acidosis that occurs when urine produced by an isolated perfused kidney is reinfused into the perfusion circuit. The addition of prostaglandin synthesis inhibitors prevented the reinfusion effect, and PGF_2-alpha, but not PGE_2, inhibited the ammoniagenic response to acidosis when given in low, but not high, doses. For those who were puzzled by the effect of reinfusion, these experiments suggest that the effect is due to prostaglandins in the urine.

The second major area of interest with regard to ammonia excretion are the mechanisms of ammonia transport. This has been an area of rapid advancement since the development of new analytic methods for ammonia. Good and DuBose[139] performed free-flow micropuncture at early and later sites along the proximal tubule, determining the total ammonia (NH_3 plus NH_4) transport first and then determining the ammonia (NH_3) concentration by measuring the total and the in situ pH. In control rats, ammonia was secreted in the early tubule, but there was apparent absorption in the later portions of the superficial proximal tubule, because the concentration of ammonia rose only slightly while considerable reabsorption of fluid occurred. In acidosis, the rate of secretion noted at the early puncture site increased sharply. The data from puncture at the later site showed further secretion. The percentage of the total ammonia composed of neutral ammonia was greater at the early site in both cases. Therefore, it appears that the early proximal tubule is the most active site of secretion, in agreement with the data with regard to bicarbonate and volume reabsorption.

Ammonia entry in the proximal tubule was also studied by Simon and Hamm,[140] in this case with *in vivo* microperfusion. An easily detectable ammonia entry was noted, which was higher when perfusate bicarbonate was low, and which also appeared to be flow dependent. Collected ammonia increased as collected total CO_2 decreased, suggesting that pH had a major effect, as is expected in diffusion trapping models. The flow dependence may indicate that flow stimulates ammonia production. If flow disrupts unstirred layers, then this can result in removal of NH_3, which could then stimulate NH_4 transport. An effect of flow on production was noted in some previous studies.[141]

Farther down the proximal tubule, Garvin *et al.*[142] examined ammonia and ammonium transport in rabbit proximal straight tubules. Spontaneous secretion of ammonia was found while bicarbonate was reabsorbed. Ammonia permeability was greater than ammonium permeability, but ammonium backleak was still possible. The rates of the backleak were similar to sodium and potassium permeability values, suggesting that ammonium backleak followed the paracellular paths. The secretory rates noted could be explained by passive permeabilities and diffusion trapping. Acetazolamide did not alter the process significantly. Finally, it is notable that ammonia gradients could occur, which diffusion trapping cannot easily produce, but no reasonable study that could prove ammonium transport occurred was forthcoming. How active transport of ammonium might occur was suggested by Kurtz and Balaban,[143] who found that ammonium can replace potassium in ATP hydrolysis by Na,K-ATPase. This could result in ammonium accumulation by cells, which might be followed by ammonium exit via the sodium–proton antiporter.

Good[144] studied the effects of potassium concentration on ammonia transport in the rat medullary thick ascending limb. Raising the potassium concentration of the perfusate to 24 meq/liter from 4 meq/liter resulted in diminished ammonia reabsorption by this segment, whether performed with or without parallel rises in bath potassium. The effect was present at both high and low flow rates. Therefore, there appears to be a strong nonmetabolic link between potassium and ammonium handling in this segment. Good and co-workers[145] also studied the movement of ammonia about the inner medulla as a whole. Micropuncture of all appropriate tubular segments as well as micropuncture of the vasa recta was performed. pH was measured with microelectrodes and ammonia by microfluorometric assays. Control and acidotic rats were used. Acidosis increased ammonia excretion, with an increase in ammonia secretion along the inner papillary collecting duct. Ammonia concentration and delivery was increased at the tip of Henle's loop, and concentrations were higher in the vasa recta as well. The concentration of ammonia at the tip of the loop was always greater than that in the collecting tubule. There were no gradients for ammonia between the vasa recta and the loop in any instance, and significant collecting duct ammonium concentrations occurred even in the absence of a marked decrease of pH in the lumen, suggesting that diffusion trapping is not the only process in evidence. The authors suggest that the combined processes that raise interstitial ammonia are of considerable importance. Since these data were obtained from all the structures involved in a direct manner, they must supersede previous estimates from clearance and *in vitro* perfusion.

The last two studies to be reported on in this section were performed by Star and colleagues[146,147] and deal with ammonia transport in isolated perfused collecting tubules. In the first of these, an intraluminal pH sensitive dye was used and ammonia entry into the lumen measured.[146] The addition of carbonic anhydrase to the perfusate was used to alter intraluminal pH. The data allowed calculation of a permeability and comparison of entry rates with those predictable from diffusion trapping. In this instance, diffusion trapping models work. The second of these studies was performed in collecting tubules from the inner and outer stripe of the outer medulla.[147] The inner stripe tubules had no disequilibrium pH in the absence of acetazolamide, despite the reports of an absence of luminal carbonic anhydrase here. A disequilibrium pH was present in the outer stripe segment. The addition of luminal carbonic anhydrase altered final pH in the inner stripe, but it did not alter ammonia entry here. This, then, appears to indicate that entry does not occur via diffusion trapping in this segment. In the outer stripe, which had a native disequilibrium, the entry of ammonium exceeded the values predicted by diffusion trapping. In the native state, then, the inner stripe follows a diffusion trapping model but the outer stripe segment secretes ammonia by some other mechanism. The disequilibrium pH also is evidence of proton secretion as the basis of bicarbonate reabsorption in this tissue, a point not well, if ever, made in the past.

9. Lactic Acidosis

In contrast to previous biennia, little work appeared that addressed experimental lactic acidosis. In the lone study we have to report, Romeh and Tannen[148] induced lactic acidosis by hypoxia and achieved a blood pH of 7.2 and a lactate concentration of 7 mM. If a hydrochloric acid infusion was given during hypoxia, blood lactate was only 2.7 mM, and if hypercarbia was superimposed, the lactate reached only 1.7 mM. When respiratory alkalosis was added to hypoxia, lactate rose. These data clearly show that lowering pH decreases production of lactate, but the authors appropriately caution against overinterpreting this for the clinical setting. Whether or not bicarbonate should be given in lactic acidosis is still an open question, and the wisest response probably remains that its use is appropriate in life-threatening acidosis because of hemodynamic effects of acidosis.

10. Miscellaneous or Global Studies of Acidification

This section has been created to include a variety of studies which, for a variety of reasons, are not easily placed into any of the preceding categories, but are of general interest. The most striking results to report here were obtained by Swenson and Maren[149] during studies of acidification of the urine by the dogfish shark. This fish routinely produces urine with a pH of 5.8, and does so regardless of diet. It has a low body temperature and maintains a low blood pCO_2, so the uncatalyzed rate of CO_2 hydration is insignificant. Increasing bicarbonate load by infusion of bicarbonate resulted in linear increases in bicarbonate reabsorption (up to 12 times baseline) without evidence of an attainable maximum. Infusion of buffers to maximally tolerable levels (above which the animals died of alkalosis) did not result in any change in urine pH, and acid excretion rose steadily. This result was obtained whether or not carbonic anhydrase inhibitors were infused. Carbonic anhydrase is essentially undetectable in these kidneys. When the possible rates of CO_2 uncatalyzed hydration are calculated, the resulting value cannot explain the acidification that occurs. The system therefore is capable of acidification of the urine in the absence of carbonic anhydrase, separating the process of acidification from the function of this enzyme. The question now is how does the shark do it?

Another study of interest was performed by Madias and Zelman.[150] These investigators repeated a classic acid feeding experiment to determine whether the earlier study missed changes in blood pH in response to nitric acid loads. In the original study, several mineral acids were fed and the effects on serum electrolytes, acid–base balance, and urinary excretion were measured. However, only preprandial measurement of blood values was obtained. The result was that despite marked differences in blood values with the varied acids, the urinary parameters were similar. In the repeat study, eight blood samples were taken at regular intervals throughout the course of the day. These animals were fed a control diet, a diet with 7 meq/kg per day hydrochloric acid, or a diet with an equal amount of nitric acid. The data show that although the hydrochloric acid group was acidemic and the nitric acid group was not in the immediate preprandial period, the nitrate group did become significantly acidotic during the course of the day. Nitric acid animals also developed hypokalemia and hyponatremia, which may have altered acid excretion. The acidosis in nitric acid feeding was not as severe as in the hydrochloric acid group, and this group excreted less chloride and more potassium. Notable was the absence of any circadian variation in acid–base status. The data thus add some explanation to the findings of the original work, but probably do not explain much else.

Two studies investigated the effects of renal ischemia on acid–base parameters in the kidney. Holloway et al.[151] induced ischemia with an arterial snare for 30 min, examined the renal pH with NMR, and followed the handling of acid, ammonia, glycine, glutamine, and bicarbonate in the postischemic period. In the postischemic period there was a surge of bicarbonate release to venous blood and urine, a decrease in ammonia in both those fluids, and a rise in renal venous glycine. Intracellular pH rose in the postischemic period as well when compared with the contralateral control kidney. Control pH was found to be 7.08. This dropped to 6.6 in ischemia and rose to 7.3 after release of the snare. There was an increase in ammoniagenesis in a later recovery period, and also an increase in glutamine synthesis. The postischemia period was also investigated by Winaver et al.[152] In this case a full hour of ischemia was induced, and measurement of renal acidification was performed via sodium sulfate infusion, urine pCO_2 measurement during bicarbonaturia, phosphate infusion, and with combinations of these procedures with amiloride infusion. Apparent acidification defects were uncovered, with a subnormal decrease in urine pH in response to sodium sulfate and a failure of urine minus blood pCO_2 to rise. Amiloride did not have its usual effects. The authors posit that there is a proton pump defect and that this may explain acidification problems in acute renal failure, but given the findings of the immediately previous paper, these conclusions are probably invalid. Acidification is likely to be low if the ischemic kidney rapidly becomes alkalemic, and if this is the case, there can hardly be said to be an acidification defect.

Ichikawa and Kon[153] presented an interesting article that addressed the mechanisms operative in the diuretic actions of carbonic anhydrase inhibitors. They measured glomerular hemodynamics in benzolamide-infused rats and found that, in spite of constancy of singular nephron glomerular filtration rate (SNGFR), hematocrit, and filtration fraction, there was a marked drop in the oncotic pressure in femoral arterial blood. Proximal reabsorption dropped as capillary hydrostatic pressure rose and capillary oncotic pressure fell. When packed red cells were infused to raise the hematocrit and thus the oncotic pressure, proximal reabsorption returned to normal, but bicarbonate reabsorption, while increasing somewhat, remained well below control. These results are similar to, but more detailed than, an earlier study by Tucker et al.[154] What the data seem to indicate is that there is more to the function of carbonic anhydrase inhibitors than the effects on proximal bicarbonate reabsorption.

The last paper to be mentioned in this section is an examination of phosphate handling in a model of the Fanconi syndrome.[155] Maleate was infused to induce the syndrome, and then a variety of phosphate-containing fluids were infused. Infusions that contained bicarbonate reduced the phosphate leak substantially. No effect of this maneuver was seen in controls. These data provide an interesting observation, but leave the underlying mechanisms unexplained.

11. Clinical Acid–Base Physiology

A wide variety of clinical acid–base papers were added to the literature, both in the form of case reports and as clinical studies. Three basic topics were well represented: studies of tubular defects, studies and reports of acid–base abnormalities in patients with normal renal function, and, finally, studies in patients with marked renal impairment with either end-stage renal failure or marked chronic renal disease. The data will be considered in that order.

11.1. Tubular Defects

Only a few papers appeared that dealt with acidification in underlying renal tubular disease. Nadler and co-workers[156] sought to uncover an underlying defect in patients who develop hyporeninemic hypoaldosterone. They found that urinary levels of 6 keto PGF_1-alpha were depressed in patients with the syndrome, and that these did not rise in response to calcium or epinephrine infusion. These results contrast with the responses noted in normal individuals and patients with similar degrees of renal insufficiency but without renin and aldosterone defects. PGE excretion was normal in the study group. Since PGF_1-alpha is a stable metabolite of PGI_2, which is a known stimulator of renin release, the postulate that the baseline defect is a prostaglandin synthesis problem can be supported. This study moves one step toward an ultimate explanation of the defect.

Pabico et al.[157] studied patients with idiopathic nephrolithiasis to determine the frequency of acidification defects. Urine pH was lowered to less than 6.0 after ammonium chloride loading, but the patients had subnormal ammonia excretion and titratable acid excretion. The data are not terribly clear, and use of 6.0 as a cutoff is high, but a defect does appear to be present.

Pizzarelli and Peacock[158] examined the effect of chronic ammonium sulfate therapy on patients with phosphatic stone disease. Both patients with and without acidification defects (defined as inability to lower urine pH to less than 5.5) were so treated. The stone recurrence data are somewhat difficult to interpret here as always, but a decline in recurrence seems to have occurred. The important point is that only one of the patients with the acidification defect had to cease therapy during the study for reasons related to acidosis. This therapy then appears to be safe even in the presence of acidification defects and deserves a wider trial.

As a last point in this section, an interesting case discussion was presented by Richardson and Halperin[159] in which the importance of urine pH in assessment of renal acidifying capacity was reconsidered. The value of the urine anion gap was stressed. If this is negative, the individual is excreting more than 80 mmoles of urinary ammonia per day; an inability to do this may be associated with acidosis despite intact ability to lower urine pH, which requires less proton excretion in the presence of low ammonia buffer.

11.2. Acid–Base Disorders in Patients with Normal Renal Function

Clinical acid–base disorders in patients with normal renal function were the topic of a fair number of reports. Several reports and studies considered the issues in diabetic ketoacidosis. Morris and co-workers[160] performed a randomized and controlled study of the effects of bicarbonate therapy in this disorder. The patients were markedly acidotic, with pH values between 6.9 and 7.14 on presentation. The nonbicarbonate group was slightly sicker to start with, but there were no differences in blood glucose, bicarbonate, pH, or ketone body concentration. The rate of drop of potassium was identical between groups. No differences in clinical outcome were noted between patients treated with or without bicarbonate. Although some question has been raised with regard to the amount of bicarbonate used, the amounts seem reasonable in our view. The impression garnered here is that bicarbonate therapy may add very little to the care of the diabetic ketoacidosis patient and should be used sparingly.

Diabetic ketoacidosis is, of course, one of the forms of acidosis marked by the presence of an increased anion gap. The size, and indeed the presence, of this gap are not absolutes, as shown by recent observations. Paulson[161] found that a tight relationship existed between the size of the anion gap and the fall in serum bicarbonate concentration in uncomplicated diabetes. While the presence of complicating factors was associated with increased variability, the basic relationship remained. The presence of renal disease resulted in a general shift to parallel curves which were related to the level of blood urea nitrogen. Volume contraction also shifted the curve. When patients deviated from the normal relationship, it was likely to be because of the presence of another acid–base disorder.

Gamblin et al.[162] described a case in which a patient presented with acidosis, positive ketones, a bicarbonate of 12, and an elevated glucose, but the anion gap was only 14. The authors described the case as ketoacidosis with normal anion gap, but whether this was the actual situation is debatable. The patient's sodium was only 132 meq/liter and the chloride was 106 meq/liter, so that correction for the dilution present reveals a corrected chloride of 114 or so. The patient therefore had a hyperchloremic acidosis, perhaps due to severe volume contraction with impaired distal delivery. The ketones may have been present due to starvation.

Methanol poisoning is yet another cause of anion gap metabolic acidosis. However, Palmisano and co-workers[163] presented a well-documented case of a 47-year-old man with a clearly defined ingestion, positive methanol levels, and an elevated osmolarity, who never developed an elevated anion gap or a bicarbonate below 20 meq/liter as he was treated with alcohol infusion and dialysis. Other similar cases from the literature were uncovered, all with rapid institution of ethanol infusion. Lactic acid generation did not become a problem despite the administration of ethanol. In this instance the positive gap acidosis was probably avoided by the ethanol, and the real message here is that ethanol infusion is efficacious and safe.

Lactic acidosis was the subject of numerous clinical discussions. Two reports were published describing cases of lactic acidosis secondary to pheochromocytoma.[164,165] Only a handful of such equivalent cases were previously known. Wang et al.[166] reviewed 21 cases of choleric acidosis to determine the etiology of the acid–base disorder usually seen. Prior to rehydration the average anion gap was 20, and this fell to 14.6 during standard fluid therapy and 11.4 in the recovery period. Ketones were not elevated, but creatinine was 2.48 mg/dl on arrival and fell to 1.7 and 1.02 in treatment and recovery periods, respectively. The pattern for serum phosphate was elevation to 8.0 mg/dl with decrease to 3.4 and 3.2 in the same periods as above. Magnesium and calcium followed similar patterns, but chloride was normal throughout. Lactate was elevated to 4.0 acutely and 1.61 in recovery. These data are interpreted as indicating that severe bicarbonate losses, hemoconcentration that raises protein concentration and thus allows for some elevation of the gap, and mild lactic acidosis are all present. Although not discussed in the article, it seems likely that some of the disorder is due to a renal acidosis caused by decreased flow through the distal tubule. Although cholera is unlikely to be seen in the United States, the paper certainly has worldwide significance.

A final note with regard to lactic acidosis is offered by Kruse and co-workers,[167] who asked whether or not the presence of underlying liver disease should alter the interpretation of elevated blood lactate in acidosis. The case records of 35 patients with liver disease and elevated lactate levels were studied. Twenty-seven admissions had notable circulatory shock, 11 did not. Blood lactate averaged 10 in shock cases and 1 in nonshock cases. There was a mild correlation between lactate level and survival. The data thus show that preexisting liver disease need not alter the clinical interpretation of elevated blood lactate.

The acidosis present during cardiopulmonary arrest was the subject of investigation by Weil and associates.[168] Making use of pulmonary artery catheters present at the time of the arrest, these clinician–investigators followed acid–base parameters in both central venous and peripheral arterial blood. The patients and their conditions were diverse. Treatment was not standardized beyond the use of usual code protocols. The results revealed that even though arterial parameters were maintained in a good range (normal pH, pCO_2 under 40, and bicarbonate between 19 and 26), the central venous values were horrid. pH there fell from 7.3 to 7.15, the pCO_2 rose from 42 mm Hg to 72, and no change in HCO_3 was apparent. Two things seem obvious: First, standard therapy was of little real use, and second, we may well be measuring the wrong samples. Whether anything better than present procedures can be developed is questionable.

One previously unreported consequence of acidosis was revealed by Eckfeldt and co-workers.[169] In a series of 32 intensive care patients with pH below 7.32 and elevation of serum amylase, the serum lipase was noted to be normal. Ketosis was not present and creatinine was under 5. Thus it appears that acidosis induces hyperamylassemia, but use of concurrent lipase levels prevents the misdiagnosis of pancreatitis.

There is just one paper to report that considers the topic of metabolic alkalosis. McAulliffe et al.[170] present seven patients with hypoproteinemia and acid–base disorders and argue that all seven individuals have metabolic alkalosis secondary to a decrease in albumin levels. They further argue that determination of serum protein and albumin concentration must be measured to perform accurate assessment of acid–base status. While the authors raise at least one important point (the common failure to consider plasma protein effects), the data shown do not prove the authors' point. Contrary to their statement that "all patients had significant 'metabolic' alkalosis," one patient had a pCO_2 of 55 torr with a pH of 7.35, and another had a pCO_2 of 47 torr in the face of alcoholic cirrhosis, clearly evidence of severe respiratory disease. Further, the paper relies to some extent on "eucapnic arterial plasma pH" measured after correction of pCO_2 to 40 torr. This maneuver may routinely show a metabolic alkalosis in patients with respiratory acidosis, but this extracorporeal posthypercapnic metabolic alkalosis is not real. The patients presented are quite complex and do not represent any simple disorder. The fact remains that there is no nomogram or system that will accurately diagnose acid–base disorders in the absence of history and sequential blood gas measurement if the patient is not in steady state.

11.3. Acid–Base Studies in Patients with Renal Impairment

A variety of electrolyte patterns are seen in patients with acid–base disorders, and the one usually associated with end-stage renal disease is an anion gap metabolic acidosis with a normal serum chloride. Wallia et al.[171] analyzed data from 70 patients with end-stage disease requiring the initiation of dialysis. Only 14 patients had this classical pattern, while 21 had low bicarbonate and high chloride, 11 had low bicarbonate, high chloride and an increased gap, 10 had low bicarbonate, normal chloride, and normal gap, and 14 had normal electrolytes. The "normal" group had lower creatinine and were mostly diabetic. In addition, they were younger than patients in the other groups. Review of the data suggests that some individuals had dialysis begun rather late (creatinine greater than 10–12 mg/dl in all but the diabetics) and had poor control of calcium and phosphate, but the data are valuable.

Lameire and Matthys[172] also studied patients near dialysis initiation. Seventeen end-stage patients were divided into two groups, those who responded to ammonium chloride loads with low urine pH and zero bicarbonaturia, and those who could not. Four patients with high fractional sodium excretion and acidosis underwent progressive sodium restriction and retesting. This maneuver resulted in improvement of bicarbonaturia and acidosis. Most of these patients had interstitial disease, and this contributed to the high incidence of salt wastage. In many ways they appear to have proximal renal tubular acidosis (RTA), and treatment with salt restriction is quite logical. These findings may be induced by the overperfusion of the few remaining nephrons at this stage.

The effects of the two forms of dialysis on body buffers were compared by Singh and associates.[173] Buffer capacity was assessed by measuring the effects of fixed amounts of ammonium chloride on serum bicarbonate and pH. Less impact of the load was seen in chronic obstructive pulmonary disease patients in comparison to hemodialysis patients, even when the former were studied in the absence of peritoneal fluid. Not discussed were such things as lean body mass and other individual differences. In the absence of these details the study is less convincing.

The debate over the choice of bicarbonate or acetate dialysis in acute situations continues. Those who believe in the superiority of bicarbonate generally recommend it because of theoretical benefits to hemodynamics. Anderson et al.[174] compared the cardiac function of six dialysis patients on acetate and bicarbonate. Cardiac function was assessed by echocardiography. In this study, no differences were noted. However, the serum bicarbonate was similar in the two groups, which is necessary for the study but which may not allow for the effects of slow acetate metabolism. In contrast to this finding, Leunissen and colleagues[175] found a significant difference when they examined the effects of the two admixtures in 12 paired studies with nine patients. Measurements here were performed with a Swan–Ganz catheter. Acetate appeared to be a cardiovascular depressant, as shown by a fall in pressure and stroke work index. The data here are strong, and the patient selection is impeccable. There is little to argue with and the point seems to be made in this instance.

Given the problems of acidosis and potassium management in the dialysis population, some have questioned the wisdom of advocating exercise in these individuals. Lundin et al.[176] put seven untrained hemodialysis patients through a moderately severe exercise protocol after screening them for coronary artery disease. In six of seven the protocol was terminated owing to leg pain. Blood pH fell from 7.39 at start to 7.33 at the point of exhaustion, 7.31 5 min later, and returned to normal in 20 min. Bicarbonate dropped and lactate rose, both remaining abnormal after 20 min of rest. The highest potassium seen was 6.0, and the level fell precipitously to 4.5 on stopping, with a slow climb to normal. The highest lactate level seen was only one-half that in untrained controls without renal disease. Latos et al.[177] presented a similar study; in this case measurements were made during exercise on dialysis days and nondialysis days in nine untrained patients. Thirty minutes of exercise was performed if tolerated. The minimal pH was about 7.3, and occurred 15 min after stopping. A moderate rise in potassium was seen during exercise, with a rapid fall thereafter. At 60% of maximal heart rate, VO_2 max was only 60% of controls. These two reports used different techniques and the timing of measurements differed as well, but the conclusions that emerged were similar. Dialysis patients exercise poorly; the reasons for this are not revealed by the studies, but clearly there were no untoward acid–base or potassium effects during exercise in these groups.

The last paper we will mention considers the effects of acidosis on the hyperphosphatemia seen in the dialysis patient. Barsotti and associates[178] measured the effect of bicarbonate infusion on serum phosphate in patients undergoing hemofiltration and in predialysis renal disease patients. The infusion of bicarbonate to the first group was shown to lower phosphate significantly, though not to normal levels. Saline infusion did not give this result. In the predialysis group, oral citrate therapy raised pH and lowered serum phosphate. It is notable that this occurred without significant changes in phosphate excretion in the few patients in whom this was measured. While the mechanism of the effect is not revealed, the effect is significant and parallels observations in animals. The result should be viewed as yet another reason for aggressive control of acidosis.

References

1. Alpern, R. J., 1985, Mechanism of basolateral membrane $H+/OH-/HCO_3-$ transport in the rat proximal convoluted tubule, *J. Gen. Physiol.* **86**:613.
2. Sasaki, S. and Berry, C. A., 1984, Mechanism of bicarbonate exit across basolateral membrane of the rabbit proximal convoluted tubule, *Am. J. Physiol.* **246**:F889.

3. Biagi, B. A. and Sohtell, M., 1986, pH sensitivity of the basolateral membrane of the rabbit proximal tubule, *Am. J. Physiol.* **250**:F261.

4. Biagi, B. A., Kubota, T., Sohtell, M., and Giebisch, G., 1981, Intracellular potentials in rabbit proximal tubules perfused *in vitro, Am. J. Physiol.* **240**:F200.

5. Biagi, B. A. and Sohtell, M., 1986, Electrophysiology of basolateral bicarbonate transport in the rabbit proximal tubule, *Am. J. Physiol.* **250**:F267.

6. Sasaki, S., Shiigai, T., Yoshiyama, N., and Takeuchi, J., 1987, Mechanism of bicarbonate exit across basolateral membrane of rabbit proximal straight tubule, *Am. J. Physiol.* **252**:F11.

7. Akiba, T., Alpern, R. J., Eveloff, J. E., Calamina, J., and Warnock, D. G., 1986, Electrogenic sodium/bicarbonate cotransport in rabbit renal cortical basolateral membrane vesicles, *J. Clin. Invest.* **78**:1472.

8. Jentsch, T. J., Matthes, H., Keller, S. K., and Wiederholt, M., 1986, Electrical properties of sodium bicarbonate symport in kidney epithelial cells (BSC-1), *Am. J. Physiol.* **251**:F954.

9. Lopes, A. G., Siebens, A. W., Giebisch, G., and Boron, W. F., 1987, Electrogenic Na/HCO_3 cotransport across basolateral membrane of isolated perfused Necturus proximal tubule, *Am. J. Physiol.* **253**:F340.

10. Krapf, R., Alpern, R. J., Rector, F. C., Jr., and Berry, C. A., 1987, Basolateral membrane Na/base cotransport is dependent on CO_2/HCO_3 in the proximal convoluted tubule, *J. Gen. Physiol.* **90**:833.

11. Burckhardt, B. C. and Fromter, E., 1987, Evidence for OH^-/H^+ permeation across the peritubular cell membrane of rat renal proximal tubule in HCO_3^--free solutions, *Pflüger's Arch. Eur. J. Physiol.* **409**:132.

12. Soleimani, M., Grassl, S. M., and Aronson, P. S., 1987, Stoichiometry of Na^+-HCO_3^- cotransport in basolateral membrane vesicles isolated from rabbit renal cortex, *J. Clin. Invest.* **79**:1276.

13. Yoshitomi, K., Burckhardt, B-C., and Fromter, E., 1985, Rheogenic sodium-bicarbonate cotransport in the peritubular cell membrane of rat renal proximal tubule, *Pflüger's Arch. Eur. J. Physiol.* **405**:360.

14. Alpern, R. J., 1987, Apical membrane chloride/base exchange in the rat proximal convoluted tubule, *J. Clin. Invest.* **79**:1026.

15. Rocco, V. K., Cragoe, E. J., Jr., and Warnock, D. G., 1987, N-ethoxycarbonyl-2-ethoxy-1,2-dihydroquinolone, amiloride analogues, and renal Na^+/H^+ antiporter, *Am. J. Physiol.* **252**:F517.

16. Goldfarb, D. and Nord, E. P., 1987, Asymmetric affinity of Na^+-H^+ antiporter for Na^+ at the cytoplasmic versus external transport site, *Am. J. Physiol.* **253**:F959.

17. Bidet, M., Tauc, M., Merot, J., Vandewalle, A., and Poujeol, P., 1987, Na^+-H^+ exchange in proximal cells isolated from rabbit kidney. I. Functional characteristics, *Am. J. Physiol.* **253**:F935.

18. Nord, E. P., Goldfarb, D., Mikhail, N., Moradeshagi, P., Hafezi, A., Vaystub, S., Cragoe, E. J., and Fine, L. G., 1986, Characteristics of the Na^+-H^+ antiporter in the intact renal proximal tubular cell, *Am. J. Physiol.* **250**:F539.

19. Kinne-Saffran, E. and Kinne, R., 1986, Proton pump activity and Mg-ATPase activity in rat kidney cortex brushborder membranes: Effect of "proton ATPase" inhibitors, *Pflüger's Arch. Eur. J. Physiol.* **407**:S180.

20. Gurich, R. W. and Warnock, D. G., 1986, Electrically neutral Na^+-H^+ exchange in endosomes obtained from rabbit renal cortex, *Am. J. Physiol.* **251**:F702.

21. Sabolic, I. and Burckhardt, G., 1986, Characteristics of the proton pump in rat renal cortical endocytotic vesicles, *Am. J. Physiol.* **250**:F817.

22. Montrose, M. H., Friedrich, T., and Murer, H., 1987, Measurements of intracellular pH in single LLC-PK1 cells: Recovery from an acid load via basolateral Na^+/H^+ exchange, *J. Membrane Biol.* **97**:63.

23. Alpern, R. J. and Chambers, M., 1987, Cell pH in the rat proximal convoluted tubule. Regulation by luminal and peritubular pH and sodium concentration, *J. Clin. Invest.* **78**:502.

24. Akiba, T., Rocco, V. K., and Warnock, D. G., 1987, Parallel adaptation of the rabbit renal cortical sodium/proton antiporter and sodium/bicarbonate cotransporter in metabolic acidosis and alkalosis, *J. Clin. Invest.* **80**:308.

25. Kurtz, I., 1987, Apical Na^+/H^+ antiporter and glycolysis-dependent H^+-ATPase regulate intracellular pH in the rabbit S3 proximal tubule, *J. Clin. Invest.* **80**:928.

26. Steels, P. S. and Boulpaep, E. L., 1987, pH-dependent electrical properties and buffer permeability of the *Necturus* renal proximal tubule cell, *J. Membrane Biol.* **100**:165.

27. Wang, W., Dietl, P., Silbernagle, S., and Oberleithner, H., 1987, Cell membrane potential: A signal to control intracellular pH and tranepithelial hydrogen on secretion in frog kidney, *Pflüger's Arch. Eur. J. Physiol.* **409**:289.

28. Adam, W. R., Koretsky, A. P., and Weiner, M. W., 1986, 31P-NMR *in vivo* measurement of renal intracellular pH: Effects of acidosis and K^+ depletion in rats, *Am. J. Physiol.* **251**:F904.

29. Henderson, R. M., Bell, P. B., Cohen, R. D., Browning, C., and Iles, R. A., 1986, Measurement of intracellular pH with microelectrodes in rat kidney *in vivo*, *Am. J. Physiol.* **250**:F203.

30. Bidet, M., Merot, J., Tauc, M., and Poujeol, P., 1987, Na^+-H^+ exchanger in proximal cells isolated from kidney. II. Short-term regulation by glucocorticoids, *Am. J. Physiol.* **253**:F945.

31. Kinsella, J. L., Cujdik, T., and Sacktor, B., 1986, Kinetic studies on the stimulation of Na^+-H^+ exchange activity in renal brush border membranes isolated from thyroid hormone-treated rats, *J. Membrane Biol.* **91**:183.

32. Nord, E. P., Howard, M. J., Hafezi, A., Moradeshagi, P., Vaystub, S., and Insel, P. A., 1987, Alpha$_2$ adrenergic agonists stimulate Na^+-H^+ antiport activity in the rabbit renal proximal tubule, *J. Clin. Invest.* **80**:1755.

33. Mellas, J. and Hammerman, M. R., 1986, Phorbol ester–induced alkalinization of canine renal proximal tubular cells, *Am. J. Physiol.* **250**:F451.

34. Pollock, A. S., Warnock, D. G., and Strewler, G. J., 1986, Parathyroid hormone inhibition of Na^+-H^+ antiporter activity in a cultured renal cell line, *Am. J. Physiol.* **250**:F217.

35. Weinman, E. J., Shenolikar, S., and Kahn, A. M., 1987, cAMP-associated inhibition of Na^+-H^+ exchanger in rabbit kidney brush border membranes, *Am. J. Physiol.* **252**:F19.

36. Harris, R. C., Brenner, B. M., and Seifter, J. L., 1986, Sodium–hydrogen exchange and glucose transport in renal microvillus membrane vesicles from rats with diabetes mellitus, *J. Clin. Invest.* **77**:724.

37. Liu, F-Y. and Cogan, M. G., 1986, Axial heterogeneity of bicarbonate, chloride, and water transport in the rat proximal convoluted tubule, *J. Clin. Invest.* **78**:1547.

38. Liu, F.-Y. and Cogan, M. G., 1987, Kinetics of bicarbonate transport in the early proximal convoluted tubule, *Am. J. Physiol.* **253**:F912.

39. Liu, F-Y. and Cogan, M. G., 1987, Angiotensin II: A potent regulator of acidification in the rat early proximal convoluted tubule, *J. Clin. Invest.* **80**:272.

40. Liu, F-Y. and Cogan, M. G., 1987, Acidification is inhibited in late proximal convoluted tubule during chronic metabolic alkalosis, *Am. J. Physiol.* **253**:F89.

41. Pastoriza-Munoz, E., Harrington, R. M., and Graber, M. L., 1987, Axial heterogeneity of intracellular pH in rat proximal convoluted tubule, *J. Clin. Invest.* **80**:207.

42. Craig, D. M., Galla, J. H., Bonduris, D. N., and Luke, R. G., 1986, Importance of the kidney in the correction of chloride-depletion alkalosis in the rat, *Am. J. Physiol.* **250**:F54.

43. Galla, J. H., Bonduris, D. N., and Luke, R. G., 1987, Effects of chloride and extracellular fluid volume on bicarbonate reabsorption along the nephron in metabolic alkalosis in the rat. Reassessment of the classical hypothesis of the pathogenesis of metabolic alkalosis, *J. Clin. Invest.* **80**:41.

44. Wall, B. M., Byrum, G. V., Galla, J. H., and Luke, R. G., 1987, Importance of chloride for the correction of chronic metabolic alkalosis in the rat, *Am. J. Physiol.* **253**:F1031.

45. Borkan, S., Northrup, T. E., Cohen, J. J., and Garella, S., 1987, Renal response to metabolic alkalosis induced by isovolemic hemofiltration in the dog, *Kidney Int.* **32**:322.

46. Maddox, D. A., and Gennari, F. J., 1986, Load dependence of proximal tubular bicarbonate reabsorption in chronic metabolic alkalosis in the rat, *J. Clin. Invest.* **77**:709.

47. Kurtz, I., Star, R., Balaban, R. S., Garvin, J. L., and Knepper, M. A., 1986, Spontaneous luminal disequilibrium pH in S3 proximal tubules. Role of ammonia and bicarbonate transport, *J. Clin. Invest.* **78**:989.

48. Atkins, J. L. and Burg, M. B., 1987, Control of steady-state pH in rabbit proximal straight tubules, *Am. J. Physiol.* **253**:F282.

49. Preisig, P. A., Ives, H. E., Cragoe, E. J., Alpern, R. J., and Rector, F. C., Jr., 1987, Role of the Na^+/H^+ antiporter in rat proximal tubule bicarbonate absorption, *J. Clin. Invest.* **80**:970.

50. Bomsztyk, K., Swenson, E. R., and Calalb, M. B., 1987, HCO_3 accumulation in proximal tubule: Roles of carbonic anhydrase, luminal buffers, and pH, *Am. J. Physiol.* **252**:F501.

51. Bomsztyk, K., 1986, Chloride transport by rat renal proximal tubule: Effects of bicarbonate absorption, *Am. J. Physiol.* **250**:F1046.

52. Baum, M., 1987, Evidence that parallel Na^+-H^+ and $Cl^- HCO_3^-$ (OH^-) antiporters transport NaCl in the proximal tubule, *Am. J. Physiol.* **252**:F338.

53. Maddox, D. A., Horn, J. F., Famiano, F. C., and Gennari, F. J., 1986, Load dependence of proximal fluid and bicarbonate reabsorption in the remnant kidney of the Munich–Wistar rat, *J. Clin. Invest.* **77**:1639.

54. Fine, L. G., Trizna, W., Bourgoignie, J. J., and Bricker, N. S., 1978, Functional profile of the uremic nephron. Role of compensatory hypertrophy in the control of fluid reabsorption by the proximal tubule, *J. Clin. Invest.* **61**:1508.

55. Cogan, M. G., 1986, Neurogenic regulation of proximal bicarbonate and chloride reabsorption, *Am. J. Physiol.* **250**:F22.

56. Bank, N., Aynedjian, H. S., and Mutz, B. F., 1986, Microperfusion study of proximal tubule bicarbonate transport in maleic acid–induced renal tubular acidosis, *Am. J. Physiol.* **250**:F476.

57. Wingo, C. S., 1986, Effect of acidosis on chloride transport in the cortical thick ascending limb of Henle perfused *in vitro, J. Clin. Invest.* **78**:1324.

58. Kondo, Y., Yoshitomi, K., and Imai, M., 1987, Effect of pH on Cl^- transport in TAL of Henle's loop, *Am. J. Physiol.* **253**:F1216.

59. Friedman, P. A. and Andreoli, T. E., 1986, Effects of $(CO_2 + HCO_3^-)$ on electrical conductance in cortical thick ascending limbs, *Kidney Int.* **30**:325.

60. Munich, G., Dietl, P., and Oberleithner, H., 1986, Chloride transport in the diluting segment of the K^+ adapted frog kidney effect of amiloride and acidosis, *Pflüger's Arch. Eur. J. Physiol.* **407**:S60.

61. Iacovitti, M., Nash, L., Peterson, L. N., Rochon, J., and Levine, D. Z., 1986, Distal tubule bicarbonate accumulation *in vivo.* Effect of flow and transtubular bicarbonate gradients, *J. Clin. Invest.* **78**:1658.

62. Capasso, G., Kinne, R., Malnic, G., and Giebisch, G., 1986, Renal bicarbonate reabsorption in the rat. I. Effects of hypokalemia and carbonic anhydrase, *J. Clin. Invest.* **78**:1558.

63. Capasso, G., Jaeger, P., Giebisch, G., Guckian, V., and Malnic, G., 1987, Renal bicarbonate reabsorption in the rat. II. Distal tubule load dependence and effect of hypokalemia, *J. Clin. Invest.* **80**:409.

64. Kunau, R. T. and Walker, K. A., 1987, Total CO_2 absorption in the distal tubule of the rat, *Am. J. Physiol.* **252**:F468.

65. Arruda, J. A. L., Wheeler, R. P., Dytko, G., and Talor, Z., 1987, Intracellular pH of the turtle bladder assessed with fluorescent probes, *Mineral Electrolyte Metab.* **13**:104.

66. Graber, M. L., Dixon, T. E., Coachman, D., Herring, K., Ruenes, A., Gardner, T., and Pastoriza-Munoz, E., 1986, Fluorescence identifies an alkaline cell in the turtle urinary bladder, *Am. J. Physiol.* **250**:F159.

67. Brem, A. S., Pacholski, M., and Lawler, R. G., 1986, Fluctuations in intracellular pH associated with vasopressin stimulation, *Am. J. Physiol.* **251**:F897.

68. Husted, R. F. and Fischer, J. L., 1987, Selectivity of basolateral anion exchange in the acidification pathway of the turtle bladder, *Am. J. Physiol.* **252**:F1022.

69. Nero, A. C., Schwartz, J. H., and Furtado, M. R. F., 1987, Characteristics of H^+ current transients induced by adverse gradient pulses in toad bladder, *Am. J. Physiol.* **253**:F606.

70. Stetson, D. L. and Steinmetz P. R., 1986, Correlation between apical intramembranous particles and H^+ secretion rates during CO_2 stimulation in turtle bladder, *Pflüger's Arch. Eur. J. Physiol.* **407**:S80.

71. Wheeler, R. P. and Arruda, J. A. L., 1987, Adaptation to metabolic acidosis by turtle urinary bladder, *Am. J. Physiol.* **252**:F256.

72. Zeidel, M. L., Silva, P., and Seifter, J. L., 1986, Intracellular pH regulation and proton transport by rabbit renal medullary collecting duct cells. Role of plasma membrane proton ATPase, *J. Clin. Invest.* **77**:113.

73. Zeidel, M. L., Silva, P., and Seifter, J. L., 1986, Intracellular pH regulation in rabbit renal medullary collecting duct cells. Role of chloride–bicarbonate exchange, *J. Clin. Invest.* **77**:1682.

74. Kleinman, J. G., Blumenthal, S. S., Wiessner, J. H., Reetz, K. L., Lewand, D. L., Mandel, N. S., Mandel, G. S., Garancis, J. C., and Cragoe, E. J., Jr., 1987, Regulation of pH in rat papillary tubule cells in primary culture, *J. Clin. Invest.* **80**:1660.

75. Wall, S. M., Muallem, S., and Kraut, J. A., 1987, Detection of a Na^+-H^+ antiporter in cultured rat renal papllary collecting duct cells, *Am. J. Physiol.* **253**:F889.

76. Diaz-Diaz, F. D., LaBelle, E. F., Eaton, D. C., and DuBose, T. D., 1986, ATP-dependent proton transport in human renal medulla, *Am. J. Physiol.* **251**:F297.

77. Koeppen, B. M., 1987, Electrophysiological identification of principal and intercalated cells in the rabbit outer medullary collecting duct, *Pflüger's Arch. Eur. J. Physiol.* **409**:138.

78. Koeppen, B. M., 1986, Conductive properties of the rabbit outer medullary collecting duct: Outer stripe, *Am. J. Physiol.* **250**:F70.

79. McKinney, T. D. and Davidson, K. K., 1987, Bicarbonate transport in collecting tubules from outer stripe of outer medulla of rabbit kidneys, *Am. J. Physiol.* **253**:F816.

80. Laski, M. E., 1987, Total CO_2 flux in isolated collecting tubules during carbonic anhydrase inhibition, *Am. J. Physiol.* **252**:F322.

81. Hays, S., Kokko, J. P., and Jacobson, H. R., 1986, Hormonal regulation of proton secretion in rabbit medullary collecting duct, *J. Clin. Invest.* **78**:1279.

82. Hays, S. R., Baum, M., and Kokko, J. P., 1987, Effects of protein kinase C activation of sodium, potassium, chloride, and total CO_2 transport in the rabbit cortical collecting tubule, *J. Clin. Invest.* **80**:1561.

83. Schuster, V. L., 1986, Cyclic adenosine monophosphate-stimulated anion transport in rabbit cortical collecting tubule. Kinetics, stoichiometry, and conductive pathways, *J. Clin. Invest.* **78**:1621.

84. Tomita, K., Pisano, J. J., Burg, M. B., and Knepper, M. A., 1986, Effects of vasopressin and bradykinin on anion transport by the rat cortical collecting duct, *J. Clin. Invest.* **77**:136.

85. Bichara, M., Mercier, O., Houllier, P., Paillard, M., and Leviel, F., 1987, Effects of antidiuretic hormone on urinary acidification and on tubular handling of bicarbonate in the rat, *J. Clin. Invest.* **80**:623.

86. Sasaki, S., Berry, C. A., and Rector, F. C., Jr., 1982, Effect of luminal and peritubular HCO_3-concentrations and PCO_2 on HCO_3- reabsorption in rabbit proximal convoluted tubules perfused *in vitro*, *J. Clin. Invest.* **70**:639.

87. Breyer, M. D., Kokko, J. P., and Jacobson, H. R., 1986, Regulation of net bicarbonate transport in rabbit cortical collecting tubule by peritubular pH, carbon dioxide tension, and bicarbonate concentration, *J. Clin. Invest.* **77**:1650.

88. McKinney, T. D. and Davidson, K. K., 1987, Effect of respiratory acidosis on total CO_2 transport by rabbit collecting tubules *in vitro*, *Clin. Res.* **35**:636A.

89. Laski, M. E., Abella, M. A., and Kurtzman, N. A., 1987, The cortical collecting tubule is the site of distal nephron adaptation to respiratory acidosis, *Clin. Res.* **35**:551A.

90. Abdelkhalek, M. B., Barlet, C., and Doucet, A., 1986, Presence of an extramitochondrial anion-stimulated ATPase in the rabbit kidney: Localization along the nephron and effect of corticosteroids, *J. Membrane Biol.* **89**:225.

91. Khadouri, C., Marsy, S., Barlet-Bas, C., and Doucet, A., 1987, Effect of adrenalectomy on NEM-sensitive ATPase along rat nephron and on urinary acidification, *Am. J. Physiol.* **253**:F495.

92. Harrington, J. T., Hulter, H. N., Cohen, J. J., and Madias, N. E., 1986, Mineralocorticoid-stimulated renal acidification: The critical role of dietary sodium, *Kidney Int.* **30**:43.

93. Stone, D. K., Seldin, D. W., Kokko, J. P., and Jacobson, H. R., 1983, Mineralocorticoid modulation of rabbit medullary collecting duct acidification: A sodium independent effect, *J. Clin. Invest.* **72**:77.

94. Mujais, S. K., Nascimento, L., Rademacher, D. R., Wilson, A., and Kurtzman, N. A., 1986, Intact ability to lower urine pH in nonacidotic adrenalectomized rats, *Mineral Electrolyte Metab.* **12:**107.

95. Bengele, H. H., Schwartz, J. H., McNamara, E. R., and Alexander, E. A., 1986, Chronic metabolic acidosis augments acidification along the inner medullary collecting duct, *Am. J. Physiol.* **250:**F690.

96. Bengele, H. H., McNamara, E. R., Schwartz, J. H., and Alexander, E. A., 1987, Inner medullary collecting duct function during rebound alkalemia, *Am. J. Physiol.* **252:**F712.

97. McKinney, T. D. and Davidson, K. K., 1987, Effect of potassium depletion and protein intake *in vivo* on renal tubular bicarbonate transport *in vitro, Am. J. Physiol.* **252:**F509.

98. Ribiero, C. and Suki, W. N., 1986, Acidification in the medullary collecting duct following ureteral obstruction, *Kidney Int.* **29:**1167.

99. Yang, W. C., Arruda, J. A. L., and Talor, Z., 1987, Na^+-H^+ antiporter in posthypercanic state, *Am. J. Physiol.* **253:**F833.

100. Winaver, J., Walker, K. A., and Kunau, R. T., 1986, Effect of acute hypercapnia on renal and proximal tubular total carbon dioxide reabsorption in the acetazolamide-treated rat, *J. Clin. Invest.* **77:**465.

101. Trivedi, B. and Tannen, R. L., 1986, Effect of respiratory acidosis on intracellular pH of the proximal tubule, *Am. J. Physiol.* **250:**F1030.

102. Verlander, J. W., Madsen, K. M., and Tisher, C. C., 1987, Effect of acute respiratory acidosis on two populations of intercalated cells in rat cortical collecting duct, *Am. J. Physiol.* **253:**F1142.

103. Bengele, H. H., Schwartz, J. H., McNamara, E. R., and Alexander, E. A., 1986, Effect of buffer infusion during acute respiratory acidosis, *Am. J. Physiol.* **250:**F115.

104. Androgue, H. J. and Madias, N. E., 1986, Renal acidification during chronic hypercapnia in the conscious dog, *Pflüger's Arch. Eur. J. Physiol.* **406:**520.

105. Batlle, D. C., Downer, M., Gutterman, C., and Kurtzman, N. A., 1985, Relationship of urinary and blood carbon dioxide tension during hypercapnia in the rat, *J. Clin. Invest.* **75:**1517.

106. May, R. C., Kelly, R. A., and Mitch, W. E., 1986, Metabolic acidosis stimulates protein degradation in rat muscle by a glucocorticoid-dependent mechanism, *J. Clin. Invest.* **77:**614.

107. May, R. C., Kelly, R. A., and Mitch, W. E., 1987, Mechanisms for defects in muscle protein metabolism in rats with chronic uremia, *J. Clin. Invest.* **79:**1099.

108. Hara, Y., May, R. C., Kelly, R. A., and Mitch, W. L., 1987, Acidosis, not azotemia, stimulates branched-chain amino acid catabolism in uremic rats, *Kidney Int.* **32:**808.

109. Carroll, J. E., Landry, A. S., Elliot, M. E., and Goodfriend, T. L., 1986, Effects of pH on adrenal angiotensin receptors and responses, *J. Lab. Clin. Med.* **108:**23.

110. Bushinsky, D. A. and Lechleider, R. J., 1987, Mechanism of proton-induced bone calcium release: Calcium carbonate dissolution, *Am. J. Physiol.* **253:**F998.

111. Kraut, J. A., Mishler, D. R., Singer, F. R., and Goodman, W. G., 1986, The effects of metabolic acidosis on bone formation and bone reabsorption in the rat, *Kidney Int.* **30:**694.

112. Orchard, C. H., Houser, S. R., Kort, A. A., Bahinski, A., Capogrossi, M. C., and Lakatta, E. G., 1987, Acidosis facilitates spontaneous sarcolasmic reticulum Ca^{++} release in rat myocardium, *J. Gen. Physiol.* **90:**145.

113. Watters, T. A., Wendland, M. F., Parmley, W. W., James, T. L., Botnivik, E. H., Wu S. T., Sievers, R., and Wikman-Coffelt, J., 1987, Factors influencing myocardial response to metabolic acidosis in isolated rat hearts, *Am. J. Physiol.* **253:**H1261.

114. Awazu, M., Berndt, T. J., and Knox, F. G., 1987, Effect of phosphate infusion on proximal tubule phosphate reabsorption in phosphate-deprived and respiratory alkalotic rats, *Mineral Electrolyte Metab.* **13:**393.

115. Levine, B. S., Kraut, J. A., Mishler, D. R., and Crooks, P. W., 1986, Effect of acute acidemia on phosphate uptake by renal proximal tubular brush-border membranes, *Am. J. Physiol.* **251:**F889.

116. Shapiro, R. J., Yong, C. K. K., and Quamme, G. A., 1987, Influence of chronic dietary acid on renal tubular handling of magnesium, *Pflüger's Arch. Eur. J. Physiol.* **409:**492.

117. Lau, K., Nichols, F. R., and Tannen, R. L., 1987, Renal excretion of divalent ions in response to chronic acidosis: Evidence that systemic pH is not the controlling variable, *J. Lab. Clin. Med.* **109:** 27.

118. Boross, M., Kinsella, J., Cheng, L., and Sacktor, B., 1986, Glucocorticoids and metabolic acidosis–induced renal transports of inorganic phosphate, calcium, and NH_4, *Am. J. Physiol.* **250:** F827.

119. Scandling, J. D. and Ornt, D. B., 1987, Mechanism of potassium depletion during chronic metabolic acidosis in the rat, *Am. J. Physiol.* **252:**F122.

120. Frick, A. and Durasin, I., 1986, Regulation of the renal transport of inorganic sulfate: Effects of metabolic changes in arterial blood pH, *Pflüger's Arch. Eur. J. Physiol.* **407:**541.

121. Atkinson, D. E. and Bourke, E., 1987, Metabolic aspects of the regulation of systemic pH, *Am. J. Physiol.* **252:**F947.

122. Atkinson, D. E. and Bourke, E., 1987, Reply, *Am. J. Physiol.* **253:**F200.

123. Knepper, M. A., Burg, M. B., Orloff, J., Berliner, R. W., and Rector, F. C., Jr., 1987, Ammonium, urea and systemic pH regulation, *Am. J. Physiol.* **253:**F199.

124. Walser, M., 1986, Roles of urea production, ammonium excretion, and amino acid oxidation in acid–base balance, *Am. J. Physiol.* **250:**F181.

125. Maren, T. H., 1987, Recovery form metabolic acidosis is a function of renal NH_4+ loss: Agreement between two models, *Am. J. Physiol.* **153:**F1308.

126. Walser, M., 1986, Ureagenesis and pH homeostasis: Reply, *Am. J. Physiol.* **250:**F1129.

127. Halperin, M. L., Chen, C. B., Cheema-Dhadli, S., West, M. L., and Jungas, R. L., 1986, Is urea formation regulated primarily by acid–base balance *in vivo? Am. J. Physiol.* **250:**F605.

128. Cheema-Dhadli, S., Jungas, R. L., and Halperin, M. L., 1987, Regulation of urea synthesis by acid–base balance *in vivo:* Role of NH_3 concentration, *Am. J. Physiol.* **252:**F221.

129. Halperin, M. L. and Bun-Chen, C., 1987, Plasma glutamine and renal ammoniagenesis in dogs with chronic metabolic acidosis, *Am. J. Physiol.* **252:**F474.

130. Kuwuhara, M., Sasaki, S., Shiigai, T., and Takeuchi, J., 1986, Glutamine transport in the rabbit proximal straight tubule: Effect of acute acid pH, *Kidney Int.* **30:**340.

131. Nagami, G. T., Sonu, C. M., and Kurokawa, K., 1987, Ammonia production by isolated mouse proximal tubules perfused *in vitro*. Effect of metabolic acidosis, *J. Clin. Invest.* **78:**124.

132. Scaduto, R. C., Jr. and Schoolwerth, A. C., 1985, Effect of bicarbonate on glutamine and glutamate metabolism by rat kidney cortex mitochondria, *Am. J. Physiol.* **249:**F573.

133. Chobanian, M. C. and Hammerman, M. R., 1987, Insulin stimulates ammoniagenesis in canine renal proximal tubular segments, *Am. J. Physiol.* **253:**F1171.

134. Chobanian, M. C. and Hammerman, M. R., 1987, Phorbol esters inhibit ammoniagenesis and gluconeogenesis in proximal tubular segments, *Am. J. Physiol.* **252:**F1073.

135. Nissim, I., Yudkoff, M., and Segal, S., 1986, Nitrogen sources for renal ammoniagenesis: Study with 15N amino acid, *Am. J. Physiol.* **251:**F995.

136. Sastrasinh, S. and Sastrasinh, M., 1986, Effect of acivicin on glutamine transport by rat renal brush border membrane vesicles, *J. Lab. Clin. Med.* **108:**301.

137. Nonoguchi, H., Takchara, Y., and Endou, H., 1986, Intra- and inter-nephron heterogeneity of ammoniagenesis in rats: Effects of chronic metabolic acidosis and potassium depletion, *Pflüger's Arch. Eur. J. Physiol.* **407:**245.

138. Tannen, R. L., and Goyal, M., 1986, Urinary inhibitor of the ammoniagenic response to acute acidosis is a prostaglandin, *J. Lab. Clin. Med.* **108:**277.

139. Good, D. W. and DuBose, T. D., 1987, Ammonia transport by early and late proximal convoluted tubule of the rat, *J. Clin. Invest.* **79:**684.

140. Simon, E. E. and Hamm, L. L., 1987, Ammonia entry along rat proximal tubule *in vivo:* Effects of luminal pH and flow rate, *Am. J. Physiol.* **253:**F760.

141. Nagami, G. T. and Kurokawa, K., 1985, Regulation of ammonia production by mouse proximal tubules perfused *in vitro*. Effect of luminal perfusion, *J. Clin. Invest.* **75:**844.

142. Garvin, J. L., Burg, M. B., and Knepper, M. A., 1987, NH_3 and NH_4+ transport by rabbit proximal straight tubules. *Am. J. Physiol.* **252:**F232.

143. Kurtz, I. and Balaban, R. S., 1986, Ammonium as a substrate for Na$^+$–K$^+$–ATPase in rabbit proximal tubules, *Am. J. Physiol.* **250:**F497.

144. Good, D. W., 1987, Effects of potassium on ammonia transport by medullary thick ascending limb of the rat, *J. Clin. Invest.* **80:**1358.

145. Good, D. W., Caflisch, C. R., and DuBose, T. D., 1987, Transepithelial ammonia concentration gradients in inner medulla of the rat, *Am. J. Physiol.* **252:**F491.

146. Star, R. A., Kurtz, I., Mejia, R., Burg, M. B., and Knepper, M. A., 1987, Disequilibrium pH and ammonia transport in isolated perfused cortical collecting ducts, *Am. J. Physiol.* **253:**F1232.

147. Star, R. A., Burg, M. B., and Knepper, M. A., 1987, Luminal pH disequilibrium ammonia transport in the outer medullary collecting duct, *Am. J. Physiol.* **252:**F1148.

148. Romeh, S. A. and Tannen, R. L., 1986, Ameliorization of hypoxia-induced lactic acidosis by superimposed hypercapnea or hydrochloric acid infusion, *Am. J. Physiol.* **250:**F702.

149. Swenson, E. R. and Maren, T. H., 1986, Dissociation of CO_2 hydration and renal acid secretion in the dogfish, *Squalus acanthias, Am. J. Physiol.* **250:**F288.

150. Madias, N. E. and Zelman, S. J., 1986, The renal response to chronic mineral acid feeding: A reexamination of the role of systemic pH, *Kidney Int.* **29:**667.

151. Holloway, J. C., Phifer, T., Henderson, R., and Welbourne, T. C., 1986, Renal acid–base metabolism after ischemia, *Kidney Int.* **29:**989.

152. Winaver, J., Agmon, D., Harari, R., and Better, O. S., 1986, Impaired renal acidification following acute renal ischemia in the dog, *Kidney Int.* **30:**906.

153. Ichikawa, I. and Kon, V., 1986, Role of peritubular capillary forces in the renal action of carbonic anhydrase inhibitor, *Kidney Int.* **30:**828.

154. Tucker, B. J., Mundy, C. A., and Blantz, R. C., 1986, Can causality be determined from proximal tubular reabsorption and peritubular physical forces? *Am. J. Physiol.* **250:**F169.

155. Shvil, Y., Wald, H., and Popovitzer, M. M., 1987, Effect of bicarbonate and phosphate on renal phosphate lead in experimental Fanconi syndrome, *Am. J. Physiol.* **252:**F310.

156. Nadler, J. L., Lee, F. O., Hsueh, W., and Horton, R., 1986, Evidence of prostacyclin deficiency in the syndrome of hyporeninemic hypoaldosteronism, *N. Engl. J. Med.* **314:**1015.

157. Pabico, R. C., McKenna, B. A., and Freeman, R. B., 1987, Renal tubular dysfunctions in patients with idiopathic calcium nephrolithiasis, *Mineral Electrolyte Metab.* **13:**462.

158. Pizzarelli, F. and Peacock, M., 1987, Effect of chronic administration of ammonium sulfate on phosphatic stone recurrence, *Nephron* **46:**247.

159. Richardson, R. M. A. and Halperin, M. L., 1987, The urine pH: A potentially misleading diagnostic test in patients with hyperchloremic metabolic acidosis, *Am. J. Kidney Dis.* **10:**140.

160. Morris, L. H., Murphy, M. B., and Kitabachi, A. E., 1986, Bicarbonate therapy in severe diabetic ketoacidosis, *Ann. Intern. Med.* **105:**836.

161. Paulson, W. D., 1987, Anion gap–bicarbonate relation in diabetic ketoacidosis, *Am. J. Med.* **81:**995.

162. Gamblin, G. T., Ashburn, R. W., Kemp, D. G., and Beuttel, S. C., 1986, Diabetic ketoacidosis presenting with a normal anion gap, *Am. J. Med.* **80:**758.

163. Palmisano, J., Gruver, C., and Adams, N. D., 1987, Absence of anion gap in metabolic acidosis in severe methanol poisoning: A case report and review of the literature, *Am. J. Kidney Dis.* **9:**441.

164. Madias, N. E., Goorno, W. E., and Herson, S., 1987, Severe lactic acidosis as a presenting feature of pheochromocytoma, *Am. J. Kidney Dis.* **10:**250.

165. Bourneman, M., Hill, S. C., and Kidd, G. S., 1986, Lactic acidosis in pheochromocytoma, *Ann. Intern. Med.* **105:**880.

166. Wang, F., Butler, T., Rabbani, G. H., and Jones, P. K., 1986, The acidosis of cholera: Contributions of hyperproteinemia, lactic acidemia, and hyperphosphatemia to an increased serum anion gap, *N. Engl. J. Med.* **315:**1591.

167. Kruse, J. A., Zaidi, S. A. J., and Carlson, R. W., 1987, Significance of blood lactate levels in critically ill patients with liver disease, *Am. J. Med.* **83:**77.

168. Weil, M. H., Rackow, E. C., Trevino, R., Grundler, W., Falk, J. L., and Griffel, M. I., 1986,

Difference in acid–base state between venous and arterial blood during cardiopulmonary resuscitation, *N. Engl. J. Med.* **315**:153.

169. Eckfeldt, J. H., Leatherman, J. W., and Levitt, M. D., 1986, High prevalence of hyperamylasemia in patients with acidemia, *Ann. Intern. Med.* **104**:362.

170. McAulliffe, J. J., Lind, L. J., Leith, D. E., and Fencl, V., 1986, Hypoproteinemic alkalosis, *Ann. Intern. Med.* **81**:86.

171. Wallia, R., Greenberg, A., Piraino, B., Mitro, R., and Puschett, J. B., 1986, Serum electrolyte patterns in end-stage renal disease, *Am. J. Kidney Dis.* **8**:98.

172. Lameire, N. and Matthys, E., 1986, Influence of progressive salt restriction on urinary bicarbonate wasting in uremic acidosis, *Am. J. Kidney Dis.* **8**(S):151.

173. Singh, S., Hong, C. D., Dale, A., and Morgan, B., 1986, Comparison of buffering capacity in patients on hemodialysis and continuous ambulatory peritoneal dialysis, *Nephron* **42**:29.

174. Anderson, L. E., Nixon, J. V., and Henrich, W. L., 1987, Effects of acetate and bicarbonate dialysate on left ventricular performance, *Am. J. Kidney Dis.* **10**:350.

175. Leunissen, K. M. L., Hoorntje, S. J., Fiers, H. A., Dekkers, W. T., and Mulder, A. W., 1986, Acetate versus bicarbonate hemodialysis in critically ill patients, *Nephron* **42**:146.

176. Lundin, A. P., Stein, R. A., Brown, C. D., LaBelle, P., Kalman, F. S., Delano, B. G., Henegan, W. F., Lazarus, N. A., Krasnow, N., and Friedman, E. A., 1987, Fatigue, acid–base and electrolyte changes with exhaustive treadmill exercise in hemodialysis patients, *Nephron* **46**:57.

177. Latos, D. L., Strimel, D., Drews, M. H., and Allison, T. G., 1987, Acid–base and electrolyte changes following maximal and submaximal exercise in hemodialysis patients, *Am. J. Kidney Dis.* **10**:439.

178. Barsotti, G., Lazzeri, M., Cristofano, C., Cerri, M., Lupetti, S., and Giovannetti, S., 1986, The role of metabolic acidosis in causing uremic hyperphosphatemia, *Mineral Electrolyte Metab.* **12**:103.

5

Mineral Metabolism

Roger A. L. Sutton and E. C. Cameron

1. Inorganic Phosphate

1.1. Renal Handling of Phosphate

There have been several excellent recent reviews of renal phosphate transport.[1-4] It has been clear for many years that inorganic phosphate reabsorption mainly occurs in the proximal tubule, and that it occurs via sodium-dependent cotransport across the brush border, energized by the sodium gradient created by the Na^+, K^+-ATPase activity in the basolateral cell membrane, with presumably passive exit of inorganic phosphate down an electrochemical gradient across the basolateral membrane. Factors known to influence phosphate excretion include parathyroid hormone (PTH), calcitonin, and acid–base disturbances. There has been particular recent interest in the effects of acid–base disturbances, with attempts to reconcile previous contradictory results. Acute metabolic acidosis has been shown to cause a direct inhibition of phosphate reabsorption in some,[5] but not in other,[6] studies. Chronic metabolic alkalosis, acute (but not chronic) respiratory acidosis, and acute metabolic alkalosis (bicarbonate infusion) have also been shown to increase phosphate excretion, whereas respiratory alkalosis decreases phosphate excretion.[4] In studies with renal brush border membrane vesicles, increasing medium pH produces an increase in sodium-coupled phosphate transport into the vesicles. One proposed mechanism for this effect of luminal alkalosis is the preferential transport of divalent phosphate (HPO_4''). However, recent studies indicate that pH may directly affect the transporter, a decrease in pH reducing the affinity of the transporter for sodium.[7]

ROGER A. L. SUTTON and E. C. CAMERON • Division of Nephrology, Vancouver General Hospital, and University of British Columbia, Vancouver, British Columbia, Canada V5Z 1M9.

It is envisaged that the transporter at the luminal surface of the brush border membrane interacts first with sodium (at least two ions), which increases the affinity of the binding site for HPO_4''. Following a conformational change, the binding sites are then exposed to the cytoplasmic surface, where sodium is released first, followed by phosphate. A rise in extracellular sodium concentration increases, but a rise in intracellular sodium concentration decreases, phosphate transport.[1] A low intravesicular pH promotes phosphate transport. This has been interpreted[1] as the result of intracellular protons reducing the affinity of the transporter for sodium on the intracellular surface, thereby promoting the unloading of sodium and phosphate, and hence increased phosphate transport. Because sensitivity to hydrogen ions is greater at a lower sodium concentration, the effects of changes in intracellular hydrogen ion concentration are more pronounced than those of extracellular hydrogen ion concentration.[1] A high dietary phosphate decreases the pH dependence of phosphate transport.[8] Numerous experiments in perfused tubules have given confusing results, though Ullrich et al.[9] did conclude that luminal alkalosis or intracellular acidification promoted phosphate transport. These processes have been studied in detail by Quamme et al.,[6,10,11] who showed that the effect of an alkaline luminal perfusate to increase phosphate transport could be modified by dietary phosphate intake or by luminal or peritubular phosphate concentration.

Phosphate transport across the basolateral membrane had been assumed to be sodium-independent. Compatible with this notion, using canine basolateral membrane vesicles in the absence of sodium, electrogenic carrier-mediated phosphate transport was demonstrated, with a capacity similar to that of sodium-dependent brush border membrane transport.[12,13] A component of this transport is inhibited by probenecid and may involve an anion exchanger. An additional sodium-stimulated component of phosphate transfer across canine basolateral membrane vesicles has been demonstrated, which involves the transfer of positive charges,[14] is of lower capacity than the brush border sodium phosphate cotransporter, and is not enhanced by increasing the pH from 6.5 to 7.5. It is suggested that this system may transfer phosphate into the cell from the blood and may be important in circumstances of inadequate phosphate supply from the lumen, for example in ureteral obstruction.[15] Evidence for a basolateral sodium-dependent phosphate transporter, different from that in the brush border membrane, has been obtained in studies using LLC-PK cells, which are believed to be of proximal tubular origin.[16]

The brush border membrane is the site for regulation of phosphate transport.[1,17-21] Regulation may be short-term or long-term.[17] The mechanisms for short-term regulation include an allosteric "regulator," changes in electrochemical driving forces, or covalent modification of the transporter, e.g., cyclic AMP-dependent phosphorylation. Long-term regulation involves changes in the number of transporters by degradation or protein synthesis.[17] Transporters may be internalized into an intracellular pool, from which they may be reinserted into the membrane. An allosteric regulator may explain the effects of pH on proximal tubular phosphate transport, as discussed above. Hormones might affect phosphate transport by influencing cellular pH.[1] The reduction of sodium-dependent phosphate transport by hexose and amino acid fluxes may result from competition for driving forces. Cyclic AMP–dependent phosphorylation and/or ADP ribosylation of brush border membrane proteins has been postulated as being involved in the PTH regulation of phosphate transport,[18] but the relationship between modified proteins and altered transport is controversial.[1] Evidence has recently been presented to suggest that PTH may activate renal tubule cells by increasing inositol triphosphate and diacylglycerol in the cells.[19] Long-term regulation, involving protein synthesis, is involved in the stimulation of sodium–phosphate cotransport by thyroxine[20,21] and by chronic phosphate depletion.[1] Glucocorticoid inhibitory effects probably involve protein synthesis and may participate in the reduction in sodium phosphate cotransport produced by chronic metabolic acidosis.[21]

Cell culture models have advantages over membrane vesicles for the study of cellular aspects of the regulation of sodium phosphate cotransport, since they may contain the complete regulatory cascade. Adaptation to medium phosphate content has been studied in LLC-PK cells derived from pig kidney.[22] Whereas the increase in phosphate transport with phosphate deprivation is protein synthesis–dependent, the decrease with phosphate feeding, and the immediate increase with reexposure to a medium of low phosphate content, are protein synthesis–independent.[22] It is suggested that these protein synthesis–independent changes result from exchanges of transporters between intracellular sites and the cell membrane (internalization and recruitment).[17,22] PTH effects have been studied in OK cells derived from the opossum kidney.[23,24] PTH reduces phosphate transport across the apical membrane, apparently not by a simple cyclic AMP–dependent reaction.[17] In LLC-PK (pig kidney) and GTC-12P3 (monkey kidney) cells, although PTH stimulates intracellular cyclic AMP, phosphate transport is not inhibited. In OK cells, PTH removal restores phosphate transport by a protein synthesis–dependent mechanism.[17] Thus PTH may cause inactivation, internalization, and permanent degradation of transporters, perhaps resulting from initial phosphorylation.

The effects of 1,25-dihydroxy vitamin D_3 [1,25(OH)$_2$D$_3$] on phosphate transport remain controversial, as a result of conflicting data from clearance and micropuncture studies.[25,26] Recent studies have suggested that 1,25(OH)$_2$D$_3$ stimulates phospholipid exchange between plasma membrane vesicles and liposomes.[27] Such phospholipid transfer *in vitro* is associated with stimulation of phosphate transport.[28] These studies suggest the possibility of a relationship between 1,25(OH)$_2$D$_3$, phosphatidylcholine biosynthesis and the regulation of renal phosphate transport. Phosphatidylcholine biosynthesis has recently been examined in proximal tubule brush border membranes from the HYP mouse—a presumed model for human X-linked hypophosphatemia.[29] These brush border membranes are deficient in phosphatidylcholine and phosphatidylethanolamine when compared with normal mice; 1,25(OH)$_2$D stimulated the transfer of phospholipid from liposomes to brush border membranes, to the same extent as in normals, and phosphate transport was stimulated, but only to the same extent as in normals. It was concluded that the abnormality of phosphatidylcholine synthesis was not the primary genetic defect in the HYP mouse.

1.2. Clinical Disorders of Renal Phosphate Transport

1.2.1. X-Linked Hypophosphatemic Rickets

In the mouse model (HYP) referred to earlier, the phosphate transport defect has been localized to the proximal tubule brush border membrane, where sodium gradient dependent phosphate transport is reduced, in association with a decrease in V_{max}, but no change in K_m.[30,31] The defect is not caused by PTH, either in the mouse or in humans.[32] There is defective adaptation to a low-phosphate diet, both in humans[33] and in the mouse, and this has recently been demonstrated in cultured renal tubule cells. In cells from the HYP mouse, there was defective adaptation to a low-phosphate environment,[34] with a failure to increase transcellular phosphate transport normally. No differences were observed in the phosphorylation or dephosphorylation of proteins in brush border membranes from control and HYP mice.[30] Recently cyclic AMP–dependent protein kinase A has been shown to be normal in renal cortical cytoplasm of the HYP mouse,[35,36] but the calcium-and-phospholipid-dependent protein kinase C activity was significantly increased in the HYP mouse.[36] Protein kinase C has been shown to inhibit phosphate transport in OK cells.[37] In addition to the impairment of phosphate transport, there is also a defect in the 1-alpha hydroxylation of vitamin D both in X-linked hypophosphatemia and in the HYP mouse, under baseline conditions and in response to PTH.[38,39] PTH stimulates the 1-alpha hydroxylase in the proximal convoluted tubule,[40] apparently via cyclic AMP, while calcitonin stimulates the 1-hydroxylase in the pars recta by an unknown mechanism.[40] The latter response has recently been shown to be normal in the HYP mouse.[41] It is not yet clear whether the defects in phosphate transport and in the 1-alpha hydroxylase in the proximal tubule are the result of a single gene abnormality. Combination therapy with 1,25-dihydroxy vitamin D and phosphate is effective for the bone disease of X-linked hypophosphatemic rickets.[42] High-dose 1,25-dihydroxy D was associated with a rise in the theoretical renal phosphate threshold (i.e., transport maximum for phosphate/glomerular filtration rate, or TMP/GFR) into the normal range. The therapy requires monitoring, and there is concern that it might intensify the joint-related problems that occur in X-linked hypophosphatemia,[43] though Polisson et al.[43] reported that periarticular calcifications (enthesiopathy) in X-linked hypophosphatemic osteomalacia were age-dependent and unrelated to previous or ongoing therapy. Recently Tenenhouse et al.[44] reported increased renal catabolism of 1,25-dihydroxy vitamin D_3 in the HYP mouse. There was increased conversion of $1,25(OH)_2D$ to 1,24,25-trihydroxy vitamin D, to 24-oxo dihydroxy D, and to 24-oxo 1,23,25-hydroxy vitamin D. Thus, in the HYP mouse, and perhaps also in human X-linked hypophosphatemic rickets, increased catabolism of 1,25-dihydroxy D may in part explain the low serum levels.

1.2.2. Hereditary Hypophosphatemic Rickets with Hypercalciuria

The new syndrome hereditary hypophosphatemic rickets with hypercalciuria was reported from the Middle East in 1985.[45] More recently, hypophosphatemia with hypercalciuria has been reported among asymptomatic relatives of these patients,[46] and it is suggested that both conditions may share the same genetic defect (renal phosphate wasting) and that the severity of the hypophosphatemia may determine whether the individual suffers from childhood rickets or merely has $1,25(OH)_2D$-mediated intestinal calcium hyperabsorption with hypercalciuria. Phosphate supplementation corrected most of the clinical and biochemical defects in this disorder. It seems possible that idiopathic hypercalciuria associated with renal phosphate wasting, which occurs among idiopathic stone-formers, may result from a similar genetic defect.

1.2.3. Oncogenous Osteomalacia

A variety of tumors have been described in association with adult-onset hypophosphatemic osteomalacia, including benign mesenchymal tumors[47] as well as prostatic, breast, and oat cell carcinomas. 1,25-Dihydroxy D levels are low and increase after tumor resection. With the recent identification of PTH-like peptides produced by a variety of malignancies associated with humoral hypercalcemia,[48–51] it will be of interest to determine whether similar factors cause oncogenous osteomalacia. Although these PTH-like factors stimulate 1,25-dihydroxy D production *in vitro*,[49] $1,25(OH)_2D$ levels are usually low in patients with humoral hypercalcemia of malignancy. In a recently reported patient with oncogenous osteomalacia complicated by hypercalcemic hyperparathyroidism, $1,25(OH)_2D$ levels were subnormal before removal of the mesenchymal tumor but increased rapidly after tumor removal.[52] TMP/GFR increased gradually over several months. The tumor factor must be a potent inhibitor of 1-alpha hydroxylation, since $1,25(OH)_2D$ levels were low despite hyperparathyroidism.

1.2.4. Vitamin D-Dependent Rickets Type 2

This uncommon variety of hereditary rickets is associated with high circulating $1,25(OH)_2D$ levels and refractoriness to treatment with $1,25(OH)_2D$. Patients without alopecia show decreased sensitivity to $1,25(OH)_2D$ but do show clinical responsiveness.[53] Patients with alopecia frequently show no response to therapy with very high doses of $1,25(OH)_2D$.[53] In one patient a response was observed to $24,25(OH)_2D$, in a dose of 2 µg/day.[53] Studies of cultured skin fibroblasts, which contain $1,25(OH)_2D$ receptors, have shown a variety of defects in responses to vitamin D,[54] including absent cytosol nuclear binding, reduced capacity or affinity of binding, and defective localization of the 1,25-receptor complex in the nucleus. In subjects with normal $1,25(OH)_2D$ binding, defective stimulation by $1,25(OH)_2D$ of the 24-hydroxylase has been documented. Responsiveness of the 24-hydroxylase to $1,25(OH)_2D$ in fibroblasts *in vitro* may be predictive of clinical responsiveness to $1,25(OH)_2D$.[55] Defects in $1,25(OH)_2D$ receptors have also been demonstrated in circulating mononuclear cells in patients with vitamin D–dependent rickets type II.[56] Recently several investigators have reported gratifying clinical responses to intravenous calcium therapy or to high-dose oral calcium therapy in patients with refractory vitamin D–dependent rickets type II.[57–60]

1.3. Role of Phosphorus and 1,25-Dihydroxy D in the Secondary Hyperparathyroidism of Renal Failure

Korkor[61] examined the hypothesis that the inhibitory effect of $1,25(OH)_2D$ on PTH release in renal failure might be reduced as a result of a decreased number of $1,25(OH)_2D$ receptors in parathyroid tissue or a decrease in the binding affinity of $1,25(OH)_2D$ to these receptors. He found that the number of receptors was reduced in hyperplastic parathyroid glands from patients with chronic renal failure, compared with patients with transplanted kidneys and patients with primary hyperparathyroidism. Thus, $1,25(OH)_2D$ binding by parathyroid tissue is reduced in renal failure and this, as well as low $1,25(OH)_2D$ levels, may contribute to the pathogenesis of secondary hyperparathyroidism in renal failure.

Following the demonstration that $1,25(OH)_2D$ directly influences PTH release,[62,63] Lopez-Hilker et al.[64] studied dogs with renal failure. As a result of a high-calcium diet, ionized calcium rose, and PTH levels also rose as $1,25(OH)_2D$ fell from 25 to 12 pg/ml. Another group of dogs was given $1,25(OH)_2D$ to prevent the fall in serum $1,25(OH)_2D$ levels, and the PTH did not rise. Two recent studies have suggested that phosphate restriction might directly reduce PTH in renal failure, independent of changes in $1,25(OH)_2D$ or in ionized calcium.[65,66] Lopez-Hilker et al. therefore studied the effects of varying phosphate intake in dogs with renal failure and found that a low-phosphate diet reduced PTH despite no change in ionized calcium or $1,25(OH)_2D$ levels. A subsequent increase in dietary phosphate intake caused severe secondary hyperparathyroidism.[67]

1.4. Hypophosphatemia

Aubier et al.[68] reported an impairment of diaphragmatic contractility in hypophosphatemic patients undergoing artificial ventilation for acute respiratory failure, many of whom were alcoholic and/or had severe infections. Diaphragmatic contractility was markedly improved after phosphate infusion. Lewis et al., using NMR spectroscopy,[69] demonstrated a metabolic lesion in skeletal muscle persisting for several weeks after correction of the phosphate deficit. The defect included abnormal intracellular acidosis on mild exertion and rapid depletion of phosphocreatine, which recovered promptly on cessation of exercise.

Profound hypophosphatemia has recently been observed in subjects who collapsed with loss of consciousness, confusion, or disorientation at the end of a marathon run. The hypophosphatemia was transient, lasting 1–2 days, and recovered spontaneously. The pathogenesis of this hypophosphatemia is uncertain.[70]

1.5. Hyperphosphatemia

Hyperphosphatemia is most commonly encountered in renal failure. Causes of hyperphosphatemia in association with a normal glomerular filtration rate include growth hormone excess, the tumor lysis syndrome, tumoral calcinosis, treatment with bisphosphonates such as disodium etidronate (EHDP), and hypophosphatasia.

In tumoral calcinosis with hyperphosphatemia, augmented renal phosphate conservation may coexist with an elevated circulating concentration of $1,25(OH)_2D_3$,[71] the opposite combination of findings to those seen in X-linked hypophosphatemia. The association of tumoral calcinosis with pseudoxanthoma elasticum had been reported prior to 1970; a further patient has recently been reported[72] with hyperphosphatemia, hypercalcemia, and elevated $1,25(OH)_2D$ levels, in whom both dietary calcium loading and glucocorticoid treatment lowered the $1,25(OH)_2D$ levels. Whyte and Rettinger[73] recently reported that all of 27 subjects with hypophosphatasia had elevated serum inorganic phosphate levels associated with elevated TMP/GFR levels, consistent with an action of alkaline phosphatase as a phosphoprotein phosphatase in the renal brush border membrane, presumably affecting renal tubular phosphate transport.

2. Calcium

2.1. Renal Handling of Calcium

The mechanism of calcium transport in the thick ascending limb of the loop of Henle has been controversial. Bourdeau and Burg[74] found calcium transport to be dependent upon the transepithelial potential difference in the cortical thick ascending limb, while PTH failed to increase transport when the PD was abolished by chloride removal from the external bathing solution.[75] Friedman[76] has recently reported studies in cortical and medullary thick ascending limbs of the mouse perfused *in vitro* with solutions of identical calcium concentration in the lumen and bath. PTH and dibutyryl cyclic AMP increased calcium transport in the cortical thick ascending limb without a change in the electrochemical driving force, indicating transcellular transport, while in the medullary thick ascending limb, which lacks PTH-activated adenyl cyclase, calcium transport was exclusively passive and voltage-dependent. It is possible that the differences between the results of Bourdeau and Burg[75] and Friedman[76] may relate to the absence of chloride in the experiments of Bourdeau and Burg. It has been suggested that calcium transport may be chloride dependent, and recently, in frog skin, Ziyadeh *et al.*[77] have shown that PTH stimulates calcium secretion and that basolateral calcium entry is chloride dependent.

The use of calcium microelectrodes *in situ* has permitted an evaluation of calcium transport in the distal convoluted tubule of the rat.[78] The ionized calcium concentration fell proportionately more than that of total calcium along the distal tubule, so that the fraction of ionized calcium fell from nearly 100% in the earliest distal tubule to approximately 10% at the end of the distal tubule.

With respect to the effects of metabolic acidosis to enhance calcium and magnesium excretion, Lau *et al.*[79] have recently shown that a comparable degree of respiratory acidosis does not induce increased calcium and magnesium excretion, indicating that the inhibition of renal tubular divalent cation reabsorption is not related to systemic pH. Intracellular pH, however, which behaves differently in chronic respiratory from metabolic acidosis,[80] may be a controlling factor. Previous studies of metabolic acidosis and alkalosis had suggested an action of bicarbonate to enhance calcium reabsorption in segments beyond the proximal tubule.[81] Recently Bomsztyk and Calalb[82] observed, in microperfusion studies, that enhanced bicarbonate reabsorption or luminal acidification in the proximal tubule of the rat was associated with a major enhancement of calcium reabsorption.

2.2. Hypercalciuria

The pathophysiology of idiopathic hypercalciuria remains controversial. While most idiopathic hypercalciuria is probably a result of primary intestinal calcium hyperabsorption, certain patients have features that would be predicted with a primary renal calcium leak, while others may have a primary renal phosphate leak, with enhanced $1,25(OH)_2D_3$ production and secondary intestinal calcium hyperabsorption (see Section 1.2.2). With respect to intestinal calcium hyperabsorption, Kaplan et al.[83] pointed out in 1977 that the hyperabsorption was greater than could be accounted for by the normal or slightly increased serum $1,25(OH)_2D$ levels. Lemann and Gray[84] have recently confirmed this finding and proposed that in absorptive hypercalciuria, calcium hyperabsorption is either independent of vitamin D, or there is some form of hypersensitivity to vitamin D, perhaps involving a receptor abnormality. Preminger and Pak[85] have recently reported that long-term thiazide therapy results in normalization of increased intestinal calcium absorption in renal hypercalciuria, whereas in absorptive hypercalciuria intestinal calcium absorption remains elevated, and the hypocalciuric effect of the thiazide eventually becomes attenuated.

There has been considerable recent interest in the role of the skeleton in idiopathic hypercalciuria. Enhanced mobilization of skeletal calcium may contribute to fasting hypercalciuria in idiopathic hypercalciuria.[86] Pacifici et al.[87] recently reported that prostaglandin inhibition with diclofenac in fasting hypercalciuria produced a marked reduction in the hypercalciuria and a rise in PTH levels, suggesting that prostaglandin-mediated bone resorption may suppress PTH levels in patients with fasting hypercalciuria.

Costanzo et al. have produced hypercalciuria in anterior pituitary implanted rats which is not mediated by prolactin.[88] The hypercalciuria is attenuated by the administration of a thiazide diuretic.[89]

2.3. Hypocalciuria

Hypocalciuria associated with a normal or only mildly reduced glomerular filtration rate occurs in a variety of disorders,[90] including familial hypocalciuric hypercalcemia, Bartter's syndrome,[91] and chronic cis-platinum nephropathy.[92] Hypocalciuria has also been described recently in preeclampsia[93] and was not attributable to changes in $1,25(OH)_2D$ levels or in filtered calcium load.

2.4. Hypercalcemia

2.4.1. Hypercalcemia of Malignancy

There have been major advances in the understanding of hypercalcemia of malignancy. There is evidence that lymphotoxin may be responsible for some or all of the osteoclast-activating activity produced by myeloma cells.[94] With respect to humoral hypercalcemia of malignancy, transforming growth factors may contribute to bone resorption.[95] Three groups of investigators[48-51] have isolated and obtained partial amino acid sequences of PTH-like peptides derived from squamous lung cancer, a renal cell cancer, and breast cancer. Kemp et al.[50] have shown that the 1-34-PTH-related peptide activates cyclic AMP in bone and kidney and stimulates bone resorption and renal calcium reabsorption and phosphaturia. Horiuchi et al.[49] also showed that the 1-34-PTH-related peptide increased $1,25(OH)_2D$ levels in thyroparathyroidectomized rats. This is of particular interest, since 1,25(OH)2D levels are generally reduced in humoral hypercalcemia of malignancy.[96] In a large clinical study of tumor-induced hypercalcemia, Harinck et al.[97] found evidence for renal calcium retention in certain types of cancer, particularly those of the kidney and lung. In this study intravenous aminohydroxypropylidene bisphosphonate was reported to be remarkably effective, in association with saline infusions, in correcting malignant hypercalcemia. In a subsequent preliminary report[98] van Holten-Verzandvoort et al. found that oral bisphosphonate produced a striking reduction in skeletal morbidity from metastatic breast cancer.

2.4.2. Primary Hyperparathyroidism

One of the clinical enigmas of primary hyperparathyroidism has been the presentation with either bone disease (osteitis fibrosa cystica), stone disease, or neither. Recently it has been recognized that $1,25(OH)_2D$ levels are inconsistently increased in primary hyperparathyroidism; part of the reason for this appears to be the dependence of $1,25(OH)_2D$ levels on 25(OH)D, as reported by LoCascio et al.[99] Patron et al.[100] recently reported that among their patients seen in Paris, those presenting with osteitis fibrosa cystica tended to have lower 1,25(OH)D levels and lower glomerular filtration rates than other patients with primary hyperparathyroidism. A substantial proportion of these patients with osteitis fibrosa were immigrants from North Africa who were vitamin D deficient. By contrast, patients with renal calculi had higher glomerular filtration rates and higher 25-hydroxy and 1,25-dihydroxy vitamin D levels, associated with much greater intestinal calcium absorption leading to hypercalciuria. Presumably the reason for the rarity of primary hyperparathyroidism presenting with osteitis fibrosa in North America is the supplementation of dairy products with vitamin D, so that nutritional vitamin D deficiency is extremely rare. In view of the recent appreciation of the direct effect of $1,25(OH)_2D$ on PTH release (discussed earlier), it is interesting to speculate[101] that vitamin D deficiency or lack of $1,25(OH)_2D$ may cause an intensification of hyperparathyroidism (as noted many years ago by Lumb and Standbury[102]) by reducing the normal feedback inhibition of $1,25(OH)_2D$ on PTH release. Furthermore, primary hyperparathyroidism itself may contribute to vitamin D deficiency by enhancing the hepatic inactivation of $25(OH)D$.[103]

Using nephrogenous cyclic AMP as an index of PTH secretion, Gardin et al.[104] have found evidence for an abnormal parathyroid set-point as well as an increased parathyroid cell mass in primary hyperparathyroidism.

Of interest, in a rat model of primary hyperparathyroidism,[105] involving chronic PTH infusion, a modest increase above physiologic levels in PTH infusion rate caused a rise in plasma $1,25(OH)_2D$ levels but no change in calcium or phosphorus levels. Higher PTH doses also produced hypercalcemia and hypophosphatemia. Thus, in the rat, increased activity of the 1-alpha hydroxylase enzyme may be the most sensitive index of PTH excess.

Brandi et al.[106] have demonstrated the presence of a factor, mitogenic for cultured bovine parathyroid cells, in plasma from patients with familial multiple endocrine neoplasia type I, which was different from plasma from normal subjects and from other conditions involving parathyroid hyperplasia (e.g., FHH and MEN type II) or from parathyroid adenoma. The mitogenic activity had an apparent molecular weight of 50,000–55,000, did not appear to originate from the parathyroids, and was demonstrable as long as 4 years after induction of hypoparathyroidism by parathyroidectomy. Schimke[107] suggests that the germinal event might be an abnormal plasma membrane receptor on the endocrine cells, while the somatic mutation might involve derepression of a primitive gene coding for a protein that promotes growth of endocrine glands.

Whereas primary parathyroid hyperplasia is multicellular (nonclonal) in origin, the issue of whether adenomas are of clonal origin has been controversial. Studies based on glucose-6-phosphate dehydrogenase enzyme content suggested a multicellular origin.[108] However, Arnold et al.[109] have recently reported alterations in restriction fragment length in the PTH gene in two parathyroid adenomas, indicating a clonal origin. Furthermore, using polymorphism in an X-linked gene (hypoxanthine phosphoribosyltransferase), six of eight adenomas from women showed monoclonality, while two gave an equivocal pattern. None of five hyperplastic glands was monoclonal.

Responsiveness of parathyroid adenomas to changes in extracellular calcium concentration has been recognized for some time. Recently Kane-Johnson et al.[110] studied responses of adenomatous parathyroid tissue to calcium levels and to beta-adrenergic agents and found a marked dissociation in secretory responses among a series of parathyroid adenomas. Tiegs et al.[111] have recently reported that calcitonin levels are normal in primary hyperparathyroidism—i.e., there is a failure of the c-cell response to sustained hypercalcemia.

The issue of whether mild asymptomatic primary hyperparathyroidism requires surgery remains unresolved. An interesting study from Sweden[112] followed 172 patients with mild hypercalcemia, identified at routine population screening, for 14 years. Mortality was significantly greater in hypercalcemic patients than controls; the difference was significant only in the under-70-year-old group. The excess mortality (56 observed vs. 39 expected deaths) was largely due to circulatory diseases. The hypercalcemic group had significantly higher blood pressures. These data might be used as an argument to support surgery for primary hyperparathyroidism, but the authors point out that parathyroid surgery has not been shown to alter mortality.

Winzelberg has reviewed the place of parathyroid imaging in patients in whom surgery is planned. In patients with previous surgery, computed-tomography scanning is probably the most useful technique.[113]

In hemodialysis patients undergoing parathyroidectomy, administration of $1,25(OH)_2D$ (2–4 μg/day) has been shown to ameliorate postoperative hypocalcemia.[114]

A recent case report[115] describes a woman with remarkably severe hypercalcemia due to primary hyperparathyroidism, who presented with the nephrotic syndrome which remitted after parathyroidectomy. Renal biopsy showed interstitial fibrosis and calcification in glomerular basement membranes, and it was speculated that calcium may have titrated the fixed negative charges in the glomerular basement membrane which normally restrain albumin.

2.4.3. Hypercalcemia Associated with Granuloma and Lymphoma

The hypercalcemia of sarcoidosis is known to be due to the presence of a 25-hydroxy vitamin D 1-alpha hydroxylase in sarcoid macrophages,[116] which differ from renal cells in that they do not appear to produce 24,25-dihydroxy vitamin D. The hypercalcemia of sarcoidosis responds to glucocorticoids and also to chloroquine.[117] Recently,[118] chloroquine has been shown to lower $1,25(OH)_2D$ levels and to correct hypercalciuria and hypercalcemia. Barre et al.[119] have also described a patient with sarcoidosis and hypercalcemia on long-term dialysis, in whom hydroxychloroquine normalized the serum calcium and $1,25(OH)_2D$ levels.

With respect to hypercalcemia in association with other granulomatous diseases, Hoffman and Korzenkowski reported a case of leprosy with elevated $1,25(OH)_2D_3$ levels,[120] whereas Ryzen and Singer reported a patient with leprosy and hypercalcemia in whom both PTH and $1,25(OH)_2D$ levels were suppressed,[121] suggesting that the hypercalcemia was not mediated by $1,25(OH)_2D$. The hypercalcemia was corrected with prednisone. Felsenfeld et al.[122] reported a patient with tuberculosis and on chronic hemodialysis who developed hypercalcemia associated with elevated $1,25(OH)_2D$ levels.

Recently, several cases of Hodgkin's disease with hypercalcemia have been described in which production of $1,25(OH)_2D$ by the lymphoma appeared to be the cause of the hypercalcemia. In one recent case report, marked elevations of $1,25(OH)_2D$ were documented during several relapses of hypercalcemia in a patient with Hodgkin's disease.[123] Hypercalcemia with an elevated $1,25(OH)_2D$ level has also been reported in a patient with a seminoma.[124]

2.4.4.   Other Causes of Hypercalcemia

Hypercalcemia has recently been reported[125] in up to 10% of patients with advanced chronic liver disease awaiting transplant, most of whom did not have liver tumors. The hypercalcemia was apparently not due to hyperparathyroidism or hypervitaminosis D, and its pathogenesis is unclear. Hypercalcemia has also been reported in 20% of patients with theophylline poisoning[126] and presumably involves a system subject to beta-adrenergic regulation, since it responded to propranolol.

Payne *et al.* studied the range of serum calcium values found within sets of siblings[127] and found a distinct clustering of calcium (and magnesium) levels, which may be important in relation to the recognition of familial hypocalciuric hypercalcemia. Bannister *et al.*[128] report the occurrence of both benign hypercalcemia and benign hypocalcemia in the same family.

Hypercalcemia has been reported to occur frequently following cardiac transplantation, apparently attributable to calcium carbonate therapy, often associated with alkalosis.[129]

Mallette and Eichhorn have examined calcium metabolism in lithium-treated patients and report a 10% incidence of hypercalcemia, which apparently results from decreased parathyroid sensitivity to calcium, as well as lithium-induced hypocalciuria.[130]

2.4.5.   Treatment of Hypercalcemia

With respect to the treatment of hypercalcemia, there have been several reports of the remarkable efficacy of the newer diphosphonates in malignant hypercalcemia.[97,98] Initial observations on the radiation protective agent WR2721 were described in the previous volume in this series.[131] WR2721 reduces renal tubular calcium reabsorption and in a recent report was observed to normalize the hypercalcemia in a rat Leydig tumor model.[132] It may prove to be useful in circumstances in which increased renal tubular calcium reabsorption contributes to an important extent to the hypercalcemia. Warrell *et al.*[133] have reported on the successful use of gallium nitrate to treat refractory hypercalcemia associated with parathyroid carcinoma. The data suggest that gallium nitrate inhibits PTH-mediated calcium release from bone.[134]

2.5.   Hypocalcemia

In hypoparathyroidism, PTH, $1,25(OH)_2D$, and serum calcium levels are usually low. A kindred with familial hypoparathyroidism has recently been described[135] in which low PTH levels were associated with normal or raised $1,25(OH)_2D$ levels and only moderate hypocalcemia, without developmental abnormalities. The authors suggest that $1,25(OH)_2D$ levels in hypoparathyroidism result from the sum of the effects of a low or normal PTH level, hypocalcemia, and hyperphosphatemia.

The cause of hypocalcemia in pancreatitis is not satisfactorily explained. In a recent case report[136] a patient with a pancreatic fistula and pancreatic ascites is described in whom hypocalcemia was associated with the accumulation of very large quantities of insoluble calcium in the ascitic fluid and with secondary hyperparathyroidism. This study indicates that the formation of calcium soaps can be the cause of severe hypocalcemia in pancreatic disease.

Hypocalcemia has been noted to occur frequently in patients with sepsis, particularly due to gram-negative organisms, and is of multifactorial origin, including parathyroid insufficiency and decreased production of $1,25(OH)_2D$, as well as unresponsiveness to $1,25(OH)_2D$.[137] Hypocalcemia is particularly associated with bacteremia and is associated with an increased mortality.[138] Zaloga et al.[139] suggest that a contributory factor in the hypocalcemia associated with critical illness could be increased calcium binding by albumin, perhaps mediated by alterations in free fatty acids which may increase the calcium binding.

Hypocalcemia associated with myocardial failure has recently been reported in a case of acute monocytic leukemia with accelerated bone formation.[140]

Breslau and Zerwekh[141] have examined the effects of estrogen and pregnancy on calcium homeostasis in pseudohypoparathyroidism. They noted that estrogen tended to lower serum calcium levels, whereas in pregnancy calcium levels were normal, PTH was suppressed, and $1,25(OH)_2D$ levels were high. They suggest that the $1,25(OH)_2D$ in pregnancy may be of placental origin. Farfel and Friedman[142] reported that mental retardation in pseudohypoparathyroidism appears to be confined to patients with deficiency of the guanine nucleotide regulatory protein, which may therefore have some role in relation to function of the central nervous system. It has recently been reported[143] that renal tubular calcium reabsorption is responsive to PTH in pseudohypoparathyroidism during treatment with $1,25(OH)_2D_3$ so that these patients do not develop the same degree of hypercalciuria as patients with idiopathic hypoparathyroidism during $1,25(OH)_2D$ therapy.

3. Vitamin D

3.1. Vitamin D Metabolism

The vitamin D endocrine system has been reviewed recently by Kumar,[144] Kurokawa,[143] and Holick.[145] The vitamin D metabolite $1,25(OH)_2D_3$ is an important steroidal hormone produced primarily by the kidney.

The initial metabolic step in this hormone system is the endogenous production of vitamin D_3 (cholecalciferol) by the skin.[144] Vitamin D_3 is produced from 7-dehydrocholesterol by exposure of the skin to ultraviolet light. Factors that have been shown to inhibit vitamin D_3 production in the skin include aging, chronic renal failure, sunscreens containing paraaminobenzoic acid, and melanin pigmentation.[145,146] Lo et al.[147] have demonstrated that though Asians require greater exposure to light than Caucasians to produce similar amounts of vitamin D_3, their total production capacity is not different. Matsuoka et al. have shown that oral exogenous administration of $1,25(OH)_2D$ does not inhibit the cutaneous synthesis of vitamin D_3 in response to acute ultraviolet light irradiation.[148]

Though the skin is the major physiologic source of vitamin D, vitamin D_2 or vitamin D_3 may also be absorbed as fat-soluble vitamins via intestinal lymphatics.[144] Vitamin D from either the skin or the gastrointestinal tract is transported in the circulation mainly bound to vitamin D binding protein (DBP) or albumin. DBP, the major carrier of vitamin D and vitamin D metabolites, is a 58,000 dalton interalpha globulin which has also been termed group-specific component.[149,150]

This glycoprotein is synthesized by the liver. The level in the blood is increased in states of estrogen excess and decreased in hypoproteinemic conditions.[149] Since the free fraction of vitamin D metabolites such as 25(OH)D has been shown to be independent of the concentration of DBP, the measurement of total serum vitamin D metabolite levels may be misleading in the evaluation of vitamin D status in patients with altered DBP levels.[151]

DBP has recently been shown to have a probable role in the sequestration and disposition of actin monomers released after tissue injury.[149,150] In addition, DBP has been demonstrated on the surface of a number of cells including circulating monocytes and human cytotrophoblasts, suggesting a role in transcellular sterol transport.[152,153]

The parent compound, vitamin D, is transported in the circulation to the liver, where it is hydroxylated to the 25(OH)D metabolite in the microsomal and mitochrondrial fractions of the hepatocytes.[144] This process is loosely regulated, so that the 25(OH)D levels in the serum are generally a good index of vitamin D reserves with the proviso that the total metabolite concentration will be affected by the concentration of DBP.[151]

In rats, chronic administration of $1,25(OH)_2D$ has been demonstrated to reduce the serum concentration of $25(OH)D_3$ by increasing its metabolic clearance rate.[154] Increased transformation of vitamin D into 25(OH)D has been found with calcium supplementation of hypocalcemic vitamin D–depleted rats.[155]

3.2. Regulation of Renal $1,25(OH)_2D$ Production

The vitamin D hormone $1,25(OH)_2D$ is produced in the mitochondria of the kidney proximal tubular cells.[143] The precursor, 25(OH)D, is enzymatically transformed into a number of metabolites. The active metabolite $1,25(OH)_2D$ is produced by the action of a cytochrome P450 mixed-function oxidase, 25(OHD) 1-alpha hydroxylase.[145]

The main activator of renal 1-alpha hydroxylase, and thus the major regulator of $1,25(OH)_2D$ secretion, is PTH.[143] This effect has been shown to be mediated through cyclic AMP and phosphorus depletion. In humans, phosphorus restriction increases production and phosphorus depletion reduces $1,25(OH)_2D$.[156]

Increased extracellular fluid calcium ion concentration may also reduce 1-alpha hydroxylase activity. This effect may have clinical significance in hyperparathyroidism with severe hypercalcemia. In this circumstance, low serum 1,25(OH)$_2$D levels may result and would not exclude the diagnosis of primary hyperparathyroidism.[157]

Kurokawa has shown that calcitonin selectively stimulates 1-alpha hydroxylase in the proximal tubule by a process different from PTH, not mediated through cyclic AMP.[143] Jaeger et al.,[158] using chronic calcitonin infusion in rats, demonstrated that calcitonin is a regulator of 1,25(OH)$_2$D production independent of calcium as well as PTH and phosphate. They demonstrated that calcitonin increased intestinal absorption by increasing circulating 1,25(OH)$_2$D levels. Hypophosphatemic mice have defective regulation of renal 1-alpha hydroxylase in response to PTH, phosphate, and calcium, but Nesbit et al.[41] demonstrated that the calcitonin-sensitive component of 1-alpha hydroxylase was not compromised in the X-linked hypophosphatemic syndrome.

A number of studies have shown that 1,25(OH)$_2$D production is reduced in the elderly.[159–162] Deficiency of substrate 25(OH)D is frequently the cause, but in addition, age-related defects in renal synthesis of the hormone have been demonstrated.[161,162]

The antimycotic agent ketoconazole has been demonstrated to decrease 1,25(OH)$_2$D production.[163] Because of the close relationship between testosterone, osteoblastic activity, and mineralization at the time of puberty, Krabbe et al.[164] studied the metabolism of vitamin D with special relation to serum testosterone during the growth spurt period. Their studies indicate that the marked increase in serum testosterone in male puberty had no significant influence on circulating vitamin D metabolite levels.

3.3. Production and Action of 24,25(OH)$_2$D

As previously stated, 25(OH)D is enzymatically transformed into a number of metabolites in the renal proximal tubular cells. 24,25(OH)$_2$D is the metabolite produced in the largest quantity.[143] Despite this fact, this metabolite does not appear to be of major physiologic importance *per se,* but is probably a degradation product similar to many other vitamin D metabolites that have been identified. Increased 1,25(OH)$_2$D concentration inhibits 1-alpha hydroxylase and stimulates 25(OH)D24 hydroxylase to produce 24,25(OH)$_2$D.

However, the search for a physiologic function for 24,25(OH)$_2$D continues to be stimulated by such findings as identification of receptors for this metabolite in parathyroid tissue.[165]

Lidor et al.,[166] in a study involving experimental fracture healing in chicks, showed that increased levels of 24,25(OH)$_2$D coincided with formation of cartilaginous tissue and that levels of 1,25(OH)$_2$D and intestinal calcium absorption were decreased, suggesting that during the process of fracture repair changes in the metabolism of vitamin D may be taking place to meet new requirements of the body.

3.4. Extrarenal Production of 1,25(OH)$_2$D

Metabolism of 25(OH)D to 1,25(OH)$_2$D has been shown to occur in extrarenal cells, including those of the placenta, bone, and neonatal keratinocytes.[145]

The extrarenal synthesis of 1,25(OH)$_2$D is well recognized to cause hypercalcemia and hypercalciuria in patients with sarcoidosis. Insogna et al.[167] demonstrated a markedly elevated 1,25(OH)$_2$D production rate in sarcoidosis patients, and no impairment of 1,25(OH)$_2$D clearance was identified. The highest production rates were found in hypercalcemic patients.

Pulmonary alveolar macrophages from patients with sarcoidosis have been shown to produce 1,25(OH)$_2$D, and recently pulmonary alveolar macrophages from normal subjects have been reported to produce 1,25(OH)$_2$D when treated with interferon-γ.[168] Studies by Reichel et al.[168] have indicated differences between the 25(OH)D metabolizing system in pulmonary alveolar macrophages and the renal metabolism of 25(OH)D. Also, studies with certain T-lymphotrophic virus–transformed lymphocytes demonstrated a 25(OH)D metabolizing system similar to, but not identical with, that of kidney cell culture systems.[169]

3.5. Actions of 1,25(OH)$_2$D

The major effect of 1,25(OH)$_2$D is to increase the active absorption of calcium from the proximal intestine.[144] This effect is mediated in the target cell through a nuclear receptor which activates transcription of specific genes and subsequently proteins, including calcium binding protein, alkaline phosphatase, and low-affinity calcium ATPase resulting in increased absorption of calcium and phosphate.[145]

One of the major developments in 1,25(OH)$_2$D physiology has been the identification of 1,25(OH)$_2$D receptors in an extremely wide variety of tissues, including the renal tubule, osteoblasts, parathyroid cells, peripheral monocytes, cells of the cerebellum, and human keratinocytes.[145] The physiologic role and importance of this hormone in a number of tissues remain to be clarified.

3.6. 1,25(OH)$_2$D, Calcium Metabolism, and the Kidney

The parathyroid gland possesses specific receptors for 1,25(OH)$_2$D and this steroidal hormone has been shown to suppress parathyroid hormone secretion.[170] In experimental uremia in rats with low circulating 1,25(OH)$_2$D levels, parathyroid 1,25(OH)$_2$D receptors have been shown to be diminished, a factor potentially relevant in the genesis of secondary renal hyperparathyroidism.[171] Recent studies using dispersed parathyroid cells indicate that 1,25(OH)$_2$D may modify membrane permeability to calcium, resulting in a rapid increase in cytosolic calcium.[170]

Receptors for 1,25(OH)$_2$D are located in the distal tubule of the kidney and appear to induce the synthesis of calcium-binding protein.[144] Both PTH and 1,25(OH)$_2$D have been shown to be necessary for normal renal tubular calcium and phosphorus reabsorption.[143] The role of 1,25(OH)$_2$D in the tubular reabsorption of phosphorus and calcium was discussed earlier.

Kurokawa[143] has proposed an intriguing scheme concerning the regulation of calcium metabolism which involves the interactions of $1,25(OH)_2D$, calcitonin, and PTH in the kidney, bone, and gastrointestinal tract. He suggests that an ingested calcium load causes an increase in extracellular fluid calcium which stimulates calcitonin secretion. The calcitonin inhibits bone resorption and activates renal tubular vitamin D production by the calcitonin pathway. He suggests that such a system may be important for calcium accumulation in the body of the growing individual.

Feinfeld and Sherwood have recently reviewed the role of parathyroid hormone and $1,25(OH)_2D$ in chronic renal failure.[172] They detail the complex interactions between $1,25(OH)_2D$, extracellular fluid phosphate levels and PTH which result from decreased nephron mass and produce secondary hyperparathyroidism. These interactions include decreased synthesis and release of $1,25(OH)_2D$ from renal tubular cells secondary to decreased cell number and phosphate retention. PTH secretion is subsequently increased secondary to low $1,25(OH)_2D$ levels and decreased ionized calcium. Turner et al.[173] have demonstrated that phosphate restriction in patients with chronic renal failure who are predialysis produced suppression of biochemical and histologic hyperparathyroidism and sustained elevation of circulating $1,25(OH)_2D$ levels.

Merke et al.[174] reviewed the possibility that because of the presence of $1,25(OH)_2D$ receptors in a wide variety of tissues, the deficiency of $1,25(OH)_2D$ in uremia may play a role in the genesis of a number of uremic dysfunctions in addition to disorders of calcium metabolism.

Aluminum toxicity is recognized to be a major etiologic factor in the development of uremic osteodystrophy.[175] Exogenously administered $1,25(OH)_2D$ increases gastrointestinal aluminum absorption as well as serum and tissue aluminum concentrations, which could be a factor in the pathogenesis of aluminum-related bone disease. In rat experiments, aluminum toxicity has been shown to produce resistance to $1,25(OH)_2D$ action in duodenal calcium transport by a mechanism that is postreceptor in origin.[176]

4. Magnesium

There have been several recent reports of renal magnesium wasting syndromes. Geven et al.[177] reported two families from the Netherlands with renal magnesium wasting of autosomal dominant inheritance and associated with striking hypocalciuria. This combination was first described by Gitelman et al.[178] and has also been reported in Bartter's syndrome[91] and in chronic cis-platinum nephropathy.[92] Geven et al. suggested that the hypocalciuria may be secondary to hypomagnesemia. However, Mavichak et al.[92] showed that correction of hypomagnesemia with magnesium infusions did not correct the hypocalciuria in cis-platinum nephropathy and suggested that the renal retention of calcium as well as the renal wasting of magnesium may be intrinsic renal tubular defects. The frequent occurrence of renal magnesium wasting has recently been documented in cyclosporine-treated renal transplant patients.[179] Similar magnesium wasting was not seen in patients treated with other immunosuppressive drugs. Renal magnesium wasting has also been reported in bone marrow transplant patients receiving cyclosporine.[180,181] The location of the renal tubular lesion leading to magnesium wasting in these disorders is uncertain; however, since the thick ascending limb of the loop of Henle is the major site of magnesium reabsorption along the nephron, it is tempting to propose a lesion at that site.

An interesting recent case report[182] describes a patient with the short bowel syndrome in whom impaired intestinal magnesium absorption was associated with renal magnesium wasting. $1,25(OH)_2D$ levels were low, perhaps owing to impaired conversion of $25(OH)D$ to $1,25(OH)_2D$ resulting from magnesium deficiency.[183] Treatment with 1-alpha $(OH)D_3$ corrected magnesium wasting, suggesting that $1,25(OH)_2D$ deficiency may impair renal magnesium reabsorption. Reports in the literature of effects of $1,25(OH)_2D$ on magnesium reabsorption are contradictory. Thus, the authors suggest that magnesium depletion may lead to impaired renal magnesium conservation, creating a vicious cycle.

Hypomagnesemic hypocalcemia, usually regarded as being due to impaired PTH release and end-organ resistance to PTH, has been reported in a parathyroidectomized patient, was refractory to $1,25(OH)_2D$, and presumably resulted from a PTH-independent impairment of calcium release from bone.[184]

References

1. Gmaj, P. and Murer, H., 1986, Cellular mechanisms of inorganic phosphate transport in kidney, *Physiol. Rev.* **66**:36–70.
2. Hammerman, M. R., 1986, Phosphate transport across renal proximal tubular cell membranes, *Am. J. Physiol.* **251**:F385–F398.
3. Jacobson, H. and Knochel, J. P., 1986, Renal handling of phosphate in health and disease, in: *The Kidney*, Volume 2 (3rd ed.), (B. M. Brenner and F. C. Rector, eds.), Saunders, Philadelphia, pp. 619–662.
4. Mizgala, C. L. and Quamme, G. A., 1985, Renal handling of phosphate, *Physiol. Rev.*, **65**:431–466.
5. Guntupalli, J., Eby, B., and Lau, K., 1982, Mechanism for the phosphaturia of NH_4Cl: Dependence on acidemia but not on diet PO_4 or PTH, *Am. J. Physiol.* **242**:F555–F560.
6. Quamme, G. A., 1985, Effects of metabolic acidosis, alkalosis and dietary hydrogen ion intake on phosphate transport in the proximal convoluted tubule, *Am. J. Physiol.* **249**:F769–F779.
7. Amstutz, M., Mohrmann, M., Gmaj, P., and Murer, H., 1985, The effect of pH on phosphate transport in rat renal brush-border membrane vesicles, *Am. J. Physiol.* **248**:F705–F710.
8. Cheng, L., Liang, C. T., and Sacktor, B., 1983, Sodium gradient–dependent phosphate transport in renal brush border membrane vesicles of rabbits adapted to high and low phosphorus diets, *Am. J. Physiol.* **245**:F175–F180.
9. Ullrich, K. J., Rumrich, G., and Kloss, S., 1978, Phosphate transport in the proximal convolution of the rat kidney, III. Effect of extracellular and intracellular pH, *Pflüger's Arch.* **377**:33–42.
10. Quamme, G. A., Mizgala, C. L., Wong, N. L. M., Whiting, S. J., 1985, Effects of intraluminal pH and dietary phosphate on phosphate transport in the proximal convoluted tubule, *Am. J. Physiol.* **249**:F759–F768.

11. Quamme, G. A. and Wong, N. L. M., 1984, Phosphate transport in the proximal convoluted tubule: effect of intraluminal pH, *Am. J. Physiol.* **249:**F323–F333.

12. Hammerman, M. R., Karl, K. A., and Hruska, K. A., 1980, Regulation of canine renal vesicle P_1 transport by growth hormone and parathyroid hormone, *Biochim. Biophys. Acta* **603:**322–335.

13. Schwab, S. J. and Hammerman, M. R., 1986, Electrogenic Na^+-independent P_1 transport in canine renal basolateral membrane vesicle, *Am. J. Physiol.* **250:**F419–F424.

14. Schwab, S. J., Klahr, S., and Hammerman, M. R., 1984, Na^+ gradient-dependent P_1 uptake in basolateral membrane vesicles from dog kidney, *Am. J. Physiol.* **246:**F663–F669.

15. Schwab, S. J., Klahr, S., and Hammerman, M. R., 1984, Uptake of P_1 in basolateral vesicles after release of unilateral ureteral obstruction, *Am. J. Physiol.* **247:**F543–F547.

16. Rabito, C. A., 1986, Sodium cotransport processes in renal epithelial cell lines, *Mineral Electrolyte Metab.* **12:**32–41.

17. Murer, H. and Malmstrom, K., 1987, How renal phosphate transport is regulated, *Int. Union Physiol. Sci, NIPS* **2:**45–48.

18. Hammerman, M. R., 1986, Phosphate transport across renal proximal tubular cell membranes, *Am. J. Physiol.* **251:**F385–398.

19. Hruska, K. A., Moskowitz, D., Esbrit, P., Civitelli, R., Westbrook, S., and Huskey, M., 1987, Stimulation of inositol trisphosphate and diacylglycerol production in renal tubular cells by parathyroid hormone, *J. Clin. Invest.* **79:**230–239.

20. Kempson, S. A. and Dousa, T. P., 1986, Current concepts of regulation of phosphate transport in renal proximal tubules, *Biochem. Pharmacol.* **35:**721–726.

21. Sacktor, B. and Kinsella, J. L., 1986, Hormonal effects on sodium cotransport systems, *Ann. NY Acad. Sci.* **456:**438–444.

22. Biber, J. and Murer, H., 1985, Na-P_1 cotransport in LLC-PK$_1$ cells: Fast adaptive response to P_1 deprivation, *Am. J. Physiol.* **249:**C430–C434.

23. Caverzasio, J., Rizzoli, R., and Bonjour, J. P., 1986, Sodium-dependent phosphate transport inhibited by parathyroid hormone and cyclic AMP stimulation in an opossum kidney cell line, *J. Biol. Chem.* **261:**3233–3237.

24. Malmstrom, K. and Murer, H., 1986, Parathyroid hormone inhibits phosphate transport in OK cells but not in LLC-PK$_1$ and JTC-12.P3 cells, *Am. J. Physiol.* **251:**C23–C31.

25. Bonjour, J-P., Caversazio, J., Muhlbauer, R., Fleisch, H., and Trechsel, U., 1979, Acute and chronic effects of vitamin D metabolites on the renal handling of phosphate, in: *Vitamin D, Basic Research and its Clinical Application* (A. W. Norman, K. Schaefer, D. V. Herrath, H-G. Grigoleit, J. W. Coburn, H. F. DeLuca, E. B. Mawer, and T. Suda, eds.), Walter de Gruyter, New York, pp. 307–314.

26. Kurnik, B. R. C. and Hruska, K. A., 1984, Effects of 1,25-dihydroxy-cholecalciferol on phosphate transport in vitamin D–deprived rats, *Am. J. Physiol.* **247:**F177–F182.

27. Kurnik, B. R. C., Huskey, M., Hagerty, D., and Hruska, K. A., 1986, Vitamin D metabolites stimulate phosphatidycholine transfer to renal brush border membranes, *Biochim. Biophys. Acta* **858:**47–55.

28. Kurnik, B. R. C., Huskey, M., and Hruska, K. A., 1987, 1,25-Dihydroxycholecalciferol stimulates renal phosphate transport by directly altering membrane phosphatidylcholine composition, *Biochim. Biophys. Acta* **917:**81–85.

29. Hruska, K. A., Robert, M., and Avioli, L. V., 1987, Membrane phospholipid (PL) metabolism and phosphate transport in X-linked hypophosphatemia (HYP-Y), *Kidney Int.* **31:**349.

30. Hammerman, M. R. and Chase, L. R., 1983, P_1 transport, phosphorylation, and dephosphorylation in renal membranes from HYP/Y mice, *Am. J. Physiol.* **245:**F701–F706.

31. Mernissi, G. E. and Doucet, A., 1985, Renal sodium transport in vitamin D resistant hypophosphatemic rickets, *Can. J. Physiol. Pharmacol.* **63:**339–1344.

32. Cowgill, L. D., Goldfarb, S., Lau, K., et al., 1979, Evidence foran intrinsic renal tubular defect in mice with genetic hypophosphatemic rickets, *Pflüger's Arch.* **371:**33–38.

33. Isogna, K. L., Broadus, A. E., and Gertner, J. M., 1983, Impaired phosphorus conservation and 1,25 dihydroxyvitamin D generation during phosphorus deprivation in familial hypophosphatemic rickets, *J. Clin. Invest.* **71:**1562–1569.

34. Kinoshita, M. G., Fukase, M., Nakada, M., et al., 1987, Defective adaptation to a low phosphate environment by cultured renal tubular cells from X-linked hypophosphatemic (HYP mice), *Biochem. Biophys. Res. Commun.* **144:**768–769.

35. Brunette, M. G., Allard, S., and Belliveau, R., 1984, Renal brush border membranes from mice with X-linked hypophosphatemia: protein composition, phosphate binding capacity, and protein kinase activity, *Can. J. Physiol. Pharmacol.* **62:**1394–1400.

36. Tenenhouse, H. S. and Henry, H. L., 1985, Protein kinase activity and protein kinase inhibitor in mouse kidney: Effect of the X-linked HYP mutation and vitamin D status, *Endocrinology* **117:** 1719–1726.

37. Nakai, M., Kinoshita, Y., Fukase, M., et al., 1987, Phorbol esters inhibit phosphate uptake in opossum kidney cells: A model for proximal renal tubular cells, *Biochem. Biophys. Res. Commun.* **145:**303–308.

38. Lobaugh, B. and Drezner, M. K., 1983, Abnormal regulation of renal 25-hydroxyvitamin D-1a-hydroxylase activity in the X-linked hypophosphatemic mouse, *J. Clin. Invest.* **71:**400–403.

39. Nesbitt, T., Drezner, M. K., and Lobaugh, B., 1986, Abnormal parathyroid hormone stimulation of 25-hydroxyvitamin D-1a-hydroxylase activity in the hypophosphatemic mouse, *J. Clin. Invest.* **77:**181–187.

40. Kawashima, H. and Kurakowa, K., 1983, Unique hormonal regulation of vitamin D metabolism in the mammalian kidney, *Mineral Elect. Metab.* **9:**227–235.

41. Nesbitt, T., Lobaugh, B., and Drezner, M. K., 1987, Calcitonin stimulation of renal 25-hydroxyvitamin D-1a-hydroxylase activity in hypophosphatemic mice, *J. Clin. Invest.* **79:**15–19.

42. Harrell, R. M., Lyles, K. W., Harrelson, J. M., Friedman, N. E., and Drezner, M. K., 1985, Healing of bone disease in X-linked hypophosphatemic rickets/osteomalacia, *J. Clin. Invest.* **75:** 1858–1868.

43. Polisson, R. P., Martinez, S., Khoury, M., et al., 1985, Calcification of entheses associated with X-linked hypophosphatemic osteomalacia, *N. Engl. J. Med.* **313:**1–6.

44. Tenenhouse, H. S., Yip, A., and Jones, G., 1988, Increased renal catabolism with 1,25 dihydroxy vitamin D_3 in murine X-linked hypophosphatemic rickets, *J. Clin. Invest.* **81:**461–465.

45. Tieder, M., Modai, D., Samual, R., Arie, R., Halabe, A., Bab, I., Gabizon, D., and Liberman, U. A., 1985, Hereditary hypophosphatemic rickets with hypercalciuria, *N. Engl. J. Med.* **312:** 611–617.

46. Tieder, M., Modai, D., Shaked, U., et al., 1987, Idiopathic hypercalciuria and hereditary hypophosphatemic rickets: Two phenotypical expressions of a common genetic defect, *N. Engl. J. Med.* **316:**125–129.

47. Weidner, N. and Santa Cruz, D., 1987, Phosphaturic mesenchymal tumors, *Cancer* **59:**1442–1554.

48. Suva, L. J., Winslow, G. A., Wettenhall, R. E. H., Hammonds, R. G., Moseley, J. M., Diefenback-Jagger, H., Rodda, C. P., Kemp, B. E., Rodriguez, H., Chen, E. Y., Hudson, P. J., Martin, T. J., and Wood, W. I., 1987, A parathyroid hormone-related protein implicated in malignant hypercalcemia: Cloning and expression, *Science* **237:**893–896.

49. Horiuchi, N., Caulfield, M. P., Fisher, J. E., Goldman, M. E., McKee, R. L., Reagan, J. E., Levy, J. J., Nutt, R. F., Rodan, S. B., Schofield, T. L., Clemens, T. L., and Rosenblatt, M., 1987, Similarity of synthetic peptide from human tumor to parathyroid hormone in vivo and in vitro, *Science* **238:**1566–1567.

50. Kemp, B. E., Moseley, J. M., Rodda, C. P., Ebeling, P. R., Wettenhall, R. E. H., Stapleton, D., Diefenbach-Jagger, H., Ure, F., Michelangeli, V. P., Simmons, H. A., Raisz, L. G., and Martin, T. J., 1987, Parathyroid hormone-related protein of malignancy: Active synthetic fragments, *Science* **238:**1568–1570.

51. Strewler, G. J., Stern, P. H., Jacobs, J. W., Eveloff, J., Klein, R. F., Leung, S. C., Rosenblatt, M., and Nissenson, R. A., 1987, Parathyroid hormonelike protein from human renal carcinoma cells: Structural and functional homology with parathyroid hormone, *J. Clin. Invest.* **80:**1803–1807.

52. Reid, I. R., Teitelbaum, S. L., Dusso, A., and Whyte, M. P., 1987, Hypercalcemic hyperparathyroidism complicating oncogenic osteomalacia, *Am. J. Med.* **83:**350–354.

53. Liberman, U. A., Eil, C., and Marx, S. J., 1986, Clinical features of hereditary resistance to 1,25-dihydroxy vitamin D (hereditary hypocalcemic vitamin D resistant rickets type II), *Adv. Exp. Med. Biol.* **196:**391–406.

54. Pike, J. W., Allergretto, E. A., Kelly, M. A., et al., 1986, 1,25-Dihydroxy vitamin D_3 receptors: altered functional domains are associated with cellular resistance to vitamin D_3, *Adv. Exp. Med. Biol.* **196:**377–390.

55. Gamblin, G. T., Liberman, U. A., Eil, C., Downs, R. W. Jr., DeGrange, D. A., and Marx, S. J. 1985, Vitamin D-dependent rickets type II, *J. Clin. Invest.* **75:**954–960.

56. Koren, R., Ravid, A., Liberman, U. A., et al., 1985, Defective binding and function of 1,25-dihydroxyvitamin D_3 receptors in peripheral mononuclear cells of patients with end-organ resistance to 1,25-dihydroxyvitamin D, *J. Clin. Invest.* **76:**2012–2015.

57. Sakati, N., Woodhouse, M. J. Y., Niles, N., et al., 1986, Hereditary resistance to 1,25-dihydroxy vitamin D: Clinical and radiological improvement during high-dose oral calcium therapy, *Hormone Res.* **24:**280–287.

58. Balsan, S., Garabedian, M., Larchet, M., et al., 1986, Long-term nocturnal calcium infusions can cure rickets and promote normal mineralization in hereditary resistance to 1,25-dihydroxyvitamin D, *J. Clin. Invest.* **77:**1661–1667.

59. Wiseman, Y., Bab, I., Gazit, D., et al., 1987, Long-term intracaval calcium infusion therapy in end-organ resistance to 1,25-dihydroxyvitamin D, *Am. J. Med.* **83:**984–990.

60. Bliziotes, M., Yergey, A. L., Nanes, M. S., Muenzer, J., Begley, M. G., Vieira, N. E., Kher, K. K., Brandi, M. L., and Marx, S. J., 1988, Absent intestinal response to calciferols in hereditary resistance to 1,25-dihydroxy vitamin D: Documentation and effective therapy with high dose intravenous calcium infusions, *J. Endocrinol. Metab.* **66:**294–300.

61. Korkor, A. B., 1987, Reduced binding of [^{3}H]1,25-dihydroxy vitamin D_3 in the parathyroid glands of patients with renal failure, *N. Engl. J. Med.* **316:**1573–1577.

62. Slatopolsky, E., Weerts, C., Thielan, J., Horst, R., Harter, H., and Martin, K. J., 1984, Marked suppression of secondary hyperparathyroidism by intravenous administration of 1,25(OH)$_2$D in uremic patients, *J. Clin. Invest.* **74:**2136–2143.

63. Silver, J., Naveh-Many, T., Mayer, H., Schmelzer, H. J., and Popovtzer, M. M., 1986, Regulation by vitamin D metabolites of parathyroid hormone gene transcription *in vivo* in the rat, *J. Clin. Invest.* **78:**1296–1301.

64. Lopez-Hilker, S., Galceran, T., Chan, Y. L., Rapp, N., Martin, K. J., and Slatopolsky, E., 1986, Hypocalcemia may not be essential for the development of secondary hyperparathyroidism in chronic renal failure, *J. Clin. Invest.* **78:**1097–1102.

65. Lucas, P. A., Brown, R. C., Woodhead, J. S., and Coles, G. A., 1986, 1-25 Dihydroxycholecalciferol and parathyroid hormone in advanced chronic renal failure: Effects of simultaneous protein and phosphorus restriction, *Clin. Nephrol.* **25:**7.

66. Schafer, K. and Herrath, D., 1987, The striking effect of ketoacids on the serum phosphate and parathyroid hormone in patients with chronic uremia, *Kidney Int.* **31:**357.

67. Lopez-Hilker, S., Dusso, A., Rapp, N., Galceran, T., Martin, K. J., and Slatopolsky, E., 1986, On the mechanism of the prevention of secondary hyperparathyroidism by phosphate restriction, *Kidney Int.* **29:**164 (Abstract).

68. Aubier, M., Murciano, D., Lecocguic, Y., Viires, N., Jacquens, Y., Squara, P., and Pariente, R., 1985, Effect of hypophosphatemia on diaphragmatic contractility in patients with acute respiratory failure, *N. Engl. J. Med.* **313:**420–424.

69. Lewis, J. F., Hodsman, A. B., Driedger, A. A., Thompson, R. T., and McFadden, R. G., 1987, Hypophosphatemia and respiratory failure: Prolonged abnormal energy metabolism demonstrated by nuclear magnetic resonance spectroscopy, *Am. J. Med.* **83:**1139–1143.

70. Dale, G. and Fleetwood, J. A., 1986, Profound hypophosphatemia in patients collapsing after a "fun run," *Br. Med. J.* **292:**447–448.

71. Zerwekh, J. E., Sanders, L. A., Townsend, J., and Pak, C. Y. C., 1980, Tumoral calcinosis: Evidence for concurrent defects in renal tubular phosphorus transport and in 1a, 25-dihydroxycholecalciferol synthesis, *Calcif. Tissue Int.* **32:**1–6.

72. Mallette, L. E. and Mechanick, J. I., 1987, Heritable syndrome of pseudoxanthoma elasticum with abnormal phosphorus and vitamin D metabolism, *Am. J. Med.* **83**:1157–1162.

73. Whyte, M. P. and Rettinger, S. D., 1987, Hyperphosphatemia due to enhanced renal reclamation of phosphate in hypophosphatasia, *J. Bone Mineral Res.* **2**(1):(Abstract #399).

74. Bourdeau, J. E. and Burg, M. B., 1979, Voltage dependence of calcium transport in the thick ascending limb of Henle's loop, *Am. J. Physiol.* **236**:F357–F364.

75. Bourdeau, J. E. and Burg, M. B., 1980, Effect of PTH on calcium transport across the cortical thick ascending limb of Henle's loop, *Am. J. Physiol.* **239**:F121–F126.

76. Friedman, P. A., 1988, Basal and hormone-activated calcium absorption in mouse renal thick ascending limbs, *Am. J. Physiol.* **254**:F62–F70.

77. Ziyadeh, F. N., Kelepouris, E., and Agus, Z. S., 1986, Relationships between calcium and chloride transport in frog skin glands, *Am. J. Physiol.* **251**:F647–F654.

78. Vick, R. S. and Costanzo, L. S., 1987, *In situ* measurement of ionized Ca concentration ($[CA^{+2}]_1$) in rat distal tubular fluid, Abstracts of the American Society of Nephrology Annual Meeting, abstract #74, p. 204A.

79. Lau, K., Nichols, R., and Tannen, R. L., 1987, Renal excretion of divalent ions in response to chronic acidosis: Evidence that systemic pH is not the controlling variable, *J. Lab. Clin. Med.* **109**: 27–33.

80. Trivedi, B. and Tannen, R. L., 1986, Effect of respiratory acidosis on intracellular pH of the proximal tubule, *Am. J. Physiol.* **250**:F1039.

81. Sutton, R. A. L., Wong, N. L. M., and Dirks, J. H., 1979, Effects of metabolic acidosis and alkalosis on sodium and calcium transport in the dog kidney, *Kidney Int.* **15**:520–533.

82. Bomsztyk, K. and Calalb, M. B., 1987, HCO_3 absorption stimulates calcium absorption in proximal tubule, Abstracts of Xth International Congress of Nephrology, London, p. 416.

83. Kaplan, R. A., Haussler, M. R., Deftos, L. J., Bone, H., and Pak, C. Y. C., 1977, The role of 1,25 dihydroxy cholecalciferol in the mediation of intestinal hyperabsorption of calcium in primary hyperparathyroidism and absorptive hypercalciuria, *J. Clin. Invest.* **59**:756–760.

84. Lemann, J. and Gray, R. W., 1987, Hypercalciuric kidney stone formers exhibit enhanced intestinal calcium absorption (Ca_A) despite only slightly elevated serum 1,25$(OH)_2$-D concentrations, Abstracts of The 20th Annual Meeting of the American Society of Nephrology, Abstract #139, p. 196A.

85. Preminger, G. M. and Pak, C. Y. C., 1987, Eventual attenuation of hypocalciuric response to hydrochlorothiazide in absorptive hypercalciuria, *J. Urol.* **137**:1104–1109.

86. Sutton, R. A. L. and Walker, V., 1986, Bone resorption and hypercalciuria in calcium stoneformers, *Metabolism* **35**:485–488.

87. Pacifici, R., Filipponi, P., Mannarelli, C., Grossi, E., Moretti, I., Tini, S., Carloni, C., Blass, A., Morucci, P., Hruska, K. H., and Avioli, L. V., 1987, Evidence for a prostaglandin mediated resorptive mechanism in fasting hypercalciuria, *J. Bone Mineral Metab.* **2**:(Abstract #397).

88. Costanzo, L. S., Smith, B., and Adler, R. A., 1987, Examination of hypercalciuria in anterior pituitary-implanted rats, *Am. J. Physiol.* **252**:F916–921.

89. Adler, R. A., Costanzo, L. S., and Stauffer, M. E., 1986, Hypercalciuria in hyperprolactinemic rats: Effect of benzthiazide, *Metabolism* **35**:668–672.

90. Sutton, R. A. L., 1986, Renal tubular disorders associated with hypocalciuria, in: *Phosphate and Mineral Homeostasis* (S. G. Marry, M. Olmer, and E. Ritz, eds.), Plenum, New York, pp. 187–192.

91. Rudin, A., Sjogren, B., and Aurell, M., 1984, Low urinary calcium excretion in Barrter's syndrome, *N. Engl. J. Med.* **310**:1190.

92. Mavichak, V., Coppin, C. M. L., Wong, N. L. M., Dirks, J. H., Walker, V., and Sutton, R. A. L., 1988, Renal magnesium wasting and hypocalciuria in chronic *cis*-platinum nephropathy in man, *Clin. Sci.* **75**:203–207.

93. Taufield, P. A., Ales, K. L., Resnick, L. M., Druzin, M. L., Gertner, J. M., and Laragh, J. H., 1987, Hypocalciuria in preeclampsia, *N. Engl. J. Med.* **316**:715–718.

94. Garrett, I. R., Durie, B. G. M., Nedwin, G. E., Gillespie, A., Bringman, T., Sabatini, M.,

Bertolini, D. R., and Mundy, G. R., 1987, Production of lymphotoxin, a bone-resorbing cytokine, by cultured human myeloma cells, *N. Engl. J. Med.* **317**:526–532.

95. Mundy, G. R., 1987, The hypercalcemia of malignancy, *Kidney Int.* **31**:142–155.
96. Stewart, A. F., Horst, R., Deftos, L. J., Cadman, E. C., Lang, R., and Broadus, A. E., 1980, Biochemical evaluation of patients with cancer-associated hypercalcemia. Evidence for humoral and nonhumoral groups, *N. Engl. J. Med.* **303**:1377–1383.
97. Harinck, H. I. J., Bijvoet, O. L. M., Plantingh, A. S. T., Body, J.-J., Elte, J. W. F., Sleeboom, H. P., Wildiers, J., and Neijt, J. P., 1987, Role of bone and kidney in tumor-induced hypercalcemia and its treatment with biphosphonate and sodium chloride, *Am. J. Med.* **82**:1133–1142.
98. van Holten-Verzandvoort, A., Harinck, H. I. J., Hermans, J., Cleton, F. J., and Bijvoet, O. L. M., 1987, Supportive bisphosphonate treatment reduces morbidity from bone lesions in breast cancer, *J. Bone Mineral Metab.* **2**(1): (Abstract #390).
99. LoCascio, V., Adami, S., Galvanini, G., Ferrari, M., Cominacini, L., and Tartarotti, D., 1985, Substrate-product relation of 1-hydroxylase activity in primary hyperparathyroidism, *N. Engl. J. Med.* **313**:1123–1125.
100. Patron, P., Gardin, J-P., and Paillard, M., 1987, Renal mass and reserve of vitamin D: Determinants in primary hyperparathyroidism, *Kidney Int.* **31**:1174–1180.
101. Kleeman, C. R., Norris, K., and Coburn, J. W., 1987, Is the clinical expression of primary hyperparathyroidism a function of the long-term vitamin D status of the patient? *Mineral Electrolyte Metab.* **13**:305–310.
102. Lumb, G. A. and Stanbury, S. W., 1974, Parathyroid function in human vitamin D deficiency and vitamin D deficiency in primary hyperparathyroidism, *Am. J. Med.* **56**:833–839.
103. Clements, M. R., Davies, M., Fraser, D. R., Lumb, G. A., Mawer, E. B., and Adams, P. H., 1987, Metabolic inactivation of vitamin D is enhanced in primary hyperparathyroidism, *Clin. Sci.* **73**:659–664.
104. Gardin, J. P., Patron, P., Fouqueray, B., Prigent, A., and Paillard, M., 1987, Maximal PTH secretory rate and set point for calcium in normal subjects and patients with primary hyperparathyroidism, *Mineral Electrolyte Metab.* **609**:1–8.
105. Jaeger, P., Jones, W., Kashgarian, M., Baron, R., Clemens, T. L., Segre, G. V., and Hayslett, J. P., 1987, Animal model of primary hyperparathyroidism, *Am. J. Physiol.* **252**:E790–E798.
106. Brandi, M. L., Aurbach, G. D., Fitzpatrick, L. A., Quarto, R., Spiegel, A. M., Bliziotes, M. M., Norton, J. A., Doppman, J. L., and Marx, S. J., 1986, Parathyroid mitogenic activity in plasma from patients with familial multiple endocrine neoplasia type 1, *N. Engl. J. Med.* **314**:1287–1293.
107. Schimke, R. N., 1986, Multiple endocrine neoplasia: Search for the oncogenic trigger, *N. Engl. J. Med.* **314**:1315–1316.
108. Fialkow, P. J., Jackson, C. E., Block, M. A., and Greenawald, K. A., 1977, Multicellular origin of parathyroid "adenomas," *N. Engl. J. Med.* **297**:696–698.
109. Arnold, A., Staunton, C. E., Kim, H. G., Gaz, R. D., and Kronenberg, H. M., 1988, Monoclonality and abnormal parathyroid hormone genes in parathyroid adenomas, *N. Engl. J. Med.* **318**:658–662.
110. Kane-Johnson, N., Strasik, L., and Orwoll, E. S., 1987, Dissociation of secretory responses to low-calcium and β-adrenergic stimulation in primary hyperparathyroidism, *Metabolism* **36**:580–584.
111. Tiegs, R. D., Body, J. J., Barta, J. M., and Hunter, H. III, 1986, Plasma calcitonin in primary hyperparathyroidism: Failure of C-cell response to substantial hypercalcemia, *J. Clin. Endocrinol. Metab.* **63**:785–788.
112. Palmer, M., Berstrom, R., Akerstrom, G., Adami, H-O., Jakobsson, S., and Ljunghall, S., 1987, Survival and renal function in untreated hypercalcaemia, *Lancet* **1**:59–62.
113. Winzelberg, G. G., 1987, Parathyroid imaging, *Ann. Intern. Med.* **107**:64–70.
114. Clair, F., Leenhardt, L., Bourdeau, A., Zingraff, J., Robert, D., Dubost, C., Sachs, E. F., and Drueke, T., 1987, Effect of calcitriol in the control of plasma calcium after parathyroidectomy, *Nephron* **46**:18–22.

115. Fellner, S. K. and Spargo, B. H., 1987, Nephrotic syndrome from hypercalcemia in a patient with primary hyperparathyroidism, *Am. J. Med.* **83**:355–358.

116. Singer, F. R. and Adams, J. S., 1986, Abnormal calcium homeostasis in sarcoidosis, *N. Engl. J. Med.* **315**:755–757 (Editorial).

117. Hunt, B. J. and Yendt, E. R., 1963, The response of hypercalcemia in sarcoidosis to chloroquine, *Ann. Intern. Med.* **59**:554–64.

118. O'Leary, T. J., Jones, G., Yip, A., Lohnes, D., Cohanim, M., and Yendt, E. R., 1986, The effects of chloroquine on serum 1,25-dihydroxyvitamin D and calcium metabolism in sarcoidosis, *N. Engl. J. Med.* **315**:727–730.

119. Barre, P. E., Gascon-Barre, M., Meakins, J. L., and Goltzman, D., 1987, Hydroxychloroquine treatment of hypercalcemia in a patient with sarcoidosis undergoing hemodialysis, *Am. J. Med.* **82**:1259–1262.

120. Hoffman, V. N. and Korzenkowski, O. M., 1986, Leprosy, hypercalcemia, and elevated serum calcitriol levels, *Ann. Intern. Med.* **105**:890–891.

121. Ryzen, E. and Singer, F. R., 1985, Hypercalcemia in leprosy, *Arch. Intern. Med.* **145**:1305–1306.

122. Felsenfeld, A. J., Drezner, M. K., and Llach, F., 1986, Hypercalcemia and elevated calcitriol in a maintenance dialysis patient with tuberculosis, *Arch. Intern. Med.* **166**:941–945.

123. Mercier, R. J., Thompson, J. M., Harmon, G. S., and Messerschmidt, G. L., 1988, Recurrent hypercalcemia and elevated 1,25-dihydroxyvitamin D levels in Hodgkin's disease, *Am. J. Med.* **84**:165–168.

124. Grote, T. H. and Hainsworth, J. D., 1987, Hypercalcemia and elevated serum calcitriol in a patient with seminoma, *Arch. Intern. Med.* **147**:221–222.

125. Gerhardt, A., Greenberg, A., Reilly, J. J., Jr., and Van Thiel, D. H., 1987, Hypercalcemia, a complication of advanced chronic liver disease, *Arch. Intern. Med.* **147**:274–277.

126. McPherson, M. L., Prince, S. R., Atamer, E. R., Maxwell, D. B., Ross-Clunis, H., and Estep, H. L., 1986, Theophylline-induced hypercalcemia, *Ann. Intern. Med.* **105**:52–54.

127. Payne, R. B., Jones, D. P., Walker, A. P., and Evans, R. T., 1986, Clustering of serum and magnesium concentrations in siblings, *Clin. Chem.* **32**:349–350.

128. Bannister, P., Sheridan, P., Dibble, J., and Payne, R. B., 1986, Benign hypercalcemia and "benign hypocalcemia" in the same family, *Ann. Intern. Med.* **105**:217–219.

129. Kafsner, P., Langsdorf, L., Marcus, R., Kraemer, F. B., and Hoffman, A. R., 1986, Milk–alkali syndrome in patients treated with calcium carbonate after cardiac transplantation, *Arch. Intern. Med.* **146**:1965–1969.

130. Mallette, L. E. and Eichhorn, E., 1986, Effects of lithium carbonate on human calcium metabolism, *Arch. Intern. Med.* **146**:770–776.

131. Sutton, R. A. L. and Cameron, E. C., 1987, Mineral Metabolism, in: *Contemporary Nephrology* (S. Klahr and S. G. Massry, eds.), Plenum Press, New York, pp. 219–282.

132. Hirschel-Scholz, S., Caverzasio, J., Rizzoli, R., and Bonjour, J. P., 1986, Normalization of hypercalcemia associated with a decrease in renal calcium absorption in Leydig cell tumor-bearing rats treated with WR-2721, *J. Clin. Invest.* **78**:319–322.

133. Warrell, R. P., Issacs, M., Alcock, N. W., and Bockman, R. S., 1987, Gallium nitrate for treatment of refractory hypercalcemia from parathyroid carcinoma, *Ann. Intern. Med.* **107**:683–686.

134. Warrell, R. P. Jr., Bockman, R. S., Coonley, C. J., Isaacs, M., and Staszewski, H., 1984, Gallium nitrate inhibits calcium resorption from bone and is effective treatment for cancer-related hypercalcemia, *J. Clin. Invest.* **73**:1487–1490.

135. Nolten, W. E., Chesney, R. W., Dabbagh, S., Lemann, J. Jr., Slatopolsky, E., Klingensmith, G. J., and DeLuca, H. F., 1987, Moderate hypocalcemia due to normal serum 1,25-dihydroxy vitamin D levels in an asymptomatic kindred with familial hypoparathyroidism, *Am. J. Med.* **82**:1157–1166.

136. Stewart, A. F., Longo, W., Kreutter, D., Jacob, R., and Burtis, W. J., 1986, Hypocalcemia

associated with calcium–soap formation in a patient with a pancreatic fistula, *N. Engl. J. Med.* **315**:496–498.

137. Zaloga, G. P. and Chernow, B., 1987, The multifactorial basis for hypocalcemia during sepsis: Studies of the parathyroid hormone-vitamin D axis, *Ann. Intern. Med.* **107**:36–41.

138. Aderka, D., Schwartz, D., Dan, M., and Levo, Y., 1987, Bacteremic hypocalcemia: A comparison between the calcium levels of bacteremic and nonbacteremic patients with infection, *Arch. Intern. Med.* **147**:232–236.

139. Zaloga, G. P., Willey, S., Tomasic, P., and Chernow, B., 1987, Free fatty acids alter calcium binding: A cause for misinterpretation of serum calcium values and hypocalcemia in critical illness, *J. Clin. Endocrinol. Metab.* **64**:1010–1014.

140. Schenkein, D. P., O'Neill, W. C., Shapiro, J., and Miller, K. B., 1986, Accelerated bone formation causing profound hypocalcemia in acute leukemia, *Ann. Intern. Med.* **105**:375–378.

141. Breslau, N. E. and Zerwekh, J. E., 1986, Relationship of estrogen and pregnancy to calcium homeostasis in pseudohypoparathyroidism, *J. Clin. Endocrinol. Metab.* **62**:45–51.

142. Farfel, Z. V. I. and Friedman, E., 1986, Mental deficiency in pseudohypoparathyroidism type IIs associated with Ns–protein deficiency, *Ann. Intern. Med.* **105**:197–199.

143. Kurokawa, K., 1987, Calcium-regulating hormones and the kidney, *Kidney Int.* **32**:760–771.

144. Kumar, R., 1986, The metabolism and mechanism of action of 1,25-dihydroxyvitamin D_3, *Kidney Int.* **30**:793–803.

145. Holick, M. F., 1987, Vitamin D and the kidney, *Kidney Int.* **32**:912–929.

146. Matsuoka, L. Y., Ide, L., Wortsman, J., MacLaughlin, J. A., and Holick, M. F., 1987, Sunscreens suppress cutaneous vitamin D_3 synthesis, *J. Clin. Endocrinol. Metab.* **64**(6):1165–1168.

147. Lo, C. W., Paris, P. W., and Holick, M. F., 1986, Indian and Pakistani immigrants have the same capacity as Caucasians to produce vitamin D in response to ultraviolet irradiation, *Am. J. Clin. Nutr.* **44**:683–685.

148. Matsuoka, L. Y., Wortsman, J., and Hollis, B. W., 1988, Lack of effect of exogenous calcitriol on the cutaneous production of vitamin D_3, *J. Endocrinol. Metab.* **66**(2):451.

149. Harper, K., McLeod, J. F., Kowalski, M. A., and Haddad, J. G., 1987, Vitamin D binding protein sequesters monomeric actin in the circulation of the rat, *J. Clin. Invest.* **79**:1365–1370.

150. Young, W. O., Goldschmidt-Clermont, P. J., Emerson, D. L., Lee, W. M., Jollow, D. J., and Galbraith, R. M., 1987, Correlation between extent of liver damage in fulminant hepatic necrosis and complexing of circulating group-specific component (vitamin D–binding protein), *J. Lab. Clin. Med.* **110**:83–90.

151. Bikle, D. D., Halloran, B. P., Gee, E., Ryzen, E., and Haddad, J. G., 1986, Free 25-hydroxyvitamin D levels are normal in subjects with liver disease and reduced total 25-hydroxy vitamin D levels, *J. Clin. Invest.* **78**:748–752.

152. McLeod, J. F., Kowalski, M. A., and Haddad, J. G., 1986, Characterization of a monoclonal antibody to human serum vitamin D binding protein (Gc globulin): Recognition of an epitope hidden in membranes of circulating monocytes, *Endocrinology* **119**:77–83.

153. Nestler, J. E., McLeod, J. F., Kowalski, M. A., Strauss, J. F. III, and Haddad, J. G., Jr., 1987, Detection of vitamin D binding protein on the surface of cytotrophoblasts isolated from human placentae, *Endocrinology* **120**:1996–2002.

154. Halloran, B., Bikle, D. D., Levens, M. J., Castro, M. E., Globus, R. K., and Holton, E., 1986, Chronic 1,25-dihydroxyvitamin D_3 administration in the rat reduces the serum concentration of 25-hydroxyvitamin D by increasing metabolic clearance rate, *J. Clin. Invest.* **78**:622–628.

155. Haddad, P., Gascon-Barre, M., Braùlt, G., and Piourde, V., 1986, Influence of calcium or 1,25-dihydroxyvitamin D_3 supplementation on the hepatic microsomal and *in vivo* metabolism of vitamin D_3 in vitamin D–depleted rats, *J. Clin. Invest.* **78**:1529–1537.

156. Portale, A. A., Halloran, B. P., Murphy, M. M., and Morris, R. C. Jr., 1986, Oral intake of phosphorus can determine the serum concentration of 1,25-dihydroxyvitamin D by determining its production rate in humans, *J. Clin. Invest.* **77**:7–12.

157. Wortsman, J., Haddad, J. G., Posillico, J. T., and Brown, E. M., 1986, Primary hyper-

parathyroidism with low serum 1,25-dihydroxyvitamin D levels, *J. Clin. Endocrinol. Metab.* **62:** 1305–1308.

158. Jaeger, P., Jones, W., Clemens, T. L., and Hayslett, J. P., 1986, Evidence that calcitonin stimulates 1,25-dihydroxyvitamin D production and intestinal absorption of calcium in vitro, *J. Clin. Invest.* **78:**456–461.

159. Bouillon, R. A., Auwerx, J. H., Lissens, W. D., and Pelemans, W. K., 1987, Vitamin D status in the elderly: Seasonal substrate deficiency causes 1,25-dihydroxycholecalciferol deficiency, *Am. J. Clin. Nutr.* **45:**755–63.

160. Lips, P., van Ginkel, F. C., Jongen, M. J. M., Rubertus, F., van der Vijgh, W. J. F., and Netelenbos, J. J. C., 1987, Determinants of vitamin D status in patients with hip fracture and in elderly control subjects, *Am. J. Clin. Nutr.* **46:**1005–1010.

161. Clemens, T. L., Zhou, X-Y., Myles, M., Endres, D., and Lindsay, R., 1986, Serum vitamin D_2 and vitamin D_3 metabolite concentrations and absorption of vitamin D_2 in elderly subjects, *J. Clin. Endocrinol. Metab.* **63:**656–660.

162. Dandona, M., Menon, R. K., Shenoy, R., Houlder, S., Thomas, M., and Mallinson, J. W., 1986, Low 1,25-dihydroxyvitamin D, secondary hyperparathyroidism, and normal osteocalcin in elderly subjects, *J. Clin. Endocrinol. Metab.* **63:**459.

163. Glass, A. R. and Eil, C., 1986, Ketoconazole-induced reduction in serum 1,25-dihydroxyvitamin D, *J. Clin. Endocrinol. Metab.* **63:**766.

164. Krabbe, S., Hummer, L., and Christiansen, C., 1986, Serum levels of vitamin D metabolites and testosterone in male puberty, *J. Clin. Endocrinol. Metab.* **62:**503–507.

165. Netelenbos, J. C., Asscheman, H., Lips, P., van der Vijgh, W. J. F., Jongen, M. J. M., van Ginkel, F., and Hackeng, W. H. L., 1986, Absence of effect of 24,25-dihydroxyvitamin D_3 in primary hyperparathyroidism, *J. Clin. Endocrinol. Metab.* **63:**246.

166. Lidor, C., Dekel, S., and Edelstein, S., 1987, The metabolism of vitamin D_3 during fracture healing in chicks, *Endocrinology* **120:**389–393.

167. Insogna, K. L., Dreyer, B. E., Mitnick, M., Ellison, A. F., and Broadus, A. E., 1988, Enhanced production rate of 1,25-dihydroxyvitamin D in sarcoidosis, *J. Clin. Endocrinol. Metab.* **66:**72–76.

168. Reichel, H., Koeffler, H. P., Barbers, R., and Norman, A. W., 1987, Regulation of 1,25-dihydroxyvitamin D_3 production by cultured alveolar macrophages from normal human donors and from patients with pulmonary sarcoidosis, *J. Clin. Endocrinol. Metab.* **65:**1201–1209.

169. Reichel, H., Koeffler, H. P., and Norman, A. W., 1987, 25-Hydroxyvitamin D_3 metabolism by human T-lymphotropic virus–transformed lymphocytes, *J. Clin. Endocrinol. Metab.* **65:**519.

170. Sugimoto, T., Ritter, C., Ried, I., Morrissey, J., and Slatopolsky, E., 1988, Effect of 1,25-dihydroxyvitamin D_3 on cytosolic calcium in dispersed parathyroid cells, *Kidney Int.* **33:** 850–854.

171. Merke, J., Hugel, U., Zlotkowski, A., Szabo, A., Bommer, J., Mall, G., and Ritz, E., 1987, Diminished parathyroid $1,25(OH)_2D_3$ receptors in experimental uremia, *Kidney Int.* **32:**350–353.

172. Feinfeld, D. A. and Sherwood, L. M., 1988, Parathyroid hormone and $1,25(OH)_2D_3$ in chronic renal failure, *Kidney Int.* **33:**1049–1058.

173. Turner, C., Compston, J., Mak, R. H. K., Vedi, S., Mellish, R. W. E., Haycock, G. B., and Chantler, C., 1988, Bone turnover and 1,25-dihydroxycholecalciferol during treatment with phosphate binders, *Kidney Int.* **33:**989–995.

174. Merke, J., Ritz, E., and Boland, R., 1986, Are recent findings on 1,25-dihydroxycholecalciferol metabolism relevant for the pathogenesis of uremia? *Nephron* **42:**277–284.

175. Sherrard, D. J., 1986, Aluminum and renal osteodystrophy, *Nephrology* **6(4):**5–11.

176. Merke, J., Lucas, P. A., Szabo, A., Helbing, F., Hugel, U., Drueke, T., and Ritz, E., 1987, $1,25(OH)_2D_3$ receptors and endorgan response in experimental aluminum intoxication, *Kidney Int.* **32:**204–211.

177. Geven, W. B., Monnens, L. A., Williams, H. L., Buijs, W. C., and ter Haar, B. G., 1987, Renal magnesium wasting in two families with autosomal dominant inheritance, *Kidney Int.* **31:**1140–1144.

178. Gitelman, H. J., Graham, J. B., and Welt, L. G., 1966, A new familial disorder characterized by hypokalemia and hypomagnesemia, *Trans. Assoc. Am. Physicians* **79**:221.

179. Barton, C. H., Vaziri, N. D., Martin, D. C., Choi, S., and Alikhani, S., 1987, Hypomagnesemia and renal magnesium wasting in renal transplant recipients receiving cyclosporine, *Am. J. Med.* **83**:693–699.

180. June, C. H., Thompson, C. B., Kennedy, M. S., Nims, J., and Thomas, E. C., 1985, Profound hypomagnesemia and renal magnesium wasting associated with the use of cyclosporine for marrow transplantation, *Transplantation* **39**:620–624.

181. June, C. H., Thompson, C. B., Kennedy, M. S., Loughran, J. P. Jr., and Deeg, H. J., 1986, Correlation of hypomagnesemia with the onset of cyclosporine-associated hypertension in marrow transplant patients, *Transplantation* **41**:47–51.

182. Fukomoto, S., Matsumoto, T., Tanaka, Y., Harada, S-I., and Ogata, E., 1987, Renal magnesium wasting in a patient with short bowel syndrome with magnesium deficiency: Effect of 1-hydroxyvitamin D_3 treatment, *J. Clin. Endocrinol. Metab.* **65**:1301–1304.

183. Rude, R. K., Adams, J. S., Ryzen, E., Endres, D. B., Niimi, H., Horst, R. L., Haddad, J. G., and Singer, F. R., 1985, Low serum concentrations of 1,25-dihydroxyvitamin D in human magnesium deficiency, *J. Clin. Endocrinol. Metab.* **61**:933–940.

184. Graber, M. L. and Schulman, G., 1986, Hypomagnesemic hypocalcemia independent of parathyroid hormone, *Ann. Intern. Med.* **104**:804–805.

6

Sodium, Calcium, and Neurogenic Factors in the Pathogenesis of Essential Hypertension

Vito M. Campese

1. Introduction

In recent years a great deal of interest has been focused on the role of sodium and calcium in the pathogenesis of hypertension. Whereas the evidence linking sodium ingestion to the genesis of hypertension in both humans and experimental animals is sufficiently convincing, serious doubts still remain as to whether abnormalities of calcium metabolism are important and, more specifically, whether reduced calcium intake and/or increased urinary calcium loss is important in the genesis of hypertension.

Since the abnormalities in calcium metabolism are more evident in salt-sensitive patients with essential hypertension, it is possible that these may be secondary to the alterations in sodium metabolism rather than primary.

In this chapter we will first deal with the evidence supporting a role of sodium in the genesis of hypertension; subsequently, we will review the controversy relating abnormalities of calcium metabolism to the pathogenesis of hypertension; final-

VITO M. CAMPESE • Division of Nephrology, LAC/USC Medical Center, Los Angeles, California 90033.

ly, we will show evidence that the abnormalities of calcium metabolism may be secondary to a defect in sodium-linked cellular calcium transport.

2. Salt and Hypertension

2.1. Epidemiologic Studies

Several epidemiologic studies suggest a relationship between dietary sodium intake and prevalence of hypertension.[1-14] Most studies of individuals within populations do not show a causal relationship.[7,15-17] These surveys are usually hampered by the small number of individuals studied, by the limited range of sodium intake, and by the large day-to-day variation in sodium intake. Within population studies of communities in which there is a larger range of salt intake, such as in Japan,[18] Korea,[15] and India,[19] a direct relationship has been observed between 24-hr urinary sodium excretion and blood pressure.

A more consistent relationship between dietary sodium intake and prevalence of hypertension has been observed in cross-sectional studies of isolated populations.[1-14] People in North America, Europe, Japan, or China, who have much higher taste for salt and availability of salt, have a greater prevalence of hypertension than populations in remote areas who do not have easy access to salt. In these unacculturated populations blood pressure also does not increase with advancing age.[20,21] When some of these people leave their villages and migrate to more acculturated regions, where the dietary sodium intake is greater, they begin eating more salt and the prevalence of hypertension increases among them.

Page et al.[2] described nomadic groups of primitive people, lean and hardworking but with high dietary sodium intake, who displayed a high prevalence of hypertension. More recently, the Intersalt Study has evaluated 10,079 men and women aged 20–59, sampled from 52 centers around the world following a highly standardized protocol.[22] Sodium excretion in these studies ranged from 0.2 mmol (Yano Mamo Indians in Brazil) to 242 mmol (North China). This study found a significant positive relationship between 24-hr urinary sodium excretion and blood pressure (both systolic and diastolic) and between individual urinary Na/K ratio and blood pressure, even when age, body mass index, and alcohol consumption were taken into account. This study also showed an inverse relationship between potassium excretion and blood pressure.

Further support for the notion of a causal relationship between sodium intake and hypertension derives from intervention studies. When subjects from African rural tribes migrate to cities, their sodium intake rises along with their blood pressure.[22] When Samburu people accustomed to low dietary sodium intake were drafted into the army of Kenya and given a diet containing a daily sodium intake of 18 g, their blood pressure increased.[23] Sodium restriction to a level of 60–90 mmol/day lowers blood pressure in a large number of hypertensive patients. The degree of fall in blood pressure observed after sodium restriction is directly related to pretreatment

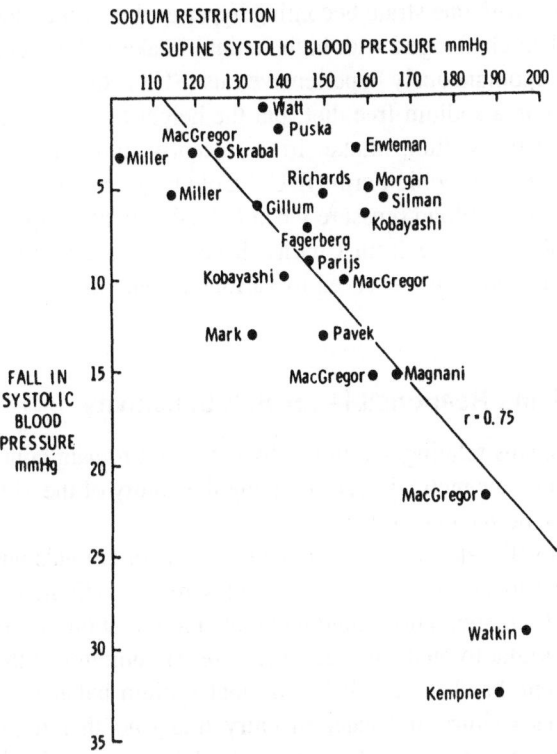

Fig. 1. Relationship between baseline systolic blood pressure and fall in systolic blood pressure following sodium restriction. (Reproduced from Ref. 24, with permission.)

levels of blood pressure: The greater the baseline blood pressure, the greater the fall in blood pressure (Fig. 1).[24]

In Japan, after reeducational campaigns between 1971 and 1981, the daily sodium consumption has fallen from 14.5 to 12.5 g. This has been associated with decreased prevalence of hypertension and of cerebrovascular accidents.[25] Similar results have been obtained in Belgium.[26]

2.2. Salt Sensitivity and Salt Resistance

Several studies have shown that not all hypertensive patients are susceptible to high dietary sodium intake. Kawasaki *et al.* classified patients with hypertension as "salt-sensitive" or "non-salt-sensitive" based on their blood pressure response to high dietary sodium intake.[27] We also found that approximately 60% of patients with essential hypertension respond to a high dietary sodium load with a rise in blood pressure equal to or greater than 10%, whereas blood pressure remained unchanged in the remaining subjects.[28]

Certain strains of rats mimic the response in humans. Dahl selectively inbred two strains of rats, with one strain becoming hypertensive, while the other remained normotensive when challenged with high sodium intake.[29] Less clear is the role of sodium intake in spontaneously hypertensive rats (SHR). In these animals hypertension can develop on a sodium-free diet, but the height to which the blood pressure rises is related to the sodium intake. More recently, however, Chen et al. have shown that SHR from Taconic Farm (IBU 3 Colony, Germantown, NY) displayed significant increases in blood pressure when fed a diet containing 8% NaCl. On the other hand, SHR purchased from Charles River were salt-resistant.[30] Thus, salt sensitivity is a phenomenon observed to various extents in several species.

2.3. Mechanisms Responsible for Salt Sensitivity

The mechanisms relating sodium to hypertension remain controversial. It has been postulated that a genetic defect involving the ability of the kidney to excrete a sodium load may be responsible.

According to Blaustein,[31] when human subjects or animals with this susceptibility are exposed to dietary sodium intake they retain sodium, which leads to an increase in blood volume. This would stimulate the secretion of a natriuretic factor with properties similar to ouabain, and, therefore, an inhibitor of the sodium pump. This factor, on one hand, reestablishes normal sodium balance, but on the other hand, it enhances sodium and calcium entry into smooth muscle cells, thereby increasing vascular contraction. The enhanced calcium penetration into sympathetic nerve terminals would also stimulate norepinephrine release and generate alterations in sodium content in red and white blood cells.

Several lines of evidence support this contention. First, isolated kidneys from Dahl's salt-sensitive prehypertensive rats excrete much less sodium than kidneys from resistant rats.[32] Second, renal cross-transplant studies in three different strains of genetically hypertensive rats have shown that hypertension is transferred with the "hypertensive kidney."[33-35] Third, normotensive siblings of hypertensive patients display a delayed excretion of an acute salt load.[36] Fourth, weanling SHR rats excrete less sodium than WKY controls despite similar sodium intakes[37]; in adult SHR, however, the ability to excrete sodium and water is diminished[38] or unaltered.[39] Fifth, Na^+,K^+-ATPase activity was higher in 5-week-old SHR than in WKY, but not in 16-week-old adult animals.[40]

Helmer[41] has suggested that the susceptibility to sodium in blacks may be related to the fact that this race, during its evolution in Africa, lived in a hot climate while the dietary sodium intake was very low. Thus, blacks have developed highly effective renal mechanisms to retain sodium. When blacks were relocated to America, their sodium intake increased while the renal mechanisms for avid sodium retention were still effective. This may have led to sodium retention and hypertension.

On the other hand, direct and indirect evidence is available to suggest that the changes in renal sodium handling in hypertension may be a consequence rather than the cause of hypertension and may be dependent on increased sympathetic activity.

According to Guyton et al., any rise in blood pressure to be sustained for a prolonged period of time requires an adaptation of the renal mechanisms for sodium handling.[42] Therefore, the change of the renal function curve could be the consequence rather than the cause of hypertension. The best demonstration in favor of this concept derives from the study of Kimura et al.[43] of two hypertensive patients with surgically correctable hypertension, one with primary aldosteronism and the other with renovascular hypertension. These investigators showed that the abnormality of the renal function curve normalized in both patients after surgery. Moreover, the slope of the renal function curve was different depending on the etiology of hypertension.

This confirms the previous observations of Guyton et al. that the renal function curves, i.e., the relationship between pressure and natriuresis, is different depending on the etiology of hypertension and the slope of this relationship tends to be flat in diseases, such as primary aldosteronism, characterized by a tendency to sodium retention.

A variety of renal intrinsic and extrinsic factors can alter the renal function curve.[44] Among the intrinsic factors are an increase in renal vascular resistance, a change in glomerular filtration coefficient, an increase in renal tubular reabsorption of sodium, and a reduction of the renal mass. Among the extrinsic factors the renin–angiotension–aldosterone and the sympathetic nervous systems are probably the most important. Both these extrinsic factors can modify the renal vascular resistance, the glomerular filtration coefficient, and the renal tubular sodium reabsorption.

We have studied the renal function curve in normal subjects, in salt-resistant, and in salt-sensitive subjects and found that the renal function curve is different in these groups of hypertensive patients, suggesting different pathogenetic mechanisms (Fig. 2).[45] In salt-resistant patients, the renal function curve is shifted to the right but it remains parallel to that of normal subjects. On the other hand, the slope of the renal function curve tends to be flat in salt-sensitive patients. In salt-resistant hypertensive patients, the shift to the right of the renal function curve could be related to an increase in renal tubular sodium reabsorption. Some investigators believe that this defect is congenital, whereas other evidence indicates that this defect may be due to extrinsic factors.

It seems unlikely that the enhanced renal tubular sodium reabsorption in salt-sensitive patients is related to increased activity of the renin–angiotensin–aldosterone system, since the plasma renin activity is usually lower in salt-sensitive patients during low-sodium diet compared with salt-resistant or normal subjects.[27,28] No difference in plasma renin activity (PRA) was present among the three groups during high dietary sodium intake. Some investigators, however, have postulated that salt sensitivity may be related to a defect of modulation of renin release and renal vascular tone.[46,47]

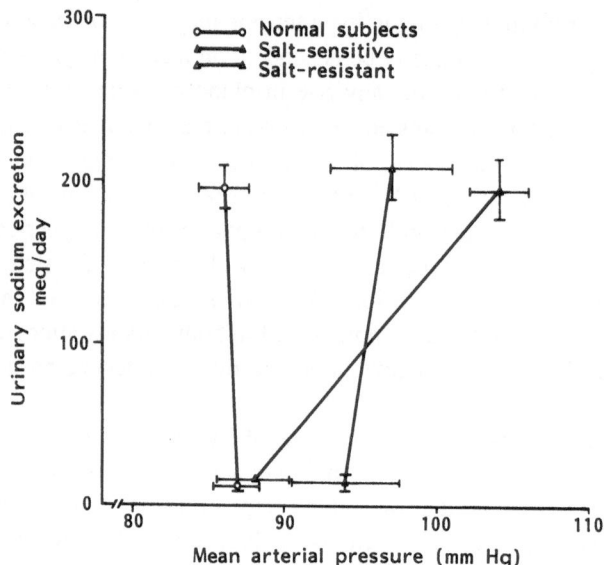

Fig. 2. The renal function curve in normal subjects, salt-resistant, and salt-sensitive patients with essential hypertension. (Reproduced from Ref. 45, with permission.)

Ample evidence is available to suggest that this defect may be related to enhanced activity of the sympathetic nervous system in response to high dietary sodium intake. During ingestion of a high-sodium diet, blood levels of norepinephrine (NE), epinephrine, and dopamine were suppressed in normal subjects, so that an inverse relationship between urinary sodium excretion and plasma levels of these amines was evident.[48] In patients with essential hypertension, this inverse relationship was not present.[28] Plasma NE levels were not different among normal subjects, or salt-resistant or salt-sensitive patients while ingesting a low-sodium diet. However, during high sodium intake, plasma NE concentration decreased significantly in normal and in salt-resistant subjects, but not in salt-sensitive patients. On the contrary, plasma NE during high sodium intake increased in the majority of patients (Fig. 3). A significant correlation was found between the changes in plasma NE and the changes in blood pressure observed during the two diets (Fig. 4). The orthostatic increments of plasma NE were also greater in salt-sensitive patients. The NE release decreased in salt-resistant but it increased in salt-sensitive patients during high sodium intake.[49] Forearm blood flow, measured by plethysmography, fell in salt-sensitive patients and increased in salt-resistant subjects during high sodium intake. These data suggest an abnormal response of the sympathetic nervous system to high sodium intake as a potential pathogenetic factor in the genesis of hypertension in a subset of patients with essential hypertension.

The increased sympathetic activity during high sodium intake may inhibit renal tubular sodium excretion and cause sodium retention and a shift of the renal func-

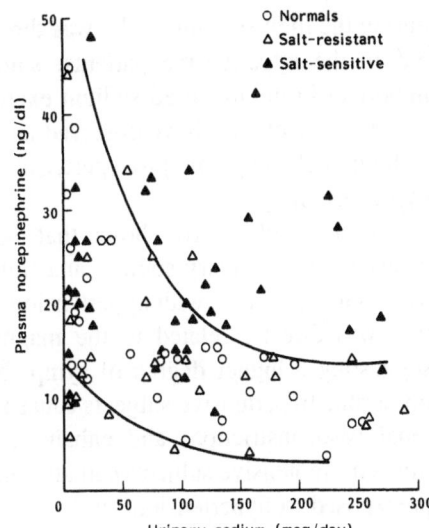

Fig. 3. Plasma norepinephrine levels in normal subjects, salt-resistant, and salt-sensitive patients with essential hypertension during low (10 meq/day) and high (200 meq/day) sodium intake. (Reproduced from Ref. 28, with permission.)

tion curve contributing to the maintenance of hypertension. Support for this concept derives from several studies in humans and animals.

Gill et al.[50] have shown that salt-sensitive subjects retain more sodium than normals and have higher plasma NE levels during high dietary sodium intake; they also observed that urinary dopamine did not increase normally in salt-sensitive patients when they were fed a high-sodium diet. The cumulative sodium retention

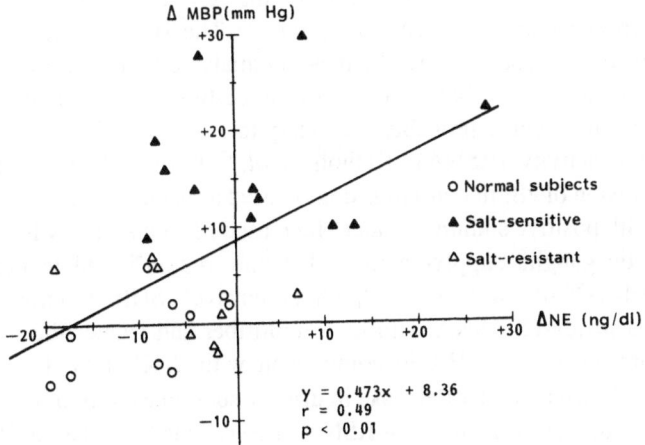

Fig. 4. Relationship between the changes in plasma norepinephrine (NE) levels and the changes in mean blood pressure observed when normal subjects or patients with essential hypertension ingest high sodium intake.

during the high sodium intake was directly related to the percent change in plasma NE in the hypertensive patients, suggesting that renal adrenergic activity was important in the impaired sodium excretion in the salt-sensitive patients.

Falkner et al.[51] have observed an abnormal sympathetic response during high sodium intake in young prehypertensive adolescents with a strong family history of hypertension.

Light et al.[52] have shown that exposure to competitive mental tasks significantly reduced urinary sodium and fluid excretion in young men with one or two hypertensive parents with hypertension. In this high-risk group, the degree of retention was directly related to the magnitude of heart rate increase during stress, suggesting a higher degree of sympathetic activation. Dietary sodium loading in borderline hypertensive subjects caused a greater fall in renal blood flow, enhanced renal vasoconstriction, and enhanced water retention during upright posture.[53] Some normotensive subjects can also display salt sensitivity, particularly if they are preexposed to hypertension.[54,55]

Skrabal et al.[54] studied the effects of moderate salt restriction in 52 male subjects aged 20–25 years with or without a family history of hypertension. They observed that subjects with a family history of hypertension were more likely to respond to sodium restriction with a significant fall in blood pressure. Salt-sensitive subjects also displayed increased pressure response to infused norepinephrine. Na,K-ATPase activity and Na–K cotransport of erythrocytes were not different between these two groups. Salt-sensitive subjects also displayed enhanced uric acid reabsorption during low-sodium diet, an indirect evidence of enhanced proximal tubular salt and water reabsorption.

Abnormalities in the relationship between sodium intake and adrenergic activity similar to those observed in humans have been observed in animal experiments. Continuous electrical stimulation of the left stellate ganglion for 7 days produced hypertension in the conscious dog.[56] The rise in blood pressure was abolished by phenoxybenzamine. In these animals sodium excretion did not increase despite the rise in blood pressure, suggesting a shift to the right of the pressure–natriuresis curve probably secondary to an increase in efferent renal sympathetic nerve activity (RSNA). Katholi et al.[57] have also shown that chronic intrarenal infusion of NE in conscious dogs caused a sustained rise in blood pressure associated with positive sodium balance. Increased nervous activity has been shown in sympathetic ganglia supplying the splanchnic region[58] and in postganglionic splanchnic fibers[59] of anesthetized ''prehypertensive'' SHR. Lundin et al.[60] have demonstrated increased RSNA with both multifiber and single fiber recordings in conscious unanesthetized SHR in comparison with WKY rats. Koepke and Di-Bona[61] have shown a greater decrease in urinary sodium excretion in concomitance with a more pronounced increase in RSNA in conscious SHR than in WKY. Renal denervation resulted in a delay of the onset of hypertension and attenuated the severity of established hypertension in SHR; this occurred concomitantly with a decrease in fractional reabsorption of sodium.[62] Lundin et al.[60] observed that SHR during air stress displayed an exaggerated decrease in urinary sodium excretion in association with a more pronounced rise in RSNA, without any alteration of effective renal blood flow (RBF) or glomerular filtration rate. The exaggerated sodium retention during stress was abolished by prior renal denervation. Recently, Ricksten et al.[63] have shown that the exaggerated natriuresis in response to intravenous infusion of isotonic saline in SHR was associated with an exaggerated inhibition of RSNA modulated via activation of cardiopulmonary baroreceptor reflexes. Even in the DOCA–salt hypertension, a classic model of salt-induced hypertension, renal denervation delayed the development of hypertension when performed prior to the start of DOCA–salt treatment and attenuated the degree of hypertension when performed in rats already treated with DOCA–salt for 3 weeks.[64] The decrease in blood pressure was associated with increased natriuresis.

All these data support the concept that increased RSNA may play an important role in the maintenance of several forms of experimental hypertension by shifting the pressure–natriuresis curve to the right, thus causing sodium retention. The efferent RSNA, however, appears to play no role in SHR or DOCA–salt hypertensive rats when the hypertension is well established.[64] Other factors, such as changes in the anatomic structure of the renal vascular bed, may become more important in far-advanced phases of hypertension. The development of salt-sensitive hypertension in Dahl's rats appears also to occur independently of measurable renal neurogenic alterations in salt and water intake.[65]

The mechanisms responsible for the greater activation of the sympathetic nervous system during high sodium intake are not clear. Winternitz and Oparil[66] have shown increased NE content in the dorsomedial and anterior hypothalamic nuclei suggesting a central mechanism. Koepke and DiBona[61] observed that high sodium intake potentiated the increase in RSNA and the decrease in urinary sodium excretion resulting from air stress in conscious SHR, suggesting a centrally mediated facilitation of sympathetic neural outflow to the kidney.

Chen et al.[30] have recently shown that a high-sodium diet in salt-sensitive SHR may elevate blood pressure by reducing noradrenergic input to depressor neurons in the anterior hypothalamus and increased noradrenergic input to neurons in the pons.

Dietz et al.,[67] on the other hand, observed that high sodium intake caused reduced reuptake of NE in the sympathetic end-terminals of stroke-prone SHR, pointing to a peripheral mechanism of activation of the sympathetic nervous system. Blaustein[31] has suggested that excessive sodium intake may stimulate the release of a ouabain-like natriuretic factor, which in turn would suppress the $Na^+–K^+$ pump, thus facilitating NE release from the sympathetic end-terminals. Finally, high sodium intake may potentiate neurogenic vasoconstriction by increasing vascular reactivity.[68]

Increased dietary intake of potassium appears to antagonize the effect of high sodium intake on sympathetic activity and on blood pressure.[69]

We have recently proposed that salt sensitivity may be related to a deranged modulation of the sympathetic and renin–angiotensin–aldosterone systems in response to high dietary sodium intake.[45] In normal subjects, normal sodium balance is maintained by increased activity of the renin–angiotensin system and of the sympathetic nervous system during a low-sodium diet and by decreased activity of these two systems during a high-sodium diet. Blood pressure does not change. In salt-resistant hypertensives, the modulatory influence of dietary sodium on the renin–angiotensin and sympathetic nervous systems remains unaltered, although reset to a greater level of blood pressure; the resetting is probably related to increased renal vascular resistance. In salt-sensitive patients, the increased renal vascular resistance causes a similar shift to the right of the pressure–natriuresis curve. However, these patients also display abnormalities in tubular reabsorption of sodium causing a depression of the slope of the pressure–natriuresis curve. The cause of this derangement in salt-sensitive patients is probably related to abnormal modulation of the renin–angiotensin and sympathetic nervous systems in response to dietary changes of sodium. On a low-sodium diet, salt-sensitive patients display less increase in plasma renin activity and plasma NE, leading to less pronounced sodium retention and to more negative sodium balance. During high dietary sodium intake, these patients display less suppression of plasma renin activity and an increase, rather than a decrease, in plasma NE levels. This would lead to blunted natriuresis and positive sodium balance. An increase in blood pressure ensues to reestablish sodium homeostasis (Fig. 5). A defect of modulation of renin release and renal vascular tone during changes in sodium balance in salt-sensitive patients has been observed by others.

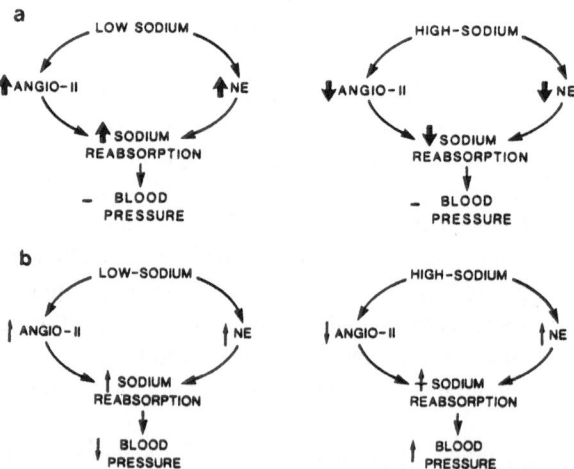

Fig. 5.   Relation between dietary sodium intake, plasma norepinephrine (NE), and angiotensin II (Angio II) levels in normal subjects, salt-resistant, and salt-sensitive subjects with essential hypertension. (a) Normal or salt-resistant subjects; (b) salt-sensitive subjects. (Reproduced from Ref. 45, with permission.)

3. Calcium and Hypertension

Calcium plays an important role in blood pressure regulation, but there is still controversy about whether abnormalities of calcium metabolism are responsible for the genesis of hypertension.

A large body of evidence indicates that both acute and chronic hypercalcemia increase blood pressure. More recently McCarron[70] has suggested that decreased dietary calcium intake and hypocalcemia can result in hypertension.

3.1. Hypercalcemia and Blood Pressure

Both acute and chronic hypercalcemia can raise blood pressure: Correction of the hypercalcemia is often followed by normalization of blood pressure. Acute administration of calcium increases blood pressure in normal human subjects,[71] as well as in rats,[72,73] and a close relationship exists between the increments in the concentration of serum calcium and the rise in blood pressure. Acute hypocalcemia, on the contrary, can lower blood pressure, particularly during upright posture.[74]

Chronic hypercalcemia associated with primary hyperparathyroidism,[75–77] secondary hyperparathyroidism (occurring in patients with chronic renal failure or renal transplantation),[78,79] vitamin D intoxication,[80] prolonged immobilization,[81] or malignancy can also cause hypertension.

Acute hypercalcemia caused a significant increase in peripheral vascular resistance without changes in cardiac index in conscious rats,[73] as well as in normal or hypertensive human subjects.[71,82]

Studies *in vitro* have shown that calcium increases arteriolar constriction in the forelimb and kidney and increases myocardial contractility.[83,84]

The vasoconstrictor action of calcium can be both direct and indirect. Ca^{2+} plays a central role in excitation–contraction coupling of vascular smooth muscle cells. Regardless of the mechanism causing cell excitation, whether it is neural, humoral, or myogenic, it results in a rise in cytosolic Ca^{2+} concentration. The increased intracellular Ca^{2+} activates the calmodulin-dependent myosin light-chain kinase, leading to formation of cross-bridges between the actin and myosin filaments and to cellular contraction.

An increase in extracellular calcium during acute or chronic hypercalcemia could enhance transcellular flux of calcium, ultimately resulting in vasoconstriction.[85] Moreover, increased extracellular concentration of Ca^{2+} may also increase the vascular responsiveness to NE, angiotensin II, or potassium,[86] whereas decreased extracellular calcium concentration or calcium antagonists reduce vascular responsiveness to NE *in vitro*.[87,88] Ca^{2+} is also important in the binding of NE to alpha-adrenergic receptors in the rabbit aorta.[89]

The effect of hypercalcemia on vascular response to NE in human subjects remains unclear and it may depend on its duration. Acute hypercalcemia did not alter the pressor response to NE or angiotensin II in normal subjects,[71] whereas chronic hypercalcemia was associated with enhanced blood pressure response to NE.[90]

Hypercalcemia could theoretically raise blood pressure through its effects on NE release from the sympathetic end-terminals and from the adrenal glands.[91-95] According to the "calcium hypothesis,"[91-93] depolarization of the sympathetic end-terminals increases Ca^{2+} influx, which stimulates NE exocytosis. It has been postulated that the endoskeleton of the sympathetic nerve terminals contains actomyosin-like neurofilaments capable of contraction when the intracellular concentration of Ca^{2+} increases. During the contraction of these neurofilaments, vesicles containing neurotransmitters migrate toward the membrane. The release of NE from the perfused cat spleen or from isolated spleen slices in response to nerve stimulation was abolished if the perfusate was calcium free,[96] and it was potentiated when the concentration of calcium was modestly increased.[97,98] However, at concentrations over 7 meq/liter calcium increased the stability of neuronal membrane and inhibited NE release.[99] On the contrary, the basal efflux of NE from mesenteric arteries in rat was stimulated by reduced concentration of Ca^{2+}.[97,100]

Very scanty and inconclusive data on the effect of Ca^{2+} on catecholamine release are available in human subjects. Marone et al.[71] have shown that intravenous administration of calcium increased plasma NE, but this occurred at a time when volume depletion was also evident. Vlachakis et al.[90] have shown increased plasma levels of NE in patients with hypercalcemia secondary to primary hyperparathyroidism, but they did not measure blood volume in their patients.

The mechanisms involved in the increase in blood pressure during acute hypercalcemia are largely independent of the renin–angiotensin system. An inverse relationship exists between intracellular Ca^{2+} and the rate of renin release. A decrease in intracellular Ca^{2+}, caused by decreased influx or increased efflux, stimulates renin secretion, while a rise in intracellular calcium inhibits renin secretion.[101,102]

On the contrary, aldosterone secretion in vitro requires calcium.[103,104] Despite these in vitro observations, studies in humans have shown no change in plasma renin or aldosterone levels during acute hypocalcemia[72] or hypercalcemia.[71]

3.2. Calcium Deficiency in Hypertension

In apparent contrast with the notion that acute or chronic hypercalcemia can cause hypertension, more recently it has been proposed that calcium deficiency may be important in the genesis of hypertension both in humans and in SHR.[70]

This hypothesis stems from the observation that a wide range of derangements in calcium balance can be observed in patients with essential hypertension or in SHR (Table I). According to this hypothesis, a decreased dietary intake of calcium and/or hypercalciuria leads to decreased serum concentration of Ca^{2+}; this derangement potentiates Ca^{2+} fluxes into smooth muscle cells, thus causing vasoconstriction.

Table 1. Derangements in Calcium Metabolism in Hypertension

---

1. Hypercalciuria
2. Decreased intestinal absorption of calcium
3. Low calcium intake
4. Reduced serum ionized calcium
5. Increased cytosolic Ca^{2+}
6. Increased serum levels of parathyroid hormone (PTH)
7. Abnormal levels of Vitamin D_3 and calcitonin
8. Hypotensive effects of oral calcium loading
9. Abnormalities in cell membrane transport of calcium

3.3. The Evidence for Hypercalciuria

Hypercalciuria has been shown both in patients with essential hypertension[105–107] and in SHR[108–110] as well as the Milan strain of SHR.[111] But the interpretation of this abnormality remains controversial. Hypercalciuria could be the consequence of increased dietary intake or of increased intestinal absorption or of a renal tubular leak of calcium, or it could be related to increased natriuresis caused by higher dietary sodium intake.

There is no evidence of increased dietary intake or of increased intestinal absorption of calcium in hypertensive subjects, and the data on intestinal calcium absorption in SHR are conflicting.[70,110,112,117]

McCarron[70] suggested that the hypercalciuria in SHR is dependent on a renal tubular calcium leak. Lau *et al.*,[110,113] on the other hand, using clearance techniques in rats with intact parathyroid glands or parathyroidectomized, were not able to detect calcium leak after an overnight fast.

One final cause of hypercalciuria in essential hypertension could be increased dietary sodium intake and natriuresis, since the urinary excretion of calcium is closely correlated with the urinary excretion of sodium.[118–120] McCarron,[70] however, has shown that hypercalciuria in essential hypertension is present at any level of urinary sodium excretion; this would indicate that hypercalcemia may occur independently of urinary sodium excretion. Despite the strong and convincing appeal of these arguments, there are equally valid counterarguments. Hypercalcemia in SHR occurs only after 15–20 weeks of age. Under steady-state conditions, hypercalciuria can be found in two models of experimental hypertension characterized by expansion of body fluid volume: the DOCA–salt[122] and the Dahl's salt-sensitive rat.[123] In Dahl's rats hypertension occurs spontaneously after exposure to high dietary sodium intake, whereas in the DOCA–salt model hypertension is experimentally induced. In the DOCA–salt model, urinary sodium excretion falls on the first day of DOCA treatment and then returns to baseline values; in contrast, urinary calcium excretion increases only after 2–3 days, probably as a consequence of volume expansion, and it persists thereafter. This suggests that volume expansion may decrease proximal tubular reabsorption of calcium and sodium and increase distal delivery. Mineralocorticoids would promote distal tubular reabsorption of sodium but not of calcium, resulting in hypercalciuria.

A further argument against the hypothesis that hypercalciuria exerts a causative role in hypertension derives from the clinical observation that patients with primary hypercalciuria do not appear to be at greater risk of developing hypertension.[124]

3.4. Intestinal Calcium Absorption in Hypertension

The data on abnormalities of intestinal calcium transport in hypertension are inconsistent and controversial. In human subjects with hypertension no systematic studies of intestinal calcium absorption have been published. The studies performed in SHR have produced conflicting results.[70,112–117] In prehypertensive (3–4 weeks old) SHR, increased intestinal absorption of calcium, positive calcium balance, and increased serum levels of 1,25(OH)2D3 have been demonstrated.[125,126] On the other hand, in the adult SHR, a decrease, no change, or an increase in intestinal calcium transport has been observed.[112–117,127] Studies of calcium balance have shown increased[110] or decreased skeletal content of calcium in SHR.[129]

3.5. Reduced Calcium Intake in Hypertension

Recently, it has been proposed that the lesser the dietary calcium intake in a given population, the greater is the probability of developing hypertension.[70] This claim is based on an analysis of the U.S. National Health and Nutrition Examination Survey I (NHANES I).[129] This analysis also found an inverse relationship between mass index and dietary calcium intake, which could indicate that overweight patients consume fewer dairy products in order to lose weight or that they may be less willing to reveal fully their dietary habits. In support of the latter possibility is the fact that the average intake of sodium was only 90 meq/day, far less than the average sodium intake in the American population.[130] Using the same data from the NHANES I survey, other investigators have reached different conclusions. Feinleib et al.[131] found no difference in dietary calcium intake between normotensive and hypertensive subjects when age and body weight were taken into account. Harlan et al.,[132] on the other hand, found an inverse correlation between dietary calcium intake and diastolic blood pressure in women but a direct correlation with systolic blood pressure in men. At least two other epidemiologic studies[133,134] have failed to show any relationship between dietary calcium intake and prevalence of hypertension. Witteman et al.,[135] on the other hand, in a survey of over 58,000 U.S. females, found an inverse relationship between dietary calcium and magnesium and hypertension independent of age, body weight, and alcohol consumption.

Finally, the prevalence of hypertension appears to be lower in unacculturated societies, despite their low calcium intake.[128]

In conclusion, there is some evidence for an inverse relationship between dietary calcium intake and prevalence of hypertension, but a cause–effect relationship remains to be proved.

Some have observed higher blood pressure in normotensive and hypertensive rats during long-term calcium deprivation[137–139]; however, these rats also developed magnesium depletion, hyperparathyroidism, and growth retardation, all variables that *per se* could affect blood pressure levels.[140,141] Mild calcium restriction within the physiologic range did not result in increased blood pressure in SHR.[142] However, more severe calcium restriction (0.25–0.5% of dietary calcium) can result in aggravation of blood pressure.[128]

3.6. The Evidence for Hypocalcemia

McCarron[143] was the first to report decreased serum concentration of ionized calcium but not of total calcium in hypertensive subjects. Resnick *et al.*, on the other hand, observed decreased ionized calcium only in patients with low renin[145] or in salt-sensitive patients,[146] but not in those with normal or high renin. Others have shown normal serum ionized calcium,[147,148] even in patients with low renin[149] or increased plasma calcium.[141–145] Finally, Harlan *et al.*[132] and Kesteloot and De Boers[151] have shown a direct relationship between serum calcium and blood pressure among patients with essential hypertension in spite of an inverse relationship between dietary calcium intake and blood pressure. The reasons for these discrepancies in serum concentration of calcium are difficult to interpret, but they could be related to the fact that multiple variables can affect serum calcium, such as serum albumin, volume–sodium status, blood pH, alcohol intake, muscular exercise, respiratory alkalosis, fasting vs. feeding, hemoconcentration, diuretic therapy, age, and sex of the patients.[156–159]

Similar inconsistencies exist in animal studies. Some have shown reduced serum ionized calcium in SHR.[70] Lau *et al.*,[110] on the other hand, considering that rats are nocturnal animals, measured serum ionized calcium in SHR at midnight, after their calcium intake with meals, and found increased levels compared with WKY. Whether this abnormality has any pathogenetic meaning or is simply the result of hypertension remains to be determined. It is significant that hypocalcemia is also observed in other forms of experimentally induced hypertension, such as in the DOCA–salt and in the 5/6 nephrectomy models.[160] These observations suggest that hypocalcemia may be a secondary rather than a primary phenomenon.

3.7. The Proposed Link between Hypocalcemia and Hypertension

Data on intracellular content calcium in platelets or leukocytes are also inconsistent. Some workers have found increased intracellular calcium and a direct correlation between content of calcium in platelets and blood pressure,[161,162] while others could not confirm these findings.[163,164] Cytosolic free calcium in neutrophils was also not different in hypertensive subjects.[165,166] Intracellular calcium has been shown to be increased in platelets, RBCs, and lymphocytes of SHR.[162,167,168]

The concentration of intracellular calcium in renal tubular cells has been shown to be increased,[169] decreased,[170] or unchanged.[171] An increase in intracellular free calcium in proximal renal tubules may downregulate production of $1,25(OH)_2D$, and account for the decreased blood levels of this vitamin in SHR.[169]

Intracellular free calcium, measured by the FURA-2 technique, was not increased in cultured vascular smooth muscle cells isolated from SHR.[172]

On the other hand, Bhalla et al.[173] observed an increase in calcium content in aortic strips of SHR of 12–16 weeks of age, but not in SHR of 31 days of age. Calcium uptake by aortic microsomes was significantly decreased in 10-day-old SHR.

Decreased activity of the magnesium–calcium–ATPase pump has been shown in vascular smooth muscle cells or in RBCs of human subjects with essential hypertension, SHR, and rats with the DOCA–salt model or hypertension.[174–176] Whether these abnormalities of calcium metabolism are primary or secondary and how they relate to the development of hypertension remain to be established.

3.8. Effect of Calcium Supplementation on Blood Pressure

If calcium deficiency were a causative factor of hypertension, adequate dietary calcium supplementations capable of maintaining a positive calcium balance should result in normalization or improvement of blood pressure. Experiments in several animal models of hypertension appear to support this notion. Calcium supplementations result in improved blood pressure control in SHR,[127,178,179] in Dahl's salt-sensitive rats,[180] in the DOCA–salt model in rat,[181] and in the two-kidney one-clip model of renovascular hypertension.[182] SHR pups fostered at birth to high-calcium (2%) SHR dams developed significantly lower blood pressure than pups fostered to low-calcium (0.01%) dams[183].

The mechanisms for the antihypertensive action of calcium supplementation in experimental animal models of hypertension are not clear. Some researchers have attributed this effect to phosphate depletion caused by high dietary calcium intake; parenteral phosphate administration reversed the antihypertensive effect of calcium in these animals.[179] However, phosphate added to the diet did not reverse the antihypertensive effect of dietary calcium.[70] Some investigators have attributed the antihypertensive action of calcium supplementation to enhanced natriuresis,[127] or to suppression of sympathetic nervous system activity.[180]

Less conclusive are the data on the effect of calcium supplementation on blood pressure in human subjects. Belizan et al.[184,185] have shown that large amounts of calcium (1 g/day) caused a significant decrease in diastolic blood pressure in normotensive subjects. McCarron and Morris,[173] however, have shown no effect of dietary calcium supplementation on blood pressure in normal subjects. However, these investigators observed a small, but significant decrease in blood pressure in untreated patients with essential hypertension, after dietary supplementation with 1 g of calcium per day for 8 weeks. The decrease in blood pressure was significant only during upright posture. Since no measurements of blood volume were obtained in these studies, and since increased dietary calcium may increase natriuresis, it is possible that the mild orthostatic changes in blood pressure caused by calcium supplementations may be related primarily to intravascular volume depletion rather than to effects on smooth muscle cell contraction.

Several other investigators have studied the effect of calcium supplementation in patients with essential hypertension, achieving conflicting results. Some found a significant reduction of blood pressure,[187-188] while others could not confirm any significant beneficial effect.[189-192] Resnick *et al.*[193] observed a significant reduction only in low-renin or in salt-sensitive patients with essential hypertension. Grobbee and Hofman showed a fall in blood pressure during oral calcium intake only in patients with low serum Ca^{2+} and high PTH levels.[194] Zemel *et al.*[195] observed that increasing dietary calcium from 356 to 934 mg/day completely reversed the rise in blood pressure caused by a high-sodium diet in six hypertensive black patients. The antihypertensive effect of calcium in these salt-sensitive patients was in part due to natriuresis and inhibition of sodium-induced volume expansion.

Therefore, studies in humans show that the antihypertensive effect of calcium supplementation is minimal and limited to the subset of salt-sensitive patients. Obviously, more studies are needed before a recommendation can be made to all hypertensive patients to increase dietary calcium intake.

4. Relation between Abnormalities of Sodium and Calcium Metabolism in Hypertension

As previously stated, abnormalities in calcium metabolism are more likely to occur in salt-sensitive and low-renin essential hypertensive subjects than in salt-resistant and normal or high-renin patients. This suggests that there may be a link between the abnormalities of sodium and those of calcium metabolism.

A current hypothesis to explain the mechanisms by which high dietary sodium intake increases blood pressure in salt-sensitive patients proposed a defect in sodium-linked cellular calcium transport, perhaps mediated in part by a hormonal inhibition of Na^+-K^+ adenosine triphosphatase activity.[94]

As a consequence of these cell membrane derangements, high dietary sodium intake could lead to increased cytosolic calcium in several organs and tissues (Fig. 6). An increase in cytosolic calcium in the juxtaglomerular cells would inhibit renin release, since Ca^{2+} is an inhibitory second messenger in the renin secretory process. Baroreceptor-mediated changes in renin secretion are modulated by depolarization-induced Ca^{2+} influx.[196] An increase in cytosolic calcium at the level of sympathetic nerve terminals could facilitate the release of norepinephrine[91-95] and explain the increase in sympathetic nervous system activity during high dietary sodium intake observed in salt-sensitive patients[28,50] and SHR.[66] Finally, increased

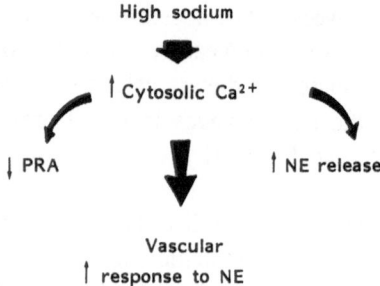

Fig. 6. Possible relationship between high dietary sodium, abnormalities of calcium metabolism, and abnormalities of renin and plasma norepinephrine (NE) levels in salt-sensitive patients with essential hypertension. PRA = plasma renin activity. (Reproduced from Ref. 45, with permission.)

intracellular Ca^{2+} in smooth muscle cells would result in greater responsiveness to pressor agonists and in increased blood pressure.[197]

References

1. Prior, I. A. M., Evans, J. G., Harvey, H. P. B., Davidson, F., and Lindsey, M., 1968, Sodium intake and blood pressure in two Polynesian populations, *N. Engl. J. Med.* **279:**515–520.
2. Page, L. B., Danion, A., and Moellering, R. C., Jr., 1974, Antecedents of cardiovascular disease in six Solomon Islands societies, *Circulation* **49:**1132–1146.
3. Oliver, W. J., Cohen, E. L., and Neel, J. V., 1975, Blood pressure, sodium intake and sodium related hormones in the Yanomamo Indians, a "no-salt" culture, *Circulation* **52:**146–151.
4. Sinnett, P. F., White, H. A., and Whyte, H. M., 1973, Epidemiological studies in a total highland population, Tuki Senta, New Guinea: Cardiovascular disease, relevant clinical, electrocardiographic radiological and biochemical findings, *J. Chronic Dis* **26:**265–290.
5. Prior, I. A. M., Grimley-Evans, J., Harvey, H. P. B., Davidson F., and Lindsey, M., 1968, Sodium intake and blood pressure in two Polynesian populations, *N. Engl. J. Med.* **279:**515–520.
6. Dahl, L. K., 1961, The possible role of chronic excess salt consumption in the pathogenesis of essential hypertension, *Am. J. Cardiol.* **8:**571–575.
7. Staessen, J., Fagard, R., Lijnen, P., Amery, A., Bulpitt, C., and Joossens, J. V., 1981, Salt and blood pressure in Belgium, *J. Epidemiol. Community Health* **35:**256–261.
8. Strazzullo, P., Trevisan, M., Farinaro, E., et al., 1983, Characteristics of the association between salt intake and blood pressure in a sample of male working population in southern Italy, *Eur. Heart J.* **4:**608–613.
9. Beevers, D. G., Hawthorne, B. M., and Padfield, P. L., 1980, Salt and blood pressure in Scotland, *Br. Med. J.* **281:**641–642.
10. Tuomilehto, J., Karppanen, H., Tanskanen, A., Tikkanen, J., and Vuori, J., 1980, Sodium and potassium excretion in a sample of normotensive and hypertensive persons in eastern Finland, *J. Epidemiol. Community Health* **34:**174–178.
11. Takamatsu, M., 1955, Figure of body fluid of farmers in the north-eastern districts viewed from angle of water and salt metabolism, *J. Sci. Lab (Rodo Kagaku)* **31:**349–370.
12. Isaacson, L. C., Modlin, M., and Jackson, W. P. U., 1963, Sodium intake and hypertension, *Lancet* **1:**946.

13. Fukuda, T., 1954, Investigation on hypertension in farm villages in Akita Schiba Igakki, Szasshi, *Chiba Med. Soc.* **29**:490–502.
14. Simpson, F. O., 1984, Salt and hypertension: Current data, attitudes and policies, *J. Cardiol. Pharmacol.* **6**:S4–S9.
15. Kesteloot, H., Park, B. C., Lee, C. S., Brems-Heyns, E., and Joossens, J. V., 1980, A comparative study of blood pressure and sodium intake in Belgium and in Korea, in *Epidemiology of Arterial Blood Pressure* (H. Kesteloot and J. V. Joossens, eds.), Martinus Nijhoff, The Hague, pp. 453–470.
16. Ljungman, S., Aurell, M., Hartford, M., Wikstrand, J., Wilhelmsen, I., and Berglund, G., 1981, Sodium excretion and blood pressure, *Hypertension* **3**:318–326.
17. Simpson, F. O., Waal-Manning, H., Bolli, P., Phelan, E. L., and Spears, G. F. S., 1978, Relationship of blood pressure to sodium excretion in a population survey, *Clin. Sci. Mod. Med.* **55** (Suppl.):373s–375s.
18. Yamori, Y., Kihara, M., Nara, Y., et al., 1981, Hypertension and diet: multiple regression analysis in a Japanese farming community, *Lancet* **1**:120.
19. Mir, M. A., Mir, F., and Khosla, T., 1984, High incidence of hypertension in heavy salt consuming population of northern Kashmir, *Circulation,* **70**(Suppl. II):II–359 (Abstract).
20. Freis, E. D., 1976, Salt volume and the prevention of hypertension, *Circulation* **53**:589–595.
21. Joossens, J. V., 1980, Dietary salt restriction: The case in favour in: *The Therapeutics of Hypertension,* Royal Society of Medicine (International Congress and Symposium Series no. 26), London, pp. 243–250.
22. Poulter, N., Khaw, K. T., Hopwood, B. E. C., Mugambi, M., Peart, W. S., and Sever, P. S., 1984, Salt and blood pressure in various populations, *J. Cardiovasc. Pharmacol.* **6**:S197–S203.
23. Shaper, A. G., Leonard, P. J., Jones, K. W., and Jones, M., 1969, Environmental effects of the body build, blood pressure and blood chemistry of nomadic warriors serving in the army of Kenya, *East Afr. Med. J.* **46**:282–289.
24. MacGregor, G. A., 1985, Sodium is more important than calcium in essential hypertension, *Hypertension* **7**:628–637.
25. *National Nutritional Survey,* 1981, Ministry of Health and Welfare, Koseisho, Japan.
26. Joossens, J. V., and Geboers, J., 1983, Salt and hypertension, *Prev. Med.* **12**:53–59.
27. Kawasaki, T., Delea, C. S., Bartter, F. C., and Smith, H., 1978, The effect of high-sodium and low-sodium intakes on blood pressure and other related variables in human subjects with idiopathic hypertension, *Am. J. Med.* **64**:193–198.
28. Campese, V. M., Romoff, M. S., Levitan, D., Saglikes, Y., Friedler, R. M., and Massry, S. G., 1982, Abnormal relationship between sodium intake and sympathetic nervous activity in salt-sensitive patients with essential hypertension, *Kidney Int.* **21**:371–378.
29. Dahl, L. K., Heine, M., and Tassinari, L., 1962, Effects of chronic salt ingestion. Evidence that genetic factors play an important role in susceptibility to experimental hypertension, *J. Exp. Med.* **115**:1173–1190.
30. Chen, Y. F., Meng, Q., Wyss, J. M., Jin, H., and Oparil, S., 1988, High NaCl diet reduces hypothalamic norepinephrine turnover in hypertensive rats, *Hypertension* **11**:55–62.
31. Blaustein, M. P., 1977, Sodium ions, calcium ions, blood pressure regulation and hypertension: A reassessment and a hypothesis, *Am. J. Physiol.* **232**:165–173.
32. Tobian, L., Lange, J., Azar, S., Iwai, J., Koop, D., Coffee, K.,, and Johnson, M. A., 1978, Reduction of natriuretic capacity and renin release in isolated blood-perfused kidneys of Dahl hypertension-prone rat, *Circ. Res.* **43**(Suppl. 1):92.
33. Dahl, L. K., and Heine, M., 1975, Primary role of renal homografts in setting blood pressure levels in rats, *Circ. Res.* **36**:692–696.
34. Kawabe, K., Watanabe, T. X., Shiono, K., and Sokabe, H., 1978, Influence on blood pressure of renal isografts between spontaneously hypertensive and normotensive rats, utilizing the F_1 hybrids, *Jpn. Heart J.* **19**:886–893.
35. Bianchi, G., Fox, U., DiFrancesco, G. F., Giovannetti, A. M., and Pagetti, D., 1974, Blood

pressure changes produced by kidney cross-transplantation between spontaneously hypertensive rats (SHR) and normotensive rats (NR), *Clin. Sci. Mol. Med.* **47**:435–448.

36. Grim, C. E., Luft, F. C., Miller, J. Z., Brown, P. L., Gannon, M. A., and Weinberger, M. H., 1979, Effects of sodium loading and depletion in normotensive first-degree relatives of essential hypertension, *J. Lab. Clin. Med.* **94**:764–771.

37. Beierwalters, W. H., Arendshorst, W., and Klemmer, P. J., 1982, Electrolytes and water balance in young spontaneously hypertensive rats, *Hypertension* **4**:908–915.

38. Roman, R. J., and Cowley, A. W., Jr., 1985, Abnormal pressure–diuresis-response in spontaneously hypertensive rats, *Am. J. Physiol.* **248**:F199–F205.

39. Vanderwalle, A., Farman, N., and Bonvalet, J. P., 1978, Renal handling of sodium in Kyto-Okamoto rats: A micropuncture study, *Am. J. Physiol.* **235**:F394–F402.

40. Cangiano, J. L., Rodriguez-Sargent, C., Opava-Stitzer, S., and Martinez-Maldonado, M., 1984, Renal Na$^+$-K$^+$-ATPase in weanling and adult spontaneously hypertensive rats, *Proc. Soc. Exp. Biol. Med.* **177**:240–246.

41. Helmer, O. M., 1967, Hormonal and biochemical factors controlling blood pressure, in: *Les concepts de Claude Bernard sur le milieu intérieur,* Librairies De L'Academie De Medecine, Paris, pp. 115–128.

42. Guyton, A. C., Coleman, T. G., Cowley, A. W., Scheel, K. W., Manning, R. D., Jr., and Norman, R. A., Jr., 1972, Arterial pressure regulation: Overriding dominance of the kidney in long-term regulation and in hypertension, *Am. J. Med.* **52**:584–594.

43. Kimura, G., Saito, F., Kojima, S., Yoshimi, H., Abe, H., Kawano, Y., Yoshida, K., Ashida, T., Kawamura, M., and Kuramochi, M., 1987, Renal function curve in patients with secondary forms of hypertension, *Hypertension* **10**:11–15.

44. Guyton, A. C., 1987, Renal function curve. A key to understanding the pathogenesis of hypertension, *Hypertension* **10**:1–6.

45. Campese, V. M., 1988, Effects of calcium antagonists on deranged modulation of the renal function curve in salt-sensitive patients with essential hypertension, *Am. J. Cardiol.* **62**:856–916.

46. Williams, G. H., and Hollenberg, N. K., 1985, Sodium-sensitive essential hypertension: Emerging insights to pathogenesis and therapeutic implications, *Contemp. Nephrol.* **3**:303–331.

47. Hollenberg, N. K., Chenitz, W. R., Adams, D. F., and Williams, G. H., 1974, Reciprocal influence of salt intake on adrenal glomerulosa and renal vascular responses to angiotensin II in normal man, *J. Clin. Invest.* **54**:34–42.

48. Romoff, M. S., Keusch, G., Campese, V. M., Wang, M. S., Friedler, R. M., Weidmann, P., and Massry, S. G., 1979, Effect of sodium intake on plasma catecholamines in normal subjects, *J. Clin. Endocrinol. Metab.* **48**:26–31.

49. Koolen, M. and VanBrummelen, P., 1984, Adrenergic activity and peripheral hemodynamics in relation to sodium sensitivity in patients with essential hypertension, *Hypertension* **6**:820–825.

50. Gill, J. R., Gullner, H. G., Lake, C. R., Lakatua, D. J., and Lan, G. 1988, Plasma and urinary catecholamines in salt-sensitive idiopathic hypertension, *Hypertension* **11**:312–319.

51. Falkner, B., Onesti, G., and Hayes, P., 1981, The role of sodium in essential hypertension in genetically hypertensive adolescents, in: *Hypertension in the Young and the Old* (G. Onesti and K. E. Kim, eds.), Grune & Stratton, New York, pp. 29–35.

52. Light, K. C., Koepke, J. P., Obrist, P. A., and Willis, P. W., IV, 1983, Psychological stress induces sodium and fluid retention in men at high risk for hypertension, *Science* **220**:429–431.

53. Lawton, W. J., Sinkey, C. A., Fitz, A. E., and Mark, A. L., 1988, Dietary salt produces abnormal renal vascoconstrictor responses to upright posture in borderline hypertensive subjects, *Hypertension* **11**:529–536.

54. Skrabal, F., Herholz, H., Neumayr, M., Hamberger, L., Ledochowski, M., Sporer, H., Hortnagl, H., Schwarz, S., and Schontzer, D., 1984, Salt sensitivity in humans is linked to enhanced sympathetic responsiveness and to enhanced proximal tubular reabsorption, *Hypertension* **6**:152–158.

55. Weinberger, M. H., 1986, Dietary sodium and blood pressure, *Hosp. Pract.* **21**:55–64.

56. Liard, J. F., Tarazi, R. L., Ferrario, C. M., and Manner, W. M., 1975, Hemodynamic and humoral characteristics of hypertension induced by prolonged stellate ganglion stimulation in conscious dogs, *Circ. Res.* **36**:455–464.

57. Katholi, R. E., Carey, R. M., Ayers, C. R., Vaughan, E. D., Yancey, M. R., and Morton, C. L., 1977, Production of sustained hypertension by chronic intrarenal norepinephrine infusion in conscious dogs, *Circ. Res.* **40**(Suppl. I):I118–I126.

58. Nakamura, K. and Nakamura, K., (1977), Selective activation of sympathetic ganglia in young spontaneously hypertensive rats, *Nature* **266**:265–266.

59. Okamoto, K., Nosako, S., Yamori, Y., and Matsumoto, M., 1967, Participation of renal factors in the pathogenesis of hypertension in the spontaneously hypertensive rat, *Jpn. Heart J.* **8**:168–180.

60. Lundin, S. and Thoren, P., 1982, Renal function and sympathetic activity during mental stress in normotensive and spontaneously hypertensive rats, *Acta Physiol. Scand.* **115**:115–124.

61. Koepke, J. P. and DiBona, G. F., 1985, High sodium intake enhances renal nerve and antinatriuretic responses to stress in spontaneously hypertensive rats, *Hypertension* **7**:357–363.

62. Winternitz, S. R., Katholi, R. E., and Oparil, S., 1980, Role of the renal sympathetic nerves in the development and maintenance of hypertension in spontaneously hypertensive rat, *J. Clin. Invest.* **66**:971–978.

63. Ricksten, S. E., Yao, T., DiBona, G. F., and Thoren, P., 1981, Renal nerve activity and exaggerated natriuresis in conscious spontaneously hypertensive rats, *Acta Physiol. Scand.* **112**:161–167.

64. Katholi, R. E., 1983, Renal nerves in the pathogenesis of hypertension in experimental animals and humans, *Am. J. Physiol.* **245**:F1–F14.

65. Osborn, J. C., Roman, R. J., and Ewens, J. O., 1988, Renal nerves and the development of Dahl salt-sensitive hypertension, *Hypertension* **11**:523–528.

66. Winternitz, S. R., and Oparil, S., 1982, Sodium–neural interactions in the development of spontaneous hypertension, *Clin. Exp. Hypertension* **4**:751–760.

67. Dietz, R., Schomig, A., Rascher, W., Strasser, R., and Kubler, W., 1980, Enhanced sympathetic activity caused by salt loading in spontaneously hypertensive rats, *Clin. Sci.* **59**:171s–173s.

68. Heistad, D. D., Abboud, F. M., and Ballard, D. R., 1971, Relationship between plasma sodium concentration and vascular reactivity in man, *J. Clin. Invest.* **50**:2022–2032.

69. Dietz, R., 1983, The role of potassium and hypotension, *Am. J. Nephrol.* **3**:100–108.

70. McCarron, D. A., 1985, Is calcium more important than sodium in the pathogenesis of essential hypertension? *Hypertension* **7**:607–627.

71. Marone, C., Beretta-Piccoli, C., and Weidmann, P., 1981, Acute hypercalcemic hypertension in man: Role of hemodynamics, catecholamines and renin, *Kidney Int.* **20**:92–96.

72. Iseki, K., Massry, S. G., and Campese, V. M., 1986, Effects of hypercalcemia and PTH on blood pressure in normal and renal failure rats, *Am. J. Physiol.* **250**:F924–F929.

73. Berl, T., Levi, M., Ellis, M., and Chaimovitz, C., 1985, Mechanism of acute hypercalcemic hypertension in the conscious rat, *Hypertension* **7**:923–930.

74. Llach, F., Weidmann, P., Reinhart, R., Maxwell, M. H., Coburn, J. W., and Massry, S. G., 1974, Effect of acute and long standing hypocalcemia on blood pressure and plasma renin activity in man, *J. Clin. Endocr. Metab.* **38**:841–847.

75. Hellstrom, J., Brike, G., and Edvall, C. A., 1958, Hypertension in hyperparathyroidism, *Br. J. Urol.* **30**:13–24.

76. Lemann, J., and Donatelli, A. S., 1964, Calcium intoxication due to primary hyperparathyroidism, *Ann. Intern. Med.* **60**:447–461.

77. Rosenthal, F. D. and Roy, S., 1972, Hypertension and Hyperparathyroidism, *Br. Med. J.* **4**:396–397.

78. Coburn, J. W., Massry, S. G., DePalma, J. R., and Shinaberger, H., 1969, Rapid appearance of hypercalcemia with initiation of hemodialysis, *JAMA* **210**:2276–2278.

79. Bennett, W. M., McDonald, W. J., Lawson, R. K., and Porter, G. A., 1974, Post-transplant hypertension; studies of cortical blood flow and the renal pressor system, *Kidney Int.* **6**:99–108.

80. Earll, J. M., Kurtzman, N. A., and Moser, R. H., 1966, Hypercalcemia and hypertension, *Ann. Intern. Med.* **64**:378–381.

81. Berliner, B. C., Shenker, I. R., and Weinstock, M. S., 1972, Hypercalcemia associated with hypertension due to prolonged immobilization, *Pediatrics* **49**:92–96.

82. Sialer, S., McKenna, D. C., and Corliss, R. J., 1967, Systemic and coronary hemodynamic effects of intravenous administration of calcium chloride, *Arch. Int. Pharmacodyn. Ther.* **169**:177–184.

83. Rasmussen, H. and Barrett, P. Q., 1984, Calcium messenger system; an integrated view, *Physiol. Rev.* **64**:938–984.

84. Morgan, J. P. and Morgan, K. G., 1984, Calcium and cardiovascular function: intracellular calcium levels during contraction and relaxation of mammalian cardiac and vascular smooth muscle as detected with aequorin, *Am. J. Med.* **77**(5A):33–46.

85. Bohr, D. F., and Webb, R. C., 1984, Vascular smooth muscle function and its changes in hypertension, *Am. J. Med.* **77**:3–16.

86. Sybertz, E. J., Vliet, G. V., and Baum, T. 1983, Analysis of the vasoconstrictor response to potassium depolarization and norepinephrine and their antagonism by differing classes of vasodilators in the perfused rat hindquarters, *J. Pharmacol. Exp. Ther.* **227**:621–626.

87. Steele, T. H., and Challoner-Hue, L., 1984, Renal interactions between norepinephrine and calcium antagonists, *Kidney Int.* **26**:719–724.

88. Golderberg, J. P. and Schrier, R. W., 1984, Effect of calcium membrane blockers on in vivo vasoconstrictor properties of norepinephrine, angiotensin II and vasopressin, *Mineral Electrocyte Metab.* **10**:178–183.

89. Ruffolo, R. R., Jr., McGreery, R. L., and Patil, P. N., 1976, A kinetic analysis of a catechol-specific binding site in the microsomal fraction from the rabbit aorta, *Eur. J. Pharmacol.* **38**:221–232.

90. Vlachakis, N. D., Frederics, R., Velasquez, M., Alexander, N., Singer, F., and Maronde, R. F., 1982, Sympathetic system function and vascular reactivity in hypercalcemia patients, *Hypertension* **4**:452–458.

91. Hukovic, S. and Muschool, E., 1962, Die Noradrenalin-abgabe aus dem isolierten Kaninchenherzen bei sympathischer Nervenreizung und ihre Pharmakologische Beeinflussung, *Naunyn-Schmiedebergs Arch. Exp. Path. Pharmakol.* **244**:81–96.

92. Rubin, R. P., 1970, The role of calcium in the release of neutrotransmitter substances and hormones, *Pharmacol. Rev.* **22**:389–427.

93. Kirpekar, J. M., Prat, J. C., and Wakade, A. R., 1975, Effect of calcium on the relationship between frequency of stimulation and release of noradrenaline from the perfused spleen of the rat, *Arch. Pharmacol.* **287**:205–212.

94. Blaustein, M. P., Ratzlaff, B. W., and Kendrick, N. K., 1978, The regulation of intracellular calcium in presynaptic nerve terminals, *Ann. NY Acad. Sci.* **307**:195–211.

95. Vanhoutte, P. M., 1978, Adrenergic neuroeffector interaction in the blood vessel wall, *Fed. Proc.* **37**:181–186.

96. Greenberg, R., 1978, The neuronal origin of prostaglandin released from the rabbit portal vein in response to electrical stimulation, *Br. J. Pharmacol.* **63**:79–85.

97. Farmer, J. B. and Campbell, I. K., 1967, Calcium and magnesium ions: Influence on the response of an isolated artery to sympathetic nerve stimulation, noradrenaline and tyramine, *Br. J. Pharmacol.* **29**:319–328.

98. Garcia, A. G., Kirpekar, S. M., and Sanchez-Garcia, P., 1976, Release of noradrenaline from the cat spleen by nerve stimulation and potassium, *J. Physiol.* **261**:301–317.

99. Vanhoutte, P. M., Verbeuren, T. J., and Webb, R. C., 1981, Local modulation of adrenergic neuroeffector interaction in the blood vessel wall, *Physiol. Rev.* **61**:151–247.

100. George, A. J. and Leach, D. G., 1975, The involvement of Ca^{2+} and Mg^{2+} in the spontaneous and drug induced release of ^3H-noradrenaline from mesenteric arteries, *Biochem. Pharmacol.* **24**:737–741.

101. Fray, J. C. S., Lush, D. J., and Valentine, A. N. D., 1983, Cellular mechanisms of renin secretion, *Fed. Proc.* **42**:3150–3154.

102. Park, C. S., Han, D. S., and Fray, J. C. S., 1981, Calcium in the control of renin secretion: Ca^{2+} influx as an inhibitory signal, *Am. J. Physiol.* **40**:F70–F74.

103. Shiffrin, E. L., Gutkowska, J., Lis, M., and Genest, J., 1982, Relative role of sodium and calcium ions in the steroidogenetic response of isolated rat adrenal glomerulosa cells, *Hypertension* **4** (Suppl. II):36–42.

104. Foster, R., Lobo, M. V., Rasmussen, H., and Marusic, E. T., 1981, Calcium: Its role in the mechanism of action of angiotensin II and potassium in aldosterone production, *Endocrinology* **109**:2196–2201.

105. McCarron, D. A., Pingree, P. A., Rubin, R. J., Gaucher, S. M., Molitch, M., and Krutzik, S., 1980, Enhanced parathyroid function in essential hypertension, a homeostatic response to a urinary calcium leak, *Hypertension* **2**:162–168.

106. Kesteloot, H. and Geboers, J., 1982, Calcium and blood pressure, *Lancet* **1**:813–815.

107. Staessen, J., Bulpitt, C., Fagard, R., Joossens, J. V., Lunen, P., and Ailery, A., 1983, Four urinary cations and blood pressure: A population study in two belgian towns, *Am. J. Epidemiol.* **117**:676–687.

108. McCarron, D. A., Yung, N. N., Ugoretz, B. A., and Krutzik, S., 1981, Disturbances of calcium metabolism in the spontaneously hypertensive rat, *Hypertension* **3**(Suppl. I):I162–I167.

109. Ayachi, S., 1979, Increased dietary calcium lowers blood pressure in the spontaneously hypertensive rat, *Metabolism* **28**:1234–1238.

110. Lau, K., Zikos, D., Spirnak, J., and Eby, B., 1984, Evidence for an intestinal mechanism in hypercalciuria of spontaneously hypertensive rats, *Am. J. Physiol.* **247**:E625–E633.

111. Bianchi, G., Ferrari, P., Salvati, P., *et al.*, 1986, A renal abnormality in the Milan hypertensive strain of rats and in humans predisposed to essential hypertension, *J. Hypertens.* **4**(Suppl. 3):S33–S36.

112. Schedl, H. P., Miller, D. L., Pape, J. M., Horst, R. L., and Wilson, H. D., 1984, Calcium and sodium transport and vitamin D metabolism in the spontaneously hypertensive rat, *J. Clin. Invest.* **73**:980–986.

113. Lucas, P. A., Brown, R. C., Drueke, T., Lacour, B., Metz, J. A., and McCarron, D. A., 1986, Abnormal vitamin D metabolism, intestinal calcium transport, and bone calcium status in the sponaneously hypertensive rat compared with its genetic control, *J. Clin. Invest.* **78**:221–227.

114. Lau, K., Langman, L. B., Gafter, V., Dudeja, P. K., and Brasitus, T. A., 1986, Increased calcium absorption in prehypertensive spontaneously hypertensive rat. Role of serum 1,25-dihydroxy vitamin D_3 levels and intestinal brush border membrane fluidity, *J. Clin. Invest.* **78**:1083–1090.

115. McCarron, D. A., Lucas, P. A., Shneidman, R. S., and Drueke, T., 1985, Blood pressure development of the spontaneously hypertensive rat following concurrent manipulation of the dietary Ca^{2+} and Na^+: Relation to intestinal Ca^{2+} fluxes, *J. Clin. Invest.* **76**:1147–1154.

116. Toraason, M. A. and Wright, G. L., 1981, Transport of calcium by duodenum of spontaneously hypertensive rat, *Am. J. Physiol.* **241**:G344–G347.

117. Gafter, U., Kathpalia, S., Zikos, D., and Lau, K., 1986, Ca^{2+} fluxes across duodenum and colon of spontaneously hypertensive rats. Effect of $1,25(OH_2)D_3$, *Am. J. Physiol.* **251**:F278–282.

118. Ackerman, G. L., 1971, Increased calcium excretion after saline administration to hypertensive subjects, *J. Lab. Clin. Med.* **77**:298–306.

119. Kleeman, C. R., Bohannan, J., Bernstein, D., Ling, S., and Maxwell, M. H., 1964, Effect of variations in sodium intake on calcium excretion in normal humans, *Proc. Soc. Exp. Biol. Med.* **115**:29–32.

120. Breslau, N. A., McGuire, J. L., Zerwekh, J. E., and Pak, C. Y. C., 1982, The role of dietary sodium on renal excretion and intestinal absorption of calcium and on vitamin D metabolism, *J. Clin. Endocrinol. Metab.* **55**:369–373.

121. McCarron, D. A., Yung, N. N., Ugoretz, B. A., and Krutzik, S., 1981, Disturbances of calcium metabolism in spontaneously hypertensive rat (SHR): Attenuation of hypertension by calcium supplementation, *Hypertension* **3**(Suppl. I):162–167.

122. Massry, S. G., Coburn, J. W., Chapman, L. W., and Kleeman, C. R., 1968, The effect of long-

term desoxycorticosterone acetate administration on the renal excretion of calcium and magnesium, *J. Lab. Clin. Med.* **71:**212–219.

123. Kurtz, T. W. and Morris, R. C., 1985, Dietary NaCl as a determinant of disordered calcium metabolism in the Dahl salt-sensitive rat, *Kidney Int.* **27:**194 (Abstract).

124. Pak, C. Y. C., 1985, Overview: Calcium and hypertension, in: *NIH Workshop on Nutrition and Hypertension.* Proceedings from a symposium (M. J. Horan, M. Blaustein, J. B. Dunbar, W. Kachadorian, N. M. Kaplan, and A. P. Simopoulos, eds.), Biochemical Information Corp., Bethesda, MD, pp. 155–165.

125. Lau, K., Langman, C. B., Grafter, U., Dudeja, P. K., and Brasitus, T. A., 1986, Increased calcium absorption in prehypertensive spontaneous hypertension. Role of serum 1,25-dihydrox-yvitamin D_3 levels and intestinal brush border membrane fluidity, *J. Clin. Invest.* **78:**1083–1090.

126. Drueke, T., Lucas, P. A., Bourgovin, P., *et al.,* 1988, Changes in calcitriol status and related parameters in the young hypertensive rat (SHR), *Kidney Int.* **33:**294.

127. Stern, N., Lee, D. B. N., Silis, V., Beck, F. W., Deftos, L., Manolagas, S. C., and Sowers, J. R., 1984, Effect of high calcium intake on blood pressure and calcium metabolism in young SHR, *Hypertension* **6:**639–646.

128. McCarron, D. A., 1988, Calcium metabolism and hypertension, *Kidney Int.* **35:**717–736.

129. McCarron, D. A., Morris, C. D., Henry, H. J., and Stanton, J. L., 1984, Blood pressure and nutrient intake in the United States, *Science* **224:**1392–1397.

130. Kaplan, N. M., 1986, *Clinical Hypertension,* 4th ed., Williams & Wilkins, Baltimore.

131. Feinleib, M., Lenfant, C., and Miller, S. A., 1984, Hypertension and calcium, *Science* **226:**384–389.

132. Harlan, W. R., Hull, A. L., Schmouder, R. L., Landis, J. R., Larkin, F. A., and Thompson, F. E., 1984, High blood pressure in older Americans: The First National Health and Nutrition Examination Survey, *Hypertension* **6:**802–809.

133. Gruchow, H. W., Sobocinski, K. A., and Barboriak, J. J., 1985, Alcohol, nutrient intake, and hypertension in U.S. adults, *JAMA* **253:**1567–1570.

134. Reed, D., McGee, D., Yano, K., and Hankin, J., 1985, Diet, blood pressure, and multi-collinearity, *Hypertension* **7:**405–410.

135. Witteman, J. C. M., Willett, W. C., Stampfer, M. J., *et al.,* 1987, Dietary calcium and magnesium and hypertension: A prospective study, *Circulation* **76**(Suppl. IV):35 (Abstract).

136. Denton, D., 1982, *The Hunger for Salt; an Anthropological and Medical Analysis,* Springer-Verlag, Berlin, Heidelberg, New York.

137. Itokawa, Y., Tanaka, C., and Fujiwara, M., 1974, Changes in body temperature and blood pressure in rats with calcium and magnesium deficiencies, *J. Appl. Physiol.* **37**(6):835–839.

138. Schleiffer, R., Pernot, F., Berthelot, A., and Gairard, A., 1984, Low calcium diet enhances development of hypertension in the spontaneously hypertension rat, *Clin. Exp. Hypertension* **6:**783–793.

139. Belizan, J. M., Pineda, O., Saniz, E., Menendez, A., and Villar, J., 1981, Rise of blood pressure in calcium-deprived pregnant rats, *Am. J. Obstet. Gynecol.* **141:**163–169.

140. Altura, B. M., Altura, B. T., and Gebrewold, A., 1984, Magnesium deficiency and hypertension: correlation between magnesium-deficient diets and microcirculatory changes *in situ, Science* **223:**1315–1317.

141. Rosenthal, F. D. and Roy, S. 1972, Hypertension and hyperparathyroidism, *Br. Med. J.* **4:**396–397.

142. Lau, K., Gafter, U., Rydell, D., *et al.,* 1986, Evidence against the role of calcium deficiency in genetic hypertension, *Hypertension* **8:**45–49.

143. McCarron, D. A., 1982, Low serum concentrations of ionized calcium in patients with hypertension, *N. Engl. J. Med.* **307:**226–228.

144. Folsom, A. R., Smith, C. L., Prineas, R. J., and Grim, R. H., 1986, Serum calcium fractions in essential hypertension and matched normotensive subjects, *Hypertension* **8:**11–15.

145. Resnick, J. M., Laragh, J. H., Sealey, J. E., and Alderman, M. H., 1983, Divalent cations in

essential hypertension: Relations between serum ionized calcium, magnesium and plasma renin activity, *N. Engl. J. Med.* **309**:888–891.

146. Resnick, L. M., DiFabio, B., Marion, R. M., and Laragh, J. H., 1987, Increased oral calcium intake prevents the pressor effects of dietary salt in essential hypertension, *Kidney Int.* **31**: 308A.

147. Kesteloot, H., Geboers, J., Math, L., and Van Hoof, R., 1983, Epidemiological study of the relationship between calcium and blood pressure, *Hypertension* **5**(Suppl.II):52–56.

148. Strazzullo, P., Nunziata, V., Cirillo, M., Giannattasio, R., Ferrara, L. A., Mattioli, P. L., and Mancini, M., 1983, Abnormalities of calcium metabolism in essential hypertension, *Clin. Sci.* **65**: 137–141.

149. Freeman, R. M., Lawton, W. J., Friedlander, M. A., and Fitz, A. E., 1985, Calcium, sodium, magnesium and renin interrelationship in hypertension, *Circulation* **72**(Suppl. III):III–421 (Abstract).

150. Bulpitt, C. J., Hodes, C., and Everitt, M. G., 1976, The relationship between blood pressure and biochemical risk factors in a general population, *Br. J. Prev. Soc. Med.* **30**:158–162.

151. Kesteloot, H. and De Boers, J., 1982, Calcium and blood pressure, *Lancet* **1**:813–815.

152. Sangal, A. K. and Beevers, D. G., 1982, Serum calcium and blood pressure, *Lancet* **2**:493.

153. Robinson, D., Bailey, A. R., and Williams, P. T., 1982, Calcium and blood pressure, *Lancet* **2**: 1215–1216.

154. Maier, H., Coroneo, M. T., Antonczyk, G., Schindler, J. G., and Heidland, A., 1980, Alterations in ionized and total calcium concentrations in parotid saliva in patients with essential hypertension, *Mineral Electrolyte Metab.* **3**:109–111.

155. Fogh-Anderson, N., Hedegaard, L., Thode, J., and Siggaard-Andersen, O., 1984, Sex-dependent relation between ionized calcium in serum and blood pressure, *Clin. Chem.* **30**:116–118.

156. Kanis, J. A. and Yates, A. J., 1985, Measuring serum calcium, *Br. Med. J.* **290**:728–729.

157. Arkwright, P. D., Beilin, L. J., Vandongen, R., Rouse, I. L., and Masarei, J. R., 1984, Plasma calcium and cortisol as predisposing factors to alcohol related blood pressure elevation, *J. Hypertension* **2**:387–392.

158. West, D. W. and Ash, O., 1984, Adult reference intervals for 12 chemistry analytes: Influences of age and sex, *Am. J. Clin. Pathol.* **81**:71–76.

159. Ljunghall, S., Joborn, H., Lundin, L., Rastad, J., Wide, L., and Akerstrom, G., 1985, Regional and systemic effects of short-term intense muscular work on plasma concentration and content of total and ionized calcium, *Eur. J. Clin. Invest.* **15**:248–252.

160. Wright, G. L., and Rankin, G. O., 1982, Concentration of ionic and total calcium in plasma of four models of hypertension, *Am. J. Physiol.* **243**:H365–H370.

161. Erne, P., Bolli, P., Burgisser, E., and Buhler, F. R., 1984, Correlation of platelet calcium with blood pressure. Effect of antihypertensive therapy, *N. Engl. J. Med.* **310**:1084–1088.

162. Bruschi, G., Bruschi, M. E., Caroppo, M., *et al.*, 1985, Cytoplasmic free [Ca^{2+}] is increased in platelets of spontaneously hypertensive rats and essential hypertensive patients, *Clin. Sci.* **68**:179–184.

163. Lenz, T., Haller, H., Ludersdorf, M., et al., 1985, Free intracellular calcium in essential hypertension: Effects of nifedipine and captopril, *J. Hypertension* **3**(Suppl. 3):S13–S15.

164. Le Quan Sang, K. H., Benlian, P., Kanawati,C., Montenay-Garestier, T., Meyer, P., and Devynck, M. A., 1985, Platelet cytosolic free calcium concentration in primary hypertension, *J. Hypertension* **3**(Suppl. 3):S33–S36.

165. Shore, A. C., Beynon, G. W., Jones, J. C., Markandu, N. D., Sagnella, G. A., and MacGregor, G. A., 1985, Mononuclear leucocyte intracellular free calcium—Does it correlate with blood pressure? *J. Hypertension* **3**:183–188.

166. Lew, P. D., Favre, L., Waldvogel, F. A., and Vallotton, M. B., 1985, Cytosolic free calcium and intracellular calcium stores in neutrophils from hypertensive subjects, *Clin. Sci.* **69**:227–230.

167. Postnov, Y. V. and Orlov, S. N., 1980, Evidence of altered calcium accumulation and calcium binding by the membranes of adipocytes in spontaneously hypertensive rats, *Pflügers Arch.* **385**: 85–87.

168. Bruschi, G., Bruschi, M. E., Caroppo, M., *et al.*, 1984, Intracellular free [Ca^{2+}] in circulating lymphocytes of spontaneously hypertensive rats, *Life Sci.* **35**:535–542.

169. Ahmed, I., Tan, S., Pesigan, M., Eby, B., and Lau, K., 1988, Increased cytosolic free Ca concentration [Ca^{2+}] in proximal tubules of spontaneously hypertensive rat: Concordance with the low 1,25(OH)$_2$D levels and responses to a high Ca diet, *Kidney Int.* **33**:291.

170. Jacobs, W. R., Brazy, P. C., and Mandel, L. J., 1987, Fura-2 measurements of intracellular free calcium in renal cortical tubules from SHR and WKY rats, *Kidney Int.* **31**:350.

171. Llibre, J., LaPointe, M., and Battle, D. C., 1987, Fura-2 measurements of cytosolic cell Ca^{2+} in renal proximal tubules and circulating lymphocytes of rats with genetic hypertension, *Kidney Int.* **31**:302.

172. Bukoski, R. D., DeWan, P., and McCarron, P. A., 1988, Intracellular Ca^{2+} in cultured aortic myocytes and mesenteric resistance vessels of spontaneously hypertensive and Wistar Kyoto rats, *FASEB J.* **2**:A503.

173. Bhalla, R. C., Webb, R. C., Singh, D., Ashley, T., and Brock, T., 1978, Calcium fluxes, calcium binding, and adenosine cyclic 3'-5'-monophosphate-dependent protein kinase activity in the aorta of spontaneously hypertensive and Kyoto–Wistar normotensive rats, *Mol. Pharmacol.* **14**:468–477.

174. Aoki, K., Yamashita, K., Tomita, N., Tazumi, K., and Hotta, K., 1974, ATPase activity and Ca^{2+} binding ability of subcellular membrane of arterial smooth muscle in spontaneously hypertensive rats, *Am. Heart J.* **15**:180–181.

175. Orlov, S. N., Pokudin, N. I., and Postnov, Y. V., 1983, Calmodulin-dependent Ca^{2+}-transport in erythrocytes of spontaneously hypertensive rats, *Pflüger's Arch.* **397**:54–56.

176. Moore, L., Hurwitz, L., Davenport, G. R., and Landon, E. J., 1975, Energy-dependent calcium uptake activity of microsomes from the aorta of normal and hypertensive rats, *Biochim. Biophys. Acta* **413**:432–443.

177. Jones, A. W. and Hart, R. G., 1975, Altered ion transport in aortic smooth muscle during deoxycorticosterone acetate hypertension in the rat, *Circ. Res.* **37**:333–341.

178. McCarron, D. A., Yung, N. N., Ugoretz, B. A., and Krutzik, S., 1981, Disturbances of calcium metabolism in the spontaneously hypertensive rat, *Hypertension* **3**(Suppl. I):I162–I167.

179. Lau, K., Chen, S., and Eby, B., 1984, Evidence for the role of PO$_4$ deficiency in antihypertensive action of high-Ca diet, *Am. J. Physiol.* **246**:H324–H329.

180. Peuler, J. D., Morgan, D. A., and Mark, A. L., 1987, High calcium diet reduces blood pressure in Dahl salt-sensitive rats by neural mechanisms, *Hypertension* **9**(Suppl. III):159–165.

181. Kurtz, T. W. and Morris, R. C., 1986, Attenuation of deoxycorticosterone-induced hypertension by supplemental dietary calcium, *J. Hypertension* **4**(Suppl. 5):S182–S191.

182. Kageyama, Y., Suzuki, H., Arima, K., and Saruta, T., 1987, Oral calcium treatment lowers blood pressure in renovascular hypertensive rats by suppressing the renin–angiotensin system, *Hypertension* **10**:375–382.

183. Muntzel, M. S., Hatton, D. C., Metz, J. A., and McCarron, D. A., 1989, Dietary calcium alters blood pressure in neonatal spontaneously hypertensive rats, *Am. J. Hypertension* **2**:158–162.

184. Belizan, J. M., Villar, J., Pineda, O., et al., 1983, Reduction of blood pressure with calcium supplementation in young adults, *JAMA* **249**:1161–1165.

185. Belizan, J. M., Villar, J., Zalazar, A., Rojas, L., Chan, D., and Bryce, G. F., 1983, Preliminary evidence of the effects of calcium supplementation on blood pressure in normal pregnant women, *Am. J. Obstet. Gynecol.* **146**:175–180.

186. McCarron, D. A. and Morris, C. D., 1985, Blood pressure response to oral calcium in persons with mild to moderate hypertension, *Ann. Intern. Med.* **103**:825–831.

187. Luft, F. C., Aronoff, G. R., Sloan, R. S., Fineberg, N. S., and Weinberger, M. H., 1986, Short-term augmented calcium intake has no effect on sodium homeostasis, *Clin. Pharmacol. Ther.* **39**:414–419.

188. Tabuchi, Y., Ogihara, T., Hashizume, K., *et al.*, 1986, Hypotensive effect of long-term oral calcium supplement in elderly patients with essential hypertension, *J. Clin. Hypertension* **3**:254–262.

189. Strazzullo, P., Siani, A., Galletti, F., *et al.*, 1985, A controlled clinical trial of long term oral calcium supplementation in arterial hypertension, in: Program of the 2nd European Meeting on Hypertension, University of Milan, Milan, (Abstract #512).

190. Singer, D. R., Markandu, N. D., Cappuccio, F. P., et al., 1985, Does oral calcium lower blood pressure. A double-blind study, *J. Hypertension* **3**:661–671.

191. Meese, R. B., Gonzalez, D. G., Casparian, J. M., Ram, C. V., Pak, C. Y., and Kaplan, N. M., 1986, Failure of calcium supplements to relieve hypertension, *Clin. Res.* **34**:218A, (Abstract).

192. Cappuccio, F. P., Markandu, N. D., Singer, D. R. J., Smith, S. J., Shore, A. C., and MacGregor, G. A., 1987, Does oral calcium supplementation lower high blood pressure? A double blind study, *J. Hypertens.* **5**:67–71.

193. Resnick, L. M., Nicholson, J. P., and Laragh, J. H., 1986, Dietary salt, calcium metabolism, and the antihypertensive efficacy of calcium channel blockade, *Kidney Int.* **29**: 257A.

194. Grobbee, D. E. and Hofman, A., 1986, Effect of calcium supplementation on diastolic blood pressure in young people with mild hypertension, *Lancet* **2**:703–707.

195. Zemel, M. B., Gualdoni, S. M., and Sowers, J. R., 1986, Sodium excretion and plasma renin activity in normotensive and hypertensive black adults as affected by dietary calcium and sodium, *J. Hypertens* **4**(Suppl. 6):S343–345.

196. Churchill, P. C., 1987, Calcium channel antagonists and renin release, *Am. J. Nephrol* **7**(Suppl. 1) :32–38.

197. Johansson, B., 1981, Vascular smooth muscle reactivity, *Annu. Rev. Physiol.* **43**:359–370.

7

Immunologic Aspects of Renal Disease

William G. Couser

1. Introduction

In this chapter, I will review information on mechanisms of immune renal diseases published only during 1986–1987, with particular attention to new directions, concepts, and processes that may have significant implications for the future. In setting this course, I inevitably exclude from review isolated observations of interest that do not blend easily into currents of the field in general. In the second half of the chapter, I will review new data on clinical entities considered in the category of immune renal disease. Whenever possible, I have linked observations on disease mechanisms made experimentally with the clinical entities that are believed to result from them.

2. Mechanisms of Immune Glomerular Injury

2.1. Glomerular Immune Deposit Formation

The study of mechanisms of immune deposit formation in glomeruli has continued, albeit at a slower rate than during the heyday of discovery of fixed antigens leading to *in situ* immune complex formation. Two excellent reviews of this area have appeared recently which summarize recent advances in considerable detail.[1,2]

WILLIAM G. COUSER • Division of Nephrology, University of Washington, Seattle, Washington 98195.

My review is organized by site of immune deposit formation within glomeruli, a variable recently shown by Feintzeig et al. to be a critical determinant of the type of lesion that results.[3] Thus deposits of a given antigen–antibody system produce a noninflammatory C5b-9-dependent lesion in a subepithelial distribution, whereas in a subendothelial or mesangial site, where deposits and the chemotactic products they generate are more accessible to circulating inflammatory cells, a much more inflammatory lesion is usually seen.[3]

2.1.1. Subepithelial Immune Complex Deposits

2.1.1.1. Fixed Glomerular Antigens. The observation several years ago that subepithelial deposits in the Heymann nephritis models of membranous nephropathy in rats result from antibody binding to a cell surface antigen (GP330), expressed in the clathrin-coated pits of the glomerular epithelial cell, led to major revisions in our concept of how subepithelial immune complex deposits form and introduced the concept of nephritis induced by antibody to glomerular cell surface antigenic epitopes.[1,2] With respect to the glomerular epithelial cell and subepithelial deposits, attention continues to focus on the Heymann nephritis models, which bear such remarkable similarity to idiopathic membranous nephropathy in humans. Although several putative antigens remain under study, the best-characterized and most-accepted antigen in Heymann nephritis remains GP330. Ronco et al. have extended the earlier observations of Kerjaschki and Farquhar to show that IgG in glomerular deposits in active Heymann nephritis is reactive with GP330, that several monoclonal antibodies to GP330 induce epimembranous deposits, that active immunization with GP330 induces subepithelial deposits and proteinuria, and that antibodies to RTE α 5, the Heymann nephritis–inducing brush border antigen identified by Edgington, Glassock, and Dixon in 1968, are also reactive with GP330.[4] Although the importance of GP330, and of deposit formation on the glomerular epithelial cell plasma membrane, has been much clarified recently, the fact that GP330 is also present in proximal tubular brush border, and that antigen derived from proximal tubular brush border (Fx1A) is conventionally used to induce Heymann nephritis, continues to stimulate work exploring the role of other brush border antigens in causing glomerular disease. However, none of these have been clearly localized to the glomerular epithelial cell, as GP330 has. A further encouragement to the study of tubular antigens is the observation that GP330 is apparently not present in human glomerular epithelial cells and that a cross-reactive antigen, GP400, is located in human and dog proximal tubular brush border[5,6] and may be the antigen that induces Heymann nephritis in rats immunized with human Fx1A.[7] Another glycoprotein antigen (GP600) with subunits weighing 150,000, 110,000, and 70,000 kd, has been identified by Singh and Makker in rat serum[8] and at the GBM–endothelial cell interface[9,10] and has been postulated to be a circulating source of nephritogenic antigen which may be taken up by clathrin-coated pits rather than synthesized at that site. Abrass has also provided evidence for a role for circulating tubular antigen in Heymann nephritis, demonstrating that a 66-kd, apparently anionic fraction of Fx1A may bind directly to glomeruli *in vivo* and *in vitro* [11] and that early AICN eluates contain antibody to this antigen, which is reactive with tubular brush border but not with glomeruli.[12] Abrass postulates that anti-idiotypic antibody to Fx1A then develops which is reactive with a second 45-kd antigen apparently expressed on glomerular cell membranes.[12]

Thus several antigen antibody systems, including both glomerular and tubular antigens, may participate in Heymann nephritis, a finding also suggested by Bagchus *et al.*, who demonstrated that absorption of anti-Fx1A with a 90-kd component in rat thymocytes reduced glomerular binding activity.[13] The use of monoclonal antibodies to identify and characterize Heymann antigens is well reviewed by Verroust *et al.* in a general review on monoclonal antibodies and glomerular antigens.[14] The exact role of each of these antigen–antibody systems in human membranous nephropathy obviously awaits further study. However, it should be emphasized that neither the absence of GP330 from human glomerular epithelial cells, nor the absence in most patients with idiopathic membranous nephropathy of antibody reactive with proximal tubular brush border by indirect immunofluorescence, excludes the presence of an autoimmune mechanism involving antibody reactive with a glomerular epithelial cell membrane antigen as the initiating event in human disease.

Apart from studies to define the antigen in Heymann nephritis, progress has also been made in understanding the cellular mechanisms of deposit formation in this model. This topic is extensively reviewed by Andres *et al.*[1] This group has shown that anti-Fx1A antibody interaction with rat glomerular epithelial cells *in vitro* is followed by antigen redistribution (capping) on the cell surface and then by shedding of immune complexes, a process requiring participation of cytoskeletal elements and calcium. Agents that prevent formation of caps by effects on the cytoskeleton also reduce formation of deposits and improve disease.[15] This cross-linking of glomerular epithelial cell membrane antigen by antibody converts the antigen from a membrane-associated form to an insoluble form bound to cytoskeleton through microfilaments.[16] When antibody to a single antigen (GP330) is used *in vivo,* this process requires formation of highly cross-linked immune complexes and hence polyclonal antibody.[16] With antibody to GP330 the formation of these immune complex deposits is initiated in the area of clathrin-coated pits along the podocyte plasmalemma lining the GBM. Following shedding of immune complexes from the cell surface, the shed immune deposits remain connected to a coated pit at some level but also become firmly attached to GBM by unknown, but probably covalent, interactions.[17] Much of this new information has been reviewed by Brown *et al.*[18] The relevance of these observations to kidney disease probably extends beyond subepithelial deposits, as suggested by recent data demonstrating the induction of glomerulonephritis by antibody to both endothelial and mesangial cell membrane antigens (see Section 2.1.2).

Studies of the immune response in Heymann nephritis indicate that it may be down-regulated by increased suppressor T cells in animals treated with mercuric chloride[19] and up-regulated by exposure to normal antigen or antibody to it which may produce antigenic release.[20] Other studies have suggested that proteolytic enzyme therapy may be effective in reducing the subepithelial immune deposits in Heymann nephritis after they are formed and also in reducing proteinuria,[21] although some of these effects may be due to a reduction in formation of deposits rather than to dissolution of previously formed deposits.

2.1.1.2. *Subepithelial Deposits Due to Exogenous Antigens.* With the focus of attention on autoimmune mechanisms and cell membrane antigens in glomerulonephritis, less attention has recently been paid to studies of serum sickness–type immune complex nephritis models. An excellent review of mechanisms of immune deposit formation involving exogenous antigens has been provided by Wener and Mannik.[2] The effect of increasing antigen dose on disease has been shown to differ with cationic and native bovine serum albumin (BSA), suggesting that these antigens produce deposit formation by different mechanisms[22,23] and that both affinity and precipitating characteristics of the inducing antibody are important.[24] An alternative factor to cationic antigen–capillary wall charge interaction in the formation of subepithelial deposits with cationic antigens is suggested by data demonstrating that cationic BSA antigen induces antibody of reduced precipitating properties and avidity, features that have long been associated with the development of predominantly membranous lesions in the chronic serum sickness models.[25] This may relate to the persistence of free antigen and antibody in the circulation facilitating *in situ* immune complex formation in these models. Other studies of charge interactions in the formation of glomerular immune deposits, predominantly subepithelial, include the observations of Chan *et al.*, who have shown very nicely that initial localization of a cationic protein that is not part of an immune complex (here cationic human IgG) can serve as a charge site for anionic antigens and then for antibodies to become localized in glomeruli, thereby facilitating *in situ* capillary wall immune complex formation.[26] Examples of such molecules may include cationic proteins derived from neutrophils and platelets, which have been shown by Camussi *et al.* to localize in glomeruli in acute serum sickness induced by native (anionic) BSA just before or concurrently with the earliest immune complex deposits.[27] Earlier observations that treatment with protamine sulfate can reduce cationic antigen localization in glomeruli have been confirmed and extended to demonstrate that treatment started after renal disease is established has little effect on proteinuria, suggesting a long-term functional defect induced by shorter-term immune injury in membranous nephropathy.[28] Factors that contribute to *in situ* glomerular immune complex formation other than charge interactions have also been explored. Ward *et al.* have confirmed, in transplant studies, that ongoing dynamic interaction of antigen and antibody with previously deposited immune complexes occurs in glomeruli of rabbits with chronic BSA serum sickness.[29] Evidence that antiidiotypic antibodies occur in immune complex nephritis and that they contribute to glomerular immune complex formation continues to accumulate. This topic has been reviewed in detail by Zanetti and Wilson[30] and Thomas and Williams.[31]

Finally, studies continue of mechanisms to remove established immune complex deposits in glomeruli in the hope that this may be of benefit, although several studies suggest that, in subepithelial deposit disease, benefits may be very limited.[28] Agodoa and Mannik have shown that excess cationic antigen is much more effective than anionic antigen in reversing or dissolving subepithelial immune complex deposits, probably because of greater access on a charge basis to the subepithelial space.[32] Removal of deposits containing charged antigen by charge competition with a polycation such as protamine was shown to be effective only with very small amounts of antibody present and is apparently not effective with the amounts of antibody present in immune complex disease.[33] Others have shown a reduction in glomerular deposits of passively administered immune complexes by systemic protease therapy, although care to distinguish between reduced deposition and dissolution of deposited complexes must be emphasized in interpreting these studies.[34]

2.1.2. Glomerulonephritis Induced by Antibodies to Glomerular Cell Membranes

The role of antibody to antigenic determinants on the glomerular epithelial cell in producing subepithelial immune complex deposits has already been discussed. This mechanism has now been extended to both mesangial and endothelial cells. A thymic antigen, Thy 1.1, has been localized to mesangial cell membranes,[35] and administration of complement-fixing polyclonal antibody to it induces an acute glomerulonephritis characterized by mesangial cell lysis and capillary aneurysm formation, followed later by mesangial cell proliferation and even crescent formation.[35-38] The lesion appears to be complement-dependent but neutrophil-independent, suggesting a role for C5b-9.[36-38] Other T-cell antigenic epitopes have been localized throughout the capillary wall and on glomerular endothelial and epithelial cells and may be relevant to nephritis induced with antithymocyte serum.[39] Mesangial immune complex deposits can also be induced by monoclonal antibodies to unique mesangial matrix antigens.[40] The relevance of each of these observations to diseases such as IgA nephropathy and mesangial proliferative glomerulonephritis remains uncertain, but the mesangial lesions produced are clearly similar to ones that may occur in these diseases. Antibody to an endothelial cell antigen (angiotensin converting enzyme) has also been shown to produce an acute glomerulonephritis in rabbits with development of subepithelial immune complex deposits that presumably derive from the endothelial cell surface.[41] Several groups have described the presence of such antibodies in patients with lupus nephritis.

2.1.3. Circulating Immune Complex Trapping

Current understanding of the factors that regulate glomerular deposition of preformed immune complexes and their role in immune complex nephritis is well reviewed by Wener and Mannik.[2] Relevant recent observations include those of Koyama *et al.* that cationized antigens have low precipitating efficiency with antibody in immune complex form and, when injected as part of immune complexes, are more likely to lead to subepithelial capillary wall deposits.[42] Whether these deposits represent deposits of preformed complexes containing cationized antigens or separate localization of antigen and antibody *in situ* is unclear. It should be noted that typical subepithelial deposits have been induced by deposition of antibody to endothelial cell surface antigens, suggesting that with an increase in capillary wall permeability, the movement of preformed immune complexes from a subendothelial site to the subepithelial space may be common.[41] Abrass and Hori have shown a reduction in mononuclear phagocyte system clearance of immune complexes in insulin-deficient diabetic rats associated with accelerated vascular deposition of immune complexes,[43] and reduced Fc receptor function in patients with several forms of active immune complex nephritis was demonstrated by others,[44] although it remains unclear whether the altered mononuclear phagocyte system function reflects cause or effect. The ability of heparan sulfate–proteoglycan–enriched anionic sites in both capillary wall and mesangium to facilitate deposition of cationic immune complexes has been established by Kanwar *et al.*[45] and of exogenous cationic protein to have a similar effect on immune complex containing anionic antigens by Chan *et al.*[26] The fact that most preformed immune complexes in humans and primates circulate bound to red blood cells via CR1 (C3b) receptors is now well established, and the potential role of alterations in the erythrocyte–immune complex clearing and processing system in the pathogenesis of immune complex nephritis is reviewed by Hebert and Cosio.[46] The demonstration of CR1 (C3b) and possibly CR2 (C3d) receptors on rat glomerular epithelial cells by Kasinath *et al.* may provide a tool for study of the possible role of such receptors in glomerular immune complex localization.[47] These authors have also recently suggested an important role for fibronectin in regulating glomerular immune complex deposits. Fibronectin is a glycoprotein present in both blood and tissues including glomerular subendothelial and mesangial areas, and fibronectin can directly bind DNA and some bacterial antigens. Fibronectin also binds to certain immune complexes by both C3b-dependent and C1q-independent mechanisms.[48] Immune complexes with fibronectin binding properties exhibit accelerated clearance and enhanced glomerular deposition as well as binding directly to glomeruli *in vitro.*[49] Several possible roles of fibronectin in renal disease have been reviewed by Schena and Pertosa.[50]

Despite continued study, evidence that antigen and antibody cause glomerular injury by depositing as preformed immune complexes from the circulation rather than by forming immune complexes *in situ* remains minimal. Direct observation of vascular immune complex formation and deposition in conjunctiva suggests that perivascular formation of immune complex deposits is accompanied by a more intense inflammatory response compared to deposition of complexes from the circulation.[51] However, Chen *et al.* have recently reported induction of both proteinuria and inflammatory changes within 2 days of injection of mice with preformed immune complexes containing monoclonal antibodies which localize predominantly in the mesangium.[52] More systematic studies of the nephritogenic potential of circulating immune complexes clearly need to be carried out.

2.1.4. Anti-Basement Membrane Antibody Disease

Another extensively studied example of *in situ* immune complex formation due to renal antigens is anti-basement membrane (anti-GBM) antibody-induced nephritis. Developments in this area have included further studies of the composition of the basement membrane itself, identification of the antigenic determinants against which anti-GBM antibody is directed and description of experimental models induced by antibody to other defined, but nontraditional, GBM antigens. Three excellent reviews of current understanding of GBM biochemistry and alterations in disease have appeared by Abrahamson, Timpl, and Uitto *et al.*[53-55] Butkowski *et al.* have extended their studies demonstrating that the Goodpasture antigen is a subunit of the noncollagenous domain of type IV collagen to characterize the chains of the M1, M2 (containing the Goodpasture epitope), and M3 subunits and have shown that the Goodpasture epitope resides in a normal, but very novel, polypeptide chain on type IV collagen.[56] Pusey *et al.* used a monoclonal antibody to collagenase soluble GBM which bound to the same bands (26 and 58 kd) as sera from 42 patients with anti-GBM disease, providing data similar to those of Butkowski and colleagues on the nature of the reactive antigen.[57] Similar antigens have been identified in alveolar and placental basement membrane.[58] However, a number of questions remain regarding the biochemical composition, distribution, and exposure of the reactive antigenic epitopes.[59]

As understanding of the molecular composition of GBM, now known to contain at least collagen IV, laminin, entactin, and heparan sulfate proteoglycans, unfolds further, investigators have studied the consequences of inducing nephritis with antibody to each of these purified components. Bygren *et al.* demonstrate that sheep with classic Steblay autoimmune glomerulonephritis induced with human basement membrane developed a broad range of anti-GBM antibodies, but the major antibody deposited in kidney is an autoantibody reactive with the M2 subunit of the globular domain of collagen IV, which contains the Goodpasture antigen.[60] Wick *et al.* reported that mice immunized with the NC1 domain itself developed linear alveolar and basement membrane deposits as well as glomerulonephritis.[61] Natori and Shibata have pursued similar studies using "nephritogenoside," an antigen separable from type IV collagen and distinct from glycoproteins such as laminin and fibronectin.[62] The nephritogenic potential of laminin has been studied by Feintzeig *et al.*, who showed that antilaminin antibody binds in the capillary wall and mesangium but fails to induce complement fixation or proteinuria, suggesting that laminin is an unlikely component of GBM antigens.[63] Of interest, autologous phase disease in this model was severe and accompanied by epithelial cell detachment, suggesting possible interference with laminin attachment protein function. Both Makino *et al.*[64,65] and Miettinen and colleagues[66] have used polyclonal antibody to core protein of heparan sulfate proteoglycan to produce a disease in rats that is characterized by exclusively subepithelial binding of IgG and C3, mild proteinuria, and selective subepithelial thickening apparently due to new basement membrane formation by glomerular epithelial cells. A similar phenomenon of subepithelial thickening and "spike" formation was described by Matsuo *et al.* in mice immunized with human glomeruli or basement membrane that developed linear/granular subepithelial deposits of IgG and C3, and the basement membrane thickening in this model was composed predominantly of laminin.[67] Using a different stimulus, induction of autoantibody by administration of mercuric chloride, Fukatsu and colleagues also showed that Brown Norway (BN) rats developed autoantibodies to laminin, collagen IV, heparan sulfate proteoglycans, and entactin, and that renal eluates from such animals react with purified laminin and collagen IV as well as with these components in cultured glomerular epithelial cells.[68] Of interest, such rats also developed substantial GBM thickening. Taken together, these results suggest that immune deposit formation near the glomerular epithelial cell surface may provide a stimulus to glomerular epithelial cell matrix production, including production of laminin and collagen IV, which results in a structurally abnormal basement membrane that may also have abnormalities in functional integrity.

2.2.   Mediators of Immune Renal Injury

This section is subdivided into those mechanisms which have been clearly shown to produce glomerular injury due to immune events—that is, antibody alone, C5b-9, inflammatory cells, and sensitized lymphocytes. Other, less clearly understood mechanisms, such as the potential nephritogenicity of resident glomerular cells, prostaglandins, and coagulation mechanisms, are also considered. Two good reviews of this topic have been published during the period covered.[69,70]

2.2.1.   Injury Induced by Antibody Alone

The ability of IgG anti-GBM antibody alone to induce glomerular injury was earlier established by us *in vivo* and in an isolated perfused rat kidney system. Boyce and Holdsworth have extended these observations in an isolated perfused rat kidney system using dextran sieving curves to demonstrate that the loss of permeability induced by anti-GBM antibody in this model may represent a loss of the charge barrier.[71] They have further shown that anti-GBM antibody deposition can activate the intrarenal renin–angiotensin system to produce a rise in renal vascular resistance and decrease in filtration rate independently of complement and other inflammatory mediators.[72] These observations may be relevant to acute antibody-induced glomerulonephritis in which C3 deposits are not seen.

2.2.2.   Injury Due to Complement Activation

Relatively little work has been recently published on complement in human renal disease. The demonstration of both C4a and C4b isotypes in the normal mesangium is of interest, although the source and function of this material are unclear.[73] In this area, most attention has been directed at the C5b-9 membrane attack complex of complement. Serum C5b-9 levels have been correlated with antimyelin antibody in dymyelinating neuropathies,[74] and cerebral spinal fluid C5b-9 has been correlated with neurologic disease in both lupus and Sjögren's syndrome.[75] Recent studies have better defined the distribution and significance of C5b-9 neoantigen deposits in human renal disease. Hinglais *et al.* described C5b-9 deposits in connective tissue and cell membranes of normal kidneys as well as at various sites associated with immune deposits in nephritic kidneys.[76] Their findings are consistent with C5b-9 activation by both immune and nonimmune mechanisms and suggest that C5b-9 formation may occur as a consequence as well as possibly a cause of renal injury. Rus *et al.* report a worse clinical prognosis in patients with primary glomerular disease who have C5b-9 deposits, which may simply reflect more severe tissue injury with subsequent C5b-9 activation.[77] Yoshioka *et al.* confirmed the presence of extensive C5b-9 deposits in sclerotic areas of glomeruli in patients with reflux nephropathy.[78] Falk *et al.* have reported the first immunoultrastructural localization of C5b-9 in human renal disease and document that much of the C5b-9 in aging and diabetic kidneys is associated with cellular debris located predominantly in the mesangium, GBM, tubular basement membrane (TBM), and vessel walls.[79] However, C5b-9 was also present in immune deposits in membranoproliferative glomerulonephritis.[79] C5b-9 appears to localize with mesangial IgA deposits in IgA nephropathy as well.[80]

Studies verifying our original observation on the nephritogenicity of C5b-9 in experimental models of immune tissue injury continue to appear. Cybulsky *et al.* have used an isolated perfused rat kidney system to demonstrate that deposits of nephritogenic amounts of antibody to glomerular epithelial cell antigen are associated with epithelial cell injury and proteinuria only when perfusate contains C6 and C8, thus permitting C5b-9 assembly, a convincing demonstration of the nephritogenic effect of C5b-9 independently of antibody.[81,82] Camussi *et al.* have used the same antibody to demonstrate C5b-9 dependent lysis of rat glomerular epithelial cells *in vitro* and to show that cellular processing of the membrane-inserted C5b-9 complex appears to occur independently of processing of the antigen–antibody complex.[83] However, the cellular mechanism of the nephritogenic C5b-9 effect that leads to increased glomerular permeability and proteinuria remains elusive since glomerular epithelial cell lysis is not a prominent feature of the most C5b-9-dependent glomerular lesions, such as experimental membranous nephropathy. Several studies now document the capacity of sublytic quantities of membrane-inserted C5b-9 to function as a stimulus to cellular production of various potential inflammatory mediators, including thromboxane B_2, by platelets[84]; thromboxane B_2, prostaglandin E_2, interleukin I, and superoxide anion by monocytes[85]; prostaglandins, interleukin 1, superoxide anion, and hydrogen peroxide by glomerular mesangial cells[86,87]; and prostaglandin E_2 and thromboxane by glomerular epithelial cells.[88] The precise role of this mechanism and of the various intracellular mediators released following C5b-9-induced cell activation, as they relate to altered glomerular permeability in glomerulonephritis, remains an area for future investigation.

2.2.3. Injury Due to Inflammatory Cells

Significant advances in this area include documentation by Feintzeig *et al.* that inflammatory cell involvement in mediating glomerular injury is very dependent on the site of immune deposit formation, with intramembranous and subendothelial (and presumably mesangial) immune deposits much more capable of eliciting an inflammatory cell response than subepithelial deposits.[3] A model of glomerulonephritis induced by *in situ* formation of IgG anti-IgG immune complexes (at several sites), which is mediated by contributions of complement, neutrophils, and monocytes, with the latter apparently requiring C3 activation to mediate injury, has been described.[89] A quantitative analysis of the infiltrating leukocytes in this model was reported by Cook *et al.* and shown to be predominantly neutrophils early and monocytes later, using FACS analysis.[90] However, most attention in this area has been focused on the role of reactive oxygen species and inflammatory cell–mediated glomerular injury. Two excellent reviews of this topic have recently appeared.[91,92] These papers review a body of earlier studies, largely by Rehan and Johnson, demonstrating that hydrogen peroxide appears to be the principal oxidant in several models of inflammatory glomerulonephritis. However, the beneficial effect of the iron chelator desferrioxamine and the hydroxyl radical scavenger dimethylthiourea in neutrophil-dependent anti-GBM nephritis in the rabbit supports a role for hydroxyl radical production as well.[93] The mechanism of hydrogen peroxide–induced glomerular injury has been further investigated by Dr. Rick Johnson in our laboratory, who has shown that physiologic concentrations of hydrogen peroxide are nephritogenic only when neutrophil-derived myeloperoxidase (MPO) is localized in the glomerular capillary wall and provided further evidence that glomerular bound MPO reacts with hydrogen peroxide in the presence of a halide to produce halogenation of basement membrane and severe histologic and functional evidence of glomerular injury.[94] Dr. Johnson's studies have further implicated the MPO–H_2O_2–halide system in glomerulonephritis by demonstrating that basement membrane halogenation occurs *in vivo* in a neutrophil-dependent model of glomerulonephritis induced by subendothelial immune complex formation and that it can be abolished by neutrophil depletion.[95] Shah *et al.* have also provided evidence that the MPO–H_2O_2–halide system of activated neutrophils can activate a latent metalloproteinase of neutrophils which has GBM-degrading properties.[96] Johnson *et al.* have also documented the capacity of physiologic concentrations of the neutrophil-derived protease elastase to cause heavy proteinuria *in vivo*.[97] Thus, both oxidants and proteases appear to be implicated in neutrophil-mediated glomerular injury and the two systems appear to interact. A further advance has been the demonstration by Johnson *et al.* that platelets are apparently required for neutrophil-mediated glomerular injury to occur.[98] The mechanism of this effect is presently unclear, but appears not to involve an effect on neutrophil chemotaxis by platelets.

2.2.4. Injury Due to Sensitized Lymphocytes

Evidence that cell-mediated immunity is involved in producing glomerulonephritis continues to accumulate, but rather slowly. Studies of T-cell subsets in human renal disease confirmed earlier findings that T cells are present in glomeruli in a variety of glomerular diseases,[99,100] that T cells and monocytes are associated,[99,100] and that T helper cells tend to be associated with proliferative glomerular lesions.[99] Hooke et al. have observed and characterized the interstitial mononuclear cell infiltrates in several forms of glomerulonephritis and demonstrated that the interstitial infiltrate correlates better with renal function than does the glomerular cellular infiltrate.[100] Using an accelerated anti-GBM antibody–induced model, Boyce et al. have shown that T lymphocytes precede macrophages in glomerular infiltrates and that the glomerular T cells produce macrophage inhibitory factor locally.[101] No recent data have emerged to further establish the ability of antibody-independent cellular mechanisms to produce glomerular injury experimentally (see also discussion of vasculitis, Section 5.1).

2.2.5. Injury Due to Resident Glomerular Cells

The availability of techniques for studying pure populations of glomerular cells in culture, as well as recognition that these cells produce a variety of growth factors and potential inflammatory mediators, has stimulated considerable ongoing work defining the cell biology of the glomerular cells and their response to injury. Because of the ease with which it can be cultured and its resemblance to circulating immune effector cells, the glomerular mesangial cell continues to receive the most attention. A summary of these data and techniques for studying glomerular cells in culture is presented by Lovett and Sterzel,[102] and Schlondorff has reviewed the data implicating the mesangial cell as a regulator of intrarenal hemodynamics.[103] Singhal et al. have provided elegant documentation and quantitation of the mesangial cell contractile response.[104] This contractile response has been shown to be stimulated by leukotrienes LTC4 and LTD4, which also induce renal vasoconstriction.[105] In addition to these mechanical phenomena, the nature of mesangial cell–derived thymocyte activating factor has been clarified by Lovett et al., who demonstrate that it closely resembles macrophage interleukin I and functions as an autocrine growth factor for mesangial cells.[106] Glomerular endothelial cells have also been shown to secrete both stimulators and a heparinlike inhibitor of mesangial cell growth.[107] The hypothesis that mesangial cell interleukin I may participate in glomerulonephritis is supported by the finding of a two- to threefold increase in kidney interleukin I mRNA from rats actively immunized to produce immune complex glomerulonephritis, although it cannot be ascertained from these data whether the mRNA studied was derived from mesangial cells.[108] Interleukin I has also been shown to stimulate mesangial cell release of vasodilatory prostaglandins.[109] Mesangial cells have also been shown to release a platelet-derived growth factor like mitogenic protein,[110] platelet activating factor,[111,112] and thrombospondin,[113] a component of extra cellular matrix analogous to fibronectin. The capacity of C5b-9 to activate mesangial cells has been commented on earlier, and a similar effect of immune complexes has been shown as measured by release of superoxide anion and has been demonstrated to be Fc receptor dependent.[114] Dietary-induced essential fatty acid deficiency has also been shown by Lefkowith and Schreiner to result in a reduction in glomerular Ia-positive mesangial cells and macrophages and in glomerular prostaglandin production,[115] effects that might substantially modify disease mediated by resident glomerular cell populations. Gurner *et al.* have provided evidence in bone marrow chimeras to show that glomerular mesangial Ia-positive cells are of bone marrow origin,[116] as previously suggested by Schreiner based on syngeneic bone marrow transplant experiments. The phagocytic activity of mesangial macrophages has been shown by Seiler *et al.* to enhance mesangial uptake of macromolecules subsequently presented to the mesangium.[117] Another study by Kimura *et al.* also suggests an important role for infiltrating macrophages rather than resident glomerular cells in the processing and degradation of mesangial macromolecules, which appear to leave the glomerulus and transport material intracellularly from the mesangium to extraglomerular areas.[118]

2.2.6. Injury Due to Coagulation Mechanisms

Most attention in this area has focused on macrophage-derived procoagulant activity, a phenomenon now thought to be related to tissue factor which can initiate fibrin deposition in glomerulonephritis by activation of the intrinsic coagulation pathway. Tipping *et al.* have shown that the increased procoagulant activity seen in several models of inflammatory glomerulonephritis correlates with glomerular macrophage infiltrates, precedes fibrin deposition, and has several functional similarities to macrophage-derived tissue factor.[119,120] Induction of macrophage procoagulant activity has been shown to parallel development of glomerulonephritis in murine lupus[121] and has also been reported in a mercuric chloride–induced model of nephritis,[122] although not associated with macrophages in the latter study. Procoagulant activity has also been measured in normal and nephritic urine by Wiggins *et al.*, where it also appears to be tissue factor–like and associated with microvesicles that may be of glomerular origin.[123,124]

Studies in humans also support a role for intraglomerular coagulation in several renal diseases. Many fibrin deposits in human kidney biopsies have been shown to represent cross-linked fibrin rather than antigens of fibrinogen or its degradation products which could be nonspecifically trapped in the kidney.[125] Although glomerular fibrin deposits were not clearly associated with macrophages or other cellular sources of tissue factor, it must be remembered that patient biopsies are usually obtained well after the acute phase of injury has occurred and subsided.

Tipping *et al.* provide evidence in two patients with rapidly progressive glomerulonephritis that glomerular procoagulant activity is generally increased and in the form of tissue factor.[126] The ability of both fibrinolytic and defibrinating agents to ameliorate early inflammatory forms of glomerulonephritis is encouraging that progress in this area may some day lead to useful therapeutic interventions in humans,[127] although experience to date with anticoagulation therapy has been distinctly disappointing.[128]

In addition to the role of macrophage-derived tissue factor in glomerular fibrin deposition, progress has also been made in elucidating the role of the platelet in glomerular disease. This area has recently been reviewed.[129,130] Platelets have been shown to be major constituents of the glomerular lesion induced by the MPO–H_2O_2–halide system[94] and in a model of subendothelial immune complex nephritis mediated by neutrophils through the MPO mechanism,[95] where they appear to be required for neutrophil oxidant injury to occur.[98] Platelet activating factor (PAF), which may derive from endothelial or mesangial cells as well as from macrophages, neutrophils, and platelets, has been shown to participate in experimental glomerulonephritis as evidenced by the reduction in injury in both nephrotoxic nephritis and *in situ* cationic IgG-induced immune complex nephritis treated with a PAF receptor antagonist.[131,132] PAF effects on the kidney have been reviewed recently by Schlondorff *et al.*[133]

2.2.7. Injury Due to Prostaglandins

Although the effects of arachidonic acid metabolites on glomerular hemodynamic responses have been well studied, and hemodynamic alterations may substantially modify various immune events, the evidence that prostaglandins themselves act as inflammatory mediators in glomerular disease has been less conclusive. Several excellent reviews of this subject have recently been published.[134−136] Stahl *et al.* report a marked enhancement of glomerular prostaglandin E_2 and thromboxane B_2 production by glomeruli from rats with experimental membranous nephropathy induced by antibody to glomerular epithelial cell antigen (passive Heymann nephritis), an effect that was dependent on glomerular complement activation.[137] Of interest, Pugliese *et al.* found that neutralization of glomerular epithelial cell polyanion also markedly increased cellular production of prostaglandin E_2, a phenomenon that may be relevant to the *in vivo* situation.[138] Administration of a thromboxane synthetase inhibitor had no effect on injury *in vivo* as assessed by the quantity of urine protein excreted.[137] Zoja *et al.* reported similar findings,[139] and Shinkai and Cameron noted that in rabbits given nephrotoxic nephritis, thromboxane synthetase inhibition made proteinuria and glomerular filtration rate worse.[140] In contrast, Cybulsky *et al.* found that thromboxane synthetase inhibition with a different agent did reduce complement-mediated proteinuria in an isolated perfused kidney variant of the passive Heymann model, suggesting a role for thromboxane in mediating injury.[141] Two studies have reported a reduction in proteinuria with indomethacin blockade of prostaglandin production in models of membranous nephropathy but have differed in interpretation regarding whether this effect was related primarily to a reduction in GFR[141] or reflected instead a mediator effect of prostaglandin.[139] At this point it appears to be generally agreed that glomerular injury, particularly if it involves complement activation, results in enhanced glomerular synthesis of prostaglandin E_2 and thromboxane and that these substances derive in part from glomerular cells. However, defining a role for these agents in causing structural rather than simply functional glomerular changes has been difficult. This is well illustrated by the findings of Ulich et al., who showed that administration of stable prostaglandin analogs results in significant reductions in both proteinuria and glomerular filtration rate (GFR) in aminonucleoside nephrosis.[142] Thus, the role played by arachidonic acid metabolites in mediating acute immune injury remains controversial.

3. Clinical Aspects of Immune Renal Disease

3.1. Introduction

Several deficiencies in our state of knowledge compromise extrapolating experimental advances easily to clinical disease. One of these is that most studies of the immunopathogenesis of glomerular disease relate only to the acute initiating phase of disease, which has often subsided at the time the patient develops sufficient clinical problems to seek medical attention. Much less studied are the probably more important issues of glomerular response to injury and factors that determine reversibility, progression, and outcome. It is unfortunate that increasing calls are now being made for abandoning the diagnostic renal biopsy in favor of empiric therapy for glomerular disease at a time when the opportunity to address these issues is rapidly expanding.[143] The call for empiric therapy comes at a time when the nonspecific immunosuppression and antiinflammatory agents advocated to treat renal disease are often of debatable efficacy. Such calls also precede and threaten an era when new techniques in cellular and molecular biology are on the verge of providing tools that will permit assessment of a number of factors, such as the role of glomerular cell–derived cytokines in producing proliferation of cells, the production of interstitial or matrix components in scarring renal diseases, and alterations in cellular phenotype in disease expression. Study of these molecular mechanisms may lead to important therapeutic advances.

Studies of the molecular biology of experimental renal disease began to appear in 1986–1987.[108] However, the application of these techniques to studying clinical renal disease is only now beginning. Several thoughtful reviews have appeared that emphasize the necessity for careful clinical pathologic correlation studies in glomerular disease and the need for more data on epidemiology and immunopathogenesis of human glomerular disease.[144–147] The need for continued work on etiology as well as immunopathogenesis of glomerular disease in order to improve therapy, particularly in diseases such as minimal-change nephrotic syndrome and idiopathic rapidly progressive glomerulonephritis (RPGN) where conventional immune mechanisms are clearly not operative, has been emphasized.[148,149] It is remarkable that in the United States in the computer age, it is not possible to determine the incidence or prevalence of clinically significant glomerulonephritis nor are any epidemiologic data being collected that would permit recognition of demographic factors important in renal disease, such as associations with geography, climate, or environmental toxins. It is hoped that the study of human glomerular diseases will continue with scientific advances rather than retreats—it seems unlikely that progress toward the goal of prevention and cure will come in any other way.

3.2. Diseases That Present as Acute Glomerulonephritis

3.2.1. Hematuria

As enthusiasm for renal biopsies has waned, evidence of the utility of careful examination of the urine sediment has increased, although it has been discouraged if reagent dip stick testing is entirely negative.[150] The association of over 10% dysmorphic red blood cells in urine sediments examined by phase microscopy with various glomerular lesions has been confirmed by some[150,151] but not by others,[152] but such studies are now generally viewed as useful in evaluating isolated hematuria. Angiographic studies in the loin pain hematuria syndrome suggest that functional intrarenal vasospasm, perhaps of autonomic origin, rather than structural vessel lesions may be important in producing hematuria.[153]

3.2.2. Postinfectious Glomerulonephritis

The incidence of postinfectious nephritis has clearly diminished over the past decade and is now well behind IgA nephropathy and other mesangial proliferative nephropathies as a cause of the acute nephritic syndrome. The subject of infection in glomerular disease has been extensively reviewed by Levy.[154] A survey in Great Britain notes that persistent infection is a rather rare cause of renal disease requiring biopsy, although the incidence is clearly higher in less developed countries.[155] The most common type of organism-specific postinfectious nephritis remains poststreptococcal glomerulonephritis, but studies of this disease now emerge primarily from developing countries, as papers from Chile,[156] India,[157] Hong Kong,[158] and Jamaica[159] point out. The rapidity with which severe disease can develop is documented in one report of a patient who went from 0 to over 80% crescents in poststreptococcal nephritis, with acute renal failure in 10 days between biopsies, but who subsequently recovered fully.[160] The higher incidence of severe congestive heart failure and the poorer prognosis in the elderly have been emphasized.[161] Several studies[156–159] confirm the usually benign course of poststreptococcal nephritis but note a low, but existent, incidence of progressive renal disease. Less than 5% of patients in a German study progressed to end-stage renal failure, although 40% of adults had residual disease.[162] In a study from India, up to 20% of adults had persistent glomerulonephritis.[157] A "garland type" immunofluorescent pattern, which appears to correspond with more severe proteinuria and glomerulosclerosis, is associated with progressive disease.[163]

No observations in humans significantly clarify the immunopathogenesis of poststreptococcal nephritis. Cross-reactivity between streptococcal cell membrane and glomerular basement membrane has been confirmed,[164] as has the relatively high incidence of IgG rheumatoid factors capable of contributing to glomerular immune deposit formation.[165] With clarification of the relatively noninflammatory potential of subepithelial immune deposits, at least in membranous nephropathy, the question of why poststreptococcal nephritis with subepithelial humps is such an inflammatory lesion remains open. It seems probable that much of the inflammation may relate to the prominent, but usually overlooked, mesangial immune complex deposits seen in this disease.

Other types of postinfectious nephritis received relatively little attention during 1986–1987. The nephritogenic potential of staphylococcal and other nonstreptococcal bacterial infections is nicely reviewed in a clinical pathologic discussion by Kassirer[166]. The presence of a nonimmunoglobulin C3 activating factor in the serum of a patient with staphylococcal endocarditis and glomerulonephritis suggests a role for complement activation on the basement membrane independent of immunoglobulin deposition in causing the glomerular lesion—a concept that may well be relevant to many patients with type 1 membranoproliferative glomerulonephritis, some of whom develop the lesion following bacterial infection.[167] The spectrum of glomerular disease in *Schistosoma mansoni* infection is reviewed by Sobh *et al.*, who report both worm antigen and antibody to it in kidneys of some patients, implicating a worm-specific immune complex mechanism in causing the lesion.[168] The relatively high incidence of progressive disease and its potential importance in undeveloped countries is emphasized. Unfortunately, no significant benefit of specific antischistosomal therapy on the course of the renal lesion has been demonstrated.[169]

With respect to viral glomerulonephritis, a review of kidney biopsies and autopsies from patients with the clinical diagnosis of cytomegaloviral glomerulopathy adds further doubt to the existence of this lesion as a clinical entity and suggests that it is more likely part of the spectrum of transplant glomerulopathies related to chronic rejection.[170] Glomerular disease in AIDS is considered in Section 4.4.

3.2.3. IgA Nephropathy

As IgA nephropathy has emerged as the most common cause of acute glomerulonephritis in developed countries, the volume of literature on this disease has expanded. Space does not permit review of most of it. An excellent symposium edited by Emancipator and Schena provides a detailed review of current understanding of clinical features and immunopathogenetic mechanisms in IgA nephropathy, with contributions from most of the prominent workers in this area.[488] The clinical features and prognostic factors in IgA nephropathy have been separately reviewed by several authors and generally document a broad clinical and histologic spectrum of disease, a relatively high rate of progression (25–50%), and an association between proteinuria exceeding 2 g, hypertension, crescents, and sclerotic glomeruli with a poor prognosis.[171–178] Debate has been waged over the prognostic significance of microscopic hematuria, but the association of microscopic hematuria and crescents with a worse prognosis seems well established. The comparison of 206 children with IgA nephropathy and 128 with Henoch–Schönlein purpura by Yoshikawa et al. again emphasizes the strong similarities between the renal manifestations and immunopathology of IgA nephropathy and Henoch–Schönlein purpura with a somewhat worse prognosis in Henoch–Schönlein purpura related to severity at outset.[179] Continued case reports of Henoch–Schönlein purpura and IgA nephropathy in the same or related patients suggest that the diseases have a similar etiology and pathogenesis.[180] Several studies of IgA nephropathy in pediatric populations confirm the more benign prognosis in children, although prognostic factors seem to be very much the same as in adults.[181–183]

The occurrence of nephrotic syndrome in IgA nephropathy has again been emphasized by several authors. Several clinical–pathologic forms can apparently be distinguished. The author would agree with Rambausek et al. that the increasing number of patients reported with steroid-responsive nephrotic syndrome, essentially normal glomeruli and IgA deposits in the mesangium, with or without hematuria, probably do not have clinically significant IgA nephropathy, but rather have minimal-change nephrotic syndrome with incidental mesangial IgA deposits.[184] Consideration of these patients in the category of IgA nephropathy only confuses attempts to clarify pathogenesis and treatment of this disease. A second group of patients have nephrotic syndrome associated with extensive IgA deposits on the glomerular capillary wall, a lesion that appears, as it does in lupus, to be associated with more severe clinical and histologic disease and a worse prognosis with little response to steroids.[185,186] Finally, Jennette et al. describe several patients with coexistent mesangial IgA deposits and subepithelial IgG deposits suggesting coincident IgA nephropathy and membranous nephropathy.[187] Other situations in which membranous nephropathy seems to develop frequently are thought to have an autoimmune basis (anti-GBM nephritis, diabetes, renal transplants, lupus nephritis), and this association, if confirmed, may be a clue to the pathogenesis of IgA nephropathy, as the authors suggest.

A second clinical manifestation of IgA nephropathy which has received recent attention is severe hypertension. Two reports emphasize the frequency of hypertension as a presenting sign in IgA nephropathy (35%) and the occurrence of malignant hypertension as a manifestation of the disease often with minimal renal abnormalities.[188,189] Not unexpectedly, patients who exhibit malignant hypertension tend to have a rather poor prognosis. Kincaid-Smith and Fairley have pointed out the very high incidence (over 60%) of hypertension in pregnant women with IgA nephropathy accompanied by decreases in renal function in 22% and a higher prevalence of crescents on biopsy.[190]

As clinical interest in IgA nephropathy has increased, so have experimental studies directed at clarifying its pathogenesis. The available animal models of IgA nephropathy, which include diseases induced by infusion of IgA containing immune complexes, immunization with dextrans, oral immunization with several agents, various forms of hepatobiliary disease, viral infection, and a spontaneous lesion in mice, and the lessons that have been learned from these models, are well reviewed by Rifai.[191] Although the lesions of mesangial cell proliferation, matrix expansion, and mesangial infiltration by circulating inflammatory cells are well described, two provocative Japanese studies have expanded knowledge of the basement membrane lesion in IgA nephropathy, which appears to be primarily responsible for the proteinuria and hematuria. These studies document "lysis of basement membrane" in the region of subepithelial deposits[192] or gaps in GBM[193] which appear to account for proteinuria and hematuria.

Of particular interest is expanding evidence for genetic factors in IgA nephropathy. A geographic clustering of cases in eastern Kentucky has been described by Wyatt et al. and suggests a role for genetic factors and perhaps for a "founder" effect in this area.[194] The reports of familial cases of IgA nephropathy have been expanded by Levy, who reviews the evidence for genetic factors in IgA nephropathy very thoroughly.[195] Welch et al. have reported a significantly increased frequency of homozygous deficiency of C4b isotype in pediatric patients with primary IgA nephropathy,[196] suggesting either a genetic basis for the disease or a selective predisposition to it in patients with C4b deficiency. Although a clear MHC linkage has not been consistently identified in IgA nephropathy outside of Japan,[197] these observations support a role for genetic factors operating in concert with immunoregulatory defects, environmental exposures, and infectious processes in producing this disease.

The nature of the humoral abnormality in IgA nephropathy has also been explored. IgA-specific B-cell hyperactivity has been documented in IgA nephropathy,[198–200] as well as increases in T helper/suppressor cell ratios,[199,201] but these have not been clearly associated with disease activity. One study documents an exaggerated IgA antibody response to oral immunization in IgA nephropathy,[202] and two studies suggest that environmental exposure to mucosal antigens such as milk and gluten may increase IgA immune complex levels and renal deposition.[203,204] The existence of elevated levels of polymeric IgA containing immune complexes in patients with IgA nephropathy has been confirmed in several studies[205–208] and sometimes correlated with hematuria, but in general, clinical correlations have not been strong. Most authors now agree that the immunoglobulins deposited in IgA nephropathy are composed primarily of polymeric IgA containing J chain, and are composed more of IgA 1 than IgA 2, but the origin (mucosal vs. plasma) of these immunoglobulins is unresolved.

With regard to the nature of the IgA antibody, some authors have reported elevated levels of polymeric IgA rheumatoid factor, usually of the IgA 1 subclass.[209–211] Antibodies to gliadin (a gluent constituent),[212] BSA,[213] and antiidiotypic antibodies to anti-BSA[214] have all been reported, as have non-IgA containing cryofibrinogens.[215] With regard to the nature of the nephritogenic antigen, herpes simplex viral antigens have been identified in glomerular deposits in a patient with tonsillitis.[216] BSA has been reported in IgA immune complex form in IgA nephropathy patients,[214] and antibody to a nuclear antigen has also been found.[217] Most studies of the nature of the immune reactants in this disease have focused very heavily on the IgA, which is not a particularly nephritogenic immunoglobulin and seems an unlikely candidate to provoke the severe inflammatory lesion along with GBM gaps which characterizes IgA nephropathy. They have also focused on exogenous antigens, although deposition of exogenous antigen containing immune complexes in the mesangium has never been shown to be a particularly nephritogenic process. None of these studies have ever provided a very convincing correlation with clinical disease. Relatively understudied, it seems to me, is the possible role of the IgG which is also usually seen in the mesangium in this disease, and the possibility of an autoantibody reacting with some mesangial cellular or matrix constituent, a process that clearly is capable of producing the type of lesions seen. Emancipator *et al.* have provided data confirming that passively injected IgA containing immune complex deposits are not associated with disease but that hematuria does occur if a complement fixing IgG component is present.[218] Rifai *et al.* also provide data that confirms the relatively limited ability of IgA immune complexes to induce mesangial complement activation but suggest than the antigenic component of the complexes may be capable of inducing complement activation and then disease.[219] Deposition of the S protein of C5b-9 and of C9 has also been reported in association with more severe disease in IgA nephropathy.[220] Clearly, the pathogenesis of IgA nephropathy remains rather poorly understood but may turn out to be more analogous to conventional antibody complement–mediated disease mechanisms that the vast IgA literature would currently suggest.

As might be anticipated from the above, progress in successfully treating IgA nephropathy has also been rather slow. Although useful information continues to accumulate, most of it is negative. No benefit was reported in long-term trials of antiplatelet agents,[221] a combination of azathioprine and anticoagulants or nonsteroidal agents,[222] and steroids.[223] Woo *et al.* report a reduction in proteinuria and decreased rate of renal deterioration with less sclerosis in patients treated prospectively with a cocktail of cyclophosphamide, dipyridamole, and Warfarin for 3 years.[224] In a later report[225] they suggest this effect can be achieved without cyclophosphamide, but present no data to support this. Similar immunosuppression–anticoagulation cocktails have been advocated in other glomerular diseases, but complications from their use have usually outweighed any apparent benefit. As it has in several other glomerular diseases, short-term cyclosporin administration has been shown to reduce proteinuria in IgA nephropathy associated with a decrease in GFR, but no long-term benefit has been documented.[226] Another prospective study compared steroids with indomethacin or dipyridamole over 19 months in patients with IgA nephropathy and between 1 and 2 g of proteinuria.[227] These authors report a reduction in proteinuria by 50% and stabilization of renal function in patients with creatinine clearances that exceeded 70 ml/min. It is unclear to what extent the nonsteroidals may have adversely affected renal function in the control group, although steroid-treated patients also received nonsteroidals after 1–3 years of prednisone therapy. A retrospective study from the same group failed to demonstrate a similar benefit in patients with more than 2 g of proteinuria.[227] Two patients with a crescentic form of IgA nephropathy are reported who appeared to benefit from plasma exchange when pulse steroids and immunosuppression had failed, but the improvements were only temporary.[228]

In total, these data, viewed in the context of many other studies of progressive, inflammatory immunologically mediated glomerulonephritis such as lupus and MPGN, suggest that steroids, and probably antiplatelet agents in selected patients, may slow deterioration of renal function, but more data are needed to determine which patients should be treated and what the complications, particularly hypertension and bleeding, are. As in most forms of glomerular disease, the treatments available are relatively toxic, work only in selected patients, and are quite nonspecific. A more specific approach to IgA nephropathy does not seem to be on the immediate horizon. Another study confirms the rather high recurrence rates for this disease in renal transplants, approaching 50% with about a 30% loss of graft function, and suggests that the recurrence rate may be much higher in living related donors (83%) compared to cadavers (14%).[229] One patient with severe recurrent disease had progressed from diagnosis to end-stage renal disease in less than 1 year.[229]

Mild forms of IgA nephropathy have now been reported in association with rheumatoid arthritis[230] and ankylosing spondylitis.[231] Several studies have addressed the entity of liver disease, mesangial IgA deposits, and hematuria.[232–234] All emphasize the frequency of glomerular abnormalities in liver disease but the relative infrequency of associated clinical findings. However, two patients with cirrhosis and acute renal failure associated with macroscopic hematuria have been reported.[234]

3.2.4. Rapidly Progressive Glomerulonephritis

3.2.4.1. Introduction. I have emphasized the clinical utility of segregating patients with RPGN into categories based on underlying immunopathologic mechanisms.[235,236] Two extensive reviews of the mechanisms underlying crescentic glomerulonephritis have appeared recently.[236,237] Perhaps the most significant developments in this area are the expanding understanding of mechanisms of crescent formation (reviewed in Ref. 237 and above) and the general evolution of the concept that the idiopathic form of RPGN (see below) is probably a form of renal or glomerular limited vasculitis.

3.2.4.2. Anti-GBM Nephritis. Studies that have clarified the nature of the GBM antigen and its localization to the noncollagenous domain of type IV collagen were reviewed earlier. Savage *et al.* have published a valuable study of 71 patients with anti-GBM disease in the British Isles studied from 1980 to 1984, which notes that 50% of patients present with glomerulonephritis alone, that many of these are older women, and that serum anti-GBM antibody levels correlate with serum creatinine at the time of presentation.[238] Treatment with cyclophosphamide for 8 weeks, prednisone, and at least 2 weeks of daily plasma exchange resulted in normalization of anti-GBM antibody levels within 8 weeks (compared to about 14 weeks without plasma exchange) and improved renal function in 21 of 27 patients with serum creatinines of <6 mg% (vs. 1 of 12 with worse renal function or on dialysis).[238] The authors continue to advocate plasma exchange for patients with anti-GBM disease who are not on dialysis and have serum creatinines of less than six. The use of plasma exchange in renal disease has been extensively reviewed by Balow.[239] The conclusion that plasma exchange is useful in anti-GBM disease has never been established by a prospective controlled study, and probably never will be. It rests largely on the observation that approximately 75% of treated patients have significant improvement compared to historical controls where less than 20% of patients survived. However, this figure of 75% is very similar to what is now achieved with immunosuppression alone in several other renal diseases (idiopathic RPGN, lupus), and there are many reasons to believe that the prognosis in anti-GBM disease has improved considerably over the past 2 decades independently of disease specific therapy. However, plasma exchange remains the treatment of choice for this disease, at least in patients with severe disease but well-preserved renal function. The general effects and complications of plasma exchange have been reviewed recently.[239-242] We have recently seen several patients with very mild disease and elevated anti-GBM antibody titers by radioimmunoassay who resolved spontaneously, a course also described by others.[243] Although classic anti-GBM disease, especially Goodpasture's syndrome, is generally self-limited with a good prognosis if glomerular destruction can be minimized while circulating antibody is present, one well-documented case of recurrent disease over 14 years has been reported.[244] Another case of graft loss at 6 months due to anti-GBM nephritis in an allograft of a patient with Alport's syndrome (which lacks the Goodpasture's antigen) is reported,[245] and this complication of transplantation in Alport's patients must be kept in mind in monitoring these patients after transplant and in selecting donors.

   3.2.4.3. Idiopathic RPGN. I define idiopathic RPGN as crescentic glomerulonephritis occurring in the absence of obvious systemic disease and without antibody deposition in glomeruli.[236] Several authors are now suggesting that this form of no-deposit RPGN is a vasculitis, a conviction that the author shares. Older studies of Serra *et al.* demonstrated that patients with focal necrotizing glomerulonephritis without immune deposits and with systemic signs of fever, malaise, or weight loss, but without histologic evidence of vasculitis, have an identical renal lesion to patients with biopsy evidence of small vessel vasculitis. Croker *et al.* provide similar data in a series of 34 patients in which no significant differences could be documented in clinical or histologic features between patients with primary necrotizing glomerulonephritis and patients with clinical and/or histologic evidence of vasculitis.[246] Furlong et al. review 20 patients and come to a similar conclusion.[247] Adu et al. review another 43 such patients from Great Britain.[248] Velosa has summarized well the case for viewing the no-deposit form of RPGN, or idiopathic crescentic glomerulonephritis, as a renal-limited form of vasculitis.[249] Patients with disease limited to the kidneys generally had a worse prognosis in these series than patients with systemic disease. This may reflect the fact that they first came to medical attention with relatively advanced renal disease.

A development of major significance in RPGN has been the popularization of measurements of antineutrophil cytoplasmic antibody (ANCA).[250] Although originally reported to to useful primarily in the diagnosis and management of Wegener's granulomatosis (see Section 5.1.5), it now appears that this assay is positive in a high percentage of patients with other forms of small vessel vasculitis including idiopathic RPGN.[251] It remains unclear whether the ANCA is a pathogenic antibody or an epiphenomenon, but the frequency with which it is present in vasculitic forms of RPGN suggests a common pathogenesis for several of these diseases. This shift in thinking may have important therapeutic implications as it suggests that the use of cyclophosphamide may be beneficial in patients with focal necrotizing glomerulonephritis and crescents, an approach to therapy that has not generally been part of the recommended therapeutic armamentarium.

Baldwin et al. have emphasized the spectrum of clinical and morphologic features in idiopathic crescentic glomerulonephritis, emphasizing the insidious onset and protracted course in some patients,[252] an observation that is timely and also perhaps accounts in part for the clearly improved prognosis in this disease over time. Although RPGN is generally considered a self-limited disease that does not require prolonged therapy, Belghiti et al. describe six cases with relapses documented by renal biopsy 6–17 months following the initial disease.[253] The extent to which pulmonary hemorrhage can dominate the clinical picture and look like Goodpasture's syndrome is emphasized in a report from Boyce and Holdsworth.[254]

Most advances in understanding the pathogenesis of idiopathic crescentic glomerulonephritis are discussed above under experimental glomerulonephritis or briefly below under vasculitis. Bolten et al. report glomerular T helper cells in RPGN that correlate with intraglomerular macrophages, but they were unable to differentiate subgroups of RPGN using T-cell subset analysis or to produce reliable prognostic information.[255] However, their findings suggest participation of cell-mediated immune mechanisms in several of these disease. The issue of how cellular crescents are formed (well reviewed in Ref. 237) is addressed by Yoshioka et al., who report predominantly glomerular epithelial cells in crescents and also note the presence of type IV collagen and laminin suggesting that synthesis of matrix components by proliferating epithelial cells may contribute to scarring and irreversibility of crescents.[256]

No significant new studies related to therapy of RPGN were published during 1986–1987.

4. Disease That Commonly Present as Nephrotic Syndrome

4.1. Nephrotic Syndrome—Physiology and Consequences

4.1.1. Measurements of Proteinuria

Increasing attention has been given to use of random urine specimens in quantitating proteinuria, thereby avoiding the inconvenience and inaccuracy of 24-hr collections. An excellent correlation between random and 24-hr urine values has been established in a broad spectrum of renal diseases when samples were collected during normal waking hours.[257] Normal values are generally less than 0.2, and values greater than 3.0 indicate urinary excretion of more than 3.0 g of protein per 24 hr.[257] The usefulness of this method for assessing postural- and exercise-induced proteinuria in adolescents and its advantage over the urinary dip stick is emphasized by Houser et al.[258] Single voided samples analyzed for albumin and creatinine also appear to be useful in assessing early renal dysfunction in diabetes.[259]

4.1.2. Mechanisms of Proteinuria

Permeability of the glomerular capillary wall to serum proteins is restricted by size- and charge-selective filtration barriers controlled by components of the capillary wall itself. Although evidence for charge-related defects in human glomerular disease is limited largely to congenital nephrotic syndrome, the charge barrier has other important functions and continues to be studied. Furness et al. used the cationic tracer polyethyleneine to study a variety of human glomerular diseases and concluded there was morphologic evidence for retention of the anionic charge sites in all of these lesions.[260] Kerjaschki et al. have identified a sialoprotein of about 140,000 kd, termed podocalyxin, as the major negatively charged sialoprotein in glomerular podocytes and have also shown it to be present in the membrane of endothelial cells.[261,262] A podocalyxin-like sialoprotein has also been identified in the glycocalyx of human visceral glomerular epithelial cells.[261] The major component of the charge barrier is probably heparan sulfate proteoglycans, although Bertolatus and Hunsicker present provocative evidence that hexadimethdrine, which causes proteinuria by binding to glomerular anionic sites, binds primarily to carboxyl groups in the glomerular basement membrane.[263] Lelongt et al. utilized antibody to heparan sulfate proteoglycan core protein to demonstrate that in aminonucleoside nephrosis heparan sulfate proteoglycans are intact, but that their charge density is increased.[264] These data are at variance with some earlier studies which suggest a defect in the charge barrier in this model of minimal-change nephrotic syndrome.

Much work has focused on the nature of the size barrier in nephrotic syndrome since this appears to be the major defect in human glomerular disease. Batsford et al. utilized cationic ferritin of various sizes to document a role for the lamina densa as an important component of the size barrier.[265] Bertolatus et al. extended earlier studies documenting that alterations in glomerular capillary wall charge are usually accompanied by defects in the size barrier as well, by demonstrating a similar phenomenon using high-molecular-weight protein markers.[266] The dependence of size-selective defects in the glomerular basement membrane on glomerular hemodynamics, presumably primarily glomerular hydraulic pressure, is illustrated by studies showing enhancement of proteinuria and alterations of glomerular membrane pore structure in nephrotic patients undergoing volume expansion with colloids.[267] The nature of this size defect is unclear and probably heterogeneous, including active rents in the capillary wall as well as other, more subtle defects, such as areas of increased hydraulic flux. However, several recent studies point to a role for the glomerular epithelial cell layer in this process. The nature of the size-selective defect in glomerular permeability induced by albumin overload was studied by Weening et al., who document increased fractional clearances of native albumin, IgG, and IgM with an apparently intact charge barrier.[268] This loss of size selectivity was accompanied by morphologic and functional evidence of an intact charge barrier and also by substantial glomerular epithelial cell degenerative changes, including swelling, epithelial foot process effacement, and occasional detachment of the epithelial cell layer from basement membrane.[268] Although these changes were attributed to proteinuria by the authors, other studies of the same model have concluded that proteinuria alone does not produce irreversible glomerular epithelial cell damage.[269] In studies of aminonucleoside nephrosis, a model induced with a glomerular epithelial cell toxin that has a large size-selective barrier defect, the development of large areas of glomerular epithelial cell detachment coincident with the onset of proteinuria has suggested that the glomerular epithelial cell layer is a significant component of the size barrier.[270] Based on these and other studies, attention has now been drawn to the epithelial cell as a major determinant of permeability defects in human nephrotic syndrome.

4.1.3. Consequences of Proteinuria

Cameron has provided a thoughtful and comprehensive review of the relationship between proteinuria and the various clinical consequences of nephrotic syndrome.[271] In particular, the uncertain relationship between urinary protein loss, serum albumin concentration, and edema formation is emphasized. The issue of whether fluid retention in nephrotic syndrome reflects reduced colloid osmotic pressure or results from intrarenal abnormalities is addressed in one study from Norway which suggests that with a reduction in colloid osmotic pressure of about 50%, abnormalities in fluid retention can be accounted for by changes in the transcapillary colloid osmotic pressure gradient and Starling forces.[272] However, Shapiro et al. report no differences in blood volumes and hormonal parameters of diminished effective blood volume in a population of patients with nephrotic syndrome and impaired water excretion and suggest that intrarenal factors, predominantly GFR, are the most important determinants of sodium and water retention.[273] Koomans et al. support this by documenting natriuresis accompanied by an increase in GFR and filtration fraction with loss of edema in steroid-responsive nephrotic syndrome before any change in serum protein concentrations can be demonstrated.[274] Another study suggests that changes in production of atrial natriuretic factor may be an important determinant of sodium and fluid retention in nephrotic syndrome.[275]

Hyperlipidemia is a common secondary manifestation of nephrotic syndrome. The mechanisms of hyperlipidemia have been extensively studied by Kaysen et al., who have shown previously that it is difficult to demonstrate a correlation between serum albumin and rates of albumin synthesis. More recently, they have studied the relationship between the rate of albumin synthesis and development of lipid abnormalities and demonstrated that triglyceride and cholesterol levels are related to the rates of albumin loss but not to albumin synthetic rates, casting doubt on the usual explanation for hyperlipidemia involving a nonspecific increase in hepatic synthesis of lipoproteins in response to reduced albumin concentration.[276] High-density-lipoprotein (HDL) subfraction studies show that total HDL cholesterol is not elevated in nephrotic syndrome but that the HDL2 subfraction, which correlates positively with ischemic heart disease, is low owing to increased urinary losses.[277] The topic of lipid abnormalities in nephrotic syndrome as they relate to subsequent development of atherosclerotic heart disease is well reviewed by Steinman in a clinical pathologic discussion.[278] Valeri et al. have examined the effect of cholesterol-lowering drugs in nephrotic syndrome and shown that colestipol and probucol induce a 20–30% reduction in cholesterol and triglyceride levels and are well tolerated.[279] However, no studies of the long-term clinical benefit of such therapy have been reported.

The phenomenon of hypercoagulation in nephrotic syndrome has also received recent attention. Mehis et al. report about a 5% incidence of thrombotic complications in children associated with more severe abnormalities in protein C, evidence of disseminated intravascular coagulation, and evidence of platelet activation similar to that seen in adults.[280] Elevated plasma fibrinogen concentrations and high-molecular-weight fibrinogen complexes have also been reported in childhood nephrotic syndrome.[281–283] Platelet hyperaggregability has been confirmed in nephrotic syndrome associated with reduced plasma antithrombin 3 and protein S deficiency.[284,285] However, none of these parameters, or other coagulation studies, demonstrate good correlation with thromboembolic complications.[286] The apparent increased requirement for heparin to anticoagulate patients with nephrotic syndrome has been attributed to decreased sensitivity to heparin.[287] A reduction in C1q, C2, factor B, C8, and C9 levels also occurs in some patients with nephrotic syndrome.[283]

Finally, several studies have addressed the efficacy of various agents in reducing protein excretion in patients with glomerular disease who do not respond to disease-specific therapy with steroids or immunosuppressive agents. Such patients with resistant nephrotic syndrome and metabolic complications thereof can be major management problems. The two classes of drugs most intensively studied are the nonsteroidal antiinflammatory agents and angiotensin converting enzyme inhibitors. Several studies confirm an antiproteinuric effect of indomethacin which appears greater than the accompanying decrease in GFR.[288-291] A reduction in proteinuria of up to 50%, exceeding the fall in GFR by a factor of over two, can occur.[289] Data suggesting that the decrease in proteinuria seen with indomethacin[288] or meclofenamate[291] may be accompanied by a significant reduction in rate of loss of GFR have also been provided. The benefits and risks (decreased renal function, allergic reactions) of treating refractory nephrotic syndrome with nonsteroidal agents are well reviewed by Velosa and Torres.[291] The mechanism of the nonsteroidal effect on proteinuria may relate to altered glomerular hemodynamics with reduced intraglomerular capillary pressure.[288,290] Another well-established way to produce a reduction in intraglomerular hydrostatic pressure is by administration of converting enzyme inhibitors. Several studies suggest that converting enzyme inhibitors are effective in reducing proteinuria in patients with refractory nephrotic syndrome. Heeg et al. report a 60% reduction in protein excretion in various diseases with lisinopril, an effect not seen with conventional antihypertensive agents.[292] Captopril reduces protein excretion in hypertensive patients.[293] Lagrue et al.[294] report a greater than 50% decrease in proteinuria in 7 of 10 patients treated with captopril who had various forms of glomerulonephritis, usually accompanied by a decrease in blood pressure. Captopril has also been reported to induce membranous nephropathy and proteinuria, although the incidence of this effect appears to be less than 1%.[293] The frequency with which nephrotic syndrome may occur as a late manifestation of hypertensive benign nephrosclerosis has also been emphasized recently.[295-297]

4.2. Minimal-Change Nephrotic Syndrome

Increasingly this entity is viewed as the mildest form of a disease process that includes mesangial proliferation and IgM deposits in a more severe form and focal glomerular sclerosis as the most severe form in which structural damage occurs and steroid responsiveness is lost. The cause of minimal-change nephrotic syndrome (MCNS) remains obscure. The occurrence of the disease as an apparent allergic reaction to nonsteroidal antiinflammatory agents continues to be reported, usually in association with interstitial nephritis, although some examples of pure MCNS have been described.[298,299] In one case, relapse of MCNS occurred without apparent further drug exposure,[300] and at least one case has been reported of apparent nonsteroidal-induced MCNS that subsequently progressed to focal sclerosis and renal failure despite discontinuation of the drug and administration of steroid therapy.[301]

The other association that continues to be reported is with malignancy. Most of these cases are with lymphoma or leukemia, particularly Hodgkin's disease, and the nephrotic syndrome may precede the diagnosis of lymphoma by several years.[302-304] These topics have been reviewed by Dabbs et al.[302] One case of MCNS with mesothelioma has been reported.[305] Although a reduction in proteinuria induced by nonsteroidals or angiotensin converting enzyme inhibitors may facilitate the management of nephrotic syndrome, no clear benefit of these agents on the long-term course of renal disease has yet been established.

An excellent review of the clinical course of MCNS in adults has been provided by Nolasco *et al.*[306] Eighty-one percent of patients eventually achieved remission with steroid therapy, although only 60% did so in 8 weeks and some required up to 16 weeks of therapy. Of the responding patients, about 25% never relapsed, 50% relapsed once, and 25% became frequent relapsers. Two-thirds of patients treated with cyclophosphamide for relapses or steroid resistance were in remission at 5 years. Six of eight patients who were untreated had spontaneous remissions. The authors conclude that compared to children, adults have a higher incidence of acute renal failure, hypertension, and reduced renal function with MCNS, respond more slowly to steroid therapy, and relapse less frequently. Allen *et al.* also report three cases of steroid-responsive MCNS in patients over 70 and emphasize the potential toxicity of steroids in the elderly as well as the utility of renal biopsy in managing these patients.[307]

With regard to the pathogenesis of MCNS, the cause of the unique glomerular lesion remains elusive. Melvin and Michael have provided a comprehensive review of current concepts of glomerular permeability and theories regarding disease mechanisms in MCNS.[308] Studies of the charge properties of serum and urine albumin in MCNS suggest relative maintenance of the charge-selective filtration barrier and a role for albumin conformational change in its excretion in this disease.[309] A defect in IgG production by B cells in active MCNS and a low serum IgG concentration with elevated IgM, IgE, and C3 are confirmed in other studies.[310,311] A potent lymphotoxin which inhibits lymphocyte blastogenesis has been identified in MCNS and in other glomerular diseases and may contribute to these impaired immune responses.[312] However, all of the changes appear to be secondary and not of pathogenic significance.

4.3. Mesangial Proliferative and IgM Nephropathy

Most authors concur that a spectrum exists among patients with idiopathic nephrotic syndrome, with one end represented by patients with pure MCNS without structural lesions and characterized by a 90% response rate to steroids, and the other end by patients with MCNS in some glomeruli but definite structural damage in others consisting of focal sclerotic lesions and a poorer response to steroids, generally 20% or less. Between these two extremes lies a group of patients who have mild glomerular morphologic abnormalities in the form of mesangial cell proliferation and/or IgM deposits, and who have an intermediate response to steroids, usually about 50%. [There is also an entity of acute glomerulonephritis associated with mesangial cell proliferation usually without mesangial immune deposits or nephrotic syndrome (mesangial proliferative glomerulonephritis). Like IgA nephropathy, this disease appears to be more common in Asian countries.] Kopolovic *et al.* report 10 patients with idiopathic nephrotic syndrome, stable renal function, and IgM deposits or mesangial cell proliferation, or both, and argue the case for classifying "IgM nephropathy" as a separate entity.[313] Lin and Chu make a similar case based on detection of elevated levels of IgM, IgM-bearing lymphocytes, and IgM-containing circulating immune complexes in 12 children with idiopathic nephrotic syndrome and IgM deposits.[314] In the absence of clues to the pathogenesis of the diffuse glomerular capillary wall lesion in these patients, it is impossible to determine whether the subgroups represent different diseases or not. However, it seems more probable that the same mechanism induces the diffuse noninflammatory increase in glomerular permeability that characterizes all patients with MCNS, focal sclerosis, IgM nephropathy, and mesangial cell proliferation, and that the focal changes seen in patients who are more resistant to steroid therapy are probably secondary developments and do not represent primary pathogenetic entities. However, other authors disagree.[315]

4.4. Focal Glomerulosclerosis

With the above considerations in mind, however, many studies continue to examine patients with focal glomerulosclerosis (FGS) as if it were a separate entity. Korbet *et al.* describe 46 patients with primary FGS.[316] They confirm results of other studies that a significant response to steroids may be seen (5 of 16 complete remissions and three partial) and demonstrate that those patients who do respond to steroids or who never develop nephrotic syndrome have a much better long-term prognosis. Miyata *et al.* point out that patients with FGS diagnosed more than 2 years after development of nephrotic syndrome appear to do better than patients with FGS in the initial biopsy, and that mesangial cell proliferation is a good predictor of steroid unresponsiveness and subsequent development of progressive renal disease.[317] A subset of patients with steroid-resistant FGS exhibit rapidly progressive renal failure with end-stage renal disease within 2.5 years.[318]

The presence of severe steroid-resistant nephrotic syndrome and mesangial cell proliferation not only predicts development of FGS and progressive renal disease, but also appears to predict the likelihood of recurrence of FGS in renal allografts.[319,320] Currently identified risk factors for recurrence of FGS include a young age, short duration of disease before transplantation (less than 3 years), mesangial cell proliferation, and perhaps the degree of histocompatibility of the allograft. Striegel *et al.* reviewed 24 patients with steroid-resistant FGS in Minnesota and described recurrent FGS in 12 (50%).[320] Proteinuria can appear within hours and early biopsies usually show MCNS. Recurrence was only 11% in patients without mesangial cell proliferation and 80% in patients with diffuse mesangial cell proliferation. These findings provide helpful guidelines for counseling patients with this disease who are considering renal transplantation.

In addition to primary FGS in idiopathic nephrotic syndrome, a very similar morphologic lesion has been reported in a variety of other conditions, usually also in association with nephrotic syndrome. FGS is again reported in 50% of patients with nephrotic syndrome and massive obesity,[321,322] where it may be associated with glomerulomegaly and suggests an analogy with the hyperfiltration, remnant kidney model of progressive FGS in rats. Gaber and Spargo point out that careful study can detect FGS in 35% of women biopsied for pregnancy-induced nephropathy, and its presence implies a higher likelihood of persistent hypertension and renal vascular disease.[323]

4.4.1. AIDS Nephropathy

Most recent attention has centered on the possible relationship between AIDS and nephrotic syndrome with FGS. There is clearly a subset of AIDS patients, perhaps 10% in some centers, who develop nephrotic syndrome and progressive renal disease.[324–326] Although a variety of lesions have been reported in these patients, FGS is the most characteristic. Other centers see a much lower incidence of this lesion,[327,328] and controversy persists with regard to whether it is specifically an AIDS-related lesion or a consequence of i.v. drug abuse, which can also be associated with FGS.[329,330] Ultrastructural studies have suggested that morphologic evidence of viral infection is more common in AIDS-associated nephropathy than it is in heroin-associated nephropathy.[325] These data, as well as recent reports of nephropathy in children with AIDS, suggest that in some patients HTLV-III infection can induce nephrotic syndrome with FGS. Thus, AIDS appears to be similar to Hodgkin's disease and nonsteroidal antiflammatory agents in providing a clue to the pathogenesis of this important disorder, although so far no one has recognized what it is.

4.4.2. Treatment of Minimal-Change Nephrotic Syndrome and Focal Glomerulosclerosis

The treatment for this disease spectrum when nephrotic syndrome is present remains oral steroids, and the data provided by Nolasco et al.[306] reconfirm the effectiveness of this treatment in adults. Cyclophosphamide remains the treatment of choice for patients with steroid-dependent or frequently relapsing clinical courses who are steroid toxic. What is needed is a therapeutic alternative to steroids that is less toxic and an agent that can be used in patients who are steroid resistant. To date, neither of these objectives has been accomplished. Two cases are reported of a measles-induced reduction in cell-mediated immunity and remission of nephrotic syndrome in MCNS.[331] Nair et al. report a response rate to alternate-day oral prednisone, 2 mg/kg, which is over 90% at 16 weeks, data very similar to those of Nolasco using daily oral prednisone, although somewhat higher doses were employed.[332] This regimen may have advantages in reducing steroid toxicity in some patients. Significant fluctuations, averaging close to 50%, are reported in urinary protein excretion in MCNS and other glomerular diseases between prednisone days on and days off in patients receiving alternate-day therapy, and this effect must be kept in mind in interpreting treatment results.[333] Garcia et al. have recently documented the effect of methylprednisolone to increase glomerular pressures and accelerate development of glomerulosclerosis in a remnant kidney model, an effect that may account for the increased proteinuria on prednisone days and needs to be considered in thinking about potential steroid toxic side effects.[334]

With regard to alternatives to prednisone therapy in MCNS, many authors have now attempted to use cyclosporine A in this disease. Tejani has reviewed this subject.[335] In general, the drug has been effective in inducing initial remissions as a substitute for prednisone and in reducing the need for steroids in some patients who are steroid dependent or frequently relapsing.[335–338] The role of cyclosporine A in treating patients who are steroid resistant is less clear. Tejani et al. report remission in three of seven patients with steroid-resistant disease and biopsy evidence of FGS.[338] Niaudet et al. found that only 1 in 10 steroid-resistant patients responded to cyclosporine.[336] Waldo and Kohaut report a partial remission in only one of six patients with steroid-resistant FGS.[339] All reports have noted short-term problems with hypertension and decreased renal function in cyclosporine-treated patients. Most studies have also noted a rather high relapse rate as soon as cyclosporine therapy is discontinued.[340] At present, it does not appear that cyclosporine adds much to the results achieved with steroids and cytotoxic agents in treating MCNS.

With regard to use of cyclophosphamide in patients with steroid-responsive disease, a German study documents the apparent benefit of 12 weeks of therapy versus 8 weeks in producing more sustained remissions (67% vs. 22%) in steroid-dependent patients.[341] The dose administered was well below the 200 mg/kg generally considered the threshold for gonadal toxicity in males. The current status of cytotoxic drug therapy in MCNS–FGS is well reviewed by Trompeter.[342]

With regard to patients with established FGS, a trial of steroid therapy is still regarded as useful. Pei et al. review 11 years of data from the Toronto glomerulonephritis registry which documents about a 40% complete remission rate with prednisone alone in both children and adults with FGS, and a considerably improved 5 year renal survival in patients who responded vs. those who did not (96% vs. 55%).[343] Despite this experience, only about one-third of adults with documented FGS received steroid therapy.[343] Griswold et al. report sustained remission in two of seven patients with steroid-resistant nephrotic syndrome and FGS treated with six doses of methylprednisolone pulse therapy and describe prolonged remissions in several responsive patients who relapsed and were then treated with cytotoxic agents.[344]

4.5. Membranous Nephropathy

Much attention continues to be directed at understanding the pathogenesis of this common cause of idiopathic nephrotic syndrome in adults, and results were reviewed in Section 2.1.1. Several additions to the clinical literature on membranous nephropathy (MN) have also appeared recently. MacTier et al. provide more data on the natural history of 37 untreated patients with idiopathic MN demonstrating that after 5 years 50% had progressive renal disease while 30% had spontaneous remissions and about 20% had persistent proteinuria while retaining normal renal function.[345] Male sex, hypertension, and proteinuria exceeding 10 g/day most reliably predicted a progressive course. These data are reasonably similar to those of other studies reported from Europe. A Japanese study reports 80% of patients had GFRs exceeding 80 ml/min at 5 years, but includes both treated and nonnephrotic patients.[346] Tornroth et al. suggest that the presence of electron-dense subepithelial immune deposits suggests active disease, whereas intramembranous lucent areas are predictive of inactive and resolving disease.[347] The controversy regarding whether or not MN is associated with malignancy is addressed in one study of 128 biopsied patients with MN that confirms an incidence of carcinoma (13%) fivefold greater than that expected in aged matched controls, particularly in patients over 40.[348] As in several other glomerular diseases, Packham and colleagues report that pregnancy in 24 patients with MN was associated with increased fetal loss, hypertension, and decreased renal function in about 10% of patients.[349] Nephrotic-range proteinuria during the first trimester was a particularly poor prognostic sign. An additional patient with MN and a superimposed crescentic glomerulonephritis with a rapidly progressive course is reported.[350] This well-recognized complication of this disease is usually associated with anti-GBM antibody and suggests a unique susceptibility to autoimmune phenomenon in these patients.

Like several other glomerular disease, MN appears to be strongly genetically influenced, with HLA B8 and DR3 prevalent in Europe and DR2 in Japan.[351,352] The association between the B8 DR3 phenotype and mononuclear phagocyte dysfunction reported in some other diseases does not appear to be present in MN.[352]

The current concepts of pathogenesis of this disease are reviewed in some detail by Couser and Abrass.[353] Recent developments in this area were reviewed earlier under mechanisms of subepithelial immune deposit formation. Verroust et al. provide another detailed review of this subject.[354] Briefly, evidence is accumulating that the disease results from autoantibody to a glomerular epithelial cell membrane antigen which produces injury by a mechanism that involves epithelial cell membrane insertion of the C5b-9 membrane attack complex of complement.[353,354] The morphologic consequences of this process include glomerular C5b-9 neoantigen deposition.[355] The basement membrane lesion that develops from this has been defined by scanning electron microscopy, which demonstrates numerous small, ridgelike projections forming trabeculae and cradlelike defects where the immune deposits are.[356] These trabeculae comprise the GBM spikes seen by light microscopy between deposits and have been shown by immunoultrastructural studies to be composed largely of laminin.[68] There is also a disruption of glomerular anionic sites, presumably heparan sulfate proteoglycans, with perhaps some diminution in total number.[357] However, studies to define the functional consequences of these defects by measuring fractional clearances of dextrans of varying sizes in human membranous nephropathy reveal that the proteinuria results from an increase in filtrate passage through a nonselective, large-pore shunt pathway which correlates in magnitude with changes in the epithelial cell layer morphologically.[358] Thus a nonrestrictive, large-pore defect in the GBM in MN appears to result from an increase in glomerular epithelial cell production of basal lamina components, particularly laminin, which follows glomerular epithelial cell C5b-9 attack, presumably induced by the binding of autoantibody to a cell membrane antigen.[353]

Progress in treating this lesion will undoubtedly eventually emerge from significant advances in understanding its pathogenesis. However, hope must be tempered by recognition that the lack of inflammatory changes and the very slowly progressive nature of this disease, as well as the defect in barrier function which is apparently due to structural alterations in basal lamina components, all result in a lesion that persists after the disease-inducing antibody is removed.[359] As a consequence, proteinuria is likely to persist for substantial periods of time after the underlying disease process is entirely eliminated, thereby complicating interpretation of results of therapy. This phenomenon is illustrated by studies in an exogenous antigen-induced model of membranous nephropathy following chronic BSA serum sickness in rats that developed membranous nephropathy, spikes, and proteinuria which persisted in the total absence of circulating antibody, antigen, or immune complexes.[360] A similar process has been well shown to occur in the autoimmune variety of experimental membranous nephropathy.

With these caveats in mind, the literature on disease-specific therapy of membranous nephropathy remains unsettled. Ponticelli et al. have reviewed these data and emphasized their own observations which suggest a beneficial effect of alternate monthly courses of methylprednisolone pulse therapy and oral chlorambucil when given to all patients.[361] Another study documents significant morphologic improvement in follow-up biopsies of patients treated with this regimen over a several-year period.[362] Ponticelli et al. and Garattini et al. review in some detail the data on beneficial effects of steroid therapy in MN which appear to have been established (but only with some difficulty) by prospective controlled studies.[361,363] Short et al. report that in 15 patients with MN and declining renal function after oral steroid therapy, pulse methylprednisolone (as used by Ponticelli) produced a sustained improvement in renal function in 10.[364] Others described two patients with idiopathic membranous nephropathy resistant to oral and pulse methylprednisolone who exhibited 2-year remissions following five to six monthly treatments with pulse cyclophosphamide.[365] Another report describes five patients resistant to the Ponticelli protocol with methylprednisolone and chlorambucil who subsequently received methylprednisolone and cyclosporine with achievement of complete remission.[366] In light of my earlier comments, it is not clear that some of these reports allowed sufficient time for initial therapies to work before moving on to other courses of therapy to which the remissions achieved have been ascribed. In one prospective controlled study enrolling only patients with idiopathic membranous nephropathy and mild renal functional impairment, 2 years of oral cyclophosphamide resulted in less proteinuria, more complete remissions, and better preservation of renal function over a 4-year follow-up period than was seen in control patients treated with steroids alone.[367] Interpretation of all of this literature remains difficult when considering the individual patient. Controversy persists regarding whether the most effective approach to idiopathic membranous nephropathy is no treatment at all because patients with relatively mild disease do well and patients with more severe disease have not been specifically shown to benefit from therapeutic intervention. Alternatively, some authors favor vigorous therapy of all patients with both steroids and cytotoxic agents. It is clear that about 50% of patients with urine protein excretions of less than 8 g, particularly if they are female, do well, and documentation of benefit in such patients will be difficult, a problem that has complicated conduct and interpretation of several large prospective studies. However, it is also clear that 50% of patients do develop progressive disease, especially those who are male and have protein excretions of over 10 g with a reduction in GFR. If therapy is effective, it must be demonstrated to be so in this group of patients which has never been specifically studied. Most of the available data suggest that steroid and immunosuppressive therapy probably is of benefit in such patients, although a prospective study is still required to demonstrate this. However, despite the frequency of this disease and the intensity with which it has been studied, no final answer is yet available on how it should best be treated.

Clues to the pathogenesis of MN are also being provided to us by the list of conditions with which it is associated. Recent publications confirm an association with hepatitis B,[368,369] although the nature of this association remains unclear. Higher hepatitis B surface antigen carrier rates are noted in several glomerular diseases as well as membranous nephropathy; the finding of glomerular hepatitis antigen deposits has not correlated well with serologic findings in these patients; and the clinical course has generally been unrelated to persistence or resolution of hepatitis B antigenemia.[369] One report of MN in a patient with an allergic reaction to nonsteroidal antiinflammatory agents has appeared,[370] and one patient with gout and nephrotic syndrome who apparently had glomerular capillary wall deposits of a proximal tubular brush border antigen has also been described.[371] MN is reported to occur in rheumatoid arthritis independently of gold or penicillamine therapy,[372] as well as consequent to gold therapy.[373] In a review of 21 patients with gold-induced MN, the insidious onset and slow resolution after discontinuation of therapy are emphasized (about 50% resolved in 12 months, but all did so by 40 months), as is the increased incidence of B8 and DR3 in these patients, the same association noted in idiopathic MN.[373] No irreversible renal functional abnormalities are reported and no therapy is apparently required.[374] One patient with lymphoma, nephrotic syndrome, and atypical fibrillary subepithelial immune deposits is described.[375] A case of MN in a patient with Guillain–Barré syndrome has also been reported.[376]

4.6. Membranoproliferative Glomerulonephritis

Relatively little new data concerning this important disease have emerged in 1986–1987. Welch *et al.* report a significant association with major histocompatibility complex antigens in MPGN type I, particularly with the extended haplotype B8, DR3 and SC01, GL02, genes encoding for the glyoxalase I enzyme located on chromosome six.[377] The data suggest both an increased initial susceptibility to MPGN associated with this haplotype, presumably representing a ''disease susceptibility gene'' located on chromosome six, as well as a worse prognosis for the disease when this haplotype is present.[377] A genetic association with MPGN I is also suggested by the report of a family in which the disease is apparently inherited as an X-linked recessive disorder.[378] The group at Cincinnati continues to provide data to support their contention that MPGN with subepithelial deposits (type III) is an entity distinct from type I MPGN.[379] They emphasize that patients with subepithelial deposits are more often detected clinically by chance, rarely have systemic symptoms in the absence of renal failure, have less glomerular proliferation, and appear to have alternate complement pathway activation as judged by the absence of early complement components in the biopsy by immunofluorescence.[379] It seems probable that MPGN I (III) is an autoimmune disease similar to systemic lupus with variations in immune response characteristics that determine the location at which immune deposits form. The occurrence of crescents and a rapidly progressive course in type I has been confirmed,[380] as has recurrence of the disease in two successive renal allografts with loss of graft function.[381] West, who has had more experience with this disease than anyone else, has detailed his reasons for advocating 2 years of alternate-day steroid therapy in treating such patients.[382] However, the data have not been obtained prospectively and the need remains for more information on the effects of steroid and immunosuppressive therapy in this disease.

The association of type II MPGN (dense-deposit disease) with partial lipodystrophy is reviewed.[377] One case in which a biopsy demonstrated a peculiar lamellation of the lamina densa several years before development of typical dense deposits is reported, suggesting that some structural defect in the capillary wall may precede the development of dense deposits.[383]

5. Glomerular Involvement in Systemic Diseases

5.1. Vasculitis

Much attention in vasculitis research has focused on observations that various inflammatory mediators may induce expression of activation antigens on endothelial cell surfaces which can, in turn, selectively elicit an immune response directed against the endothelial cell. Thus, a leukocyte adhesion molecule is induced on endothelial cells by lymphotoxin, tumor necrosis factor, and interleukin I, which can then promote lymphocyte and inflammatory leukocyte adherence and inflammation.[384] A similar sequence has been reported *in vivo* in patients treated with interleukin II who develop a vascular leak syndrome associated with endothelial cell activation and leukocyte adhesion molecule expression.[385] Moreover, in Kawasaki syndrome, a childhood illness with systemic vasculitis involving medium-sized arteries and venules, IgG and IgM antibodies have been found which can cause complement-mediated lysis of interleukin I or tumor necrosis factor–stimulated endothelial cells, suggesting that the vascular lesions may be mediated by antibody to cell activation antigens.[386] These observations may represent major advances in understanding the pathogenesis of vasculitis and the reasons for differential effects on different-sized vessels. The concept of idiopathic crescentic glomerulonephritis as a renal limited variant of vasculitis suggests that these concepts may be particularly relevant to that disease. The observation of elevated levels of antineutrophil cytoplasmic antibody in several forms of vasculitis also suggests a common mechanism.[251]

Moyer *et al.* have done sequential studies on an apparently cell-induced form of vasculitis in autoimmune MRL/l pr mice and show initial T helper cell vasculitic infiltrates without neutrophils suggesting an initiating cell-mediated immune reaction in this model.[387]

5.1.1. Large Vessel Vasculitis

Adu *et al.* review 43 patients with classical polyarteritis nodosa and note that virtually all of them have evidence of small vessel disease as well.[388]

5.1.2. Small Vessel Vasculitis

5.1.2.1. Renal Vasculitis. Most of the new information on this entity, which is now regarded as present in patients who have focal necrotizing glomerulonephritis with crescents and no other systemic disease, was discussed earlier under idiopathic crescentic glomerulonephritis or under vasculitis. Confusion in terminology in discussing such cases is illustrated by the review of Adu *et al.*, who described 41 patients with renal vasculitis under the title "Polyarteritis and the Kidney."[388] Again, the importance of segmental necrotizing glomerular lesions in making a diagnosis of vasculitis is emphasized, most patients did not have glomerular immune deposits, and age and initial renal function were the most important prognostic factors.[388]

A number of additional cases of small vessel vasculitis involving the kidney have been reported including associations with hypocomplementemic urticarial vasculitis.[389] A segmental necrotizing glomerulonephritis with loss of renal function was reported in four patients with rheumatoid arthritis.[390] Chang-Miller *et al.* report 29 cases with relapsing polychondritis and renal involvement, many of which had vasculitis and systemic necrotizing glomerulonephritis with crescents and without immune deposits.[391] Finally, renal involvement was present in one case of a paraneoplastic vasculitis with cutaneous vasculitis and arthritis associated with a myeloproliferative disorder.[392]

5.1.2.2. Systemic Lupus Erythematosus

5.1.2.2.1. Clinical Lupus Nephritis. The current state of understanding of lupus nephritis has been extensively reviewed in an NIH conference moderated by Balow,[393] as well as in other papers.[394] The NIH conference reviews again data from this group which suggest that analysis of the renal biopsy to both classify the type of glomerular lesion in lupus and to quantitate activity and chronicity is useful in selecting therapy. A number of studies have supported the utility of renal biopsy, at least in patients with severe lupus nephritis, as a useful guide to prognosis and therapy. Leaker *et al.* report a series of 135 biopsied patients with lupus nephritis and demonstrate a close correlation between the severity of disease as judged by crescent formation, the evidence of chronicity on biopsy, and a poor prognosis.[395] However, their results did not confirm data from the NIH associating male sex and age less than 24 with a poor prognosis.[395] Rush *et al.* also found that histologic assessment of chronicity, particularly measurements of glomerular sclerosis and interstitial fibrosis, was a useful predictor of clinical course in 20 children with diffuse proliferative lupus nephritis.[396] However, the chronicity index appears to be useful only in diffuse proliferative lupus nephritis, whereas patients with less severe glomerular lesions seem to do well even with high chronicity indices.[393,395] Lewis *et al.* comment on the difficulty of analyzing clinical pathologic correlations in this disease and include an analysis of the number of glomeruli that must be present in a biopsy to have 95% confidence that more than 50% of glomeruli are abnormal (more than 20 glomeruli must be present).[397] These investigators, who have recently completed a large prospective study of the role of plasma exchange in diffuse proliferative lupus nephritis, also have studied the prognosis of severe segmental glomerular lesions (more than 50% involvement) compared to patients with diffuse disease and shown them to be extremely similar (actuarial 5-year survival 59 vs. 53%).[398] It is further noted that patients with severe lupus nephritis histologically have about a 10% chance of developing end-stage renal disease within a year despite having a normal serum creatinine at the time of diagnosis.[399] Ponticelli *et al.* report a kidney survival rate of 79% at 10 years in patients with diffuse proliferative lupus nephritis.[400] Both of these studies of short- and long-term prognosis in severe lupus nephritis demonstrate markedly improved patient and renal survival rates compared to data from 15–20 years ago. Henry *et al.* note that patients with severe rapidly progressive lupus nephritis may have acute tubular necrosis as a cause of their acute renal failure and subsequently experience remarkable recovery.[401]

Font *et al.* report 15 cases of systemic lupus erythematosus (SLE) without clinical renal involvement, nine of whom had class II–III disease on biopsy, but provide no data to support their contention that this finding on biopsy necessitates therapy or that patients profit from therapy.[402] Park *et al.* review tubulointerstitial disease in lupus and point out that extensive tubulointerstitial nephritis is present in 33% of patients, correlates well with the severity of glomerular disease, has some prognostic significance, and, surprisingly, does not correlate with immune complex deposits on either tubular basement membrane or interstitial vessels.[403]

Much attention has been devoted recently to the issue of pregnancy in lupus, particularly the association between the so-called lupus anticoagulant and spontaneous abortion. The lupus anticoagulant is an IgG autoantibody to phospholipids which inhibits generation of the prothrombin activation complex, is measured by prolongation of the partial thromboplastin time and Russell viper venom time, and is directly related to the incidence of thrombotic events, particularly vascular occlusion and spontaneous abortion. It is present in 7–25% of patients, depending on assay conditions. Measurement of anticardiolipin activity represents a related antiphospholipid antibody and may be a more sensitive assay for the lupus anticoagulant.[402–407] Continued reports of a positive association between anticardiolipin antibody and spontaneous miscarriage in lupus have appeared[408,409] and raise the issue of whether such patients should be treated with antiplatelet agents, immunosuppression, or even plasma exchange during pregnancy, an issue that cannot be resolved by data available at this point.[410] Bobie et al. report on 213 pregnancies in patients with lupus nephritis, of whom 34% had exacerbation of lupus activity during pregnancy, and note the improved prognosis if pregnancy occurs during a remission in disease activity.[410]

The relative infrequency of recurrent lupus nephritis in allografts is emphasized by Roth et al., who found biopsy abnormalities in only 2 of 15 patients, including eight with HLA identical grafts.[411] Another recurrence without graft loss was reported by Kumano et al.[412] The Australian–New Zealand experience confirms the good prognosis of patients with end-stage renal disease secondary to lupus nephritis treated with either hemodialysis or renal transplantation.[413] However, Rodby et al. point out in eight patients followed prospectively after initiation of pertioneal dialysis that clinical and serologic manifestations of disease activity did not seem to diminish when end-stage renal disease developed.[414]

5.1.2.2.2. *Pathogenesis of Lupus Nephritis.* The current status of anti-DNA antibodies and DNA-containing immune complexes in lupus is reviewed by Emlen et al.[415] The NZB mouse model continues to be a mainstay of research on the pathogenesis of nephritis and autoimmunity in SLE. Several studies document the presence of only a few anti-DNA antibody idiotypes in contributing to the development of nephritis in both mice and people. Hahn and Ebling show that three idiotypes emerge with age in NZB mice and two of these account for the bulk of the glomerular antibody deposits.[416] Gavalchin et al. report that the restricted idiotypes of anti-DNA antibody seen in glomerulonephritis-susceptible F_1 hybrids of NZB mice are uniquely cationic and that these cationic antibodies also predominate in glomerular deposits.[417] Madaio et al. have shown that one of the restricted idiotypes present in lupus serum is also present in the small amounts of anti-DNA antibody detectable in normal people, suggesting that the B-cell clone which expands to produce pathogenic anti-DNA antibody in lupus may also be present, but inactive, in normal individuals.[418] These authors have also shown that certain monoclonal anti-DNA antibodies from MRL/lpr mice can bind directly to non-DNA glomerular antigens to form glomerular immune deposits, indicating that DNA and anti-DNA antibody may not be critical components of the antibodies that produce renal disease in murine lupus.[419] Further evidence for the importance of this anti-DNA antibody polyreactivity in producing lupus nephritis is provided by studies showing that antibody eluted from glomerular deposits demonstrates more polyreactivity than simultaneously obtained serum IgG.[420]

Other than anti-DNA antibodies, antibodies with other specificities have also been noted in lupus associated with glomerulonephritis. Hashemi et al. confirm the presence of antiendothelial cell antibodies in lupus.[421] These have clearly been shown to capable of causing glomerulonephritis experimentally.[41] A negative association between IgM rheumatoid factor and lupus nephritis is reported by Helin *et al.*[422] Anti-RNA polymerase I antibody has been isolated from glomeruli in NZB mice and shown to correlate with the severity of the glomerular disease.[423]

Several studies of interest have emerged regarding the nature and role of immune complexes in lupus. Cosio *et al.* have characterized the role of the erythrocyte CR1 receptor system in clearing DNA-containing immune complexes in nonhuman primates.[424] Horgan and Emlen described complement activation by very small (12–22S), DNA-containing immune complexes, which do not bind to red cell CR1 receptors and may therefore escape rapid clearance.[425] Similar independence from the erythrocyte clearing mechanism is described for IgG anti-ds DNA immune complexes.[426] Although many previous studies have failed to demonstrate much correlation between circulating complex levels measured by various techniques and renal disease in lupus nephritis, Greisman *et al.* report that the presence of a 64-kd component of C1q in circulating complexes was correlated with impairment of complement-dependent immune complex clearance and development of renal disease.[427] However, Uwatoko *et al.* have provided convincing evidence that the C1q binding activity usually present in lupus serum does not represent soluble immune complexes, but rather the presence of an autoantibody to a collagenlike region on C1q.[428]

The current status of the idiotypic network and its relationship to autoimmunity is lucidly reviewed by Zanetti,[429] and problems with the study and interpretation of anti-DNA antibodies are discussed by Eilat.[430] Of particular interest with regard to the polyreactivity of anti-DNA antibody is the observation of Jacob *et al.* that a monoclonal anti-DNA antibody also reacts with five apparently non-DNA cell membrane proteins referred to as lupus-associated membrane proteins (LAMP).[431] LAMP are present in normal human glomeruli. However, the exact nature and relationship of anti-LAMP antibodies to lupus nephritis remain to be defined. Although multiple other studies related to the autoimmune basis of lupus were published during 1986–1987, most of these do not bear directly on the pathogenesis of lupus nephritis.

5.1.2.2.3. Treatment of Lupus Nephritis. The current status of immunosuppressive drug therapy for lupus nephritis is well reviewed by Balow,[393,432] and the latter paper provides useful details of the protocols for cytotoxic drug therapy now utilized at the NIH. Other reviews by Miescher[433] and Steinberg[434] also contain useful information on pathogenetic and therapeutic aspects of lupus nephritis. The major new data to emerge during this period, which are also reviewed in several of the articles cited earlier,[432–434] are the findings of Austin *et al.* from the NIH.[435] This paper updates the status of 107 patients with lupus nephritis in long-term, randomized therapeutic trials at the NIH and reports that patients treated every 3 months with an intravenous pulse dose of cyclophosphamide combined with low-dose (0.5 mg/kg per day) prednisone had better preservation of renal function than patients treated concurrently with high-dose (1 mg/kg per day) oral prednisone, particularly if they were in a high-risk group defined as having a chronicity index of greater than one on initial biopsy.[435] Comparisons of other immunosuppressive drug programs (oral azathioprine, cyclophosphamide, or combined azathioprine and cyclophosphamide) did not demonstrate significant improvement over steroids alone. However, the rather tenuous statistical significance of the data reported by Austin (significance would be lost if one patient in the i.v. cyclophosphamide group developed renal insufficiency) has been noted.[436] At present the balance of evidence suggests that in patients with diffuse proliferative lupus nephritis and evidence of activity and chronicity on biopsy, treatment with a cytotoxic agent is probably more efficacious in preserving renal function than treatment with steroids alone. Available evidence also suggests that administration of cyclophosphamide as an intravenous pulse dose every 1 or 3 months may be somewhat safer than daily oral cyclophosphamide, but no strong case can be made for cyclophosphamide vs. other immunosuppressive agents in the treatment of lupus nephritis.

Although isolated reports of apparent responses to plasma exchange in patients with severe, often resistant, lupus nephritis continued to appear,[437,438] the results of a large, prospective controlled study of plasma exchange in severe lupus nephritis show no benefit of this therapy on renal function.[439,440] Pulse methylprednisolone therapy is also still advocated by some as a useful way to initiate high-dose steroid therapy in severe, progressive lupus nephritis. A small, controlled study from England compared pulse methylprednisolone at a dose of 100 mg/day vs. 1000 mg/day and demonstrated no difference between the two programs.[441] Although cyclosporine has been used in murine SLE to reduce autoantibody levels[442] and improve glomerulonephritis,[443] its use in clinical lupus nephritis has generally been disappointing and complicated by problems with nephrotoxicity. However, one study reports apparent benefit with low-dose cyclosporine (5 mg/kg per day) in lupus nephritis.[444] The group at Stanford has reported prolonged remission and reduced renal disease in murine lupus nephritis treated with total lymphoid irradiation[445] and has updated their previously published clinical experience with total lymphoid irradiation in humans to include 15 patients followed for up to 6 years with remarkable and apparently sustained improvements in renal function and proteinuria.[446] Wofsy has provided a very thorough and objective analysis of the current literature on the use of cytotoxic drugs, methylprednisolone pulse therapy, plasma exchange, and total lymphoid irradiation in lupus nephritis with some guidelines for selection of therapy that are as reasonable as any.[447]

Finally, several studies suggest possible new directions for therapeutic initiatives in lupus nephritis. Several specific immunomodulating approaches may be possible. Therapy with anti-Ia antibodies has previously been shown to prevent lupus nephritis in NZB mice, and more recently shown to directly affect autoantibody production by B cells rather than altering immune regulation.[448] Anti-idiotypic antibody to anti-DNA reduces anti-DNA antibody production in vitro.[449]

DMSO retards development of renal disease in NZB mice apparently without altering autoantibody levels and may act by stimulating prostaglandin production.[450] Similarly, a fish oil diet significantly retards development of the renal lesion in NZB mice, although it is unclear whether this effect is due to a reduction in the local inflammatory response or to alteration of the systemic immune response.[451] It is hoped that the rapid advances in understanding the molecular basis for autoimmunity will lead to additional progress and new ideas for therapy in this area.

5.1.3. Henoch–Schönlein Purpura

Lee *et al.* review the clinical and morphologic features of 17 adults with Henoch–Schönlein purpura (HSP) and glomerulonephritis.[452] Although the prognosis in HSP in adults is generally considered to be worse than it is in children, these patients did quite well, with 10 recovering completely and five exhibiting persistent proteinuria but no loss of renal function. Most patients had relatively mild renal disease and all were treated with steroids. Another 17 patients are reviewed by Walker *et al.* with similar conclusions.[453] These authors emphasize the frequency of preceding bacterial infections in precipitating episodes of HSP, a point also made by the description of HSP in a patient with endocarditis[454] and following a streptococcal infection.[455] Pulmonary hemorrhage may occur in HSP and be a presenting feature of the illness.[455] A case of recurrent HSP with disease in a renal transplant is reported, with the disease apparently contributing to graft failure.[456] No significant contributions to advancing therapy of the renal disease in HSP appeared during 1986–1987.

5.1.4. Cryoglobulinemia

Several excellent reviews of renal involvement in dysproteinemias and in cryoglobulinemia in particular appeared during 1986–1987.[457–459] The frequency of positive hepatitis B antigenemia, IgM rheumatoid factor, low levels of early complement components C1q and especially C4 with normal CH50, and fibrillary deposits by electron microscopy are emphasized by all authors. Most authors agree that in patients with severe renal involvement with decreased complement and nephrotic syndrome, methylprednisolone pulse therapy and plasma exchange are probably indicated. Although most reports have described use of cytotoxic drugs with plasma exchange, in one study of nine patients with progressive nephropathy treated with several weeks of plasma exchange with low-dose steroids and no immunosuppression, renal function improved significantly in five.[460] A case of type II cryoglobulinemia with glomerulonephritis associated with small lymphocytic lymphoma is notable for the absence of typical glomerular immune deposits and the presence of extensive glomerular mononuclear cell infiltrates early in the renal disease.[461] Alpers *et al.* describe seven patients with mild glomerulonephritis associated with fibrillar deposits in the mesangium and along capillary walls that stain for IgG and kappa chains. Most patients had hypertension, nephrotic syndrome, and progressive renal disease, but none had clinical or morphologic evidence of amyloid.[462]

5.1.5. Wegener's Granulomatosis

The utility of the antineutrophil cytoplasmic antibody test in the diagnosis and management of Wegener's was emphasized earlier under vasculitis.[251] A well-documented case of anti-GBM disease occurring in the same patient with Wegener's granulomatosis suggests possible common features, perhaps genetic, in the pathogenesis of these disorders.[463] The occasional utility of trimethoprim–sulfamethoxazole in the management of Wegener's granulomatosis is pointed out in one report of a positive response to this treatment in a patient who apparently failed to respond to cyclophosphamide,[464] a phenomenon that has been commented on in older studies.

5.2. Glomerulonephritis in Renal Transplants

Relatively little new material about recurrent glomerulonephritis in transplants was provided during 1986–1987. However, Habib *et al.* provide a comprehensive review of glomerular pathology in 410 children undergoing renal transplantation.[465] They describe recurrent glomerulonephritis in 40 of 140 patients with glomerular disease, *de novo* glomerulonephritis in 52, and transplant glomerulopathy in 29. Recurrent disease was particularly notable in focal glomerular sclerosis (34%), Henoch–Schönlein purpura (88%), IgA nephropathy (75%), type I membranoproliferative glomerulonephritis (70%), and type II membranoproliferative glomerulonephritis (100%). As in many previous studies, most of the patients reported did not suffer adverse clinical consequences of the morphologic recurrence of their disease. In this study, patients with recurrent focal sclerosis were generally older than 6, had a shorter duration of disease prior to transplantation, and exhibited more mesangial proliferation in their biopsies. Several patients with recurrent focal sclerosis apparently responded to methylprednisolone pulse therapy or to cyclosporine and one had a spontaneous remission.[465] Recurrent Henoch–Schönlein purpura was most prominent in patients with a short duration of disease (less than 15 months), a phenomenon noted in all of the other recurrent diseases as well. Sixteen percent of all patients who received transplants develop *de novo* disease and 10% developed *de novo* membranous nephropathy, but nephrotic syndrome and graft loss were rare. A rather high incidence of *de novo* anti-GBM disease was noted (4.5%), although the effect of the antibody on graft function was usually minimal. None of these patients had hereditary nephritis. This report using current morphologic and immunopathologic criteria for diagnosis by an experienced group does not provide any data to suggest that recurrent glomerulonephritis is much different in children than it is in adults and represents an excellent review and updating of the topic.

5.3. Thrombotic Microangiopathy (Hemolytic Uremic Syndrome and Thrombotic Thrombocytopenic Purpura)

Several important contributions to understanding this common and important group of diseases appeared during 1986–1987. The topic in general has been well reviewed by several authors, including Neild,[466] Kaplan and Proesmans,[467] and Remuzzi.[468] It is becoming increasing apparent that the bloody diarrhea that often precedes clinical cases of hemolytic uremic syndrome (HUS) is usually caused by *Escherichia coli* 0157, which produces verotoxin in both children[469,470] and adults.[471] In one reported outbreak of hemorrhaghic colitis in a nursing home, HUS developed in 22% of elderly patients, most of whom died.[472] Antibiotic therapy was associated with increased risk of infection and a higher mortality rate.[472] In the Puget Sound area the disease associated with 0157 hemorrhagic colitis appears to be endemic and increasing in frequency.[469] In addition to endotheliotropic *E. coli*, other stimuli can clearly produce HUS, including other bacterial and viral infections[466–468] and several drugs, particularly cyclosporine in both liver and bone marrow transplant recipients[473,474] and mitomycin C in patients with malignancy.[475,476] Successful treatment of the disease with plasma exchange has been reported in one case of thrombotic thrombocytopenic purpura (TTP) apparently induced by cyclosporine.[473] All of these agents appear to have direct toxic effects on the vascular endothelium which presumably initiates the platelet aggregation. The exact nature of the endothelial lesion is still controversial. Speculation continues that thrombotic microangiopathy may result from a deficiency in plasma factors required for endothelial cell synthesis of prostacyclin (PGI_2) with consequent local platelet aggregation.[477] Demonstration of reduced fatty acid content of red cell membranes in HUS,[478] elevated plasma levels of the PGI_2 metabolite 6 keto PGF1 alpha,[479] and occasional responses to prostacyclin therapy are consistent with this hypothesis.[479] However, most of these changes could also be secondary to endothelial cell injury from other causes rather than primary factors. Remuzzi provides a comprehensive discussion of the data on the pathogenesis of HUS–TTP and its possible interpretations.[468] Intravascular release of platelet mitogens has also been reported as a possible contributing factor to vascular proliferative lesions in HUS.[480] Fibronectin is depressed in the serum in HUS, is present along with fibrinogen and platelet antigens in glomeruli, and may also contribute to the development of this lesion.[481] Although these diseases are generally thought of as self-limited, recurrent HUS has been reported without obvious precipitating cause in adults,[482] and recurrence seems to be rather common in TTP.[483] Recurrence of HUS in renal transplant patients is well described.[484] The use of cyclosporine and antilymphocyte globulin may predispose to recurrence and should probably be avoided, but no good predictive factors for recurrence in these patients have emerged.[484]

Current therapeutic approaches to thrombotic microangiopathies are well reviewed elsewhere.[466–468] The use of plasma infusion and plasma exchange in TTP is reviewed by Shepard and Bukowski, who concluded that plasma exchange with fresh frozen plasma and use of steroids and antiplatelet agents represent the most promising approach to therapy.[485] Clinical trials are currently in progress to attempt to ascertain which component of this cocktail is the most efficacious. A reduction in mortality from TTP from 41% to 17% between 1975–1980 and 1980–1985 at the hospital of the University of Pennsylvania associated with the advent of plasma exchange therapy suggests a beneficial effect from this treatment.[486] Based on studies showing inhibition of platelet aggregating activity in TTP by normal IgG, high-dose immunoglobulin infusion has been employed successfully in one patient with TTP resistant to plasma exchange.[487]

References

1. Andres, G., Brentjens, J. R., Caldwell, P. R. B., Camussi, G., and Matsuo, S., 1986, Biology of disease. Formation of immune deposits and disease, *Lab. Invest.* **55:**510–520.
2. Wener, M. H. and Mannik, M., 1986, Mechanisms of immune deposit formation in renal glomeruli, *Springer Semin. Immunopathol.* **9:**219–235.
3. Feintzeig, I. D., Dittmer, J. E., Cybulsky, A. V., and Salant, D. J., 1986, Antibody, antigen, and glomerular capillary wall charge interactions: Influence of antigen location on in situ immune complex formation, *Kidney Int.* **29:**649–657.
4. Ronco, P., Neale, T. J., Wilson, C. B., Galceran, M., and Verroust, P., 1986, An immunopathologic study of A 330-kD protein defined by monoclonal antibodies and reactive with anti-RTEα 5 antibodies and kidney eluates from active Heymann nephritis, *J. Immunol.* **136:**125–130.
5. Kerjaschki, D., Horvat, R., Binder, S., Susani, M., Dekan, G., Ojha, P. P., Hillemanns, P., Ulrich, W., and Donini, U., 1987, Identification of a 400-kd protein in the brush borders of human kidney tubules that is similar to gp330, the nephritogenic antigen of rat Heymann nephritis, *Am. J. Pathol.* **129:**183–191.
6. Behar, M., Katz, A., and Silverman, M., 1986, Biochemical investigation of the pathogenesis of Heymann nephritis, *Kidney Int.* **30:**9–15.
7. Natori, Y., Hayakawa, I., and Shibata, S., 1987, Heymann nephritis in rats induced by human renal tubular antigens: characterization of antigen and antibody specificities, *Clin. Exp. Immunol.* **69:**33–40.
8. Singh, A. K. and Makker, S. P., 1986, Circulatory antigens of Heymann nephritis I. Identification and partial characterization, *Immunology* **57:**467–472.
9. Singh, A. K. and Schwartz, M. M., 1986, Circulatory antigen of Heymann nephritis. II. Isolation of a 70,000 MW antigen from normal rat serum which cross-reacts with Heymann nephritis antigen, *Immunology* **59:**451–458.
10. Makker, S. P. and Makker, D. M., 1986, A simple technique for detecting the antigen of Heymann nephritis in glomeruli by immunofluorescence, *Clin. Exp. Immunol.* **64:**615–622.
11. Abrass, C. K. and Cohen, A. H., 1986, The role of circulating antigen in the formation of immune deposits in experimental membranous nephropathy, *Proc. Soc. Exp. Biol. Med.* **183:**348–357.
12. Abrass, C. K., 1986, Evaluation of sequential glomerular eluates from rats with Heymann nephritis, *J. Immunol.* **137:**530–535.
13. Bagchus, W. M., Vos, J. T. W. M., Hoedemaeker, Ph. J., and Bakker, W. W., 1986, The specificity of nephritogenic antibodies. III. Binding of anti-Fx1A antibodies in glomeruli is dependent on dual specificity, *Clin. Exp. Immunol.* **63:**639–647.
14. Verroust, P., Ronco, P. M., and Chatelet, F., 1986, Monoclonal antibodies and identification of glomerular antigens, *Kidney Int.* **30:**649–655.
15. Camussi, G., Noble, B., Van Liew, J., Brentjens, J. R., and Andress, G., 1986, Pathogenesis of passive Heymann glomerulonephritis: chlorpromazine inhibits antibody-mediated redistribution of cell surface antigens and prevents development of the disease, *J. Immunol.* **136:**2127–2135.

16. Allegri, L., Brianti, E., Chatelet, F., Manara, G. C., Ronco, P., and Verroust, P., 1986, Polyvalent antigen–antibody interactions are required for the formation of electron-dense immune deposits in passive Heymann's nephritis, *Am. J. Pathol.* **126:**1–6.

17. Kerjaschki, D., Miettinen, A., and Farquhar, M. G., 1987, Initial events in the formation of immune deposits in passive Heymann nephritis, gp330-anti-gp330 immune complexes from in epithelial coated pits and rapidly become attached to the glomerular basement membrane, *J. Exp. Med.* **166:**109–128.

18. Brown, D., McCluskey, R. T., and Ausiello, D. A., 1987, The cell biology of Heymann nephritis: A model of human membranous glomerulonephritis, *Am. J. Kidney Dis.* **5:**74–76.

19. Pelletier, L., Galceran, M., Pasquier, R., Ronco, P., Verroust, P., Bariety, J., and Druet, P., 1987, Down modulation of Heymann's nephritis by mercuric chloride, *Kidney Int.* **32:**227–232.

20. Barabas, A. Z., Cornish, J., and Lannigan, R., 1986, Stimulation of circulating autoantibody levels in the rat with established progressive passive Heymann nephritis, *Clin. Exp. Immunol.* **65:** 34–41.

21. Nakazawa, M., Emancipator, S. N., and Lamm, M. E., 1986, Proteolytic enzyme treatment reduces glomerular immune deposits and proteinuria in passive Heymann nephritis, *J. Exp. Med.* **164:**1973–1987.

22. Furness, P. N. and Turner, D. R., 1987, An assessment of the influence of antigen dose in two new models of chronic serum sickness glomerulonephritis in the rat, *Br. J. Exp. Path.* **68:**527–538.

23. Yamamoto, T., Miyazaki, S., Kawasaki, K., Yaoita, E., and Kihara, I., 1986, Rat bovine serum albumin (BSA) nephritis. VI. The influence of chemically altered antigen, *Clin. Exp. Immunol.* **65:** 51–56.

24. Noble, B., Steward, M. W., Vladutiu, A., and Brentjens, J. R., 1987, Relationship of the quality and quantity of circulating anti-BSA antibodies to the severity of glomerulonephritis in rats with chronic serum sickness, *Clin. Exp. Immunol.* **67:**277–282.

25. Koyama, A., Inage, H., Kobayashi, M., Narita, M., and Tojo, S., 1986, Effect of chemical cationization of antigen on glomerular localization of immune complexes in active models of serum sickness nephritis in rabbits, *Immunology* **58:**529–534.

26. Chan, E. K. L., Boyd, N. D., Alexander, F., Barabas, A. Z., and Lanningan, R., 1986, Effect of cationic proteins on the glomerular deposition of anionic proteins and immune complexes, *Nephron* **43:**93–104.

27. Camussi, G., Tetta, C., Meroni, M., Torri-Tarelli, L., Roffinello, C., Alberton, A., Deregibus, C., and Sessa, A., 1986, Localization of cationic proteins derived from platelets and polymorphonuclear neutrophils and local loss of anionic sites in glomeruli of rabbits with experimentally-induced acute serum sickness, *Lab. Invest.* **55:**56–62.

28. Oite, T., Shimizu, F., Batsford, S. R., and Vogt, A., 1986, The effect of protamine sulfate on the course of immune complex glomerulonephritis in the rat, *Clin. Exp. Immunol.* **64:**318–322.

29. Ward, D. M., Lee, S., and Wilson, C. B., 1986, Direct antigen binding to glomerular immune complex deposits, *Kidney Int.* **30:**706–711.

30. Zanetti, M. and Wilson, C. B., 1986, A role for antiidiotypic antibodies in immunologically mediated nephritis, *Am. J. Kidney Dis.* **7:**445–451.

31. Thomas, M. A. B. and Williams, D. G., 1987, Idiotypes and antiidiotypic antibodies in health and disease, *Q. J. Med.* **65:**883–888.

32. Agodoa, L. Y. C. and Mannik, M., 1987, Removal of subepithelial immune complexes with excess unaltered or cationic antigen, *Kidney Int.* **32:**13–18.

33. Raj, A. S., Tuscan, M., Shapiro, B., Glatfelter, A., Kunkel, R., and Wiggins, R. C., 1986, Amount of antibody is critical for immune complex displacement by charge competition from both rabbit glomeruli and anionic beads, *Clin. Exp. Immunol.* **64:**629–637.

34. Nakazawa, M., Emancipator, S. N., and Lamm, M. E., 1986, Removal of glomerular immune complexes in passive serum sickness nephritis by treatment in vivo with proteolytic enzymes, *Lab. Invest.* **55:**551–556.

35. Yamamoto, T., Yamamoto, K., Kawasaki, K., Yaoita, E., Shimizu, F., and Kihara, I., 1986, Immunoelectron microscopic demonstration of thy-1 antigen on the surfaces of mesangial cells in the rat glomerulus, *Nephron* **43**:293–298.
36. Bagchus, W. M., Hoedemaeker, Ph. J., Rozing, J., and Bakker, W. W., 1986, Glomerulonephritis induced by monoclonal anti-thy 1.1 antibodies. A sequential histological and ulstrastructural study in the rat, *Lab. Invest.* **55**:680–687.
37. Yamamoto, T. and Wilson, C. B., 1987, Complement dependence of antibody-induced mesangial cell injury in the rat, *J. Immunol.* **138**:3758–3765.
38. Yamamoto, T. and Wilson, C. B., 1987, Quantitative and qualitative studies of antibody-induced mesangial cell damage in the rat, *Kidney Int.* **32**:514–525.
39. Bagghus, W. M., Donga, J., Rozing, J., Hoedemaeker, Ph. J., and Bakker, W. W., 1986, The specificity of nephritogenic antibodies, *Transplantation* **41**:739–745.
40. Mendrick, D. L. and Rennke, H. G., 1986, Immune deposits formed in situ by a monoclonal antibody recognizing a new intrinsic rat mesangial matrix antigen, *J. Immunol.* **137**:1517–1526.
41. Matsuo, S., Fukatsu, A., Taub, M. L., Caldwell, P. R. B., Brentjens, J. R., and Andres, G., 1987, Glomerulonephritis induced in the rabbit by antiendothelial antibodies, *J. Clin. Invest.* **79**:1798–1811.
42. Koyama, A., Inage, H., Kobayashi, M., Ohta, Y., Narita, M., Tojo, S., and Cameron, J. S., 1986, Role of antigenic charge and antibody avidity on the glomerular immune complex localization in serum sickness mice, *Clin. Exp. Immunol.* **64**:606–614.
43. Abrass, C. K. and Hori, M. T., 1987, Alterations in plasma clearance and tissue localization of model immune complexes in rats with streptozotocin-induced diabetes, *Immunology* **60**:331–336.
44. Roccatello, D., Coppo, R., Martina, G., Rollino, C., Basolo, B., Frattasio, C., Fasano, M. E., Amoroso, A., Picciotto, G., Bajardi, P., Cordonnier, D., and Piccoli, G., 1987, Fc-receptor function of the mononuclear phagocyte system in glomerulonephritis secondary to some multisystem diseases, *Am. J. Nephrol.* **7**:85–92.
45. Kanwar, Y. S., Caulin-Glaser, T., Gallo, G. R., and Lamm, M. E., 1986, Interaction of immune complexes with glomerular heparan sulfate–proteoglycans, *Kidney Int.* **30**:842–851.
46. Hebert, L. A. and Cosio, F. G., 1987, The erythrocyte–immune complex–glomerulonephritis connection in man, *Kidney Int.* **31**:877–885.
47. Kasinath, B. S., Maaba, M. R., Schwartz, M. M., and Lewis, E. J., 1986, Demonstration and characterization of C3 receptors on rat glomerular epithelial cells, *Kidney Int.* **30**:852–861.
48. Cosio, F. G. and Bakaletz, A. P., 1986, Binding of human fibronectin to antigen–antibody complexes, *J. Lab. Clin. Med.* **107**:453–458.
49. Cosio, F. G. and Bakaletz, A. P., 1987, Role of fibronectin on the clearance and tissue uptake of antigen and immune complexes in rats, *J. Clin. Invest.* **80**:1270–1279.
50. Schena, F. P. and Pertosa, G., 1988, Fibronectin and the kidney, *Nephron* **48**:177–182.
51. Meyer, P. A. R., 1987, The observation of immune complex formation and deposition in the eyes of living rabbits, *Clin. Exp. Immunol.* **69**:166–178.
52. Chen, X-M., Tanaka, T., Kobayashi, Y., Shigematsu, H., and Okumura, K., 1987, Experimental glomerulonephritis induced by immune complexes of monoclonal antibodies produced by immunoglobulin class-switch variants, *Lab. Invest.* **57**:665–672.
53. Abrahamson, D. R., 1986, Recent studies on the structure and pathology of basement membranes, *J. Pathol.* **149**:257–278.
54. Timpl, R., 1986, Recent advances in the biochemistry of glomerular basement membrane, *Kidney Int.* **30**:293–298.
55. Uitto, J., Murray, L. W., Blumberg, B., and Shamban, A., 1986, Biochemistry of collagen in disease, *Ann. Intern. Med.* **105**:740–756.
56. Butkowski, R. J., Langeveld, J. P. M., Wieslander, J., Hamilton, J., and Hudson, B. G., 1987, Localization of the Goodpasture epitope to a novel chain of basement membrane collagen, *J. Biol. Chem.* **262**:7874–7877.

57. Pusey, C. D., Dash, A., Kershaw, M. J., Morgan, A., Reilly, A., Rees, A. J., and Lockwood, C. M., 1987, A single autoantigen in Goodpasture's syndrome identified by a monoclonal antibody to human glomerular basement membrane, *Lab. Invest.* **56:**23–31.

58. Weber, M., Kohler, H., Manns, M., Baum, H-P., and Meyer Zum Buschenfelde, K-H, 1987, Identification of Goodpasture target antigens in basement membranes of human glomeruli, lung, and placenta, *Clin. Exp. Immunol.* **67:**262–269.

59. Kefalides, N. A., 1987, The Goodpasture antigen and basement membranes: The search must go on, *Lab. Invest.* **56:**1–3.

60. Bygren, P., Wieslander, J., and Heinegard, D., 1987, Glomerulonephritis induced in sheep by immunization with human glomerular basement membrane, *Kidney Int.* **31:**25–31.

61. Wick, G., Von Der Mark, H., Dietrich, H., and Timpl, R., 1986, Globular domain of basement membrane collagen induces autoimmune pulmonary lesions in mice resembling human Goodpasture disease, *Lab. Invest.* **55:**308–317.

62. Natori, Y. and Shibata, S., 1986, Comparison of nephritogenic glycopeptide, nephritogenoside, isolated from rat glomerular basement membranes with other basement membrane components, *Connect. Tissue Res.* **15:**245–255.

63. Feintzeig, I. D., Abrahamson, D. R., Cybulsky, A. V., Dittmer, J. E., and Salant, D. J., 1986, Nephritogenic potential of sheep antibodies against glomerular basement membrane laminin in the rat, *Lab. Invest.* **55:**531–541.

64. Makino, H., Gibbons, J. T., Reddy, M. K., and Kanwar, Y. S., 1986, Nephritogenicity of antibodies to proteoglycans of the glomerular basement membrane I, *J. Clin. Invest.* **77:**142–156.

65. Makino, H., Lelongt, B., and Kanwar, Y. S., 1988, Nephritogenicity of proteoglycans II a model of immune complex nephritis, *Kidney Int.* **34:**195–208.

66. Miettinen, A., Stow, J. L., Mentone, S., and Farquhar, M. G., 1986, Antibodies to basement membrane heparan sulfate proteoglycans bind to the laminae rarae of the glomerular basement membrane (GBM) and induce subepithelial GBM thickening, *J. Exp. Med.* **163:**1064–1084.

67. Matsuo, S., Brentjens, J. R., Andres, G., Foidart, J-M., Martin, G. R., and Martinez-Hernandez, A., 1986, Distribution of basement membrane antigens in glomeruli of mice with autoimmune glomerulonephritis, *Am. J. Pathol.* **122:**36–49.

68. Fukatsu, A., Matsuo, S., Killen, P. D., Martin, G. R., Andres, G. A., and Brentjens, J. R., 1988, The glomerular distribution of type IV collagen and laminin in human membranous glomerulonephritis, *Hum. Pathol.* **19:**64–68.

69. Emancipator, S. N., 1986, Pathways of tissue injury initiated by humoral immune mechanisms, *Lab. Invest.* **54:**475–478.

70. Hruby, Z., Lowry, R. P., Forbes, R. D. C., and Marghesco, D., 1986, Immune mechanisms and molecular mediators of glomerular injury in experimental nephritis: Summary of current results and continuing studies, *Transplant. Proc.* **18:**664–666.

71. Boyce, N. W. and Holdsworth, S. R., 1986, Direct antiGBM antibody induced alterations in glomerular permselectivity, *Kidney Int.* **30:**666–672.

72. Boyce, N. W. and Holdsworth, S. R., 1987, Intrarenal hemodynamic alterations induced by anti-GBM antibody, *Kidney Int.* **31:**8–14.

73. Feucht, H. E., Jung, C. M., Gokel, M. J., Riethmuller, G., Zwirner, J., Brase, A., Held, E., and O'Neil, G. J., 1986, Detection of both isotypes of complement C4, C4A and C4B, in normal human glomeruli, *Kidney Int.* **30:**932–936.

74. Koski, C. L., Sanders, M. E., Swoveland, P. T., Lawley, T. J., Shin, M. L., Frank, M. M., and Joiner, K. A., 1987, Activation of terminal components of complement in patients with Guillain–Barré syndrome and other demyelinating neuropathies, *J. Clin. Invest.* **80:**1492–1497.

75. Sanders, M. E., Alexander, E. L., Koski, C. L., Frank, M. M., and Joiner, K. A., 1987, Detection of activated terminal complement (C5b-9) in cerebrospinal fluid from patients with central nervous system involvement of primary Sjögren's syndrome or systemic lupus erythematosus, *J. Immunol.* **138:**2095–2099.

76. Hinglais, N., Kazatchkine, M. D., Bhakdi, S., Appay, M-D., Mandet, C., Grossetete, J., and Bariety, J., 1986, Immunohistochemical study of the C5b-9 complex of complement in human kidneys, *Kidney Int.* **30:**399–410.

77. Rus, H. G., Niculescu, F., Nanulescu, M., Cristea, A., and Florescu, P., 1986, Immunohistochemical detection of terminal C5b-9 complement complex in children with glomerular diseases, *Clin. Exp. Immunol.* **65:**66–72.

78. Yoshioka, K., Takemura, T., Matsubara, K., Miyamoto, H., Akano, N., and Maki, S., 1987, Immunohistochemical studies of reflux nephropathy, *Am. J. Pathol.* **129:**223–231.

79. Falk, R. J., Sisson, S. P., Dalmasso, A. P., Kim, Y., Michael, A. F., and Vernier, R. L., 1987, Ultrastructural localization of the membrane attack complex of complement in human renal tissue, *Am. J. Kidney Dis.* **9:**121–128.

80. Rauterberg, E. W., Lieberknecht, H-M., Wingen, A-M., and Ritz, E., 1987, Complement membrane attack (MAC) in idiopathic IgA-glomerulonephritis, *Kidney Int.* **31:**820–829.

81. Cybulsky, A. V., Rennke, H. G., Feintzeig, I. D., and Salant, D. J., 1986, Complement-induced glomerular epithelial cell injury: The role of the membrane attack complex in rat membranous nephropathy, *J. Clin. Invest.* **77:**1096–1104.

82. Cybulsky, A. V., Quigg, R. J., and Salant, D. J., 1986, The membrane attack complex in complement-mediated glomerular epithelial cell injury: Formation and stability of C5b-9 and C5b-7 in rat membranous nephropathy, *J. Immunol.* **137:**1511–1516.

83. Camussi, G., Salvidio, G., Biesecker, G., Brentjens, J., and Andres, G., 1987, Heymann antibodies induced complement-dependent injury of rat glomerular visceral epithelial cells, *J. Immunol.* **139:**2906–2914.

84. Betz, M., Seitz, M., and Hansch, G. M., 1987, Thromboxane B_2 synthesis in human platelets induced by the late complement components C5b-9, *Int. Arch. Allergy Appl. Immun.* **82:**313–316.

85. Hansch, G. M., Seitz, M., and Betz, M., 1987, Effect of the late complement components C5b-9 on human monocytes: Release of prostanoids, oxygen radicals and of a factor inducing cell proliferation, *Int. Arch. Allergy Appl. Immun.* **82:**317–320.

86. Adler, S., Baker, P. J., Johnson, R. J., Ochi, R. F., Pritzl, P., and Couser, W. G., 1986, Complement membrane attack complex stimulates production of reactive oxygen metabolites by cultured rat mesangial cells, *J. Clin. Invest.* **77:**762–767.

87. Lovett, D. H., Haensch, G-M., Goppelt, M., Resch, K., and Gemsa, D., 1987, Activation of glomerular mesangial cells by the terminal membrane attack complex of complement, *J. Immunol.* **138:**2473–2480.

88. Hansch, G. M., Betz, M., Gunther, J., Rother, K. O., and Sterzel, B., 1988, The complement membrane attack complex stimulates the prostanoid production of cultured glomerular epithelial cells, *Int. Arch. Allergy Appl. Immun.* **85:**87–93.

89. Thaiss, F., Batsford, S., Mihatsch, M. J., Heitz, P. U., Bitter-Suermann, D., and Vogt, A., 1986, Mediator systems in a passive model of in situ immune complex glomerulonephritis, *Lab. Invest.* **54:**624–635.

90. Cook, H. T., Smith, J., and Cattell, V., 1987, Isolation and characterization of inflammatory leukocytes from glomeruli in an in situ model of glomerulonephritis in the rat, *Am. J. Pathol.* **126:** 126–136.

91. Baud, L., and Ardailiou, R., 1986, Reactive oxygen species: production and role in the kidney, *Am. J. Physiol.* **251:**F765–F776.

92. Canavese, C., Stratta, P., and Vercellone, A., 1987, Oxygen free radicals in nephrology, *Int. J. Artificial Organs.* **10:**379–389.

93. Boyce, N. W. and Holdsworth, S. R., 1986, Hydroxyl radical mediation of immune renal injury by desferrioxamine, *Kidney Int.* **30:**813–817.

94. Johnson, R. J., Couser, W. G., Chi, E. Y., Adler, S., and Klebanoff, S. J., 1987, New mechanism for glomerular injury. Myeloperoxidase–hydrogen peroxide–halide system, *J. Clin. Invest.* **79:**1379–1387.

95. Johnson, R. J., Klebanoff, S. J., Ochi, R. F., Adler, S., Baker, P., Sparks, L., and Couser, W. G., 1987, Participation of the myeloperoxidase–H_2O_2–halide system in immune complex nephritis, *Kidney Int.* **32:**342–349.

96. Shah, S. V., Baricos, W. H., and Basci, A., 1987, Degradation of human glomerular basement membrane by stimulated neutrophils, *J. Clin. Invest.* **79:**25–31.

97. Johnson, R. J., Couser, W. G., Alpers, C. E., Vissers, M., Schulze, M., and Klebanoff, S. J., The human neutrophil serine proteinases, elastase and cathepsin G, can mediate glomerular injury in vivo, *J. Exp. Med.* **168:**1169–1174.

98. Johnson, R. J., Alpers, C. E., Pritzl, P., Schulze, M., Baker, P., Pruchno, C., and Couser, W. G., 1988, Platelets mediate neutrophil-dependent immune complex nephritis in the rat, *J. Clin. Invest.* **82:**1225–1235.

99. Nolasco, F. E. B., Cameron, J. S., Hartley, B., Coelho, A., Hildreth, G., and Reuben, R., 1987, Intraglomerular T cells and monocytes in nephritis: Study with monoclonal antibodies, *Kidney Int.* **31:**1160–1166.

100. Hooke, D. H., Gee, D. C., and Atkins, R. C., 1987, Leukocyte analysis using monoclonal antibodies in human glomerulonephritis, *Kidney Int.* **31:**964–972.

101. Boyce, N. W., Tipping, P. G., and Holdsworth, S. R., 1986, Lymphokine (MIF) production by glomerular T-lymphocytes in experimental glomerulonephritis, *Kidney Int.* **30:**673–677.

102. Lovett, D. H. and Sterzel, R. B., 1986, Cell culture approaches to the analysis of glomerular inflammation, *Kidney Int.* **30:**246–254.

103. Schlondorff, D., 1987, The glomerular mesangial cell: An expanding role for a specialized pericyte, *Fed. Proc.* **1:**272–281.

104. Singhal, P. C., Scharschmidt, L. A., Gibbons, N., and Hays, R. M., 1986, Contraction and relaxation of cultured mesangial cells on a silicone rubber surface, *Kidney Int.* **30:**862–873.

105. Simonson, M. S. and Dunn, M. J., 1986, Leukotriene C_4 and D_4 contract rat glomerular mesangial cells, *Kidney Int.* **30:**524–531.

106. Lovett, D. H., Szamel, M., Ryan, J. L., Sterzel, R. B., Gemsa, D., and Resch, K., 1986, Interleukin 1 and the glomerular mesangium. I. Purification and characterization of a mesangium cell-derived autogrowth factor, *J. Immunol.* **136:**3700–3705.

107. Castellot, J. J., Hoover, R. L., and Karnovsky, M. J., 1986, Glomerular endothelial cells secrete a heparin like inhibitor and a peptide stimulator of mesangial cell proliferation, *Am. J. Pathol.* **125:**493–500.

108. Werber, H. I., Emancipator, S. N., Tykocinski, M. L., and Sedor, J. R., 1987, The interleukin 1 gene is expressed by rat glomerular mesangial cells and is augmented in immune complex glomerulonephritis, *J. Immunol.* **138:**3207–3212.

109. Lovett, D. H., Resch, K., and Gemsa, D., 1987, Interleukin I and the glomerular mesangium. II. Monokine stimulation of mesangial cell prostanoid secretion, *Am. J. Pathol.* **129:**543–551.

110. Abboud, H. E., Poptic, E., and DiCorleto, P., 1987, Production of platelet-derived growth factorlike protein by rat mesangial cells in culture, *J. Clin. Invest.* **80:**675–683.

111. Schlondorff, D., Goldwasser, P., Neuwirth, R., Satriano, J. A., and Clay, K. L., 1986, Production of platelet-activating factor in glomeruli and cultured glomerular mesangial cells, *Am. J. Physiol.* **250:**F1123–F1127.

112. Lianos, E. A. and Zanglis, A., 1987, Biosynthesis and metabolism of 1-O-alkyl-2-acetyl-sn-glycero-3-phosphocholine in rat glomerular mesangial cells, *J. Biol. Chem.* **292:**8990–8993.

113. Raugi, G. J. and Lovett, D. H., 1987, Thrombospondin secretion by cultured human glomerular mesangial cells, *Am. J. Pathol.* **129:**364–372.

114. Sedor, J. R., Carey, S. W., and Emancipator, S. N., 1987, Immune complexes bind to cultured rat glomerular mesangial cells to stimulate superoxide release, *J. Immunol.* **138:**3751–3757.

115. Lefkowith, J. B. and Schreiner, G., 1987, Essential fatty acid deficiency depletes rat glomeruli of resident macrophages and inhibits angiotensin II–induced eicosanoid synthesis, *J. Clin. Invest.* **80:**947–956.

116. Gurner, A. C., Smith, J., and Cattell, V., 1987, The origin of Ia antigen–expressing cells in the rat kidney, *Am. J. Pathol.* **127:**342–347.
117. Seiler, M. W., Terrell, C. H., Finnegan, A., Sterzel, R. B., and Hoyer, J. R., 1986, Studies of glomerular mesangial uptake and processing of macromolecules. I. Effect of polyvinyl alcohol-induced macrophages on uptake of iron dextran, *Lab. Invest.* **54:**616–623.
118. Kimura, M., Nagase, M., Hishida, A., and Honda, N., 1987, Intramesangial passage of mononuclear phagocytes in murine lupus glomerulonephritis, *Am. J. Pathol.* **127:**149–156.
119. Tipping, P. G., Worthington, L. A., and Holdsworth, S. R., 1987, Quantitation and characterization of glomerular procoagulant activity in experimental glomerulonephritis, *Lab. Invest.* **56:**155–159.
120. Tipping, P. G. and Holdsworth, S. R., 1986, The participation of macrophages, glomerular procoagulant activity, and factor VIII in glomerular fibrin deposition. Studies on anti-GBM antibody–induced glomerulonephritis in rabbits, *Am. J. Pathol.* **124:**10–17.
121. Cole, E. H., Sweet, J., and Levy, G. A., 1986, Expression of macrophage procoagulant activity in murine systemic lupus erythematosus, *J. Clin. Invest.* **78:**887–893.
122. Kanfer, A., DeProst, D., Guettier, C., Nochy, D., Le Floch, V., Hinglais, N., and Druet, P., 1987, Enhanced glomerular procoagulant activity and fibrin deposition in rats with mercuric chloride–induced autoimmune nephritis, *Lab. Invest.* **57:**138–143.
123. Wiggins, R. C., Glatfelter, A., Kshirsagar, B., and Brukman, J., 1986, Procoagulant activity in normal human urine associated with subcellular particles, *Kidney Int.* **29:**591–597.
124. Wiggins, R., Glatfelter, A., Kshirsager, B., and Beals, T., 1987, Lipid microvesicles and their association with procoagulant activity in urine and glomeruli of rabbits with nephrotoxic nephritis, *Lab. Invest.* **56:**264–272.
125. Takemura, T., Yoshioka, K., Akano, N., Miyamoto, H., Matsumoto, K., and Maki, S., 1987, Glomerular deposition of cross-linked fibrin in human kidney diseases, *Kidney Int.* **32:**102–111.
126. Tipping, P. G., Dowling, J. P., and Holdsworth, S. R., 1988, Glomerular procoagulant activity in human proliferative glomerulonephritis, *J. Clin. Invest.* **81:**119–125.
127. Tipping, P. G., Thomson, N. M., and Holdsworth, S. R., 1986, A comparison of fibrinolytic and defibrinating agents in established experimental glomerulonephritis, *Br. J. Exp. Pathol.* **67:**481–491.
128. Wardle, E. N., 1986, Anticoagulation in renal diseases: 20 years on and what is the outcome? *Nephron* **44:**81–84.
129. Capron, A., Joseph, M., Ameisen, J. C., Capron, M., Pancre, V., and Auriault, C., 1987, Platelets as effectors in immune and hypersensitivity reactions, *Int. Arch. Allergy Appl. Immun.* **82:**307–312.
130. Nath, K. A., 1987, Platelet participation in renal diseases, *Kidney* **20:**1–6.
131. Camussi, G., Pawlowski, I., Saunders, R., Brentjens, J., and Andres, G., 1987, Receptor antagonist of platelet activating factor inhibits inflammatory injury induced by *in situ* formation of immune complexes in renal glomeruli and in the skin, *J. Lab. Clin. Med.* **110:**196–206.
132. Bertani, T., Livio, M., Macconi, D., Morigi, M., Bisogno, G., Patrono, C., and Remuzzi, G., 1987, Platelet activating factor (PAF) as a mediator of injury in nephrotoxic nephritis, *Kidney Int.* **31:**1248–1256.
133. Schlondorff, D., Detlef, S., and Neuwirth, R., 1986, Platelet-activating factor and the kidney, *Am. J. Physiol.* **251:**F1–F11.
134. Stahl, R. A. K. and Thaiss, F., 1987, Eicosanoids: Biosynthesis and function in the glomerulus, *Renal Physiol.* **10:**1–13.
135. Rahman, M. A., Stork, J. E., and Dunn, M. J., 1987, The roles of eicosanoids in experimental glomerulonephritis, *Kidney Int.* **32:**S40–S48.
136. Ardaillou, R., Baud, L., and Sraer, J., 1987, Role of arachidonic acid metabolites and reactive oxygen species in glomerular immune–inflammatory process, *Springer Semin. Immunopathol.* **9:**371–385.

137. Stahl, R. A. K., Adler, S., Baker, P. J., Chen, Y-P., Pritzl, P. M., and Couser, W. G., 1987, Enhanced glomerular prostaglandin formation in experimental membranous nephropathy, *Kidney Int.* **31:**1126–1131.

138. Pugliese, F., Singh, A. K., Kasinath, B. S., Kreisberg, J. I., and Lewis, E. J., 1987, Glomerular epithelial cell, polyanion neutralization is associated with enhanced prostanoid production, *Kidney Int.* **32:**57–61.

139. Zoja, C., Benigni, A., Verroust, P., Ronco, P., Bertani, T., and Remuzzi, G., 1987, Indomethacin reduces proteinuria in passive Heymann nephritis in rats, *Kidney Int.* **31:**1335–1343.

140. Shinkai, Y. and Cameron, S., 1987, Rabbit nephrotoxic nephritis: Effect of a thromboxane synthesis inhibitor on evolution and prostaglandin excretion, *Nephron* **47:**211–219.

141. Cybulsky, A. V., Lieberthal, W., Quigg, R. J., Rennke, H. G., and Salant, D. J., 1987, A role for thromboxane in complement-mediated glomerular injury, *Am. J. Pathol.* **128:**45–51.

142. Ulich, T. R., Meline, J. A., Ni, R-X., Keys, M., and Wu, C. H., 1987, Stable analogs of prostaglandins E_1 and $F_2\alpha$ ameliorate the proteinuria of aminonucleoside-of-puromycin nephrosis in Lewis rats, *Am. J. Pathol.* **129:**133–139.

143. Levey, A. S., Lau, J., Pauker, S. G., and Kassirer, J. P., 1987, Idiopathic nephrotic syndrome, puncturing the biopsy myth, *Ann. Intern. Med.* **107:**697–713.

144. Mallick, N. P., Short, C. D., and Hunt, L. P., 1987, How far since Ellis? The Manchester study of glomerular disease, *Nephron* **46:**113–124.

145. Katafuchi, R., Takebayashi, S., Taguhi, T., and Harada, T., 1987, Structural–function correlations in serial biopsies from patients with glomerulonephritis, *Clin. Nephrol.* **28:**169–173.

146. Tiebosch, A., Wolters, J., Frederik, P., VanDerWiel, T., Zeppenfeldt, E., and van Brenda Vriesman, P., 1987, Epidemiology of idiopathic glomerular disease: A prospective study, *Kidney Int.* **32:**112–116.

147. Date, A., Raghavan, R., John, T. J., Richard, J., Kirubakaran, M. G., and Shastry, J. C. M., 1987, Renal disease in adult indians: A clinicopathological study of 2827 patients, *Q. J. Med.* **64:** 729–737.

148. Lockwood, C. M., 1986, New advances in understanding the treatment of glomerulonephritis, *Clin. Nephrol.* **26:**S76–S80.

149. Glassock, R. J., 1987, Clinical aspects of glomerular disease, *Am. J. Kidney Dis.* **10:**181–185.

150. De Santo, N. G., Nuzzi, F., Capodicasa, G., Lama, G., Caputo, G., Rosati, P., and Giordano, C., 1987, Phase contrast microscopy of the urine sediment for the diagnosis of glomerular and nonglomerular bleeding-data in children and adults with normal creatrinine clearance, *Nephron* **45:**35–39.

151. Stapleton, F. B., 1987, Morphology of urinary red blood cells: A simple guide in localizing the site of hematuria, *Pediatr. Clin. North Am.* **34:**561–569.

152. Raman, G. V., Pead, L., Lee, H. A., and Maskell, R., 1986, A blind controlled trial of phasecontrast microscopy by two observers for evaluating the source of haematuria, *Nephron* **44:**304–308.

153. Bergroth, V., Konnttinen, Y., Nordstrom, D., and Laasonen, L., 1987, Loin pain and haematuria syndrome: Possible association with intrarenal arterial spasms, *Br. Med. J.* **294:**1657.

154. Levy, M., 1986, Infections and glomerular disease, *Clin. Immun. Allerg.* **6:**405–435.

155. Jones, J. M. B., and Davison, A. M., 1986, Persistent infection as a cause of renal disease in patients submitted to renal biopsy: A report from the glomerulonephritis registry of the United Kingdom MRC, *Q. J. Med.* **58:**123–132.

156. Berrios, X., Quesney, F., Morales, A., Blazquez, J., Lagomarsino, E., and Bisno, A. L., 1986, Acute rheumatic fever and poststreptococcal glomerulonephritis in an open population: Comparative studies of epidemiology and bacteriology, *J. Lab. Clin. Med.* **108:**535–542.

157. Chugh, K. S., Malhotra, H. S., Sakhuja, V., Bhusnurmath, S., Singhal, P. C., Unni, V. N., Singh, N., Pirzada, R., and Kapoor, M. M., 1987, Progression to end stage renal disease in poststreptococcal glomerulonephritis (PSGN)-Chandigarh study, *Int. J. Art. Organs* **10:**189–194.

158. Leung, D. T. Y., Tseng, R. Y. M., Go, S. H., French, G. L., and Lam, C. W. K., 1987, Post-streptococcal glomerulonephritis in Hong Kong, *Arch. Dis. Childhood* **62**:1075–1076.

159. Williams, W., 1987, Poststreptococcal glomerulonephritis: How important is it as a cause of chronic renal diseases, *Transplant. Proc.* **14**:97–100.

160. Fairley, C., Mathews, D. C., and Becker, G. J., 1987, Rapid development of diffuse crescents in post-streptococcal glomerulonephritis, *Clin. Nephrol.* **28**:256–260.

161. Melby, P. C., Musick, W. D., Luger, A. M., and Khanna, R., 1987, Poststreptococcal glomerulonephritis in the elderly, *Am. J. Nephrol.* **7**:235–240.

162. Vogl, W., Renke, M., Mayer-Eichberger, D., Schmitt, H., and Bohle, A., 1986, Long-term prognosis for endocapillary glomerulonephritis of poststreptococcal type in children and adults, *Nephron* **44**:58–65.

163. Sorger, K., Gessler, M., Hubner, F. K., Kohler, H., Olbing, H., Schulz, W., Thoenes, G. H., and Thoenes, W., 1987, Follow-up studies of three subtypes of acute postinfections glomerulonephritis ascertained by renal biopsy, *Clin. Nephrol.* **27**:111–124.

164. Lange, C. F., Weber, M., and Nayyar, R. P., 1986, Age-effects on the reactivity of antistreptococcal cell membrane antisera to murine glomerular basement membrane, *Renal Physiol.* **9**:148–159.

165. Sesso, R. C. C., Ramos, O. L., and Pereira, A. B., 1986, Detection of IgG-rheumatoid factor in sera of patients with acute poststreptococcal glomerulonephritis and its relationship with circulating immunecomplexes, *Clin. Nephrol.* **26**:55–60.

166. Scully, R. E., Mark, E. J., McNeely, W. F., and McNeely, B. U., 1987, Case records of the Massachusetts General Hospital: Case 26-1987, *N. Engl. J. Med.* **316**:1642–1651.

167. Craddock, C. F., Richards, N. P., Powell, R. J., and Morgan, A. G., 1987, Novel C3 nephritic factor activity in the glomerulonephritis of staphylococcal endocarditis, *Q. J. Med.* **65**:895–898.

168. Sobh, M. A., Moustafa, F. E., El-Housseini, F., Basta, M. T., Deelder, A. M., and Ghoniem, M. A., 1987, Schistosomal specific nephropathy leading to end-stage renal failure, *Kidney Int.* **31**:1006–1011.

169. Martinelli, R., Perreijra, L. J., and Rocha, H., 1987, The influence of anti-parasitic therapy on the course of the glomerulopathy associated with *Schistosomiasis mansoni*, *Clin. Nephrol.* **27**:229–232.

170. Herrara, G. A., Alexander, R. W., Cooley, C. F., Luke, R. G., Kelly, D. R., Curtis, J. J., and Gockerman, J. P., 1986, Cytomegalovirus glomerulopathy: A controversial lesion, *Kidney Int.* **29**:725–733.

171. Magil, A. B. and Ballon, H. S., 1987, IgA nephropathy, *Nephron* **47**:246–252.

172. Bene, M. C. and Faure, G., 1987, IgA nephropathy, *Springer Semin. Immunopathol.* **9**:387–398.

173. Bennett, W. M., Nicholls, K., and Kincaid-Smith, P., 1987, Clinicopathological associations in mesangial IgA nephropathy, *Am. J. Nephrol.* **7**:166–167.

174. Boyce, N. W., Hodsworth, S. R., Thompson, N. M., and Atkins, R. C., 1986, Clinicopathological associations in mesangial IgA nephropathy, *Am. J. Nephrol.* **6**:246–252.

175. Clarkson, A. R., Woodroffe, A. J., Aarons, I., Hiki, Y., and Hale, G., 1987, IgA Nephropathy, *Annu. Rev. Med.* **38**:157–168.

176. D'Amico, G., 1987, The commonest glomerulonephritis in the world: IgA nephropathy, *Q. J. Med.* **64**:709–727.

177. D'Amico, G., Minetti, L., Ponticelli, C., Fellin, G., Ferrario, F., Barbiano Di Belgioioso, G., Imbasciati, E., Ragni, A., Bertoli, S., Fogazzi, G., and Duca, G., 1986, Prognostic indicators in idiopathic IgA mesangial nephropathy, *Q. J. Med.* **59**:363–378.

178. Lee, H. S., Koh, H. I., Lee, H. B., and Park, H. C., 1987, IgA nephropathy in Korea: A morphological and clinical study, *Clin. Nephrol.* **27**:131–140.

179. Yoshikawa, N., Ito, H., Yoshiya, K., Nakahara, C., Yoshiara, S., Hasegawa, O., Matsuyama, S., and Matsuo, T., 1987, Henoch–Schoenlein nephritis and IgA nephropathy in children: A comparison of clinical course, *Clin. Nephrol.* **27**:233–237.

180. Thorner, P. S., Farine, M., Arbus, G. S., Poucell, S., and Baumal, R., 1986, IgA nephropathy:

Henoch–Schönlein purpura and Berger's disease in one patient, *Int. J. Pediatr. Nephrol.* **7**:131–136.

181. Yoshikawa, N., Ito, H., Yoshiara, S., Nakahara, C., Yoshiya, K., Hasegawa, O., and Matsuo, T., 1987, Clinical course of immunoglobulin A nephropathy in children, *J. Pediatr.* **110**:555–560.

182. Kusumoto, Y., Takebayashi, S., Taguchi, T., Harada, T., and Naito, S., 1987, Long-term prognosis and prognostic indices of IgA nephropathy in juvenile and in adult Japanese, *Clin. Nephrol.* **28**:118–124.

183. Yoshikawa, N., Ijima, K., Maehara, K., Yoshiara, S., Yoshiya, K., Matsua, T., and Okada, S., 1987, Mesangial changes in IgA nephropathy in children, *Kidney Int.* **32**:585–589.

184. Rambausek, M., Waldherr, R., Rauterberg, W., Andrassy, K., and Ritz, E., 1987, Mesangial IgA nephropathy and idiopathic nephrotic syndrome, *Nephron* **47**:190–193.

185. Yoshimura, M., Kida, H., Abe, T., Takeda, S., Katagiri, M., and Hattori, N., 1987, Significance of IgA deposits on the glomerular capillary walls in IgA nephropathy, *Am. J. Kidney Dis.* **9**:404–409.

186. Andreoli, S., Yum, M. N., and Bergstein, J. M., 1986, IgA nephropathy in children: significance of glomerular basement membrane deposition of IgA, *Am. J. Nephrol.* **6**:28–33.

187. Jennette, J. C., Newman, J., and Diaz-Buxo, J. A., 1987, Overlapping IgA and membranous nephropathy, *Am. J. Clin. Pathol.* **88**:74–78.

188. Perez-Fontan, M., Miguel, J. L., Picazo, M. L., Martinez-Ara, J., Selgas, R., and Sicilia, L. S., 1986, Idiopathic IgA nephropathy presenting as malignant hypertension, *Am. J. Nephrol.* **6**:482–486.

189. Lubias, R., Botley, A., Darnell, A., Montoliu, J., and Revert, L., 1987, Malignant or accelerated hypertension in IgA nephropathy, *Clin. Nephrol.* **27**:1–7.

190. Kincaid-Smith, P. and Fairley, K. F., 1987, Renal disease in pregnancy, three controversial areas: Mesangial IgA nephropathy, focal glomerular sclerosis (focal and segmental hyalinosis and sclerosis), and reflux nephropathy, *Am. J. Kidney Dis.* **9**:328–333.

191. Rifai, A., 1987, Experimental models for IgA-associated nephritis, *Kidney Int.* **31**:1–7.

192. Yoshikawa, N., Yoshiara, S., Yoshiya, K., and Matsua, T., 1986, Lysis of the glomerular basement membrane in children with IgA nephropathy and Henoch-Schonlein nephritis, *J. Pathol.* **150**:119–126.

193. Terasaki, T., Sano, M., Narita, M., and Tojo, S., 1986, Ultrastructural study of gaps of the glomerular basement membrane in IgA nephropathy, *Am. J. Nephrol.* **6**:443–449.

194. Wyatt, R. J., Rivas, M. L., Julian, B. A., Quiggins, P. A., Woodford, S. Y., McMorrow, R. G., and Baehler, R. W., 1987, Regionalization in hereditary IgA nephropathy, *Am. J. Hum. Genet.* **41**:36–50.

195. Levy, M., 1987, Do genetic factors play a role in Berger's disease? *Pediatr. Nephrol.* **1**:447–454.

196. Welch, T. R., Berry, A., and Beischel, L. S., 1987, C4 isotype deficiency in IgA nephropathy, *Pediatr. Nephrol.* **1**:136–139.

197. Naito, S., Kohara, M., and Arakawa, K., 1987, Association of class II antigens of HLA with primary glomerulopathies, *Nephron* **45**:111–114.

198. Hale, G. M., McIntosh, S. L., Hiki, Y., Clarkson, A. R., and Woodroffe, A. J., 1986, Evidence for IgA-specific B cell hyperactivity in patients with IgA nephropathy, *Kidney Int.* **29**:718–724.

199. Feehally, J., Beattie, T. J., Brenchley, P. E. C., Coupes, B. M., Mallick, N. P., and Postlethwaite, R. J., 1986, Sequential study of the IgA system in relapsing IgA nephropathy, *Kidney Int.* **30**:924–931.

200. Schena, F. P., Mastrolitta, G., Fracasso, A. R., Pastore, A., and Ladisa, N., 1986, Increased immunoglobulin-secreting cells in the blood of patients with active idiopathic IgA nephrology, *Clin. Nephrol.* **26**:163–168.

201. Lai, K. N., Lai, F. M., Chui, S. H., Chan, Y. M., Tsao, G. S. W., Leung, K. N., and Lam, C. W. K., 1987, Studies of lymphocyte subpopulations and immunoglobulin production in IgA nephropathy, *Clin. Nephrol.* **28**:281–287.

202. Leinikki, P. O., Mustonen, J., and Pasternack, A., 1987, Immune response to oral polio vaccine in patients with IgA glomerulonephritis, *Clin. Exp. Immunol.* **68:**33–38.
203. Russell, M. W., Mestecky, J., Julian, B. A., and Galla, J. H., 1986, IgA-associated renal diseases: Antibodies to environmental antigens in sera and deposition of immunoglobulins and antigens in glomeruli, *J. Clin. Immunol.* **6:**74–86.
204. Coppo, R., Basolo, B., Rollino, C., Roccatello, D., Martina, G., Amore, A., Bongiorno, G., and Piccoli, G., 1986, Mediterranean diet and primary IgA nephropathy, *Clin. Nephrol.* **26:**72–82.
205. Lozano, L., Garcia-Hoyo, R., and Egido, J., 1987, IgA nephropathy: Association of a history of macroscopic hematuria episodes with increased production of polymeric IgA, *Nephron* **45:**98–103.
206. Davin, J. C., Foidart, J. B., and Mahieu, P. R., 1987, Relation between biological IgA abnormalities and messangial IgA deposits in isolated hematuria in childhood, *Clin. Nephrol.* **28:**73–80.
207. Hernando, P., Edigo, J., de Nicolas, R., and Sancho, J., 1986, Clinical significance of polymeric and monomeric IgA complexes in patients with IgA nephropathy, *Am. J. Kidney Dis.* **8:**410–416.
208. Yagame, M., Miura, T. M., Tanigaki, T., Suga, T., Nomoto, Y., and Sakai, H., 1987, Detection of IgA-class circulating immune complexes (CIC) in sera from patients with IgA nephropathy using a solid-phase anti-C3 Facb enzyme immunoassay (EIA), *Clin. Exp. Immunol.* **67:**270–276.
209. Julian, B. A., Czerkinsky, C., Russell, M. W., Galla, J. H., Koopman, W. J., Mestecky, J., Moldoveanu, Z., and Jackson, S., 1987, Striking elevation of serum IgA, IgA-containing immune complexes, and IgA rheumatoid factor in clinically silent dermatitis herpetiformis, *Am. J. Kidney Dis.* **10:**378–384.
210. Czerkinsky, C., Koopman, W., Jackson, S., Collins, J., Crago, S., Schrohenloher, R. E., Julian, B. A., Galla, J. H., and Mestecky, J., 1986, Circulating immune complexes and immunoglobulin A rheumatoid factor in patients with mesangial immunoglobulin A nephropathies, *J. Clin. Invest.* **77:**1931–1938.
211. Sinico, R. A., Fornasieri, A., Oreni, N., Benuzzi, S., and D'Amico, G., 1986, Polymeric IgA rheumatoid factor in idiopathic IgA mesangial nephropathy (Berger's disease), *J. Immunol.* **137:**536–541.
212. Fornasieri, A., Sinico, R. A., Maldifassi, P., Bernasconi, P., Vegni, M., and D'Amico, G., 1987, IgA-Antigliadin antibodies in IgA mesangial nephropathy (Berger's disease), *Br. Med. J.* **295:**78–80.
213. Yap, H. K., Sakai, R. S., Woo, K. T., Lim, C. H., and Jordan, S. C., 1987, Detection of bovine serum albumin in the circulating IgA immune complexes of patients with IgA nephropathy, *Clin. Immunol. Immunopathol.* **43:**395–402.
214. Gonzalez-Cabrero, J., Egido, J., Sancho, J., and Moldenhauer, F., 1987, Presence of shared idiotypes in serum and immune complexes in patients with IgA nephropathy, *Clin. Exp. Immunol.* **68:**694–702.
215. Nagy, J., Ambrus, M., Paal, M., Trinn, C., and Burger, T., 1987, Cryoglobulinaemia and cryofibrinogenaemia in IgA nephropathy: A follow-up study, *Nephron* **46:**337–342.
216. Tomino, Y., Yagame, M., Omata, F., Nomoto, Y., and Sakai, H., 1987, A case of IgA nephropathy associated with adeno- and herpes simplex viruses, *Nephron* **47:**258–261.
217. Nomoto, Y., Suga, T., Miura, M., Nomoto, H., Tomino, Y., and Sakai, H., 1986, Characterization of an acidic nuclear protein recognized by autoantibodies in sera from patients with IgA nephropathy, *Clin. Exp. Immunol.* **65:**513–519.
218. Emancipator, S. E., Ovary, Z., and Lamm, M. E., 1987, The role of mesangial complement in the hematuria of experimental IgA nephropathy, *Lab. Invest.* **57:**269–276.
219. Rifai, A., Chen, A., and Imai, H., 1987, Complement activation in experimental IgA nephropathy: An antigen-mediated process, *Kidney Int.* **32:**838–844.
220. Tomino, Y., Yagame, M., Eguchi, K., Nomato, Y., and Sakai, H., 1987, Immunofluorescent studies on S-protein in glomeruli from patients with IgA nephropathy, *Am. J. Pathol.* **129:**402–406.
221. Chan, M. K., Kwan, S. Y. L., Chan, K. W., and Yeung, C. K., 1987, Controlled trial of antiplatelet agents in mesangial IgA glomerulonephritis, *Am. J. Kidney Dis.* **4:**417–421.

222. Belovexhdov, N. and Robeva, R., 1987, Clinical and therapeutic studies in mesangial immunoglobulin A glomerulonephritis, *Int. Urol. Nephrol.* **19:**341–345.

223. Lai, K. N., Lai, F. M., and Chan, K. W., 1986, Corticosteroid therapy in IgA nephropathy with nephrotic syndrome: A long-term controlled trial, *Clin. Nephrol.* **26:**174–180.

224. Woo, K. T., Edmondson, R. P. S., Yap, H. K., Wu, A. Y. T., Chiang, G. S. C., Lee, E. J. C., Pwee, H. S., and Lim, C. H., 1987, Effects of triple therapy on the progression of mesangial proliferative glomerulonephritis, *Clin. Nephrol.* **27:**56–64.

225. Woo, K. T., et al., 1987, Letter to the editor, *Clin. Nephrol.* **27:**304–306.

226. Lai, K. N., Lai, F. M., Li, P. K. T., and Vallance-Owen, J., 1987, Cyclosporin treatment of IgA nephropathy: A short term controlled trial, *Br. Med. J.* **295:**1165–1168.

227. Kobayashi, Y., Fujii, K., Hiki, Y., and Tateno, S., 1986, Steroid therapy in IgA nephropathy: A prospective pilot study in moderate proteinuric cases, *Q. J. Med.* **61:**935–943.

228. Lai, K. N., Lai, F. M., Leung, A. C. T., Ho, C. P., and Vallance-Owen, J., 1987, Plasma exchange in patients with rapidly progressive idiopathic IgA nephropathy: A report of two cases and review of literature, *Am. J. Kidney Dis.* **10:**66–70.

229. Bachman, U., Biaza, C., Amend, W., Feduska, N., Melzer, J., Salvatierra, O., and Vincenti, F., 1986, The clinical course of IgA-nephropathy and Henoch–Schönlein purpura following renal transplantation, *Transplantation* **42:**511–515.

230. Helin, H., Korpela, M., Mustonen, J., and Pasternack, A., 1986, Mild mesangial glomerulopathy—A frequent finding in rheumatoid arthritis patients with hematuria or proteinuria, *Nephron* **42:**224–230.

231. Shu, K. H., Lian, J. D., Yang, Y. F., Lu, Y. S., Wang, J. Y., Lan, J. L., and Chou, G., 1986, Glomerulonephritis in ankylosing spondylitis, *Clin. Nephrol.* **25:**169–174.

232. Newell, G. C., 1987, Cirrhotic glomerulonephritis: Incidence, morphology, clinical features, and pathogenesis, *Am. J. Kidney Dis.* **9:**183–190.

233. Kawaguchi, K., and Koike, M., 1986, Glomerular lesions associated with liver cirrhosis: An immunohistochemical and clinicopathologic analysis, *Hum. Pathol.* **17:**1137–1143.

234. Praga, M., Costa, J. R., Shandas, G. J., Martinez, M. A., Miranda, B., and Rodicio, J. L., 1987, Acute renal failure in cirrhosis associated with macroscopic hematuria of glomerular origin, *Arch. Intern. Med.* **147:**173–174.

235. Couser, W. G., 1986, Chapter 100, Glomerular diseases, in: *Textbook of Medicine. A Systematic Approach*, 2nd ed. (J. Stein et al. eds.), Little Brown, Boston, pp. 834–861.

236. Couser, W. G., 1988, Rapidly progressive glomerulonephritis. Classification and treatment, *Am. J. Kidney Dis.* **11:**449–464 (In-depth Review.)

237. Salant, D. J., 1987, Immunopathogenesis of crescentic glomerulonephritis and lung purpura, *Kidney Int.* **32:**408–425.

238. Savage, C. O., Pusey, C. D., Bowman, C., Rees, A. J., and Lockwood, C. M., 1986, Anti-glomerular basement membrane antibody mediated disease in the British Isles 1980–4, *Br. Med. J.* **292:**301–304.

239. Balow, J. E., 1986, Plasmapheresis: Development and application in treatment of renal disorders, *Artificial Organs* **101:**324–330.

240. Jones, J. V., 1986, Response to apheresis: Problems of assessment in immune disease, *Clin. Nephrol.* **26:**S70–S75.

241. Vangelista, A., Frasca, G. M., and Bonomini, V., 1986, Parameters for indication of plasmapheresis and the interpretation of results, *Clin. Nephrol.* **26:**S64–S69.

242. Gajdos, P., Pourrat, J., Elkharrat, D., and Terre, C., 1987, National register for plasma exchange—The French Society for Hemapheresis. Results for 1985, *Plasma Ther. Technol.* **8:**137–141.

243. Nilssen, D. E., Talseth, T., and Brodwall, E. K., 1986, The many faces of Goodpasture's syndrome, *Acta. Med. Scand.* **220:**489–491.

244. Mehler, P. S., Brunvand, M. W., Hutt, M. P., and Anderson, R. J., 1987, Chronic recurrent Goodpasture's syndrome, *Am. J. Med.* **82:**833–835.

245. Teruel, J. L., Liano, F., Mampaso, F., Moreno, J., Serrano, A., Quereda, C., and Ortuno, J., 1987, Allograft antiglomerular basement membrane glomerulonephritis in a patient with Alport's syndrome, *Nephron* **46**:43–44.

246. Croker, B. P., Lee, T., and Gunnells, J. C., 1987, Clinical and pathologic features of polyarteritis nodosa and its renal-limited variant: Primary crescentic and necrotizing glomerulonephritis, *Hum. Pathol.* **18**:39–44.

247. Furlong, T. J., Ibels, L. S., and Eckstein, R. P., 1987, The clinical spectrum of necrotizing glomerulonephritis, *Medicine* **66**:192–201.

248. Adu, D., Howie, A. J., Scott, D. G. I., Bacon, P. A., McGonigle, R. J. S., and Michael, J., 1987, Polyarteritis and the kidney, *Q. J. Med.* **62**:221–237.

249. Velosa, J. A., 1987, Idiopathic crescentic glomerulonephritis or systemic vasculitis? *Mayo Clin. Proc.* **62**:145–147.

250. Savage, C. O., Jones, S., Winearls, C. G., Marshall, P. D., and Lockwood, C. M., 1987, Prospective study of radioimmunoassay for antibodies against neutrophil cytoplasm in diagnosis of systemic vasculitis, *Lancet* **20**:1389–1393.

251. Falk, R. J. and Jennette, J. C., 1988, Anti-neutrophil cytoplasmic autoantibodies with specificity for myeloperoxidase in patients with systemic vasculitis and idiopathic necrotizing and crescentic glomerulonephritis, *N. Engl. J. Med.* **318**:1651–1657.

252. Baldwin, D. S., Neugarten, J., Feiner, H. D., Gluck, M., and Spinowitz, B., 1987, The existence of a protracted course in crescentic glomerulonephritis, *Kidney Int.* **31**:790–794.

253. Belghiti, D., Levy, Y., Rifle, G., Ottavioli, J., Rickelynck, J., Wolf, C., Chalopin, J., and Sobel, A., 1987, Relapses of idiopathic diffuse crescentic glomerulonephritis without immune deposits: Report of 6 cases, *Am. J. Nephrol.* **7**:22–27.

254. Boyce, N. W. and Holdsworth, S. R., 1986, Idiopathic Goodpasture's syndrome, *Nephron* **44**:22–25.

255. Bolton, W. K., Innes, D. J., Sturgill, B. C., and Kaiser, D. L., 1987, T cells and macrophages in rapidly progressive glomerulonephritis: Clinicopathologic correlations, *Kidney Int.* **32**:869–876.

256. Yoshioka, K., Takemura, T., Akano, N., Miyamoto, H., Iseki, T., and Maki, S., 1987, Cellular and non-cellular compositions of crescents in human glomerulonephritis, *Kidney Int.* **32**:284–291.

257. Schwab, S. J., Christensen, R. L., Dougherty, K., and Klahr, S., 1987, Quantitation of proteinuria by the use of protein-to-creatinine ratios in single urine samples, *Arch. Intern. Med.* **147**:943–944.

258. Houser, M. T., Jahn, M. F., Kobayashi, A., and Walburn, J., 1986, Assessment of urinary protein excretion in the adolescent: Effect of body position and exercise, *J. Pediatr.* **109**:556–561.

259. Nathan, D. M., Rosenbaum, C., and Protasowicki, V. D., 1987, Single-void urine samples can be used to estimate quantitative microalbuminuria, *Diabetes Care* **10**:414–418.

260. Furness, P. N., Turner, D. R., and Cotton, R. E., 1986, Basement membrane charge in human glomerular disease, *J. Pathol.* **150**:267–278.

261. Kerjaschki, D., Poczewski, H., Dekan, G., Horvat, R., Balzar, E., Kraft, N., and Atkins, R. C., 1986, Identification of a major sialoprotein in the glycocalyx of human visceral glomerular epithelial cells, *J. Clin. Invest.* **78**:1142–1149.

262. Horvat, R., Hovarka, A., Dekan, G., Poczewski, H., and Kerjaschki, D., 1986, Endothelial cell membranes contain podocalzxin—The major sialoprotein of visceral glomerular epithelial cells, *J. Cell Biol.* **102**:484–491.

263. Bertolatus, J. A. and Hunsicker, L. G., 1987, Polycation binding to glomerular basement membrane: Effect of biochemical modification, *Lab. Invest.* **56**:170–179.

264. Lelongt, B., Makino, H., and Kanwar, Y. S., 1987, Status of glomerular proteoglycans in aminonucleoside nephrosis, *Kidney Int.* **31**:1299–1310.

265. Batsford, S. R., Rohbach, R., and Vogt, A., 1987, Size reduction in the glomerular capillary wall: Importance of lamina densa, *Kidney Int.* **31**:710–717.

266. Bertolatus, J. A., Abuyousef, M., and Hunsicker, L. G., 1987, Glomerular sieving of high molecular weight proteins in proteinuric rats, *Kidney Int.* **31**:1257–1266.

267. Shemesh, O., Deen, W. M., Brenner, B. M., McNeely, E., and Myers, B. D., 1986, Effect of colloid volume expansion on glomerular barrier size-selectivity in humans, *Kidney Int.* **29**:916–923.

268. Weening, J. J., Guldener, C. V., Daha, M. R., Klar, N., Van Der Wal, A., and Prins, F. A., 1987, The pathophysiology of protein-overload proteinuria, *Am. J. Pathol.* **129**:64–73.

269. Schwartz, M. M., Bidani, A. K., and Lewis, E. J., 1986, Glomerular epithelial cell structure and function in chronic proteinuria induced by homologous protein-load, *Lab. Invest.* **55**:673–679.

270. Messina, A., Davies, D. J., Dillane, P. C., and Ryan, G. B., 1987, Glomerular epithelial abnormalities associated with the onset of proteinuria in aminonucleoside nephrosis, *Am. J. Pathol.* **126**:220–229.

271. Cameron, J. S., 1987, The nephrotic syndrome and its complications, *Am. J. Kidney Dis.* **10**:157–171.

272. Fadnes, H. O., Pape, J. F., and Sundsfjord, J. A., 1986, A study on oedema mechanisms in nephrotic syndrome, *Scand. J. Clin. Lab. Invest.* **46**:533–538.

273. Shapiro, M. D., Nicholls, K. M., Groves, B. M., and Schrier, R. W., 1986, Role of glomerular filtration rate in the impaired sodium and water excretion of patients with the nephrotic syndrome, *Am. J. Kidney Dis.* **8**:81–87.

274. Koomans, H. A., Boer, W. H., and Mees, E. J. D., 1987, Renal function during recovery from minimal lesions nephrotic syndrome, *Nephron* **47**:173–178.

275. Tulassay, T., Rascher, W., Lang, R. E., Seyberth, H. W., and Scharer, K., 1987, Atrial natriuretic peptide and other vasocative hormones in nephrotic syndrome, *Kidney Int.* **31**:1391–1395.

276. Kaysen, G. A., Gambertoglio, J., Felts, J., and Hutchison, F. N., 1987, Albumin synthesis, albuminuria and hyperlipemia in nephrotic patients, *Kidney Int.* **31**:1368–1376.

277. Short, C. D., Durrington, P. N., Mallick, N. P., Hunt, L. P., Tetlow, L., and Ishola, M., 1986, Serum and urinary high density lipoproteins in glomerular disease with proteinuria, *Kidney Int.* **29**: 1224–1228.

278. Scully, R. E., Mark, E. J., McNeely, W. F., and McNeely, B. U., 1987, Case records of the Massachusetts General Hospital: Case 14-1987, *N. Engl. J. Med.* **316**:860–869.

279. Valeri, A., Gelfand, J., Blum, C., and Appel, G. B., 1986, Treatment of the hyperlipidemia of the nephrotic syndrome: A controlled trial, *Am. J. Kidney Dis.* **8**:388–396.

280. Mehis, O., Addrassy, K., Koderisch, J., Herzog, U., and Ritz, E., 1987, Hemostasis and thromboembolism in children with nephrotic syndrome: Differences from adults, *J. Pediatr.* **110**:862–867.

281. Alkjaersig, N., Fletcher, A. P., Narayanan, M., and Robson, A. M., 1987, Course and resolution of the coagulopathy in nephrotic children, *Kidney Int.* **31**:772–780.

282. Bennett, A., and Cameron, J. S., 1987, Platelet hyperaggregability in the nephrotic syndrome which is not dependent on arachidonic acid metabolism or on plasma albumin concentration, *Clin. Nephrol.* **27**:182–188.

283. Strife, C. F., Jackson, E. C., Forristal, J., and West, C. D., 1986, Effect of the nephrotic syndrome on the concentration of serum complement components, *Am. J. Kidney Dis.* **8**:37–42.

284. Mori, R., Triolo, L., De Stefano, V., Giusti, B. P., De Sole, P., and Leone, G., 1988, Plasma levels and loss of antithrombin III in chronic ambulatory peritoneal dialysis and nephrotic patients, *Nephron* **48**:213–216.

285. Vigano-D'Angelo, S., D'Angelo, A., Kaufman, C. E., Sholer, C., Esmon, C. T., and Comp, P. C., 1987, Protein S deficiency occurs in the nephrotic syndrome, *Arch. Intern. Med.* **107**:42–47.

286. Robert, A., Olmer, M., Sampol, J., Gugliotta, J., and Casanova, P., 1987, Clinical correlation between hypercoagulability and thrombo-embolic phenomenon, *Kidney Int.* **31**:830–835.

287. Vermylen, C. G., Levin, M., Lanham, J. G., Hardisty, R. M., and Barratt, T. M., 1987, Decreased sensitivity to heparin in vitro in steroid-responsive nephrotic syndrome, *Kidney Int.* **31**: 1396–1401.

288. Vriesendorp, R., Donker, A. J. M., de Zeeuw, D., de Jong, P. E., van der Hem, G. K., and

Brentjens, J. R. H., 1986, Effects of nonsteroidal antiinflammatory durgs on proteinuria, *Am. J. Med.* **81**:84–94.

289. Alavi, N., Lianos, E. A., Venuto, R. C., Mookerjee, B. K., and Bentzel, C. J., 1986, Reduction of proteinuria by indomethacin in patients with nephrotic syndrome, *Am. J. Kidney Dis.* **8**:397–403.

290. Vriesendorp, R., de Zeeuw, D., de Jong, P. E., Donker, A. J. M., Pratt, J. J., and van der Hem, G. K., 1986, Reduction of urinary protein and prostaglandin E$_2$ excretion in the nephrotic syndrome by non-steroidal anti-inflammatory drugs, *Clin. Nephrol.* **25**:105–110.

291. Velosa, J. A. and Torres, V. E., 1986, Benefits and risks of nonsteroidal antiinflammatory drugs in steroid-resistant nephrotic syndrome, *Am. J. Kidney Dis.* **8**:345–350.

292. Heeg, J. E., de Jong, P. E., van der Hem, G. K., and de Zeeuw, D., 1987, Reduction of proteinuria by angiotensin converting enzyme inhibition, *Kidney Int.* **32**:78–83.

293. Lewis, E. J., 1987, Angiotensin-converting enzyme inhibitors: Considerations regarding proteinuria, *Am. J. Kidney Dis.* **10**:30–38.

294. Lagrue, G., Robeva, R., and Laurent, J., 1987, Antiproteinuric effect of captopril in primary glomerular disease, *Nephron* **46**:99–100.

295. Rapola, J., 1987, Congenital nephrotic syndrome, *Pediatr. Nephrol.* **1**:441–446.

296. Morduchowicz, G., Boner, G., Ben-Basset, M., and Rosenfeld, J. B., 1986, Proteinuria in benign nephrosclerosis, *Arch. Intern. Med.* **146**:1513–1516.

297. Narvarte, J., Prive, M., Saba, S. R., and Ramirez, G., 1987, Proteinuria in hypertension, *Am. J. Kidney Dis.* **10**:408–416.

298. Hannedouche, T., Fournier, J. F., Moore, N., Godin, M., and Fillastre, J. P., 1986, Letters to the editor: Nephrotic syndrome due to isolated minimal change glomerular disease in a patient taking pirprofen, *Clin. Nephrol.* **25**:314.

299. Beun, G. D. M., Leunissen, K. M. L., Van Brenda Vriesman, P. J. C., and Van Hooff, J. P., 1987, Isolated minimal change nephropathy associated with diclofenac, *Br. Med. J.* **295**:182–183.

300. Schwartzman, M. and D'Agati, V., 1987, Spontaneous relapse of naproxen-related nephrotic syndrome, *Am. J. Med.* **82**:329–332.

301. Artinano, M., Etheridge, W. B., Stroehlein, K. B., and Barcenas, C. G., 1986, Progression of minimal-change glomerulopathy to focal glomerulosclerosis in a patient with Fenoprofen nephropathy, *Am. J. Nephrol.* **6**:353–357.

302. Dabbs, D. J., Striker, L., Mignon, F., and Striker, G., 1986, Glomerular lesions in lymphomas and leukemias, *Am. J. Med.* **80**:63–70.

303. Huisman, R. M., de Jong, P. E., de Zeeuw, D., van Imhoff, G. W., and van der Hem, G. K., 1986, Nephrotic syndrome preceding Hodgkin's disease by 42 months, *Clin. Nephrol.* **26**:311–313.

304. Orman, S. V., Schechter, G. P., Whang-Peng, J., Guccion, J., Chan, C., Schulof, R. S., and Shalhoub, R. J., 1986, Nephrotic syndrome associated with a clonal T-cell leukemia of large granular lymphocytes with cytotoxic function, *Arch. Intern. Med.* **146**:1827–1829.

305. Schroeter, N. J., Rushing, D. A., Parker, J. P., and Beltaos, E., 1986, Minimal-change nephrotic syndrome associated with malignant mesothelioma, *Arch. Intern. Med.* **146**:1834–1836.

306. Nolasco, F., Cameron, J. S., Heywood, E. F., Hicks, J., Ogg, C., and Williams, D. G., 1986, Aduot-onset minimal change nephrotic syndrome: A long-term follow-up, *Kidney Int.* **29**:1215–1223.

307. Allen, M. J., Thomas, A. C., and Eastwood, J. B., 1987, Minimal change glomerulonephritis in the elderly—The role of renal biopsy, *Clin. Nephrol.* **28**:99–101.

308. Melvin, T. and Michael, A. F., 1986, New insights into the pathogenesis of minimal change disease, *Clin. Immunol. Allergy* **6**:369–390.

309. Ghiggeri, G. M., Candiano, G., Ginevri, F., Gusmano, R., Ciardi, M. R., Perfumo, F., Delfino, G., Cuniberti, C., and Queirolo, C., 1987, Renal selectivity properties towards endogenous albumin in minimal change nephropathy, *Kidney Int.* **32**:69–77.

310. Yokoyama, H., Kida, H., Abe, T., Koshino, Y., Yoshimura, M., and Hattori, N., 1987, Impaired

immunoglobulin G production in minimal change nephrotic syndrome in adults, *Clin. Exp. Immunol.* **70:**110–115.

311. Chan, M. K., Chan, K. W., and Jones, B., 1987, Immunoglobulins (IgG, IgA, IgM, IgE) and complement components (C_3, C_4) in nephrotic syndrome due to minimal change and other forms of glomerulonephritis, a clue for steroid therapy? *Nephron* **47:**125–130.

312. Thomson, N. P. and Kraft, N., 1987, Normal human serum also contains the lymphotoxin found in minimal change nephropathy, *Kidney Int.* **31:**1186–1193.

313. Kopolovic, J., Shvil, Y., Pomeranz, A., Ron, N., Rubinger, D., and Oren, R., 1987, IgM nephropathy: Morphological study related to clinical findings, *Am. J. Nephrol.* **7:**275–280.

314. Lin, C. and Chu, C., 1986, Studies of circulating immune complexes and lymphocyte subpopulations in childhood IgM mesangial nephropathy, *Nephron* **44:**198–203.

315. Border, W. A., 1988, Distinguishing minimal-change disease from mesangial disorders, *Kidney Int.* **34:**419–434.

316. Korbet, S. M., Schwartz, M. M., and Lewis, E. J., 1986, The prognosis of focal segmental glomerular sclerosis of adulthood, *Medicine* **65:**304–311.

317. Miyata, J., Takebayashi, S., Taguchi, T., Naito, S., and Harada, T., 1986, Evaluation and correlation of clinical and histological features of focal segmental glomerulosclerosis, *Nephron* **44:** 115–120.

318. Claris-Appiani, A., Galato, R., Marra, G., Assael, B. M., and Seveso, M., 1986, Prediction of the progression of renal failure in adult and in pediatric patients with malignant focal glomerulosclerosis, *Clin. Nephrol.* **26:**87–90.

319. Verani, R. R., and Hawkins, E. P., 1986, Recurrent focal segmental glomerulosclerosis: A pathological study of the early lesion, *Am. J. Nephrol.* **6:**263–270.

320. Striegel, J. E., Sibley, R. K., Fryd, D. S., and Mauer, S. M., 1986, Recurrence of focal segmental sclerosis in children following renal transplantation, *Kidney Int.* **30:**S44–S50.

321. Kasiske, B. L. and Crosson, J. T., 1986, Renal disease in patients with massive obesity, *Arch. Intern. Med.* **146:**1105–1109.

322. Jennette, J. C., Charles, L., and Grubb, W., 1987, Glomerulomegaly and focal segmental glomerulosclerosis associated with obesity and sleep-apnea syndrome, *Am. J. Kidney Dis.* **10:**470–472.

323. Gaber, L. W. and Spargo, B. H., 1987, Pregnancy-induced nephropathy: The significance of focal segmental glomerulosclerosis, *Am. J. Kidney Dis.* **9:**317–323.

324. Rao, T. K. S., Friedman, E. A., and Nicastri, A. D., 1987, The types of renal disease in the acquired immunodeficiency syndrome, *N. Engl. J. Med.* **316:**1062–1068.

325. Chander, P., Soni, A., Suri, A., Bhagwat, R., Yoo, J., and Tresar, G., 1987, Renal ultrastructural markers in AIDS-associated nephropathy, *Am. J. Pathol.* **126:**513–526.

326. Pardo, V., Meneses, R., Ossa, L., Jaffe, D. J., Strauss, J., Roth, D., and Bourgoignie, J. J., 1987, AIDS-related glomerulopathy: Occurrence in specific risk groups, *Kidney Int.* **31:**1167–1173.

327. Humphreys, M. H. and Schoenfeld, P. Y., 1987, Renal complications in patients with the acquired immune deficiency syndrome (AIDS), *Am. J. Nephrol.* **7:**1–7.

328. Humphreys, M. H. and Schoenfeld, P. Y., 1987, AIDS and renal disease, *Kidney* **20:**7–12.

329. Nurse, H., 1987, Heroin and nephropathy, *Transplant. Proc.* **14:**56.

330. May, D. C., Helderman, J. H., Eigenbrodt, E. H., and Silva, F. G., 1986, Chronic sclerosing glomerulopathy (heroin-associated nephropathy) in intravenous T's and blues abusers, *Am. J. Kidney Dis.* **8:**404–409.

331. Lin, C. and Hsu, H., 1986, Histopathological and immunological studies in spontaneous remission of nephrotic syndrome after intercurrent measles infection, *Nephron* **42:**110–115.

332. Nair, R. B., Date, A., Kirubakaran, M. G., and Shastry, J. C. M., 1987, Minimal-change nephrotic syndrome in adults treated with alternate-day steroids, *Nephron* **47:**209–210.

333. Wetzels, J. F. M., Gerlag, P. G. G., Sluiter, H. E., Hoitsma, A. J., and Koene, R. A. P., 1986, prednisone-induced fluctuations of proteinuria in patients with a nephrotic syndrome, *Nephron* **44:** 344–350.

334. Garcia, D. L., Rennke, H. G., Brenner, B. M., and Anderson, S., 1987, Chronic glucocorticoid therapy amplifies glomerular injury in rats with renal ablation, *J. Clin. Invest.* **80**:867–874.

335. Tejani, A., 1987, Relapsing nephrotic syndrome, *Nephron* **45**:81–85.

336. Niaudet, P., Habib, R., Tete, M., Hinglais, N., and Broyer, M., 1987, Cyclosporin in the treatment of idiopathic nephrotic syndrome in children, *Pediatr. Nephrol.* **1**:566–573.

337. Tejani, A., 1987, Cyclosporine treatment in patients with primary glomerular disease, *Int. J. Pediatr. Nephrol.* **8**:1–3.

338. Tejani, A., Butt, K., Trachtman, H., Suthanthiran, M., Rosenthal, C. J., and Khawar, M. R., 1987, Cyclosporine-induced remission of relapsing nephrotic syndrome in children, *J. Pediatr.* **111**:1056–1062.

339. Waldo, F. B. and Kohaut, E. C., 1987, Therapy of focal segmental glomerulosclerosis with cyclosporine A, *Pediatr. Nephrol.* **1**:180–182.

340. Hoyer, P. F., Krull, J., and Brodehl, J., 1986, Letters to the editor: Cyclosporine in frequently relapsing minimal change nephrotic syndrome, *Lancet* **9**:335.

341. Oemar, B. S. and Brodehl, J., 1987, Cyclophosphamide treatment of steroid dependent nephrotic syndrome: Comparison of eight weeks with 12 week course, *Arch. Dis. Childhd.* **62**:1102–1106.

342. Trompeter, R. S., 1986, Minimal change nephrotic syndrome and cyclophosphamide, *Arch. Dis. Childhood* **61**:727–729.

343. Pei, Y., Cattran, D., Delmore, T., Katz, A., Lang, A., and Rance, P., 1987, Evidence suggesting under-treatment in adults with idiopathic focal segmental glomerulosclerosis, *Am. J. Med.* **82**:938–944.

344. Griswold, W. R., Tune, B. M., Tune, B. M., Reznik, V. M., Vazquez, M., Prime, D. J., Brock, P., and Mendoza, S. A., 1987, Treatment of childhood prednisone-resistant nephrotic syndrome and focal segmental glomerulosclerosis with intravenous methylprednisolone and oral alkylating agents, *Nephron* **46**:73–77.

345. MacTier, R., Jones, J. M. B., Payton, C. D., and McLay, A., 1986, The natural history of membranous nephropathy in the west of Scotland, *Q. J. Med.* **60**:793–802.

346. Kida, H., Asamoto, T., Yokoyama, H., Tomosugi, N., and Hattori, N., 1986, Long-term prognosis of membranous nephropathy, *Clin. Nephrol.* **25**:64–69.

347. Tornroth, T., Honkanen, E., and Pettersson, E., 1987, The evolution of membranous glomerulonephritis reconsidered: new insights from a study on relapsing disease, *Clin. Nephrol.* **28**:107–117.

348. Brueggemeyer, C. D. and Ramirez, G., 1987, Membranous nephropathy: A concern for malignancy, *Am. J. Kidney Dis.* **9**:23–26.

349. Packham, D. K., North, R. A., Fairley, K. F., Whitworth, J. A., and Kincaid-Smith, P., 1987, Membranous glomerulonephritis and pregnancy, *Clin. Nephrol.* **28**:56–64.

350. Abreo, K., Abreo, F., Mitchell, B., and Schloemer, G., 1986, Idiopathic crescentic membranous glomerulonephritis, *Am. J. Kidney Dis.* **8**:257–261.

351. Papiha, S. S., Pareek, S. K., Rodger, R. S. C., Morley, A. R., Wilkinson, R., Roberts, D. F., and Kerr, D. N. S., 1987, HLA-A, B, and Bf allotypes in patients with idiopathic membranous nephropathy (IMN), *Kidney Int.* **31**:130–134.

352. Roccatello, D., Coppo, R., Amoroso, A., Curtoni, E. S., Martina, G., Basolo, B., Amore, A., Rollino, C., Picciotto, G., Cordonnier, D., Sena, L., and Piccoli, G., 1987, Failure to relate mononuclear phagocyte system function to HLA-A, B, C, DR, DQ antigens in membranous nephropathy, *Am. J. Kidney Dis.* **9**:470–475.

353. Couser, W. G. and Abrass, C. K., 1988, Pathogenesis of membranous nephropathy, *Am. Rev. Med.* **39**:517–530.

354. Verroust, P., Ronco, P., and Chatelet, F., 1987, Antigenic targets in membranous glomerulonephritis, *Springer Semin. Immunopathol.* **9**:341–358.

355. Cosyns, J. P., Katatchkine, M. D., Bhakdi, S., Mandet, C., Grossetete, J., Hinglais, N., and Bariety, J., 1986, Immunohistochemical analysis of C3 cleavage fragments, factor H, and C5b-9 terminal complex of complement in de novo membranous glomerulonephritis occurring in patients with renal transplant, *Clin. Nephrol.* **26**:203–208.

356. Weildner, N. and Lorentz, W. B., 1986, Scanning electron microscopy of the acellular glomerular basement membranes in idiopathic membranous glomerulopathy, *Lab. Invest.* **154**:84–92.

357. Okada, K., Kawakami, K., Miyao, M., and Oite, T., 1986, Ultrastructural alterations of glomerular anionic sites in idiopathic membranous glomerulonephritis, *Clin. Nephrol.* **26**:7–14.

358. Shemesh, O., Ross, J. C., Deen, W. M., Grant, G. W., and Myers, B. D., 1986, Nature of the glomerular capillary injury in human membranous glomerulopathy, *J. Clin. Invest.* **77**:868–877.

359. Couser, W. G., 1988, Pathogenesis and theoretical basis for treatment of membranous nephropathy, in: *Nephrology,* Volume 2 (A. M. Davison, ed.), Bailliere Tindall, London, pp. 701–713.

360. Noble, B., Van Liew, J. B., and Brentjens, J. R., 1986, A transition from proliferative to membranous glomerulonephritis in chronic serum sickness, *Kidney Int.* **29**:841–848.

361. Ponticelli, C., Zucchelli, P., and Passerini, P., 1987, Therapy of idiopathic membranous nephropathy, *Springer Semin. Immunopathol.* **9**:431–440.

362. Zucchelli, P., Cagnoli, L., Pasquali, S., Casanova, S., and Donini, U., 1986, Clinical and morphologic evolution of idiopathic membranous nephropathy, *Clin. Nephrol.* **25**:282–288.

363. Garattini, S., Bertani, T., and Remuzzi, G., 1987, What is the basis for the use of steroids in the treatment of idiopathic membranous nephropathy? *Nephron* **45**:1–6.

364. Short, C. D., Solomon, L. R., Gokal, R., and Mallick, N. P., 1987, Methylprednisolone in patients with membranous nephropathy and declining renal function, *Q. J. Med.* **65**:929–940.

365. Grekas, D., Kalekou, H., Tsakalos, N., and Tourkantonis, A., 1987, Can cyclophosphamide pulse therapy change the natural course of idiopathic glomerulopathy resistant to steroids? *Nephron* **47**:236–237.

366. DeSanto, N. G., Capodicasa, G., and Giordano, C., 1987, Treatment of idiopathic membranous nephropathy unresponsive to methylprednisolone and chlorambucil with cyclosporin, *Am. J. Nephrol.* **7**:74–76.

367. West, M. L., Jindal, K. K., Bear, R. A., and Goldstein, M. B., 1987, A controlled trial of cyclophosphamide in patients with membranous glomerulonephritis, *Kidney Int.* **32**:579–584.

368. Makker, S. P., 1986, Hepatitis B associated membranous glomerulonephropathy, *Indian J. Pediatr.* **53**:317–325.

369. Editorial, 1987, HBV and glomerulonephritis, *Lancet* **1**:252–253.

370. Sennesael, J., Van den Houte, K., and Verbeelen, D., 1986, Reversible membranous glomerulonephritis associated with ketoprofen, *Clin. Nephrol.* **26**:213–215.

371. Yokoyama, H., Kida, H., Asamato, T., Abe, T., Koshino, Y., and Hattori, N., 1986, Gouty kidney associated with membranous nephropathy: Participation of renal tubular epithelial antigen, *Nephron* **44**:361–364.

372. Higuchi, A., Suzuki, Y., and Okado, T., 1987, Membranous glomerulonephritis in rheumatoid arthritis unassociated with gold or penicillamine treatment, *Ann. Rheumat. Dis.* **46**:488–490.

373. Hall, C. L., Fothergill, N. J., Blackwell, M. M., Harrison, P. R., MacKenzie, J. C., and MacIver, A. G., 1987, the natural course of gold nephropathy: Long term study of 21 patients, *Br. Med. J.* **295**:745–748.

374. Collins, A. J., 1987, Glod treatment for rheumatoid arthritis: Reassurance on protein uria, *Br. Med. J.* **295**:739–740.

375. Rosenmann, E., Brisson, M. L., Bercovitch, D. D., and Rosenberg, A., 1988, Atypical membranous glomerulonephritis with fibrillar subepithelial deposits in a patient with malignant lymphoma, *Nephron* **48**:226–230.

376. Murphy, B. F., Gonzales, M. F., Ebeling, P., Fairley, K. F., and Kincaid-Smith, P., 1986, Membranous glomerulonephritis and Landry–Guillain–Barré syndrome, *Am. J. Kidney Dis.* **8**:267–270.

377. Welch, T. R., Beischel, L., Balakrishnan, K., Quinlan, M., and West, C. D., 1986, Major-histocompatibility-complex extended haplotypes in membranoproliferative glomerulonephritis, *N. Engl. J. Med.* **314**:1476–1481.

378. Stutchfield, P. R., White, R. H. R., Cameron, A. H., Thompson, R. A., Mackintosh, P., and Wells, L., 1986, X-linked mesangiocapillary glomerulonephritis, *Clin. Nephrol.* **26**:15–156.

379. Jackson, E. C., McAdams, A. J., Strife, C. F., Forristal, J., Welch, T. R., and West, C. D., 1987, Differences between membranoproliferative glomerulonephritis types I and III in clinical presentation, glomerular morphology, and complement perturbation, *Am. J. Kidney Dis.* **9:**115–120.

380. Korzets, Z., Bernheim, J., and Bernheim, J., 1987, Rapidly progressive glomerulonephritis (crescentic glomerulonephritis) in the course of type I idiopathic membranoproliferative glomerulonephritis, *Am. J. Kidney Dis.* **10:**56–61.

381. Glicklich, D., Matas, A. J., Sablay, L. B., Senitzer, D., Tellis, V. A., Soberman, R., and Veith, F. J., 1987, Recurrent membranoproliferative glomerulonephritis type I in successive renal transplants, *Am. J. Nephrol.* **7:**143–149.

382. West, C. D., 1986, Childhood membranoproliferative glomerulonephritis: An approach to management, *Kidney Int.* **29:**1077–1093.

383. Sato, H., Saito, T., Seino, J., Ootaka, T., Kyogoku, Y., Furuyama, T., and Yoshinaga, K., 1987, Dense deposit disease: Its possible pathogenesis suggested by an observation of a patient, *Clin. Nephrol.* **27:**41–45.

384. Pober, J. S., Lapierre, L. A., Stolpen, A. H., Brock, T. A., Springer, T. A., Fiers, W., Bevilacqua, P., Mendrick, D. L., and Gibrone, M. A. Jr., 1987, Activation of cultured human endothelial cells by recombinant lymphotoxin: Comparison with tumor necrosis factor and interleukin 1 species, *J. Immunol.* **138:**3319–3324.

385. Cotran, R. S., Pober, J. S., Gimbrone, M. A. Jr., Springer, T. A., Wiebke, E. A., Gaspari, A. A., Rosenberg, S. A., and Lotze, M. T., 1987, Endothelial activation during interleukin 2 immunotherapy: A possible mechanism for the vascular leak syndrome, *J. Immunol.* **139:**1883–1888.

386. Leung, D. Y. M., Geha, R. S., Newburger, J. W., Burns, J. C., Fiers, W., Lapierre, L. A., and Pober, J. S., 1986, Two monkines, interleukin 1 and tumor necrosis factor, render cultured vascular endothelial cells subsceptible to lysis by antibodies circulating during Kawasaki syndrome, *J. Exp. Med.* **164:**1958–1972.

387. Moyer, C. F., Strandberg, J. D., and Reinisch, C. L., 1987, Systemic mononuclear-cell vasculitis in MRL/Mp-lpr/lpr mice: A histological and immunocytochemical analysis, *Am. J. Pathol.* **127:**229–242.

388. Adu, D., Howie, A. J., Scott, D. G. I., Bacon, P. A., McGonigle, R. J. S., and Michael, J., 1987, Polyarteritis and the kidney, *Q. J. Med.* **62:**221–237.

389. Ramirez, G., Saba, S. R., and Espinoza, L., 1987, Hypocomplementemic vasculitis and renal involvement, *Nephron* **45:**147–150.

390. Kuznetsky, K. A., Schwartz, M. M., Lohmann, L. A., and Lewis, E. J., 1986, Necrotizing glomerulonephritis in rheumatoid arthritis, *Clin. Nephrol.* **26:**257–264.

391. Chang-Miller, A., Okamura, M., Torres, V. E., Michet, C. J., Wagoner, R. D., Donadio, J. V., Offord, K. P., and Holley, K. E., 1987, Renal involvement in relapsing polychondritis, *Medicine* **66:**202–217.

392. Longley, S., Caldwell, J. R., and Panush, R. S., 1986, Paraneoplastic Vasculitis: Unique syndrome of cutaneous angiitis and arthritis associated with myeloproliferative disorders, *Am. J. Med.* **80:**1027–1030.

393. Balow, J. E., Austin, H. A., Tsokos, G. C., Antonovych, T. T., Steinberg, A. D., and Klippel, J. H., 1987, Lupus nephritis, *Ann. Intern. Med.* **106:**79–94.

394. Dillard, M. G., 1987, Systemic lupus erythematosus—The nephrologist's viewpoint, *Transplant. Proc.* **19:**57–59.

395. Leaker, B., Fairley, K. F., Dowling, J., and Kincaid-Smith, P., 1987, Lupus nephritis: Clinical and pathological correlations, *Q. J. Med.* **62:**163–179.

396. Rush, P. J., Baumal, R., Shore, A., Balfe, J. W., and Schreiber, M., 1986, Correlation of renal histology with outcome in children with lupus nephritis, *Kidney Int.* **29:**1066–1071.

397. Lewis, E. J., Kawala, K., and Schwartz, M. M., 1987, Histologic features that correlate with the prognosis of patients with lupus nephritis, *Am. J. Kidney Dis.* **10:**192–197.

398. Schwartz, M. M., Kawala, K. S., Corwin, H. L., and Lewis, E. J., 1987, The prognosis of segmental glomerulonephritis in systemic lupus erythematosus, *Kidney Int.* **32:**274–279.

399. Kasinath, B. S., Nielson, E. G., Hebert, L., Schwartz, M. M., Lewis, E. J., *et al.*, 1986, Short-term prognosis of severe proliferative lupus nephritis, *Am. J. Kidney Dis.* **8:**239–243.

400. Ponticelli, C., Zucchelli, P., Morini, G., Cagnoli, L., Banfi, G., and Pasquali, S., 1987, Long-term prognosis of diffuse lupus nephritis, *Clin. Nephrol.* **28:**263–271.

401. Henry, R., Williams, A. V., McFadden, N. R., and Pilia, P. A., 1986, Histopathologic evaluation of lupus patients with transient renal failure, *Am. J. Kidney Dis.* **8:**417–421.

402. Font, J., Torras, A., Cervera, R., Darnell, A., Revert, L., and Ingelmo, M., 1987, Silent renal disease in systemic lupus erythematosus, *Clin. Nephrol.* **27:**283–288.

403. Park, M. H., Agati, V. D., Appel, G. B., and Pirani, C. L., 1986, Tubulointerstitial disease in lupus nephritis: relationship to immune deposits, interstitial inflammation, glomerular changes, renal function, and prognosis, *Nephron* **44:**309–319.

404. Averbuch, M., Koifman, B., and Levo, Y., 1987, Lupus anticoagulant, thrombosis and thrombocytopenia in systemic lupus erythematosus, *Am. J. Med. Sci.* **393:**1–5.

405. Norberg, R., Nived, O., Sturfelt, G., Unander, M., and Arfors, L., 1987, Anticardiolipin and complement activation: relation to clinical symptoms, *J. Rheumatol.* **14:**149–153.

406. Lenzi, R., Rand, H. J., and Spiera, H., 1986, Anticardiolipin antibodies in pregnant patients with systemic lupus erythematosus, *N. Engl. J. Med.* **314:**1392–1393.

407. Petri, M., Rheinschmidt, M., Whiting-O'Keefe, Q., Hellmann, D., and Corash, L., 1987, The frequency of lupus anticoagulant in systemic lupus erythematosus. A study of sixty consecutive patients by activated partial thromboplastin time, Russell viper venom time, and anticardiolipin antibody level, *Ann. Intern. Med.* **106:**524–531.

408. Lockshin, M. D., Druzin, M. L., Goei, S., Qamar, T., Magid, M. S., Jovanovic, L., and Ferenc, M., 1985, Antibody to cardiolipin as predictor of fetal distress or death in pregnant patients with systemic lupus erythematosus, *N. Engl. J. Med.* **313:**152–156.

409. Howard, M. A., Firkin, B. G., Healy, D. L., and Choong, S-C. C., 1987, Lupus anticoagulant in women with multiple spontaneous miscarriage, *Am. J. Hematol.* **26:**175–178.

410. Bobie, G., Liote, F., Houillier, P., Grunfeld, J. P., and Jungers, P., 1987, Pregnancy in lupus nephritis and related disorders, *Am. J. Kidney Dis.* **9:**339–343.

411. Roth, D., Milgrom, M., Esquenazi, V., Strauss, J., Zilleruelo, G., and Miller, J., 1987, Renal transplantation in systemic lupus erythematosus: one center's experience, *Am. J. Nephrol.* **7:**367–374.

412. Kumano, K., Sakai, T., Mashimo, S., Endo, T., Koshiba, K., Elises, J. S., and Iitaka, K., 1987, A case of recurrent lupus nephritis after renal transplantation, *Clin. Nephrol.* **27:**94–98.

413. Pollock, C. A. and Ibels, L. S., 1987, Dialysis and transplantation in patients with renal failure due to systemic lupus erythematosus. The Australian and New Zealand experience, *Aust. NZ J. Med.* **17:**321–325.

414. Rodby, R. A., Korbet, S. M., and Lewis, E. J., 1987, Persistence of clinical and serologic activity in patients with systemic lupus erythematosus undergoing peritoneal dialysis, *Am. J. Med.* **83:**613–618.

415. Emlen, W., Pisetsky, D. S., and Taylor, R. P., 1986, Antibodies to DNA, a perspective, *Arthritis Rheum.* **29:**1417–1426.

416. Hahn, B. H. and Ebling, F. M., 1987, Idiotype restriction in murine lupus; high frequency of three public idioptypes on serum IgG in nephritic NZB/NZW F_1 mice, *J. Immunol.* **138:**2110–2118.

417. Gavalchin, J., Seder, R. A., and Datta, S. K., 1987, The NZB × SWR model of lupus nephritis, *J. Immunol.* **138:**128–137.

418. Madaio, M. P., Schattner, A., Shattner, M., and Schwartz, R. S., 1986, Lupus serum and normal human serum contain anti-DNA antibodies with the same idiotypic marker, *J. Immunol.* **137:**2535–2540.

419. Madaio, M. P., Carlson, J., Cataldo, J., Ucci, A., Migliorini, P., and Pankewycz, O., 1987,

Murine monoclonal anti-DNA antibodies bind directly to glomerular antigens and form immune deposits, *J. Immunol.* **138**:2883–2889.

420. Pankewycz, O. G., Migliorini, P., and Madaio, M. P., 1987, Polyreactive autoantibodies are nephritogenic in murine lupus nephritis, *J. Immunol.* **139**:3287–3294.

421. Hashemi, S., Smith, C. D., and Izaguirre, C. A., 1987, Anti-endothelial cell antibodies: Detection and characterization using a cellular enzyme-linked immunosorbent assay, *J. Lab. Clin. Med.* **109**: 434–440.

422. Helin, H., Korpela, M., Mustonen, J., and Pasternack, A., 1986, Rheumatoid factor in rheumatoid arthritis associated renal disease and in lupus nephritis, *Ann. Rheum. Dis.* **45**:508–511.

423. Stetler, D. A. and Cavallo, T., 1987, Anti-RNA polymerase I antibodies: Potential role in the induction and progression of murine lupus nephritis, *J. Immunol.* **138**:2119–2123.

424. Cosio, F. G., Hebert, L. A., Birmingham, D. J., Dorval, B. L., Bakaletz, A. P., Kujala, G. A., Edberg, J. C., and Taylor, R. P., 1987, Clearance of human antibody/DNA immune complexes and free DNA from the circulation of the nonhuman primate, *Clin. Immunol. Immunopathol.* **42**:1–9.

425. Horgan, C. and Emlen, W., 1987, Complement fixation by small, DNase-resistant DNA-anti-DNA immune complexes, *Mol. Immunol.* **24**:109–116.

426. Taylor, R. P., Edberg, J. C., Kujala, G. A., and Sloman, A. J., 1987, The interaction of antibody/DNA immune complexes with complement, *Arthritis Rheum.* **30**:176–185.

427. Greisman, S. G., Redecha, P. B., Kimberly, R. P., and Christian, C. L., 1987, Differences among immune complexes: Association of C1q in SLE immune complexes with renal disease, *J. Immunol.* **138**:739–745.

428. Uwatoko, S., Aotsuka, S., Okawa, M., Egusa, Y., Yokohari, R., Aizawa, C., and Suzuki, K., 1987, C1q solid-phase radioimmunoassay: Evidence for detection of antibody directed against the collagen-like region of C1q in sera from patients with systemic lupus erythematosus, *Clin. Exp. Immunol.* **69**:98–106.

429. Zanetti, M., 1986, New concepts in autoimmunity, *Immunol. Invest.* **15**:287–310.

430. Eilat, D., 1986, Anti-DNA antibodies: Problems in their study and interpretation, *Clin. Exp. Immunol.* **65**:215–222.

431. Jacob, L., Lety, M-A., Bach, J-F., and Louvard, D., 1986, Human systemic lupus erythematosus sera contain antibodies against cell-surface protein(s) that share(s) epitope(s) with DNA, *Immunology* **83**:6970–6974.

432. Balow, J. E., 1986, Lupus nephritis: Natural history, prognosis and treatment, *Clin. Immunol. Allergy* **6**:391–404.

433. Miescher, P. A., 1986, Treatment of systemic lupus erythematosus, *Springer Semin. Immunopathol.* **9**:271–282.

434. Steinberg, A. D., 1986, The treatment of lupus nephritis, *Kidney Int.* **30**:769–787.

435. Austin, H. A., Klippel, J. H., Balow, J. E., Le Riche, N. G. H., Steinberg, A. D., Plotz, P. H., and Decker, J. L., 1986, Therapy of lupus nephritis controlled trial of prednisone and cytotoxic drugs, *N. Engl. J. Med.* **314**:614–619.

436. Felson, D. T. and Anderson, J., 1986, Treatment of lupus nephritis, *N. Engl. J. Med.* **315**:458–459.

437. Schroeder, J. O., Euler, H. H., and Loffler, H., 1987, Synchronization of plasmapheresis and pulse cyclophosphamide in severe systemic lupus erythematosus, *Ann. Intern. Med.* **107**:344–346.

438. Jordan, S. C., Ho, W., Ettenger, R., Salusky, I. B., and Fine, R. N., 1987, Plasma exchange improves glomerulonephritis of systemic lupus erythematosus in selected pediatric patients, *Pediatr. Nephrol.* **1**:276–280.

439. Hebert, L., Nielsen, E., Pohl, M., Lachin, J., Hunsicker, L., and Lewis, E. J., 1987, Clinical course of severe lupus nephritis during the controlled clinical trial of plasmapheresis therapy (PPT), *Kidney Int.* **31**:201 (Abstract).

440. Lewis, E. J. and Lachin, J., 1987, Primary outcomes in the controlled trial of plasmapheresis

therapy (PPT) in severe lupus nephritis, Collaborative Study Group (LNCSG), *Kidney Int.* **31:**208 (Abstract).

441. Edwards, J. C. W., Snaith, M. L., and Isenberg, D. A., 1987, A double blind controlled trial of methylprednisolone infusions in systemic lupus erythematosus using individualised outcome assessment, *Ann. Rheum. Dis.* **46:**773–776.

442. Gunn, H. C., 1986, Successful treatment of autoimmunity in (NZB × NZW) F_1 mice with cyclosporin and (Nva²)-cyclosporin: I. Reduction of autoantibodies, *Clin. Exp. Immunol.* **64:**225–233.

443. Gunn, H. C. and Ryffel, B., 1986, Successful treatment of autoimmunity in (NZB × NZW)F_1 mice with cyclosporin and (Nva²)-cyclosporin: II. Reduction of glomerulonephritis, *Clin. Exp. Immunol.* **64:**234–242.

444. Miescher, P. A., Favre, H., Chatelanat, F., and Mihatsch, M. J., 1987, Combined steroid-cyclosporin treatment of chronic autoimmune diseases, *Klin. Wochenschr.* **65:**727–736.

445. Kotzin, B. L., Arndt, R., Okada, S., Ward, R., Thach, A. B., and Strober, S., 1986, Treatment of NZB/NZW mice with total lymphoid irradiation: Long-lasting suppression of disease without generalized immune suppression, *J. Immunol.* **136:**3259–3271.

446. Strober, S., Farinas, C., Field, E. H., Solovera, J. J., Kiberd, B. A., Myers, B. D., and Hoppe, R. T., 1987, Lupus nephritis after total lymphoid irradiation: Persistent improvement and reduction of steroid therapy, *Ann. Intern. Med.* **107:**689–690.

447. Boushey, H. A., Warnock, D. G., and Smith, L. H., 1987, New approaches to treating systemic lupus erythematosus, *West J. Med.* **147:**181–186.

448. Klinman, D. M,. Lefkowitz, M. D., Raveche, E. S., and Steinbert, A. D., 1986, Effect of anti-Ia treatment on the production of anti-DNA antibody by NZB mice, *Eur. J. Immunol.* **16:**939–944.

449. Epstein, A., Greenberg, M., Diamond, B., and Grayzel, A. I., 1987, Suppression of anti-DNA antibody synthesis *in vitro* by a cross-reactive antiidiotypic antibody, *J. Clin. Invest.* **79:**997–1000.

450. Milner, L. S., De Chadarevian, J-P., Goodyer, P. R., Mills, M., and Kaplan, B. S., 1987, Amelioration of murine lupus nephritis by dimethylsulfoxide, *Clin. Immunol. Immunopathol.* **45:**259–267.

451. Alexander, N. J., Smythe, N. L., and Jokinen, M. P., 1987, The type of dietary fat affects the severity of autoimmune disease in NZB/NZW mice, *Am. J. Pathol.* **127:**106–121.

452. Lee, H. S., Koh, H. I., Kim, M. J., and Rha, H. Y., 1986, Henoch–Schoenlein nephritis in adults: A clinical and morphological study, *Clin. Nephrol.* **26:**125–130.

453. Walker, R. J., Bailey, R. R., Lynn K. L., and Swainson, C. P., 1986, Henoch-Schonlein nephritis, *NZ Med. J.* **99:**534–535.

454. Montoliu, J., Miro, J. M., Campistol, J. M., Trilla, A., Mensa, J., Torras, A., and Revert, L., 1987, Henoch–Schönlein purpura complicating staphylococcal endocarditis in a heroin addict, *Am. J. Nephrol.* **7:**137–139.

455. Shichiri, M., Tsutsumi, K., Yamamoto, I., Ida, T., and Iwamoto, H., 1987, Diffuse intrapulmonary hemorrhage and renal failure in adult Henoch–Schönlein purpura, *Am. J. Nephrol.* **7:**140–142.

456. Nast, C. C., Ward, H. J., Koyle, M. A., and Cohen, A. H., 1987, Recurrent Henoch–Schönlein purpura following renal transplantation, *Am. J. Kidney Dis.* **9:**39–43.

457. Smolens, P., 1987, The kidney in dysproteinemic states, *AKF Nephrol. Letter* **40:**27–42.

458. Cordonnier, D. J., Renversez, J. C., Vialtel, P., and Dechelette, E., 1987, The kidney in mixed cryoglobulinemias, *Springer Semin. Immunopathol.* **9:**395–415.

459. Perez, G. O., Pardo, V., and Fletcher, M-A., 1987, Renal involvement in essential mixed cryoglobulinemia, *Am. J. Kidney Dis.* **10:**276–280.

460. Ferri, C., Moriconi, L., Gremignai, G., Migliorini, P., Paleologo, G., Fosella, P. V., and Bombardieri, S., 1986, Treatment of the renal involvement in mixed cryoglobulinemia with prolonged plasma exchange, *Nephron* **43:**246–253.

461. Jacquot, C., Nochy, D., D'Auzac, C., Durandy, A., Regnier, A., Lemann, M., Druet, P. H., and

Bariety, J., 1987, Glomerulonephritis, B monoclonal small lymphocytic lymphoma and mixed cryoglobulinemia, *Clin. Nephrol.* **27**:263–268.

462. Alpers, C. E., Rennke, H. G., Hopper, J., and Biava, C. G., 1987, Fibrillary glomerulonephritis: An entity with unusual immunofluorescence features, *Kidney Int.* **31**:781–789.

463. Wahls, T. L., Bonsib, S. M., and Schuster, V. L., 1987, Coexistent Wegener's granulomatosis and anti-glomerular basement membrane disease, *Hum. Pathol.* **18**:202–205.

464. West, B. C., Todd, J. R., and King, J. W., 1987, Wegener granulomatosis and trimethoprim-sulfamethoxazole, *Ann. Intern. Med.* **106**:840–842.

465. Habib, R., Antignac, C., Hinglais, N., Gagnadoux, M-F., and Broyer, M., 1987, Glomerular lesions in the transplanted kidney in children, *Am. J. Kidney Dis.* **10**:198–207.

466. Neild, G., 1987, The haemolytic uraemic syndrome: a review, *Q. J. Med.* **63**:367–376.

467. Kaplan, B. S. and Proesmans, W., 1987, The hemolytic uremic syndrome of childhood and its variants, *Semin. Hematol.* **24**:148–160.

468. Remuzzi, G., 1987, HUS and TTP: Variable expression of a single entity, *Kidney Int.* **32**:292–308.

469. Tarr, P. I. and Hickman, R. O., 1987, Hemolytic uremic syndrome epidemiology: A population-based study in King County, Washington, 1971 to 1980, *Pediatrics* **80**:41–45.

470. Taylor, C. M., White, R. H. R., Winterborn, M. H., and Rowe, B., 1986, Haemolytic–uraemic syndrome:Clinical experience of an outbreak in the West Midlands, *Br. Med. J.* **292**:1513–1516.

471. White, D. J., Yong, F., and McKendrick, M. W., 1988, Haemolytic uraemic syndrome in adults, *Br. Med. J.* **296**:899.

472. Carter, A. O., Borczyk, A. A., Carlson, J. A. K., Harvey, B., Hockin, J. C., Karmali, M. A., Krishnan, C., Korn, D. A., and Lior, H., 1987, A severe outbreak of *Escherichia coli* 0157:H7-associated hemorrhagic colitis in a nursing home, *N. Engl. J. Med.* **317**:1496–500.

473. Dzik, W. H., Goergi, B. A., Khettry, U., and Jenkins, R. L., 1987, Cyclosporine-associated thrombotic thrombocytopenic purpura following liver transplantation-successful treatment with plasma exchange, *Transplantation* **44**:570–572.

474. Craig, J. I. O. and Sheehan, T., 1987, The haemolytic uraemic syndrome and bone marrow transplantation, *Br. Med. J.* **295**:887.

475. Jain, S. and Seymour, A. E., 1987, Mitomycin C associated hemolytic uremic syndrome, *Pathology* **19**:58–61.

476. Hostetter, A. L., Tubbs, R. R., Ziegler, T., Gephardt, G. N., McMahon, J. T., and Schreiber, M. L., 1986, Chronic glomerular microangiopathy complicating metastatic carcinoma, *Hum. Pathol.* **18**:342–348.

477. Remuzzi, G., Zoja, C., de Gaetano, G., and Rossi, E. C., 1987, Prostacyclin and hemolytic uremic syndrome: From the laboratory to an international registry, *Int. J. Artificial Organs* **10**:337–340.

478. Powell, H. R., Groves, V., McCredie, D. A., Yong, A., and Pitt, J., 1987, Low red cell arachidonic acid in hemolytic uremic syndrome, *Clin. Nephrol.* **27**:8–10.

479. Hautekeete, M. L., Nagler, J. M., Cuykens, J. J., Parizel, G., Laekeman, G. M., and Herman, A. G., 1986, 6-keto-PGF1α levels and prostacyclin therapy in 2 adult patients with hemolytic–uremic syndrome, *Clin. Nephrol.* **26**:157–159.

480. Levin, M., Walters, M. D. S., Waterfield, M. D., Stroobant, P., Cheng, D. J., and Barratt, T. M., 1986, Platelet-derived growth factors as possible mediators of vascular proliferation in the sporadic haemolytic uraemic syndrome, *Lancet* **2**:830–833.

481. Cosio, F. G., Eddy, A., Mentser, M. I., and Bergstein, J. M., 1985, Decreased plasma fibronectin levels in children with hemolytic–uremic syndrome, *Am. J. Med.* **78**:549–554.

482. Meroni, M., Volpi, A., Battini, G., Conte, F., Ferrario, G., Giordano, F., Tarelli, L. T., Tommasi, A., and Sessa, A., 1986, Recurrent hemolytic uremic syndrome: case report, *Nephron* **44**:263–264.

483. Rose, M. and Eldor, A., 1987, High incidence of relapses in thrombotic thrombocytopenic purpura, *Am. J. Med.* **83**:437–444.

484. Hebert, D., Sibley, R. K., and Mauer, S. M., 1986, Recurrence of hemolytic uremic syndrome in renal transplant recipients, *Kidney Int.* **30:**S51–S58.

485. Shepard, K. V. and Bukowski, R. M., 1987, The treatment of thrombotic thrombocytopenic purpura with exchange transfusions, plasma infesions, and plasma exchange, *Semin. Hematol.* **24:** 178–193.

486. Lichtin, A. E., Schreiber, A. D., Hurwitz, S., Willoughby, T. L., and Silberstein, L. E., 1987, Efficacy of intensive plasmapheresis in thrombotic thrombocytopenic purpura, *Arch. Intern. Med.* **147:**2122–2126.

487. Finn, N. G., Wang, J. C., and Hong, K. J., 1987, High-dose intravenous γ-immunoglobulin infusion in the treatment of thrombotic thrombocytopenic purpura, *Arch. Intern. Med.* **147:**2165–2167.

488. Emancipator, S. M. and Schena, F. P., 1987, IgA nephropathy, *Seminars in Nephrology* **7:**274–318.

8

Acute Renal Failure and Toxic Nephropathy

H. David Humes and Joseph M. Messana

1. General Aspects

Recent prospective studies of hospital-acquired acute renal failure have revealed it to be a serious illness.[1,2] The development of hospital-acquired acute renal failure is associated with a sixfold increase in risk of dying. In fact, patients who develop an elevation of serum creatinine concentration greater than 3 mg/dl have a mortality rate of 64%. Development of this condition also has a marked impact on the length of stay of a patient in hospital. One recent report demonstrated that the development of acute renal failure increased a patient's length of stay in the hospital an average of 13–23 days. The most common etiologies of hospital-acquired acute renal failure include aminoglycoside nephrotoxicity, radiocontrast exposure, volume depletion, and septic shock. These etiologies highlight the role of both toxic and ischemic processes in clinically relevant acute renal failure. Prevention of hospital-acquired acute renal failure is, therefore, critically important, not only to diminish the mortality rate associated with this disease process, but also to limit the cost of hospital care. For example, a carefully done retrospective analysis of 1756 patients receiving aminoglycosides was undertaken to determine the economic impact of aminoglycoside associated nephrotoxicity.[3] An incidence rate of 7% in these patients was identified for aminoglycoside-associated nephrotoxicity. In this study, the additional cost of treating this complication in these patients totaled approximately $2500 per episode.

H. DAVID HUMES and JOSEPH M. MESSANA • University of Michigan Medical School, and Veterans Administration Medical Center, Ann Arbor, Michigan 48105.

Mechanisms responsible for development of acute renal failure in humans have recently been shown to be similar to pathophysiology of ischemic acute renal failure in experimental animal models.[4] Ten patients who developed protracted acute renal failure after cardiac surgery were evaluated using differential clearance of various markers of glomerular filtration. Results demonstrated that human acute renal failure is characterized by transtubular backleak of glomerular filtrate and by sluggish tubular fluid flow rates, strongly supporting the existence of severe and generalized intraluminal tubule obstruction as the major nephronal determinants of excretory failure in this clinical disorder.

This chapter further examines recent literature regarding the pathophysiology and clinical aspects of the most relevant forms of clinically recognized acute renal failure, including aminoglycoside nephrotoxicity, radiocontrast nephrotoxicity, and ischemic acute renal failure. In addition, because of the developing importance in understanding cyclosporine (CsA) nephrotoxicity, detailed discussion of this clinical process is also included in this review.

2. Cyclosporine

Nephrotoxicity is the most frequent and clinically most important complication associated with CsA use. A dose-related decline in glomerular filtration rate (GFR) with elevated levels of blood urea nitrogen (BUN) and serum creatinine concentrations occurs in nearly all CsA-treated patients, including transplant recipients and those with autoimmune diseases.

2.1. Clinical Features

2.1.1. Nephrotoxicity

There are differences in the definition of CsA nephrotoxicity. These differences are summarized in Table I. In most clinical disease states in which CsA is used, there are two primary forms of nephrotoxicity: (1) acute drug-induced toxicity, which occurs within the first several months; and (2) chronic (late) drug-induced toxicity, which occurs after several months of CsA use. The acute form most often responds to CsA dose reductions, whereas the chronic form often does not. In the setting of renal transplantation there are three forms of CsA nephrotoxicity: (1) acute (initial posttransplant dysfunction); (2) subacute (early posttransplant dysfunction); and (3) chronic (late-use dysfunction). As noted in Table I, the "acute" and "subacute" forms of nephrotoxicity may, in fact, be overlapping and also properly labeled as instances of "acute drug toxicity," but certain clinical situations in the renal transplantation experience may predispose the recipient to an immediate form of CsA nephrotoxicity, which appears to be distinctly different from the less acute, or subacute, form of toxicity.

An acute decline in renal function may occur immediately following or during the first week after transplantation. This initial, acute form of nephrotoxicity in the

Table I. Definition of Cyclosporine Nephrotoxicity

Renal transplantation	Other disease processes
1. Acute Initial or immediate dysfunction More prolonged ATN with CsA use in setting of renal transplant	1. Acute Early CsA
2. Subacute Early dysfunction Functional reduction of GFR Arteriolopathy	
3. Chronic Late dysfunction (interstitial fi- brosis)	2. Chronic Late CsA use (inter- stitial fibrosis)

renal transplant setting has been reported to occur more frequently in patients who have received cadaveric renal allografts with prolonged warm ischemia time or prolonged (24 hr or more) machine perfusion preservation or in patients in whom surgical completion of the renal vascular anastomosis of the patients in whom surgical completion of the renal vascular anastomosis of the transplanted organ required 45 min or more.[5,6] This interaction between CsA and renal ischemia has been documented in a recent experimental animal study.[7] In this study, a CsA dose of 5 mg/kg potentiated renal excretory dysfunction in a rat model of renal ischemic injury. Of note, CsA potentiated the renal dysfunction induced by 30–45 min of a two-kidney clamp model of renal ischemia only if it was administered after, but not prior to, the ischemic event. This initial graft nonfunction or delayed graft function in the presence of CsA therapy has resulted in a significant decrease in 3-month graft survival compared to grafts without delayed function. In addition, CsA treatment in patients with delayed graft function results in significant increases in the number of dialyses required or time needed for the recipient patient to recover from acute tubular necrosis (ATN) during the posttransplant period compared to azathioprine (Aza)-treated patients.

A subacute, or later form of acute, CsA nephrotoxicity is frequently seen in the first few weeks or months following renal transplantation.[8] This form of toxicity can present in one of two ways. The most common presentation is characterized by a mild to moderate, but nonprogressive, reduction in glomerular filtration rate and an increase in serum creatinine concentration rarely above 2.5 mg/dl. This alteration may occur as early as 2 weeks after initiation of therapy. Reduction of CsA dose usually results in reversal of the decline in renal function. A less common presentation is a renal vasculopathy that may develop within the first 4 months following initiation of CsA therapy.[9] This form of toxicity presents with a rapid deterioration of renal function. The histologic picture is one of intimal proliferation, fibrin deposition, and thrombotic occlusion of the arcuate and interlobular arteries of the renal cortex. Renal failure is usually progressive despite discontinuation of CsA and conversion to Aza and can be accompanied by moderate thrombocytopenia and a microangiopathic hemolytic anemia. These histologic alterations are not accompanied by changes associated with acute rejection and are very similar to those seen in the hemolytic–uremic syndrome.

Finally, a chronic form of CsA nephrotoxicity appears to develop in a sub-population of renal transplant recipients. This form of toxicity is characterized by slow, but progressive declines in renal excretory function as reflected by slow progressive elevations in BUN and serum creatinine concentrations. Dose reduction may reverse a component of the decline in renal function, but in some circum-stances the lower dose required to improve renal function may not provide sufficient immunosuppression. Since chronic rejection has clinical and histologic features similar to those used to define this type of nephrotoxicity, the existence of chronic CsA nephrotoxicity characterized by interstitial fibrosis in the renal transplant was initially debated. Experience with the drug in patients not receiving renal allografts has demonstrated the development of renal interstitial fibrotic processes in patients receiving long-term CsA. There is now little doubt as to the existence of this form of chronic toxicity.[10,11]

The definition of the chronic form of CsA toxicity has been most notable. In the clinical setting of heart transplantation, a CsA-related chronic progressive de-cline in renal function leading, in some patients, to chronic renal failure requiring dialytic support has been described.[10] This renal process is characterized histo-logically by a diffuse interstitial fibrosis and focal glomerulosclerosis. Morphologic alterations consisting of areas of interstitial fibrosis, tubular atrophy, and mild interstitial cell infiltration have also been described in patients treated long term with CsA for autoimmune uveitis.[11] The severity of the morphologic abnormalities in these patients with uveitis did not correlate with the average or cumulative dose of CsA. Elevations of serum creatinine concentration in this group of patients followed on average for 2 years was 2.4 mg/dl.

The experience of long-term CsA use in cardiac transplantation deserves spe-cial comment in view of a recent report detailing the follow-up of cardiac allograft recipients who have been treated with CsA for as long as 48 months.[12] These cardiac transplant recipients receiving CsA had a plateauing of GFR to approx-imately 50 ml/min between 24 and 48 months after transplantation. These GFR values were one-half the values observed in Aza-treated historical controls. How-ever, on renal biopsy, a progressive picture consisting of progressive glomerular sclerosis and collapse of glomerular capillaries, progressive interstitial fibrosis, and tubular atrophic changes was observed despite this plateauing of the GFR. This histologic progression suggests that a progressive injury pattern can develop in transplant recipients treated with CsA which is not adequately reflected by declines in GFR. The mechanism of this process is presently unclear and is not seen con-sistently in noncardiac transplant recipients, specifically those receiving renal or liver transplants. The difference in incidence may well be due to the striking hypertension that develops in cardiac transplant recipients treated with CsA. Both diastolic and systolic blood pressures averaged 10–15 mm Hg higher in CsA-treated allograft recipients, compared to levels seen in the historical Aza group. This increase in blood pressure was observed even though these patients were treated with appropriate antihypertensive regimens. Thus, the glomerular and interstitial changes observed in this subset of transplant patients may well be due to the exaggerated hypertensive side effect of this drug.

Five of the one hundred CsA- treated patients who were included in this report developed end-stage renal disease, although the initial large doses of CsA used in this study may have led to overestimation of the occurrence of this process. Although 5 patients of the original 100 CsA-treated patients developed end-stage renal disease, 23 additional patients survived 24 months or longer with the institution of this CsA program, compared to the group of 100 previous cardiac transplant recipients treated with Aza and prednisone. This regimen was also associated with lower maintenance prednisone dose requirements. This report clearly indicates the major effect of CsA to improve survival rates in cardiac transplant patients. This increase in survival rate is certainly more advantageous than the 5% risk of developing end-stage renal disease with the use of this agent at 24–48 months follow-up. Whether this same progressive toxic process will develop in other clinical situations in which CsA is used is unclear, especially in view of the high incidence of hypertension developing in these cardiac transplant patients upon institution of CsA therapy. Certainly, better characterization of the course and dose dependency of this potential chronic toxicity of CsA is required both in patients receiving transplant allografts as well as those with immunologically mediated diseases.

2.1.2. Other Toxic Complications

Besides a decline in GFR, other forms of CsA-related renal abnormalities have been described, including hyperkalemia and hypomagnesemia.

Renal transplant recipients treated with CsA have been shown to have higher serum potassium levels than patients receiving Aza.[13] In fact, hyperkalemia requiring treatment has been reported to occur in as many as 25% of patients receiving CsA.[14] This abnormality cannot be explained by a change in GFR, preexisting diabetes mellitus, diuretics, or the administration of either potassium-sparing or beta-adrenergic blocking agents. Most patients also develop hypercholoremic metabolic acidosis with normal urine-acidifying ability.[15] When measured, plasma aldosterone levels are routinely low for the degree of hyperkalemia, and plasma renin activity is either low or low normal in these patients. In addition, when these patients are given a potassium load, they excrete less potassium than normal individuals despite a similar rise in plasma aldosterone levels, thereby suggesting a renal tubule resistance to aldosterone.[16] This complex of clinical findings is highly reminiscent of hyporeninemic hypoaldosteronism, which is often seen in patients with chronic tubulointerstitial disease, a morphologic abnormality associated with chronic CsA nephrotoxicity.

Hypomagnesemia has also been reported as a common complication associated with CsA therapy. One study has reported that 11 of 24 patients treated with CsA after undergoing bone marrow transplantation developed either serum magnesium levels less than 1 meq/liter or symptomatic hypomagnesemia requiring magnesium replacement.[17] This disorder could not be explained by the administration of other drugs, such as amminoglycosides and amphotericin, which are also known to induce hypomagnesemia. In these patients, urinary magnesium excretion was increased in the presence of low serum magnesium concentrations, suggesting renal magnesium wasting. A more recent prospective evaluation described the effect of CsA on serum and urinary magnesium content in 27 renal transplant recipients treated with CsA and prednisone.[18] The hypomagnesemia that occurred by week 2 or 3 was dependent on allograft function. If good allograft function was present, a substantial drop in serum magnesium developed. Almost all patients among the 27 studied during the 5- to 6-month interval required magnesium supplementation to maintain serum magnesium levels above 1.6 mg/dl. Despite this supplementation, moderate to severe hypomagnesemia developed in 5 of the 27 patients. Two of these five showed overt signs and symptoms of magnesium depletion. Supplemental oral magnesium in the form of oral magnesium oxide (750 mg/day) was generally adequate to raise serum magnesium levels to the low-normal range (1.6 mg/dl) in the majority of patients. Three patients, however, required much larger doses (1.5 g/24 hr of magnesium oxide). Renal magnesium wasting appeared to be a major contribution to the observed hypomagnesemia. Inadequate dietary intake, malabsorption, gastrointestinal losses, or the use of various drugs, including furosemide, did not appear to be the major factor. Fecal magnesium excretion, however, was not measured, so firm exclusion of this possibility as a contributing factor could not be ruled out.

2.1.3. Hypertension

Hypertension is an important side effect of CsA therapy, both in transplant and in nontransplant patients. Its occurrence after cardiac transplant is especially striking.[19] The mechanism of this abnormality is presently unclear. Although CsA has been demonstrated to stimulate renin production in rat kidney cortex slices[20] and to raise plasma renin activity in experimental animals after several days,[21] CsA therapy has not been shown to stimulate plasma renin activity in humans.[19] Both low and normal serum aldosterone levels have been reported in patients receiving CsA. The renin–angiotensin–aldosterone system does not appear to play a causal role in this complication.[19] Urinary catecholamine levels have also been within normal limits. Neurogenic and direct vascular mechanisms for CsA-induced hypertension have been suggested but not proven,[22] although a recent report suggest a direct effect of CsA to promote alterations in intracellular calcium levels which would favor greater contractile responses in smooth muscle cells.[48]

A recent report has also shed some light on the difficulty of precisely identifying the effect of CsA-induced hypertension in the renal transplant recipient population.[23] This study demonstrated that CsA can elevate blood pressure in recipients of renal transplants, since blood pressure in this transplanted group fell after discontinuation of CsA. This rise in blood pressure appeared to correlate with the alterations in renal excretory function, since the improvement in blood pressure control after conversion from CsA to conventional therapy correlated significantly with a decline in plasma creatinine. Of note, along with a decline in blood pressure in these patients after conversion from CsA to Aza, fewer antihypertensive drugs were required to attain a normotensive state compare to the number of agents required in conventionally treated patients who received azothioprine and prednisone. This finding suggests that the administration of higher amounts of steroids during the first 3 months after transplantation in the Aza-treated patients may be an additional cause for persistently elevated blood pressures in patients undergoing renal transplantation. The mechanisms of these effects are unknown but certainly suggest that CsA has an effect on blood pressure in the renal transplant patient and that the use of steroid therapy may play as important a role in the persistent elevations in blood pressure after renal transplantations. This study points out the difficulty of specifically delineating the role of CsA on blood pressure after transplantation of various organs because of the prominent use of concomitant steroid therapy. Further studies are obviously required to elucidate the precise role of CsA in blood pressure regulation.

2.1.4. Drug Interactions

Numerous drugs have been shown either to affect the metabolism of CsA or to alter the nephrotoxic potential of CsA (see Table II). These drug interactions result in alterations in the therapeutic efficacy or incidence of toxic complications of CsA. Thus, the knowledge of these potential interactions will prevent inadequate immunosuppression or toxic overdosage.

Table II. Drug Interactions with Cyclosporine

Elevated cyclosporine serum levels
Erythromycin
Ketoconazole
Metaclopramide
Anabolic steriods (methyltestosterone, danazol)
Oral contraceptive
Calcium channel blockers (diltiazem, nicardipine, verapamil)
Decreased cyclosporine serum levels
Rifampin
Phenytoin
Nafcillin
Potentiation of nephrotoxicity
Amphotericin B
Aminoglycosides
Melphalan

Drugs have been shown to increase the serum or blood levels of CsA during a stable and consistent dosing schedule either by decreasing hepatic metabolism or by increasing its gastrointestinal absorption. Since CsA is metabolized by the hepatic cytochrome P-450 system,[24] drugs that decrease the activity of this metabolic detoxification system will increase CsA serum or blood levels. To this date, the antibiotic erythromycin[25] and the antifungal agent ketoconazole[26] are the only well-proven compounds that inhibit the P-450 enzyme system and increase circulating CsA levels, resulting in enhanced toxicity with potentiated immunosuppression and nephrotoxicity. Since CsA is used to suppress immunologic responses, these drug interactions among CsA and antibacterial and antifungal agents are of substantial clinical importance because of the possible use of these antibiotics to treat infectious complications in the immunosuppressed patient.

The coadministration of CsA with metoclopramide has also been reported to increase CsA blood levels.[39] Since metoclopramide has been shown to hasten gastric emptying and since CsA is absorbed primarily in the small intestine, the mechanism of this interaction appears to be increased bioavailability of CsA secondary to potentiated oral absorption. Other drugs have the ability to increase hepatic cytochrome P-450 activity and have the potential to decrease circulating CsA levels, resulting in diminished therapeutic efficiency. Rifampin[27] and phenytoin[28] are inducers of hepatic P-450 activity and have been demonstrated to lower serum and blood CsA levels. This interaction results in subtherapeutic CsA levels, with the risk of diminished immunosuppressive effect and graft rejection of a transplanted organ. A recent single case report has also implicated the antibiotic nafcillin to lower CsA levels to subtherapeutic levels during concomitant therapy.[29] Further studies are necessary to confirm this single case report. Similarly, androgens, such as danazol and methyltestosterone, inhibit hepatic drug metabolism, and oral contraceptive steroids are weak inhibitors of hepatic microsomal enzymes. These may be the mechanisms by which these drugs have been reported to increase cyclosporine levels.[30-32] The calcium channel blocking agents also have the potential to inhibit cytochrome P-450-mediated drug metabolism.[33] Accordingly, several of the agents, including verapamil, diltiazem, and nicardipine, have been demonstrated to raise CsA serum and blood levels.[34-36] This effect of calcium channel blocking agents to elevate CsA levels, however, may not be associated with increasing nephrotoxicity, since these agents may also ameliorate the effect of CsA to lower renal blood flow, thereby reducing the severity of CsA-induced nephrotoxicity.[37] Of note, the H_2 antagonist cimetidine is also a well-documented inhibitor of the hepatic P-450 system,[38] but enhancement of CsA blood or serum levels with increased toxicity has yet to be reported in the clinical literature.

Various drugs that either are nephrotoxins or influence renal hemodynamics have the potential to aggravate CsA nephrotoxicity. Amphotericin B, which promotes both renal vasoconstriction and toxic renal tubule cell injury, is commonly used in the transplant population to treat fungal infections. The concomitant use of this antibiotic with CsA has been clearly shown to increase the incidence of nephrotoxicity.[40] undoubtedly owing to the combined renal vascular effects of this antifungal agent and CsA. Dose adjustments of either agent may help prevent this complication. Other drugs, especially aminoglycoside antibiotics, and Melphalan have also been reported to increase cyclosporine nephrotoxicity[41,42] and should be used with care while administering CsA. Drugs that inhibit prostaglandin synthesis, including aspirin and other nonsteroidal antiinflammatory agents, are well known to decrease renal blood flow (RBF) in disease states in which vasodilatory prostaglandins are required to maintain RBF. Prostaglandin inhibition with these agents may further potentiate the declines in RBF produced by CsA, although careful clinical conformation of this potential intervention has not been published.

Finally, several reports have suggested that the use of trimethoprim and trimethoprim/sulfamethoxazole promotes significant elevations in serum creatinine levels when used with CsA.[43] This rise in serum creatinine, however, has been associated with no change in serum or blood CsA levels. These agents have been shown to inhibit creatinine secretion by the renal tubule in normal individuals, thereby leading to diminished creatinine clearance and increases in serum creatinine levels under normal circumstances. A similar process appears to occur in patients treated with CsA, so that it is presently felt that this particular drug interaction does not reflect a true deterioration of renal excretory function secondary to a potentiation of CsA nephrotoxicity.

2.2. Pathogenesis

A large number of experimental studies have demonstrated a functional hemodynamic basis for acute and subacute forms of CsA nephrotoxicity. CsA has been clearly demonstrated to produce dose-dependent increases in renal vascular resistance resulting in declines in RBF and GFR both acutely after intravenous administration and subacutely after several days of parenteral or oral administration.[44,45] This persistent, modest decline in RBF is consistent with the clinical observations that CsA produces a mild to moderate reduction in GFR that is acutely reversible after discontinuation or dose reduction, and that is, in most instances, nonprogressive.

It has been suggested that direct stimulation of adrenergic renal nerves producing vasoconstriction plays an important role in these renal hemodynamic effects of CsA.[46] A more direct effect on vascular tissue has been suggested by reports of a direct effect of CsA to induce contraction in isolated aorta strips from the rat.[47] This effect was blunted by the noncompetitive alpha-adrenergic antagonist phenoxybenzamine, suggesting that CsA may induce contraction by stimulating release of norepinephrine from sympathetic nerve terminals within the aortic strip. The calcium antagonist verapamil blunted this contractile response, further suggesting a role for calcium entry into vascular smooth muscle to produce this effect.

In fact, further studies using an *in vitro* system of cultured smooth muscle cells to measure intracellular calcium transients induced by angiotensin II and their relationship to pretreatment with CsA has been recently reported.[48] These experiments demonstrated that pretreatment of smooth muscle cells with CsA increased

Table III. Pathogenetic Features of
Cyclosporine Nephrotoxicity

Acute
  Renal vasoconstriction
    Increased sympathetic nerve activity
    Alterations in prostaglandin metabolism
    Direct arterial smooth muscle effects
  Vasculopathy
    Direct endothelial cell damage
    Platelet aggregation
Chronic
  Interstitial fibrosis
    Fibroblast activation
  Interstitial cell proliferation
    Mononuclear cell infiltration

---

the amplitude and duration of the angiotensin II-induced rise in intracellular calcium concentration. This increase in intracellular calcium concentration induced by angiotensin II appears to be due to both an increase in the hormone-inducible mobilization of calcium from intracellular stores and an increase in calcium flux into cells from the extracellular space. The half-maximal effects of CsA on this angiotensin II-induced rise in intracellular calcium was approximately 1.7 μM, somewhat higher than the optimal plasma levels of CsA on the immunosuppressive effect in humans, which is in the range of 200 nM–1 μM.

The precise role of the renin–angiotensin system in the CsA-induced decline in renal blood flow is not clearly defined. Recent micropuncture studies have evaluated the effects of CsA on single-nephron GFR (SNGFR) determinants.[49] Using rats with glomeruli that are accessible by micropuncture techniques, this report demonstrated that CsA promoted a decline in SNGFR due to both a decrease in glomerular plasma flow as well as a decline in the glomerular ultrafiltration coefficient (K_f). Of interest, this decline in RBF appeared to be dependent, in part, on the renin–angiotensin system and calcium channel entry, but was not influenced by prostaglandin inhibition. The effect of captopril to blunt the CsA effect on RBF and GFR suggests that the renin–angiotensin system may participate in this renal vascular effect, but this effect has not always been consistently demonstrated in the literature.

A recent comprehensive study using micropuncture, whole kidney, and whole animal balance studies may explain the previous inconsistent findings relating to the role of the renin–angiotensin system in the CsA-induced decline in RBF[50] reported in the literature. In this study, whole kidney clearance parameters demonstrated that GFR was significantly lower in the CsA-treated group compared to controls, but that mean systemic blood pressure was not affected. SNGFR showed similar declines. This reduction in SNGFR could not be attributed to tubuloglomerular feedback promoted by an increase in distal fluid delivery in CsA-treated animals. Renal blood flow was significantly reduced in the CsA-treated animals compared to controls and was associated with significant elevations in renal vascular resistance as well. Treatment of these two animal groups with captopril, an angiotensin converting enzyme inhibitor, and saralasin, a specific angiotensin II antagonist, normalized the increased renal vascular resistance, but systemic blood pressure fell significantly in CsA-treated rats. Since the decrease in renal vascular resistance following the inhibition of the renin–angiotensin system may have been due to autoregulatory vasodilation secondary to systemic hypotension, the renal blood flow autoregulatory response before and after captopril administration was assessed. This maneuver demonstrated that autoregulation of RBF was impaired in the CsA-treated animals but not in controls, and that most of the captopril-induced decline in renal vascular resistance resulted from the residual autoregulatory vasodilation response to systemic hypotension in the CsA-treated rats. Further results demonstrated that both RBF and GFR in CsA-treated animals could be improved by renin–angiotensin system inhibition when blood pressure was held constant, but because similar improvements were also seen in control animals not receiving CsA, inhibition of the renin–angiotensin system did not play a major role in the CsA-induced deficits in RBF and GFR compared to untreated controls. Therefore, despite the significant improvement in renal function following renin–angiotensin system blockade, the impaired RBF and GFR in CsA-treated animals was still present. These data do not support the hypothesis that renin-angiotensin is a primary mediator of the vasoconstriction in CsA nephrotoxicity.

There is increasing evidence that alterations in renal prostaglandin metabolism may contribute to the renal hemodynamic alterations produced by CsA. CsA administration consistently increases renal production of the vasoconstrictor prostanoid thromboxane in both experimental animals and humans.[51−53] This effect appears to be due to an effect of CsA to alter the activity of the phospholipase responsible for the release of the free fatty acid arachidonic acid, which is the precursor of prostaglandins.[52] Lowering renal thromboxane production leads to partially improved CsA-induced declines in RBF and GFR in both clinical and experimental settings.[51,53] The effect of CsA on renal production of other prostaglandins, including PGI_2 and PGE_2, has been controversial. Further support for an important role for prostaglandins in the renal vascular response to CsA has been demonstrated by substituting fish oil rich in eicosapentaenoic acid (EPA) for the conventional olive oil CsA vehicle.[53] This maneuver ameliorated the decline in GFR and RBF in animals receiving daily doses of CsA. This amelioration was associated with a decline in renal cortex synthesis of thromboxane (Tx) B_2, a stable metabolite of the vasoconstrictor prostanoid TxA_2. These results suggest that an increase in renal biosynthesis of the vasoconstrictor thomboxane, with or without a decrease in vasodilator prostaglandins, mediates, in part, the hemodynamic effects of CsA. Effects of CsA on prostaglandin metabolism of vascular tissue have also been demonstrated.[54] Cultured rat aorta smooth muscle cells were preincubated with CsA. CsA inhibited both basal prostaglandin E_2 (PGE_2) release and PGE_2 release stimulated by angiotensin II, arginine vasopressin, and the calcium ionophore ionomycin. This effect, once again, appears to be due to an interference of the activity of phospholipase to release free arachidonic acid from phospholipid stores within the membrane.

The vasculopathy reported with CsA use is characterized by prominent fibrin deposition and thrombotic occlusion of glomerular capillaries.[8] This process may be a consequence of direct toxic injury to endothelial cells promoted by CsA.[55] In addition, a recent study has also demonstrated an effect of CsA to promote platelet aggregation.[56] This multidimensional study examined both *in vitro* and *in vivo* effects of CsA on platelet aggregation in response to various aggregating agents. A dose-responsive increase in platelet aggregation was found *in vitro*, with a threshold effect at approximately 125 ng/ml, a clinically achievable level. Furthermore, both normal individuals and renal transplant recipients showed a CsA-related increase in platelet aggregation. This CsA-induced increase in platelet aggregation was also suggested by a trend toward normal platelet aggregation when patients were converted from CsA to azathioprine. Of note, the platelet release of thromboxane A_2 was also enhanced in platelets of allograft recipients taking CsA as well. Since thromboxane is a local renal vasoconstrictor, this enhanced release may suggest a further mechanism by which CsA produces renal vasoconstriction.

The mechanism of CsA-induced chronic interstitial fibrosis is not well understood at present. Animal data suggest that CsA has the potential to induce an interstitial process characterized by interstitial cell proliferation and fibrosis.[44] Of note, a recent report demonstrated that long-term CsA administration to the rat at a dose of 20 mg/kg every other day led to a major reduction to 30% of control levels of GFR as measured by inulin clearance, but no change in RBF as measured by para-aminohippurate (PAH) clearance.[57] This finding is in striking contrast to the acute effects of CsA administration on both RBF and GFR. The effects on GFR in this model, however, did not occur until 3 months of therapy. After several months of CsA treatment, focal interstitial fibrosis developed in these rats. These results suggest that the decline in GFR in this animal model of chronic CsA nephrotoxicity occurred without any change in RBF and thus does not appear to be attributable to a reduction in RBF and an increase in renal vascular resistance, as has been suggested by more acute studies. Further experiments are necessary to define the precise mechanism of this renal interstitial process by determining its dose dependency and its relationship to the renal vascular alterations produced by CsA.

2.3. Treatment

The approach to treatment of CsA nephrotoxicity is primarily dose adjustment to minimize the adverse renal effects of this agent. It is now widely accepted that a relationship exists between the serum levels of CsA and its immunosuppressive and toxic effects. Because of the considerable inter- and intrapatient variability in CsA levels achieved with any given dose, serum drug level monitoring is useful in determining dosage modification to lower the potential nephrotoxic complications of this agent.

Based on the clinical experience of many transplant centers, certain recommendations can be made regarding the basic strategy for CsA dosage with achievement of specific optimum serum levels. Owing to variability in absorption and time to reach peak concentrations, the measurement of serum trough levels (24 hr after a dose of CsA and prior to the next dose) is recommended rather than peak levels. The simplest assay is the radioimmunoassay performed on plasma/serum or whole blood, and the values outlined below are based on this assay. High-pressure liquid chromatography (HPLC) can also be used for assessment of CsA levels but is more difficult to establish. Although more complex, the HPLC technique has a clear advantage over radioimmunoassay (RIA) due to its specificity in measuring native unmetabolized CsA. Therefore, the values obtained from HPLC are lower since they represent only unmodified drug, whereas RIA levels detect CsA and its metabolites.[58] Extensive investigations are presently being carried out to identify specific toxic metabolites, so that toxicity may be better predicted and/or prevented by monitoring the serum or whole blood by HPLC techniques for this metabolite.

During the first few weeks posttransplant, trough plasma/serum levels of 150–250 ng/ml or whole blood levels of 450–750 ng/ml appear adequate. At 3 months posttransplant and with maintenance doses of CsA, trough plasma/serum levels of 75–150 ng/ml or whole blood levels of 225–450 ng/ml appear sufficient to maintain graft function and limit nephrotoxicity. These levels are only guidelines and usually correlate with immunosuppressive efficacy and/or toxicity. The correlation is not complete since toxicity has been observed with low levels and rejection events occurring in the face of adequate CsA levels. Clinical evaluation is, therefore, essential in the appropriate and safe use of CsA in transplant recipients.

A better understanding of CsA nephrotoxicity has resulted in several modifications in the early CsA-alone or CsA-plus-prednisone drug regimens. The rationale behind these modifications is either to avoid acute CsA nephrotoxicity during the early postoperative phase or to provide more effective immunosuppression by adding other immunosuppressive agents working through different mechanisms of action in order to reduce the overall CsA dosage. Experience indicates that the use of CsA immediately following renal transplantation can potentiate the degree of, and time for recovery from, acute tubular necrosis (ATN) that may be present due to surgical or mechanical difficulties such as extensive warm ischemia time or prolonged machine preservation. Because of this potentiation of delayed graft function, one approach has been to delay CsA therapy until renal excretory function has recovered to a specified level, such as a serum creatinine concentration of less than 3 mg/dl. This approach, however, eliminates the important beneficial effects of CsA on the recognitive phase of the immune response and is probably not the best strategy to address acute CsA nephrotoxicity in allografts with ATN. In this regard, many transplant centers have elected to treat these patients with antithymocyte globulin plus Aza during this early critical phase, followed by conversion from Aza to CsA once renal function has improved. This approach has had excellent early results.[59] If CsA is used initially and if renal failure and oliguria persist for more than 3 weeks, however, conversion from CsA to Aza therapy may be indicated, since recovery of renal function with continued CsA therapy is unlikely. On the other hand, an increased risk of graft rejection has been associated with conversion of CsA therapy to Aza.[60,61] Consequently, a compromise approach consisting of a marked reduction in CsA dosage and addition of Aza to convert from double (prednisone and CsA) to triple (prednisone, lower dose CsA, and Aza) therapy may be the best alternative.[62,63]

3. Aminoglycosides

3.1. Clinical Features

Identification of risk factors for aminoglycoside nephrotoxicity has recently been undertaken in a prospective, randomized, double-blind controlled fashion in 214 patients, by Moore and associates.[64] These patients were hospitalized on a general medicine service and received at least nine doses of either tobramycin or gentamicin in combination with standard doses of methicillin, nafcillin, or cephalothin. Estimates of creatinine clearance were based on the serum creatinine, age, weight, and sex of a given subject. Nephrotoxicity occurred in 14% of patients, and the potential roles of various risk factors in the development of nephrotoxicity were examined by both univariate analysis and multivariate discriminant analysis. When considered by univariate analysis, the following factors were significantly associated with the onset of nephrotoxicity: dose and trough aminoglycoside levels, liver disease, shock, female sex, and normal creatinine clearance. Stepwise, multi-variant discriminant analysis revealed identical results; however, the initial trough aminoglycoside level was not a significant factor in the multivariate equation. Discriminant analysis based only on factors identifiable before the onset of therapy, including sex, age, liver disease, and calculated creatinine clearance, led to a less complete prediction of clinical outcome. The addition of information on peak aminoglycoside levels and the presence or absence of hypotension led to more thorough discrimination between the toxic and nontoxic patient. An unexpected finding in this study was the apparent adverse influence of a normal GFR on the development of aminoglycoside nephrotoxicity. These authors speculated that increased luminal drug delivery in the nephrotoxic group may be the factor underlying nephrotoxicity, although the actual pretreatment functional differences between the groups were small. Duration of treatment, total administered dose, concomitant sepsis, urinary tract infection, and cephalothin administration did not significantly add to the predictive power of the equation. Aminoglycoside peak plasma level was the most important variable in this study. Interestingly, the presence of liver disease and being female were significant risks.[65,66]

3.2. Comparative Clinical Nephrotoxicity of the Aminoglycosides

Clinically relevant comparisons regarding aminoglycoside nephrotoxicity can be made most usefully in hospitalized patients requiring these drugs. The precise incidence of aminoglycoside-associated nephrotoxicity depends on both functional criteria for nephrotoxicity and the nature of the population examined. Other critically important factors in this determination are the random assignment of patients to control and treatment groups and adherence to a double-blind evaluation protocol.[67]

Kahlmeter and Dahlager analyzed 144 published clinical aminoglycoside trials concerning nearly 10,000 patients.[68] This review underscores the difficulties inherent in comparing relative drug nephrotoxicities by pooling data from multiple studies. The striking variation in the incidence of nephrotoxicity in prospective comparative trials emphasizes the need for rigorously defined nephrotoxicity criteria, patient randomization, concurrent controls, and double-blind evaluations. Overall, gentamicin and tobramycin appeared to be of equal nephrotoxicity and were slightly more nephrotoxic than amikacin and netilmicin; amikacin and netilmicin appeared to be equally nephrotoxic. When prospective comparative trials were considered separately, gentamicin appeared to be the most nephrotoxic drug, followed in order of decreasing nephrotoxicity by tobramycin, amikacin, and netilmicin. An interesting and unexplained finding was that the incidence of gentamicin nephrotoxicity was greater in compared trials with netilmicin than the incidence observed when gentamicin was compounded with tobramycin. A similar phenomenon has been observed with gentamicin by Smith and Lietman.[67] Gentamicin, in a comparative trial with tobramycin, appeared to be more nephrotoxic than an earlier comparative trial by this same group with amikacin. These authors have attributed this effect, in part, to a lengthening of the observation period for nephrotoxicity and to the exclusion of patients with possible nephrotoxicity from the denominator of the incidence ratio. An early, prospective, comparative study of gentamicin and amikacin in small numbers of patients suggested a significantly higher incidence of nephrotoxicity among gentamicin-treated patients.[69] This study involved small numbers of patients, was not double-blind, and demonstrated poorer pretreatment renal function in the group destined to receive gentamicin. Later, prospective, randomized studies have confirmed that amikacin is significantly less nephrotoxic than gentamicin.[68,70] Holm and colleagues[70] prospectively studied 135 patients with serious gram-negative infections and noted a 20% nephrotoxicity incidence in gentamicin-treated patients compared to a 6% incidence in amikacin-treated patients. Although overall antibacterial efficacies were similar between the drugs, pharmacokinetic studies revealed that serum amikacin levels exceeded the minimal inhibitory capacity for cultured organisms by 10-fold for 75% of a 12-hr therapy period, compared to 40% for gentamicin. Morphologic and biochemical effects of amikacin in the kidney do appear to be different than those produced by gentamicin or tobramycin. In a comparative, retrospective study of patients undergoing nephrectomy for hypernephroma, DeBroe and colleagues[71] compared the effects of three parenterally administered aminoglycosides on cortical drug levels, morphology, lysosomal alterations, and in vitro phospholipase A_1 inhibition. Gentamicin, tobramycin, and amikacin each induce an early cortical phospholipidosis of similar magnitude. Administration of gentamicin and tobramycin produced similar levels of tissue accumulation, ultrastructural lysosomal alterations, and phospholipase A_1 inhibition. While renal cortical amikacin levels were higher than those achieved by gentamicin or tobramycin injection, amikacin induced significantly less change in lysosomal volume and structural alterations and no loss of phospholipase A_1 activity.

Early experimental animal studies by Luft et al.[72] and by Soberon et al.[73] suggested that netilmicin, the N-1-ethyl derivative of sisomicin, possessed only mild nephrotoxic properties in rodents. In a multicenter, randomized, prospective, blinded clinical comparative trial, patients with serious gram-negative infections were assigned to receive netilmicin–ticarcillin or tobramycin–ticarcillin.[74] Although nephrotoxicity occurred in 4% of tobramycin-treated patients and 1% of netilmicin-treated patients, the difference was not statistically significant. Clinical and antibacterial efficacy were similar between the two regimens. Daschner and coinvestigators, using an identical protocol, demonstrated a 15% incidence of nephrotoxicity with the combination tobramycin–ticarcillin and no cases of nephrotoxicity in patients treated with netilmicin–ticarcillin.[75] In summary, then, reviews of comparative trials of clinically relevant aminoglycosides by others have suggested that gentamicin possesses the greatest clinical nephrotoxic potential, followed in decreasing order by tobramycin, amikacin, and netilmicin.[68]

3.3. Pathogenesis

The pathogenesis of the toxic effects of aminoglycosides on renal epithelium have focused most recently on the effect of these antibiotics on phospholipid metabolism. Specific alterations in cellular phospholipids occur in clinical, whole animal, and cell culture models of aminoglycoside nephrotoxicity.[71,76,77] These changes are tissue specific and consist of preferential increases in phosphatidylinositol, phosphatidylcholine, and phosphatidylserine.[76,77] Available evidence suggests that these alterations in lipid composition involve all cellular organelles and probably result from drug inhibition of multiple phospholipases of varying substrate specificity and cellular location as well as from redirection of glycerolipid biosynthesis.[76,77] Although a precise causal relationship between cellular phospholipidosis and injury remains to be demonstrated, evidence suggests that the nephrotoxic potential of a given aminoglycoside, the degree of phospholipidosis, and the potency of phospholipase inhibition are closely related.[71]

The basis of this effect of aminoglycosides on phospholipids appears to be due to the binding between aminoglycosides and membrane phospholipids, which involves the electrostatic interaction of the cationic, polybasic antibiotic and the acidic phospholipids, particularly the phosphoinositides.[78,79] Importantly, the polyphosphoinositides are known to occur in relatively large amounts in mammalian kidney.[80] Marche et al. have carefully studied the effect of aminoglycosides on phosphoinositide metabolism in rat erythrocyte membrane ghosts.[81] Under the experimental conditions employed, only the polyphosphoinositide phospholipids incorporated the ^{32}P label. Under basal control conditions, erythrocyte ghost membranes incorporated four times more radioactivity into phosphatidylinositol biphosphate (TPI) than into phosphatidylinositol monophosphate (DPI). The presence of 0.3 mM neomycin or greater in membrane incubations led to a reversal of the distribution of radioactivities associated with TPI and DPI; importantly, total ^{32}P incorporated into the polyphosphoinositides remained unchanged. The lack of an effect of neomycin on phosphatidylinositol (PI) kinase activity or on TPI phosphomonoesterase activity suggested that this reversal of radioactive labeling is due to an effect on DPI kinase. In this regard, the neomycin effect is similar to the effect observed in incubations containing 40 mM $MgCl_2$, a concentration known to inhibit DPI kinase in this system. Decreases in TPI and DPI ^{32}P labeling at neomycin concentrations greater than 1 mM suggested a possible effect on PI kinase activity. Marche *et al.* observed that the rank order of potency among the aminoglycosides for this phosphoinositide effect was neomycin/gentamicin/dibekacin/kanamycin/amikacin/streptomycin and paralleled whole animal nephrotoxic potential and relative cationicity of these antibiotics.

The polyphosphoinositides occupy a central role in the cell surface receptor transduction preceding calcium mobilization, protein kinase C activation, arachidonic acid release, and guanylate cyclase activation.[82] Given the rapidity of polyphosphoinositide turnover, any drug effect on the enzymes catalyzing phosphoinositide interconversions may potentially result in significant alterations in membrane structure and function. Transport or permeability alterations uniquely accompanying these changes have not yet been demonstrated. These results do not, however, exclude a role for less well-defined acidic phospholipid moieties in the membrane binding and, possibly, toxicity of aminoglycosides.[83] Competitive binding studies of both brush-border membrane vesicles and liposomes with various aminoglycosides and polyamines lend further support for a predominant role of anionic phospholipids in drug binding. Competitive inhibition of tissue drug accumulation has been observed among aminoglycosides and between aminoglycosides and organic polycations. Such drug-binding data, however, from whole animal and whole kidney studies are hazardous to interpret.[84] In this regard, renal cortical amikacin levels exceeded tobramycin levels for a given dose during *in vivo* drug infusion despite the greater *in vitro* binding of tobramycin to renal brush-border membranes. This greater *in vitro* binding of tobramycin is expected, based on simple charge considerations. This molecule has five ionizable amino groups and an approximate net charge of 3.1 at pH 7.4, compared to a predicted net charge of 2.4 for amikacin. Similarly, studies of *in vitro* drug-binding interactions fail to completely predict whole organ nephrotoxicity.[78,84]

In this regard, more refined analyses of aminoglycoside–membrane interactions have suggested significant effects on binding by amino group orientation and by hydrophobic interactions.[85] Brasseur *et al.* have demonstrated that increments in synthetic liposomal phosphatidylinositol led to a cooperative increase in aminoglycoside binding and that a small, but consistent, amount of any aminoglycoside remains membrane-bound at neutral pH and high-ionic-strength incubation conditions, suggesting the involvement of more than electrostatic forces. These authors used a computer-linked conformational analysis and an energy minimization procedure to predict the most likely conformation of aminoglycoside and phos-phatidylinositol moieties in a mixed monolayer after :epwise interaction with up to four phosphatidylinositols. Using the 2-deoxystreptamine ring as a reference plane, dibekacin and gentamicin penetrate deeply into the lipid layer above the position of the inositol phosphorus through the hydrophobic interaction of phosphatidylinositol fatty acyl chains and the $2',6'$-diaminodeoxyglycosyl moiety. Tobramycin pene-trates less deeply into the lipid layer, but three of five amino groups of gentamicin, dibekacin, and tobramycin ($N'2, N 3, N1$) interact electrostatically with the phospho groups of four phosphtidylinositols. It is probable that the inositol moiety is able to move freely over the deeply engaged aminoglycosides. In distinction to gentamicin and tobramycin, the kanamycin A and amikacin conformations associated with minimal interactional energies establish lipid–drug hydrophobic interactions with the $3''$-deoxy-$3''$-aminoglucosyl moiety. It is predicted that the $6'$-hydroxy-$6'$-ami-noglucosyl moiety is slightly above the inositol phospho groups (kanamycin A) or below them (amikacin). The vertical disposition of amikacin in the monolayer is stabilized by the 4-amino-2-hydroxy-1-oxobutyl side chain. For kanamycin A and amikacin, only two amino groups ($N3, N^16$) are available for meaningful interaction with the phospho groups of phosphotidylinositol, and inositol mobility over those antibiotics is restricted. The weakly binding streptomycin is attached through two guanidinium groups on the same glycosyl moiety, with weak hydrophobic interac-tions provided by the 2-deoxy-2-methylaminoglycosyl moiety, with resulting re-strictions on inositol mobility. In general, inhibition of *in vitro* phospholipase activity is associated with a more negative interactional energy and deeper penetra-tion into the lipid layer.[21] Such sophisticated physical approaches may allow greater insight into biochemical mechanisms of aminoglycoside nephrotoxicity, the cre-ation of less nephrotoxic drugs, and an explanation for the failure of simple elec-trostatic formulations to predict binding and toxicity.

A role of aminoglycoside-induced mitochondrial dysfunction has also been suggested to be important in the pathogenesis of aminoglycoside nephrotoxicity. The aminoglycosides have specific effects on the inner mitochondrial membrane to disrupt efficient bionergetic transformation processes.[86,87] These alterations in mi-tochondrial membrane alterations appear to relate, at least in part, to ami-noglycoside-induced stimulation of the generation of reactive oxygen metabolites by renal cortical mitochondria.[88] In fact, the importance of the generation of reac-tive oxygen metabolites in aminoglycoside nephrotoxicity has recently been sup-ported by the finding that administration of scavengers of the hydroxyl radical ameliorate gentamicin nephrotoxicity, and maneuvers that enhance hydroxyl radical formation potentiate gentamicin-induced renal dysfunction in the rat model.[89]

3.4. Modification of Experimental Aminoglycoside Nephrotoxicity

Approaches that may ameliorate aminoglycoside nephrotoxicity are promising. The most exciting strategy consists of identifying compounds that are competitive inhibitors of aminoglycoside membrane binding. Small organic polycations were initially tested, but these had appreciable nephrotoxicity of their own.[90] Because calcium is an effective competitive inhibitor of aminoglycoside binding to biologic membranes,[91] oral calcium supplementation was used to increase delivery of the ion to the kidney. Oral calcium loading markedly protected against gentamicin nephrotoxicity as measured by both renal functional and biochemical indices of renal cell injury.[91,92] However, the protective effect of calcium was not accompanied by a change in either peak renal cortical gentamicin levels or the time taken to reach them. Thus, it is possible that the effects of calcium are mediated either by the inhibition of gentamicin's action within renal cells rather than on their surfaces, or other, as yet unidentified, metabolic alterations might occur during oral calcium loading. Because of the large amounts of calcium required to achieve this protective effect, this maneuver probably is not clinically applicable.

This type of therapeutic approach has been extended to the use of various polyamino acids, including polylysine, polyasparagine, and polyaspartic acid, as detailed in Figure 1.[93] These compounds inhibit aminoglycoside binding to renal brush-border membranes. Furthermore, these agents, when coadministered with aminoglycosides to rats, completely protect against nephrotoxicity but have no effect on the antibacterial activity of these antibiotics *in vitro*. These findings

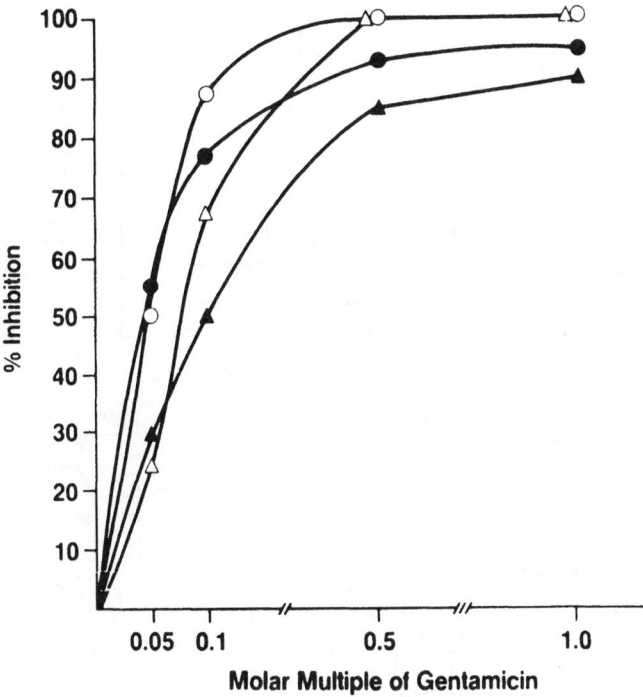

Fig. 1. *In vitro* and *in vivo* responses of polyamino acid inhibition of membrane binding and nephrotoxocity of gentamicin. ▲ = polyasparagine membrane-binding inhibition; △ = polyasparagine nephrotoxicity inhibition; ● = polyaspartic acid membrane-binding inhibition; ○ = polyaspartic acid nephrotoxicity inhibition. These data demonstrate that these polyamino acids both inhibit gentamicin binding to isolated renal brush-border membranes and protect against gentamicin nephrotoxicity at similar molar ratios. (Reprinted from Ref. 93.)

demonstrate that interventions have been identified which ameliorate nephrotoxicity in animal models which may be eventually applicable to the clinical situation.

4. Radiocontrast Agent Nephrotoxicity

4.1. Chemistry of Radiocontrast Agents

4.1.1. Traditional Ionic Media

The most commonly used ionic agents are triiodinated derivatives of benzoic acid, including the sodium and meglumine salts of diatrizoate and iothalamate (Fig. 2). Ionic media dissociate in solution, and for every three iodine atoms responsible

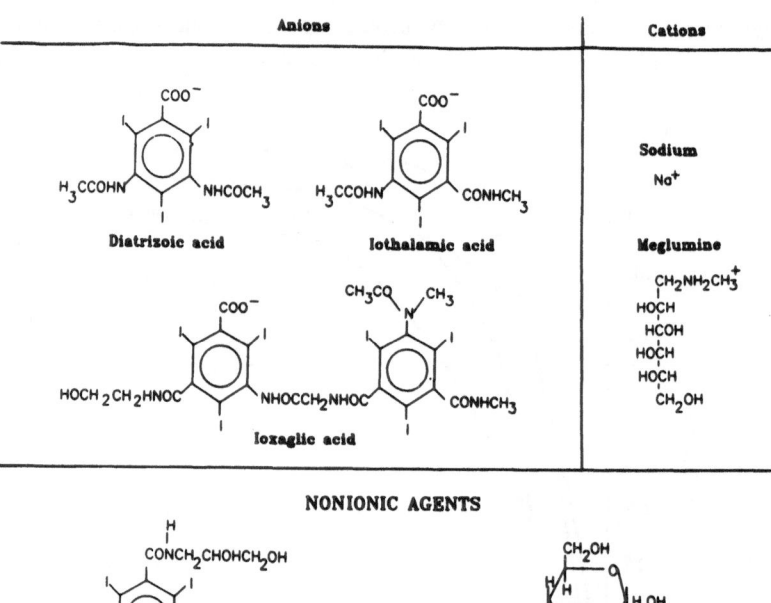

Fig. 2. Chemical structures of clinically available radiocontrast agents.

Table IV. Physical Properties of Equiiodine Concentrations of Selected Nonionic and Ionic Contrast Media

Agent	Iodine (m/ml)	Osmolality (mOsm/kg)
Ionics		
Diatrizoate	292	1511
Meglumine 52%		
Sodium 8%		
Ioxaglate	320	600
Meglumine 39.3%		
Sodium 19.6%		
Nonionics		
Iohexol	300	672
Iopamidol	300	616

for radiographic opacity, two osmotically active particles are formed: a radiopaque anion and a cation. The osmolalities of ionic agents may exceed the osmolality of blood by a ratio ranging from 5:1 to 7:1, depending on the particular iodine concentration and cationic ratio needed for specific radiologic studies (Table IV). Most adverse reactions of the traditional ionic media are due to their cationic chemotoxicity and hyperosmolality.[94,95] In order to reduce these side effects, efforts were made to develop nonionic, water-soluble contrast agents with an increased iodine-to-osmotic particle ratio. These endeavors resulted in the formulation of two distinct categories of low-osmolality media: the ionic–dimeric agents and the nonionic agents.

4.1.2. Ionic–Dimeric Media

The ionic–dimeric media involve the polymerization of two triiodobenzoic acid derivatives to form a single dimeric anion. When formulated with meglumine and/or with a sodium cation, six iodine atoms and two osmostic particles are formed, as in ioxaglate meglumine/sodium (Fig. 2). Although ioxaglate offers lower osmolality than the traditional ionic media per given degree of opacification, it can, because of its cationicity, interfere with normal neuroelectrical activity and is therefore contraindicated in myelography.

4.1.3. Nonionic Media

Another approach to lower osmolality and reduce inherent toxicity has been the development of a nonionic medium, which does not dissociate in solution and includes three iodine atoms for every osmotic particle. This development was accomplished by replacing the carboxyl group and the noniodine side chains of an ionic medium with nonionizing polyhydroxyalkyl groups (Fig. 2). The newer approach (e.g., metrizamide, iohexol, and iopamidol) completely eliminates the sodium and meglumine cations that accompany both the ionic and the ionic–dimeric agents. In theory, the ionic–dimeric and the nonionic contrast media could be expected to reduce the osmolality exhibited by equivalent iodine concentrations of the traditional ionic media by 50%. As can be seen in Table IV, however, the actual decrease in osmolality of the two categories of radiocontrast agents is greater than 50%, owing to the aggregation of the respective molecules in solution.[95]

Metrizamide, the first nonionic medium to become commercially available, is a derivative of metrizoic acid, a traditional ionic agent (Fig. 2). The carboxyl group of metrizoate is covalently attached to glucosamine, a glucose derivative, thus providing water solubility without ionic dissociation. Even though metrizamide seems to produce less intravascular and subarachnoid toxicity in both animals and humans than the traditional ionic media, its use is usually confined to myelography because of its instability. Metrizamide is unstable in solution, requires on-site reconstitution from lyophilized powder, and is also unstable when exposed to heat or sterilized by autoclaving.

The newer nonionic agents iohexol and iopamidol were formulated to improve stability and further reduce toxicity (Fig. 2). As they can be sterilized by heat and remain stable in solution, they are much more convenient than metrizamide. Furthermore, clinical and experimental studies have demonstrated that the subarachnoid toxicity of both iohexol and iopamidol is even lower than that of metrizamide.[96,97] All these factors have contributed to a current trend toward replacing metrizamide with these nonionic agents in myelography and toward employing the nonionic compounds intravascularly as well.

4.2. Pathogenesis

As discussed in Volume 4 of *Contemporary Nephrology*,[98] the following contributing mechanisms appear to be involved in radiocontrast-induced nephrotoxicity: (1) hemodynamic alterations—an initial brief increase in RBF followed by a longer period of vasoconstriction is produced following radiocontrast administration; (2) intrarenal/tubular obstruction, resulting from interactions between the contrast agent and the proteinaceous debris within the lumen of the renal tubule; and (3) toxic injury to renal proximal tubule cells, produced directly by the contrast agent. The deleterious effects of the three mechanisms are simultaneous and probably synergystic. Predisposing clinical factors for the development of radiocontrast-induced acute renal failure include preexisting renal insufficiency, long-standing diabetes mellitus, multiple myeloma, dehydration, high doses and/or repeated administration of contrast media, advanced age, atherosclerosis.[98]

Since the nephrotoxic potential of a contrast agent is dependent on the magnitude of its effects on each of these three factors, a comparison of the relative nephrotoxicity of two agents must include assessment of each agent's effects on each of these processes. In this regard, results from recent animal and *in vitro* studies suggest that iopamidol has significantly less deleterious effects on each of the pathogenic mechanisms mentioned previously than does diatrizoate. The pathophysiology of the renal vasoconstrictive response to radiocontrast administration appears to be related directly to the osmolality of the administered compound and to the resulting osmotic diuresis. This increase delivery to the distal nephron promoted by this osmotic diuresis promotes tubuloglomerular feedback and renal arteriolar vasoconstriction.[99] Consequently, the less hypertonic the contrast solution, the lower the degree of renal vasoconstriction. As iopamidol is less hyertonic than diatrizoate-containing preparations, it could be predicted that the radiocontrast-induced vasoconstrictive response would be milder after the administration of iopamidol than after diatrizoate. Indeed, recent experiments in dogs have revealed that the decline in RBF following intravenous iopamidol injection is only one-half the decline from baseline value observed after the administration of diatrizoate.[100,101]

The direct toxicity of the nonionic agent diatrizoate and of the newer, nonconventional ionic derivative iopamidol to renal proximal tubule cells has recently been compared.[102] Suspensions enriched in rabbit tubule segments were exposed to equal and clinically achievable concentrations of the conventional diatrizoate or of iopamidol, with or without a short period of hypoxia. Renal tubule viability parameters, including basal and uncoupled respiratory rates as well as potassium, calcium, and ATP contents, were then measured. Under oxygenated conditions, exposure of renal tubule suspensions to either 25 mM of iopamidol or of diatrizoate produced greater metabolic alterations than those observed under control conditions. Furthermore, the toxicity produced by diatrizoate, as measured by basal respiratory rate and calcium content, was greater than that produced by iopamidol under these oxygenated conditions. During a short period of hypoxia concomitant with contrast media exposure, the alterations in the renal tubule suspensions exposed to 25 mM of diatrizoate were significantly greater than in those exposed to 25 mM of iopamidol. Iopamidol had less of a detrimental effect on renal tubule calcium content, ATP depletion, and uncoupled respiratory rate than did diatrizoate. Thus, diatrizoate was more toxic to rabbit renal proximal tubule cells than iopamidol and this *in vitro* difference in toxicity was enhanced by hypoxia.

Further results suggest that iopamidol is less likely than diatrizoate to interact with urinary proteins or cellular membrane fragments of renal tubules.[103] This agent is, therefore, less likely than diatrizoate to produce a dense protein complex that may accumulate within the tubular lumina and produce intratubular, intrarenal obstruction.

All these experimental studies indicate that, compared to diatrizoate, iopamidol has less deleterious effects on renal hemodynamics, less direct toxicity on renal proximal tubule cells, and less propensity for interaction with renal membranes and urinary proteins that may result in damage and deposition of intratubular debris. In fact, whole animal experiments have demonstrated that the degree of acute tubular necrosis, as measured histologically, induced by *in vivo* renal ischemia followed by intravenous contrast administration was much less when iopamidol was used than when diatrizoate was infused.[104] These results confirm the *in vivo* correlates of relative nephrotoxicity of these two agents predicted by the *in vitro* experiments. These *in vitro* and *in vivo* experimental findings suggest that the newer nonionic contrast agents may be efficacious in reducing the incidence of radiocontrast-induced acute renal failure. Accordingly, these nonionic agents may prove to be useful alternatives to conventional ionic contrast agents in patients at risk for radiocontrast nephrotoxicity. Further clinical evaluation to demonstrate clinical relevance of these experimental findings is necessary before conclusions can be drawn about the relative nephrotoxic potential of these agents.

5. Ischemic Acute Renal Failure

Postischemic acute renal failure is one of the most dramatic clinical syndromes. It occurs abruptly and results in the failure of the kidney as an excretory organ, but under most circumstances is a reversible disease process, with renal function returning to normal within several days to several weeks. Ischemic acute renal failure continues to be a major cause of morbidity and mortality in severely ill individuals. The study of this disorder, therefore, continues to be an important area of nephrologic research.

It is now widely accepted that the development of fixed structural ischemic acute renal failure, or acute tubular necrosis, is due to renal tubular cell injury.[105,106] The majority of *in vivo* experiments suggest that the proximal tubule segment is most susceptible to ischemic injury, but more recent *in vitro* experiments, using the isolated perfused kidney model, have emphasized a contribution of the loop of Henle to this process.[107]

5.1. Importance of Adenosine Triphosphate

An understanding of ischemic acute renal failure, like an understanding of the pathogenesis of ischemic injury to any other organ, is based on a knowledge of the processes determining cellular injury. A simple, but extremely useful, approach to the understanding of cell injury is to consider this process as a dynamic interplay between degradative and synthetic events. Under normal circumstances, a cell maintains its viability by a carefully balanced interplay between synthetic and degradative events, as detailed in Figure 3. Cell injury develops when synthetic processes cannot keep pace with degradative events. Ischemia leads to cell injury because of both activation of critical degradative processes and a decline in synthetic function due to a decrease in availability of high-energy compounds promoted by the ischemic state. Under this formulation, not only are degradative processes important, but a critical role for depletion of cellular energy stores, predominantly in the form of adenosine triphosphate (ATP), is considered.

Much recent work has focused on a variety of degradative events that occur during ischemia and reperfusion, including phospholipase activation, cellular cal-

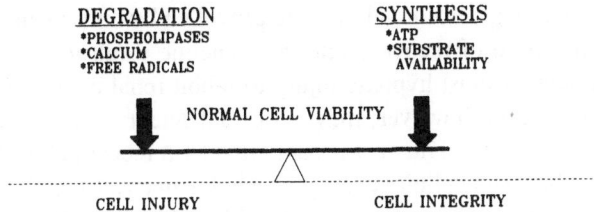

Fig. 3. Dynamic interplay between synthetic and degradative events. Cell injury develops if this balance is weighted toward more degradative or less synthetic processes.

cium overload, and free radical and oxygen metabolite generation.[108,109] These degradative processes promote damage to cellular and subcellular membranes, critical events which determine the course of cellular injury. The pathogenesis of ischemic cell injury can thus be viewed as the simultaneous derangement of several metabolic processes that act in concert to produce a cascade of events that finally lead to plasma and subscellular membrane dysfunction incompatible with the maintenance of cell viability.

Ischemia directly leads to declines in the rate of oxidative phosphorylation due to a lack of oxygen availability. A fall in cellular ATP levels develops, especially in the renal proximal tubule cell, which is almost completely dependent on oxidative phosphorylation for energy production. Ischemia also promotes redistribution of intracellular calcium pools that results in phospholipase activation and phospholipid degradation. When phospholipid degradation occurs, concominantly with the decline in levels of high-energy phosphate compounds, phospholipid synthesis cannot keep pace with phospholipid degradation and net membrane phospholipid loss occurs with accumulation of potentially toxic lipid by-products, including free fatty acids and lysophospholipids. An increase in plasma membrane calcium permeability develops, and the influx of calcium down its electrochemical gradient from extracellular to intracellular compartments occurs. This calcium is taken up and sequestered in mitochondria and causes further alterations in mitochondrial structure and function leading to further declines in cellular ATP content. Therefore, a vicious cycle of progressive cellular membrane deterioration, accumulation of toxic lipid byproducts, cellular energy store depletion, and deranged cellular bioenergetics develops until reparative and synthetic processes cannot keep pace with degradative events. Free radicals and oxygen metabolite production during ischemia and reoxygenation of ischemic tissues may be instrumental in these events by contributing, in a critical manner, to membrane alterations. Of importance, ATP depletion plays a key central role in this formulation.

A variety of experiments have supported this important role for ATP in ischemic injury. Maneuvers that inhibit cell energy utilization, such as intracellular acidosis and inhibition of Na,K-ATPase with ouabain, protect against the degree of cell injury induced by an ischemic or hypoxic stress.[110,111] Maneuvers that increase cell energy utilization, such as increasing membrane permeability with amphotericin B, potentiate hypoxic or ischemic cell injury.[112] ATP–$MgCl_2$ infusion protects against the degree of renal damage provoked by an ischemic insult as well as enhancing the speed of recovery after an ischemic insult *in vivo*.[113–115] ATP–MgCl$_2$ also protects against hypoxic injury to rabbit renal proximal tubule cells *in vitro*.[116] ATP depletion, however, may not be sufficient as an only determinant of renal epithelial cell injury. This fact is supported by a recent publication looking at the relationships between cellular energy thresholds in a renal epithelial cell culture line, LLC-PK$_1$, and development of irreversible cell injury.[117] In this study, oxidative phosphorylation and glycolysis were inhibited by the addition of various inhibitors and/or glucose deprivation to achieve stepwise ATP depletion. These results identified a very low threshold for ATP levels at approximately 5–10% of normal values which preserve the viability of LLCPK$_1$ cells. Thus, ATP depletion to this degree was not sufficient to induce irreversible cell injury. However, in the face of ATP depletion and increasing degradative processes that may be provoked by ischemia or hypoxia, substantial cell injury may occur even with modest declines in ATP content. In this regard, a recent report assessed the affect of exogenous phospholipase A$_2$ to promote injury in freshly isolated rabbit renal proximal tubule cells.[118] Exogenous phospholipase A$_2$ did not produce any significant changes in metabolic parameters, which are quantitative of cell injury, in nonhypoxic renal proximal tubule preparations, despite significant alterations in phospholipid levels. In contrast, exogenous phospholipase A$_2$ treatment of mildly hypoxic tubules resulted in a severe degree of cell injury. This injury was associated with significant phospholipid alterations with marked declines in phosphotidylcholine and phosphotidylethanolamine and significant rises in lysophosphotidylcholine and phosphotidylethanolamine. These injurious metabolic effects occurring during simultaneous exogenous phospholipase A$_2$ and hypoxia exposure were blocked, in a dose-dependent manner, with addition of exogenous ATP–MgCl$_2$ to the preparation. This protective affect of ATP was associated with improvement of phospholipid levels and declines in potentially toxic lipid by-products. These results are, thus, consistent with the thesis that activation of phospholipase by ischemia or hypoxia produces proximal renal tubule cell injury only when cell ATP levels decline. This dependency is most likely due to the fact that phospholipid resynthesis in the face of ATP depletion cannot keep pace with phospholipid degradation. These findings further support the notion that the balance between degradative and synthetic forces within a cell is critical in maintaining cell viability.

The importance of ATP in maintaining cell viability is also supported by the recent demonstration of the ability of exogenously administered ATP to dissociate the degree of cell injury from cell calcium overload in freshly isolated renal proximal tubule cells.[119] In this report, supplementation of rabbit renal proximal tubule suspensions with 2 mM ATP–MgCl$_2$ resulted in fivefold increases in both total cell and mitochondrial calcium content. Despite this major calcium overload, indicators of tubule viability remained normal. Furthermore, 45 min of hypoxia resulted in substantial tubule cell injury, but exogenous ATP supplementation resulted in significant improvement of tubule cell viability despite causing four- to sixfold increases in cell calcium content. ATP supplementation, therefore, appears to limit the degree of irreversible cell injury developing after hypoxia and reoxygenation. ATP depletion appears, thus, to be necessary for the development of calcium-induced mitochondrial dysfunction under hypoxic conditions. Excessive cell calcium overload in the presence of supraphysiologic concentrations of ATP can, therefore, be dissociated from decreased cell viability. The importance of ATP in the preservation of mitochondrial function has also been clearly demonstrated in isolated mitochondrial preparations.[120]

5.2. Mitochondrial Dysfunction

Mitochondria are critical for the production and maintenance of cellular ATP levels. During ischemia, the functional capacity of mitochondria is relatively unimportant since the availability of oxygen, which is the final necessary component of oxidative phosphorylation, is severely limited. Impaired mitochondrial function, however, becomes of critical importance when the oxygen supply to a tissue or cell is restored and the capacity for repair requires replenishment of the cellular high energy phosphate supply, a function almost entirely dependent on intact mitochondrial oxidative phosphorylation in the proximal tubule cell. For this reason much attention has been focused on mitochondrial functional changes during ischemic injury and during the reperfusion or reoxygenation stage following ischemia.

A critical role for mitochondrial calcium uptake and overload in the development of mitochondrial dysfunction during the reperfusion or reoxygenation stage has been demonstrated.[124] The understanding of the interrelationships of calcium and mitochondrial function is, therefore, critical in the understanding of developing ischemic cell injury. In this regard, mitochondria are able to take up and to retain calcium up to certain levels without deleterious effects.[121] Above these levels, greater calcium uptake produces spontaneous release of mitochondrial calcium. This calcium efflux occurs via both ruthenium-red-sensitive, i.e., via the electrophoretic uniport, and ruthenium-red-insensitive pathways. This release is accompanied by loss of other mitochondrial cations, of adenine nucleotides, and of the ability of mitochondria to maintain a membrane potential.[121,122] These alterations in mitochondrial permeability induced by calcium uptake appear to occur via pathophysiologic and not via physiologic pathways. Of importance, lesser amounts of calcium uptake are required to produce these permeability changes when calcium is taken up by mitochondria in the presence of the organic hydroperoxide tert-butyl hydroperoxide[121,122] and these calcium-induced alterations can be ameliorated by the presence of adenine nucleotides or oxidizable substrates.[120,124]

Calcium uptake by mitochondria provokes these mitochondrial membrane alterations and damage in large part by activating mitochondrial phospholipases, which leads to hydrolysis of phospholipids[126,127] and production of free fatty acids and lysophospholipids.[120,121] These derivatives of phospholipid breakdown alter the permeability of the inner mitochondrial membrane, resulting in functional deterioration.

The role for free radicals or oxygen metabolites in mitochondrial damage promoted by calcium uptake and overload is presently not clearly defined. Recent studies have demonstrated that calcium and free radicals produced by exogenous generating systems work in concert to promote injury to mitochondria between site 1 and 2 of the electron transport chain with complete uncoupling of oxidative phosphorylation.[129] Similar synergistic damaging effects of free radicals and calcium on rat brain mitochondria have also been reported.[130]

These additive effects of free radicals and calcium to promote mitochondrial damage may relate to the fact that free radicals stimulate endogenous phospholipase activity.[131] It is unclear, however, at this time whether this effect of free radicals to stimulate membrane phospholipases occurs indirectly by promoting release of free calcium ions from subcellular organelles[132] or directly due to the increased susceptibility of membrane-peroxidized phospholipids to the action of phospholipases[133,134] or to the physical changes within the membrane bilayer resulting from free-radical injury.

Free-radical and oxygen metabolite generation may produce membrane dysfunction not only indirectly by potentiating phospholipase activity, but directly by promoting lipid peroxidation. Unsaturated fatty acids are especially prone to this degradative process of lipid peroxidation.[135] Since the mitochondrial membrane is rich in phospholipids containing large amounts of unsaturated fatty acids, mitochondria are especially susceptible to lipid peroxidative damage. Mitochondria are also at risk for peroxidative damage since the process of electron transport by the cytochromes, most notably the semiquinones, produces oxygen.[136] Furthermore, potentiation of free-radical–induced lipid peroxidative injury by products of activated CoA, palmitoyl–carnitine, and lysophosphotidylcholine has been demonstrated in isolated membranes.[137] Thus, not only do free radicals promote phospholipase activity, but the by-products of phospholipase activation also promote free-radical–induced oxidative damage.

6. Role of Reactive Oxygen Species in Postischemic Renal Injury

Recent advances in our understanding of ischemia-induced organ dysfunction implicate an important role for the reperfusion period in the development of both morphologic and functional derangements previously attributed to ischemia alone. Oxygen-derived free radicals and other reactive oxygen species (ROS) are generated in abundance during oxygenated reperfusion and most likely mediate the bulk of reperfusion-induced injury after ischemia. Biologically important ROS include superoxide anion (O_2^-), hydroxyl free radical (OH), hydrogen peroxide (H_2O_2), hypochlorous acid (HOCl), and singlet oxygen ($^1O_2$).[138–142]

Several biochemical defenses against oxidant stress are common to virtually all aerobic organisms (Fig. 4). They include the enzymes superoxide dismutase,[144]

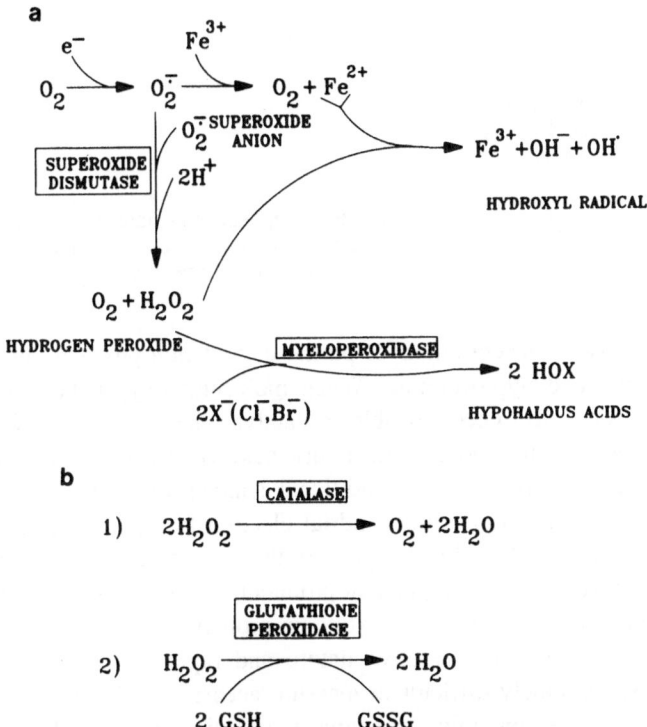

Fig. 4. Important chemical reactions in the generation of reactive oxygen species. (a) The central role of hydrogen peroxide; (b) metabolism of hydrogen peroxide.

catalase,[142,143] and glutathione peroxidase,[145–148] as well as water-soluble factors such as ascorbic acid and glutathione and lipid-soluble antioxidants (e.g., vitamin E or D-tocopherols).[149,156] During ischemia, however, supplies of endogenous scavengers may be depleted, permitting cellular injury by free radicals during the reperfusion period.[150,151]

Reactive oxygen metabolites are produced in small quantities as a result of normal cell metabolism. The profound alterations of cell metabolism that occur during ischemia and reperfusion result in a marked increase in ROS production. The major source of superoxide generation in postischemic tissue appears to be the enzyme xanthine oxidase (XO or type O).[152] The enzyme is synthesized as xanthine dehydrogenase (XD and type D) and under normal conditions accounts for approximately 90% of total activity. XD cannot transfer electrons to molecular oxygen to form superoxide. XO activity appears in ischemic tissue and is most likely the result of partial proteolytic degradation of the XD enzyme.[153] Recent evidence suggests that elevated cytosolic free calcium concentrations that occur during ischemia may activate a calcium-dependant protease which results in conversion from type D to type O activity.[152] Concomitantly, the catabolism of cell ATP during ischemia

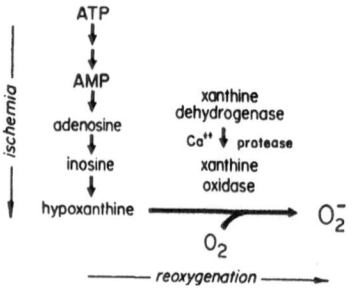

Fig. 5. Proposed mechanism for ischemia-induced production of superoxide and hydrogen peroxide. (Reprinted from McCord, with permission[152].)

results in increased concentrations of purine degradation products, including adenosine, inosine, and hypoxanthine. When molecular oxygen becomes available during reperfusion, XO becomes able to catalyze the one-electron oxidations of hypoxanthine to xanthine and xanthine to uric acid with the generation of a superoxide anion at each step (Fig. 5). Additional sources of ROS generation during reperfusion include aberrant mitochondrial electron transport[154] and, potentially, activation of peripheral blood leukocytes. In this regard, activated phagocytic neutrophils and macrophages are capable of producing a variety of ROS which contribute to their known bactericidal and cytotoxic properties.[155,156]

ROS, because of their reactive nature and rapid interaction with biologic molecules, are extremely difficult to measure accurately. Our knowledge of oxidant-induced damage, including ischemia–reperfusion injury, is largely based on observations of the effects of electrophilic ROS on cell constituents, including lipid peroxidation, glutathione oxidation, and correlation of these values with functional parameters. Development of a cohesive theory that incorporates the known facts about ROS-induced tissue injury has been hampered by the effects of ROS on multiple biologic systems and the limited techniques so far available with which to study these phenomena. Potential mechanisms for ROS-induced cell injury include lipid peroxidation of plasma and subcellular organelle phospholipid membranes, oxidation of protein sulfhydryl groups, and nucleic and acid damage.[149,158,159]

Peroxidation of membrane phospholipid components results in dramatic alterations in membrane structure and function by loss of membrane lipids, production of toxic lipid byproducts,[160] peroxidative damage to adjacent lipoproteins, and activation of membrane phospholipases.[161] Phospholipase activation by lipid peroxides may be particularly damaging because free fatty acids liberated by the action of phospholipases may be more susceptible to further peroxidation and enhanced autocatalytic propagation of lipid peroxidation. The uncontrolled peroxidation of cellular membranes can thus lead to profound effects on membrane structure and function and may be sufficient to cause cell death.[149,159,162,163]

Although lipid peroxidation can be an important pathway leading to cell injury, free radicals can cause oxidation of protein and nonprotein thiol groups, leading to additional changes in cellular enzyme activity. Various oxidants (t-butyl hydroperoxide, menadione) have been shown to cause disruption of calcium homeostasis due to a decline of plasma membrane Ca^{2+}-ATPase activity and inhibition of ATP-dependent microsomal calcium sequestration,[164,165] resulting in a rise in cytosolic free calcium content and loss of cell viability.[166] The injurious effects of these compounds have been linked to depletion of both soluble and protein-bound thiols and were prevented by the sulfhydryl protective agent dithioerythritol.[164,165,167]

Several recent *in vivo* studies support a major role for ROS in the pathogenesis of postischemic renal injury.[168–178] Paller and co-workers[168] evaluated the effects of the superoxide radical scavenger SOD and the hydroxyl radical scavenger dimethylthiourea on renal function after 60-min *in vivo* renal artery occlusion in rats. Each of these agents provided partial protection against renal excretory dysfunction following ischemia and reperfusion. The XO inhibitor allopurinol also provided protection against postischemic acute renal failure when given before the onset of ischemia. Baker and co-workers[170] have subsequently confirmed the protective effects of SOD administered immediately before reperfusion in a similar rat model. In this study, heat-inactivated SOD or SOD administered before ischemia had no protective effect on renal function or rat mortality. SOD has been reported to provide similar protection in a canine kidney warm ischemia model.[169]

Paller and Hebbel[171] have extended earlier observations in the rat renal artery clamp model of ischemia. Using a closed rebreathing apparatus, they measured exhaled ethane as an index of lipid peroxidation after ischemia alone and after ischemia and reperfusion. Ethane production was not significantly increased after ischemia alone, but exhibited striking increases within 10 min of reperfusion after ischemia. The renal source of ethane production was illustrated by subjecting animals to ischemia followed by nephrectomy and demonstrating no postsurgical increase in ethane production in these animals. Allopurinol, 40 mg/kg given before ischemia, completely abolished the reperfusion-induced increase in ethane production. Similarly, SOD, given before ischemia and again before reperfusion, reduced the reperfusion-associated ethane production. Paller[172] has also shown that surgically induced hypothyroidism, as well as exogenous glutathione infusion, both of which result in increased renal glutathione content, partially protected against 60 min of ischemia with reperfusion in this model.

Similar protective effects of allopurinol or SOD treatment have been reported in a swine cold-ischemia model of renal transplantation.[173] Furthermore Green *et al.*[174,175] have reported evidence of ROS-mediated reperfusion injury in rabbit kidneys after 24 hr of cold-ischemia. Deferroximine, mannitol, or uric acid, all of which scavenge ROS, reduced the amount of lipid peroxidation in their model. Unfortunately, correlation of renal functional parameters with lipid peroxidation data was not reported in their studies. The protective effect of ROS scavengers on renal transplant function in another animal model was observed after 24° cold perfusion via an *ex vivo* shunt, but not after the more common clinical practice of flush cooling.[176]

Linas and co-workers[177,178] have studied the impact of ROS during ischemia and reperfusion using graded periods of warm ischemia *in situ* with reperfusion by the isolated perfused kidney technique, measuring renal function and renal cortical glutathione levels following 20, 30, or 45 min of ischemia and 60 min of reperfusion. Increasing duration of ischemia was associated with decreased GFR and tubular Na^+ reabsorption, as well as decreasing cortical glutathione content. Reperfusion with DMTU or dimethylsulfoxide (DMSO)-containing solutions, both effective ROS scavengers, prevented glutathione consumption and attenuated reperfusion-induced renal injury after 20 or 30 min of ischemia. Renal function was not improved after 45 min of ischemia, although glutathione consumption was prevented by DTMU or DMSO. Control experiments using perfusate containing hydrogen peroxide, either preformed or generated by glucose oxidase/glucose, confirmed the specific effect of ROS to deplete renal cortical glutathione concomitantly with functional deterioration. Perfusion with collagenase or elastase produced similar degrees of injury without reducing renal cortical glutathione content.

Treatment with the hypoxanthine oxidase inhibitor allopurinol in renal ischemia models *in vitro* has yielded largely negative results. Negative protective effects with allopurinol have been found during *in vitro* study of isolated proximal tubule segments and in preserved cadaveric kidneys,[179,180] in contrast to positive results in *in vivo* experiments.[168,173,181–183] These findings suggest that the protective effects of allopurinol noted in *in vivo* models of renal ischemia may be due to effects on nephronal processes rather than directly related to its effect on ROS generation.

Most studies of the role of ROS in mediating renal cell injury after ischemia have been accomplished *in vivo,* in which both humoral and hemodynamic factors can influence the outcome of the studies. Recent reports have documented the effects of hypoxia and reoxygenation on isolated renal proximal tubules.[184] Thirty minutes of hypoxia resulted in depletion of cell glutathione, without evidence for increased lipid peroxidation as measured by tubule malondialdehyde (MDA) content. Within 15 min of reoxygenation, however, MDA levels were significantly elevated compared to controls. Functional viability parameters, including potassium and ATP content and respiratory rate, decreased after hypoxia and then gradually returned to control values, while MDA levels remained elevated. In this model, supplementation of tubule suspensions with exogenous glutathione ameliorated injury after hypoxia and reoxygenation, but effected only marginal declines in tubule MDA levels.[185] Furthermore, glutathione depletion did not potentiate the degree of cell injury produced by hypoxia and reoxygenation.[106] These *in vitro* studies suggest that ROS are generated by renal tubule epithelia during reoxygenation after hypoxia, but their pathogenetic role in renal tubular dysfunction after ischemia and reperfusion remains uncertain.

In summary, much recent evidence suggests that reactive oxygen species are generated in renal tissue during reperfusion after ischemia. Discrepant results from *in vivo* and *in vitro* studies, however, cast doubt on the specific role of ROS in the pathophysiology of postischemic acute renal failure. Further studies, both *in vivo* and *in vitro,* are required to clarify the magnitude and specific location of ROS-induced renal cell injury after ischemia and reperfusion, and to assess the specific hemodynamic and humoral effects of these reactive molecules on renal tissue.

References

1. Shusterman, N., Strom, B. L., Murray, T. G., Morrison, G., West, S. L., and Maislin, G., 1987, Risk factors and outcome of hospital-acquired acute renal failure, *Am. J. Med.* **83:**65–71.
2. Hou, S. H., Bushinsky, D. A., Wish, J. B., Cohen, J. J., and Harrington, J. T., 1983, Hospital-acquired renal insufficiency: A prospective study, *Am. J. Med.* **74:**243–248.
3. Eisenberg, J. M., Koffer, H., Glick, H. A., Connell, M. L., Loss, L. E., Talbot, G. H., Shusterman, N. H., and Strom, B. L., 1987, What is the cost of nephrotoxicity associated with aminoglycosides? *Ann. Intern. Med.* **107:**900–909.
4. Moran, S. M. and Myers, B. D., 1985, Pathophysiology of protracted acute renal failure in man, *J. Clin. Invest.* **76:**1440–1448.
5. The Canadian Multicentre Transplant Study Group, 1986, A randomized clinical trial of cyclosporine in cadaveric renal transplantation, *N. Engl. J. Med.* **314:**1219–1225.
6. Flechner, S. M., Payne, W. D., Van Buren, C., Kerman, R., and Kahan, B. D., 1983, The effect of cyclosporine on early graft function in human renal transplantation, *Transplantation* **36:**268–272.
7. Bia, M. J. and Tyler, K. A., 1987, Effect of cyclosporine on renal ischemic injury, *Transplantation* **43:**800–804.
8. Kahan, B. D. (ed.), 1985, Cyclosporine-associated renal injury, *Transpl. Proc.* **17:**185–196.
9. Sommer, B. G., Innes, J. T., Whitehurst, R. M., Sharma, H. M., and Ferguson, R. M., Cyclosporine-associated renal arteriopathy resulting in loss of allograft function, *Am. J. Surg.* **149:** 756–764.
10. Myers, B. D., Ross, J., Newton, L., Luetscher, J., and Perlroth, M., 1984, Cyclosporine-associated chronic nephrology, *N. Engl. J. Med.* **311:**699–705.
11. Palestine, A. G., Austin, H. A., III, Balow, J. E., Antonovych, T. T., Sabnis, S. G., Preuss, H. G., and Nussenblatt, R. B., 1986, Renal histopathologic alterations in patients treated with cyclosporine for uveitis, *N. Engl. J. Med.* **314:**1293–1298.
12. Myers, B. D., Sibley, R., Newton, L., Tomlanovich, S. J., Boshkos, C., Stinson, E., Luetscher, J. A., Whitney, D. J., Krasny, D., Coplon, N. S., and Perlroth, M. G., 1988, The long-term course of cyclosporine-associated chronic nephropathy, *Kidney Int.* **33:**590–600.
13. European Multicentre Trial, 1982, Cyclosporine A as sole immunosuppressive agent in recipients of kidney allografts from cadaver donors, *Lancet* **2:**57–60.
14. Najarian, J. S., Strand, M., Fryd, D. S., *et al.,* 1983, Comparison of cyclosporine versus azathioprine-antilymphocyte globulin in renal transplantation, *Transpl. Proc.* **15:**438–441.
15. Adu, D., Turney, M. J., *et al.,* 1983, Hyperkalemia in cyclosporine-treated renal allograft recipients, *Lancet,* **2:**370–372.
16. Bantle, J. P., Nath, K. A., Sutherland, D. E. R., Najarian, J. S., and Ferris, T. F., 1985, Effect of cyclosporine on the renin–angiotensin system and potassium excretion in renal transplant recipients, *Arch. Intern. Med.* **145:**505–508.
17. June, C. H., Thompson, C. B., Kennedy, M. S., Nims, J., and Thomas, E. D., 1985, Profound hypomagnesemia and renal magnesium wasting associated with the use of cyclosporine for marrow transplantation, *Transplantation* **39:**620–624.
18. Barton, C. H., Vaziri, N. D., Martin, D. C., *et al.,* 1987, Hypomagnesemia and renal magnesium wasting in renal transplant recipients receiving cyclosporine, *Am. J. Med.* **83:**693–699.
19. Bellet, M., Carbol, C., Sassano, P., Leger, P., Corvol, P., and Menard, J., 1985, Systemic hypertension after cardiac transplantation: Effect of cyclosporine on the renin-angiotensin-aldosterone system, *Am. J. Cardiol.* **56:**927–931.
20. Baxter, C. R., Duggin, G. G., Willis, N. S., Hall, B. M., Horvath, J. S., and Tiller, D. J., 1982, Cyclosporine A-induced increases in renin storage and release, *Res. Commun. Chem. Pathol. Pharmacol.* **37:**305–312.
21. Murray, B. M., Paller, M. S., and Ferris, T. F., 1985, Effect of acute and chronic cyclosporine administration on renal hemodynamics in conscious rats, *Kidney Int.* **28:**767–774.

22. Thompson, M. E., Shapiro, A. P., Johnson, A. M., Reeves, R., Itzkoff, J., Ginchereau, E., Hardesty, R. L., Griffith, B. L., Bahnson, H. T., and McDonald, R., Jr., 1983, New onset of hypertension following cardiac transplantation: A preliminary report and analysis, *Transpl. Proc.* **15:**2573–2577.

23. Chapman, J. R., Marcen, R., Arias, M., Raine, A. E. G., Dunnill, M. S., and Morris, P. J., 1987, Hypertension after renal transplantation, *Transplantation* **43:**860–864.

24. Maurer, G., Loosli, H. R., Schrier, E., and Keller, B., 1984, Disposition of cyclosporine in several animal species and man. Structural elucidation of its metabolites, *Drug. Disposal Metab.* **12:**120–126.

25. Jensen, C. W. B., Flechner, S. M., Van Buren, C. T., Frazier, O. H., Cooley, D. A., Lorber, M. I., and Kahan, B. D., 1987, Exacerbation of cyclosporine toxicity by concomitant administration of erythromycin, *Transplantation* **43:**263–270.

26. White, D. J. G., Blatchford, N. R., and Cauwenbergh, G., 1984, Cyclosporine and ketoconazole, *Transplantation* **37:**214–215.

27. Modry, D. L., Stinson, E. B., Oyer, P. E., Jamieson, S. W., Baldwin, J. C., *et al.*, 1985, Acute rejection and massive cyclosporine requirements in heart transplant recipients treated with rafampin, *Transplantation* **39:**313–314.

28. Freeman, D. J., Laupacis, A., Keown, P. A., Stiller, C. R., and Carruthers, S. G., 1984, Evaluation of cyclosporin-phenytoin interaction with observations on cyclosporin metabolites, *Br. J. Clin. Pharmacol.* **18:**887–893, 1984.

29. Veremus, S. A., Maddux, M. S., Pollak, R., and Mozes, M. F., 1987, Subtherapeutic cylosporine concentrations during nafcillin therapy, *Transplantation* **43:**913–915.

30. Ross, W. B., Roberts, D., Griffin, P. J. A., and Salaman, J. R., 1986, Cyclosporine interaction with danazol and norethisterone, *Lancet* **2:**330.

31. Moller, B. B. and Ekelund, B., 1985, Toxicity of cyclosporine during treatment of androgens, *N. Engl. J. Med.* **313:**1416.

32. Maurer, G., 1985, Metabolism of cyclosporine, *Transplant Proc.* **17**(Suppl. 1):19–26.

33. Renton, K. W., 1985, Inhibition of hepatic microsomal drug metabolism by the calcium channel blockers diltiazem and verapamil, *Biochem. Pharmacol.* **34:**2, 549–553.

34. Grino, J. M., Sebate, I., Castelao, A. M., and Alsina, J., 1986, Influence of diltiazem on cyclosporine clearance, *Lancet* **1:**1387.

35. Bourbigot, B., Guiserix, J., Bressollette, L., Morin, J. F., and Cledes, J., 1986, Nicardipine increases cyclosporine blood levels, *Lancet* **1:**1447.

36. Lindholm, A. and Henricsson, S., 1987, Verapamil inhibits cyclosporine metabolism, *Lancet* **1:** 1262–1263.

37. Iaina, A., Herzog, D., Cohen, D., *et al.*, 1986, Calcium entry-blockade with verapamil in cyclosporine A plus ischemia induced acute renal failure in rats, *Clin. Nephrol.* **25**(Suppl. 1): S168–S170.

38. Puurunen, J. and Pelkonen, O., 1984, Cimetidine inhibits microsomal drug metabolism in the rat, *Eur. J. Pharmacol.* **5:**214–215.

39. Wadhwa, N. K., Schroeder, T. J., O'Flaherty, E., Pesce, A. J., Myre, S. A., and First, M. R., 1987, The effect of oral metoclopramide on the absorption of cyclosporine, *Transplantation* **43:** 211–213.

40. Kennedy, M. S., Deeg, H. J., Siegel, M., Crowley, J. J., Storb, R., and Thomas, E. D., 1983, Acute renal toxicity with combined use of amphotericin B and cyclosporine after marrow transplantation, *Transplantation* **35:**211–215.

41. Whiting, P. H., Simpson, J. G., Davidson, R. J. L., and Thomson, A. W., 1982, The toxic effects of combined administration of cyclosporin A and gentamicin, *Br. J. Exp. Pathol.* **63:**554–561.

42. Dale, B. M., Sage, R. E., Norman, J. E., Barber, S., and Kotasek, D., 1985, Bone marrow transplantation following treatment with high-dose melphalan, *Transplant Proc.* **17**(2):1711–1713.

43. Thompson, J. F., Chalmers, D. H. K., Hunnisett, A. G. W., Wood, R. F. M., and Morris, P. J., 1983, Nephrotoxicity of trimethoprim and cotrimoxazole in renal allograft recipients treated with cyclosporin, *Transplantation* **36:**204–206.

44. Jackson, N. M., Hsu, C. H., Visscher, G. E., Venkatachalam, M. A., and Humes, H. D., 1987, Alterations in renal structure and function in a rat model of cyclosporine nephrotoxicity, *J. Pharmacol. Exp. Ther.* **242:**749–756.

45. Murray, B. M., Paller, M. S., and Ferris, T. F., 1985, Effects of cyclosporine administration on renal hemodynamics in conscious rats, *Kidney Int.*, **28:**767–774.

46. Moss, N. G., Rowell, S. L., and Falk, R. J., 1985, Intravenous cyclosporine activates afferent and efferent renal nerves and causes sodium retention in innervated kidneys in rats, *Proc. Natl. Acad. Sci. USA* **82:**8222–8226.

47. Xue, H., Bukoski, R. D., McCarron, D. A., and Bennett W. M., 1987, Induction of contraction in isolated rat aorta by cyclosporine, *Transplantation* **43:**715–718.

48. Pfeilschifter, J. and Ruegg, U. T., 1987, Cyclosporin A augments angiotensin II-stimulated rise in intracellular free calcium in vascular smooth muscle cells, *Biochem. J.* **248:**883–887.

49. Barros, E. J. G., Boim, M. A., Ajzen, H., Ramos, O. L., and Schor, N., 1987, Glomerular hemodynamics and hormonal participation on cyclosporine nephrotoxicity, *Kidney Int.* **32:**19–25.

50. Kaskel, F. J., Devarajan, P., Arbeit, L. A., Partin, J. S., and Moore, L. C., 1987, Cyclosporine nephrotoxicity: Sodium excretion, autoregulation, and angiotensin II, *Am. J. Physiol.*, **252** (Renal Fluid Electrolyte Physiol. **21**):F733–F744.

51. Perico, N., Benigni, A., Zoja, C., Delaini, F., and Remuzzi, G., 1986, Functional significance of exaggerated renal thromboxane A_2 synthesis induced by cyclosporine A, *Am. J. Physiol.* **251** (*Renal Fluid Electrolyte Physiol.* **20**):F581–F587.

52. Coffman, T. M., Carr, D. R., Yarger, W. E., and Klotman, P. E., 1987, Evidence that renal prostaglandin and thromboxane production is stimulated in chronic cyclosporine nephrotoxicity, *Transplantation* **43:**282–285.

53. Elzinga, L., Kelley, V. E., Houghton, D. C., and Bennett, W. M., 1987, Modification of experimental nephrotoxicity with fish oil as the vehicle for cyclosporine, *Transplantation* **43:**271–274.

54. Kurtz, A., Pfeilschifter, J., Kuhn, K., and Koche, K. M., 1987, *Biochem. Biophys. Res. Commun.* **147:**542–549.

55. Zoja, C., Furci, L., Ghilardi, F., Zilio, P., Benigni, A., and Remuzzi, G., 1986, Cyclosporine-induced endothelial cell injury, *Lab. Invest.* **55:**455–462, 1986.

56. Grace, A. A., Barradas, M. A., Mikhaildis, D. P., Jeremy, J. Y., Moorhead, J. F., Sweny, P., and Dandona, P., 1987, Cyclosporine A enhances platelet aggregation, *Kidney Int.* **32:**889–895.

57. Bertani, T., Perico, N., Abbate, M., Battaglia, C., and Remuzzi, G., 1987, Renal injury induced by long-term administration of cyclosporine A to rats, *Am. J. Pathol.* **127:**569–579.

58. Huang, W. Y., Lipsey, A. I., and Cheng, M. H., 1987, Comparison of cyclosporine determinations in whole blood by three different methods, *Am. J. Clin. Pathol.* **87:**528–532.

59. Diethelm, A. G., 1986, Clinical diagnosis and management of the renal transplant recipient with cyclosporine nephrotoxicity, *Transpl. Proc.* **18:**82–87.

60. Carpenter, C. B., Milford, E. L., Kirkman, R. L., Strom, T. B., Lazarus, J. M., and Tilney, N. L., 1985, Stability of renal allograft recipients after conversion from cyclosporine to azathioprine, *Transpl. Proc.* **17:**261–265.

61. Flechner, S. M., Lorber, M., Van Buren, C., Kerman, R., and Kahan, B. D., 1985, The case against conversion to azathoprine in cyclosporine-treated renal recipients, *Transpl. Proc.* **17:**276–281.

62. Simmons, R. L., Canafax, D. M., Strand, M., Ascher, N. L., Payne, W. S., Sutherland, D. E. R., and Najarian, J. S., 1985, Management and prevention of cyclosporine nephrotoxicity after renal transplantation: Use of low doses of cyclosporine, azathioprine, and prednisone, *Transpl. Proc.* **17:**266–275.

63. Lorber, M. I., Flechner, S. M., Van Buren, C. T., Sorensen, K., Kerman, R. H., and Kahan, B., 1987, Cyclosporine Toxicity: The effect of combined therapy using cyclosporine, azathioprine and prednisone, *Am. J. Kidney Dis.* **9:**476–484.

64. Moore, R. D., Smith, C. R., Lipsky, T. J., Mellits, E. D., and Lietman, P. S., 1984, Risk factors for nephrotoxicity in patients treated with aminoglycosides, *Ann. Intern. Med.* **100:**352–357.

65. Cabrera, J. Arroyo, V., Ballesta, A., Rimola, A., Gual, J., Elena, M., and Rodes, J., 1982, Aminoglycoside nephrotoxicity in cirrhosis. Value of urinary B_2-microglobulin to discriminate functional renal failure from acute tubular damage, *Gastroenterology* **82:**97–105.

66. Kourilsky, O., Solez, K., Morel-Maroger, L., Whelton, A., Duhoux, P., and Sraer, J. D., 1982, The pathology of acute renal failure due to interstitial nephritis in man, with comments on the role of interstitial inflammation and sex in gentamicin nephrotoxicity, *Medicine* **61:**258–268.

67. Lietman, P. S. and Smith, C. R., 1983, Aminoglycoside nephrotoxicity in humans, *Rev. Infect. Dis.* **5:**S284.

68. Kahlmeter, G. and Dahlager, J., 1984, Aminoglycoside toxicity—A review of clinical studies published between 1975 and 1982, *J. Antimicrob. Chemother.* **13**(Suppl. A):9–22.

69. Lerner, S. A., Seligsohn, R., and Matz, G. J., 1977, Comparative clinical studies of ototoxicity and nephrotoxicity of amikacin and gentamicin, *Am. J. Med.* **62:**919.

70. Holm, S. E., Hill, B., Lowestad, R., Maller, R., and Vikerfors, T. A., 1983, A prospective randomized study of amikacin and gentamicin in serious injections with focus on efficacy, toxicity and duration of serum levels above the MIC, *J. Antimicrob. Chemother.* **12:**393–402.

71. DeBroe, M. E., Paulus, G. J., Verprooten, G. A., Roels, F., Buyssens, N., Weden, R., VanHoot, F., and Tulkens, P. M., 1984, Early effects of gentamicin, tobramycin and amikacin on the human kidney, *Kidney Int.* **25:**643–652.

72. Luft, F. C., Yum, M. N., and Kleit, S. A., 1976, Comparative nephrotoxicities of netilmicin and gentamicin in rats, *Antimicrob. Agents Chemother.* **10:**845–849.

73. Soberon, L., Bowman, R. L., Pasoriza-Munoz, E., and Kaloyanides, G. J., 1979, Comparative nephrotoxicities of gentamicin, netilmicin and tobramycin in the rat, *J. Pharmacol. Exp. Ther.* **210:**334–343.

74. Lerner, A. M., Cone, L. A., Jansen, W., Reyes, M. P., Blair, D. C., Wright, G. E., and Lorber, R. R., 1983, Randomized, controlled trial of the comparative efficacy, auditory toxicity and nephrotoxicity of tobramycin and netilmicin, *Lancet* **1:**1123–1126.

75. Daschner, F. D., Just, A. M., Jansen, W., and Lorber, R., 1984, Netilmicin versus tobramycin and multicentre studies, *J. Antimicrob. Chemother.* **13**(A):37–45.

76. Knauss, T. C., Weinberg, J. M., and Humes, H. D., 1983, Alterations in renal cortical phospholipid content induced by gentamicin: Time course, specificity and subcellular localization, *Am. J. Physiol.* **224:**F535–F546.

77. Schwertz, D. W., Kreisberg, J. I., and Venkatachalam, M. A., 1984, Effects of aminoglycosides on proximal tubule brush border membrane phosphatidylinositol-specific phospholipase C, *J. Pharmacol. Exp. Ther.* **231:**48.

78. Sastrasinh, M., Knauss, T. C., Weinberg, J. M., and Humes, H. D., 1982, Identification of the aminoglycoside binding site in rat renal brush border membranes, *J. Pharmacol. Exp. Ther.* **222:**350–358.

79. Schacht, J., 1979, Isolation of an aminoglycoside receptor from guinea pig inner ear tissues and kidney, *Arch. Otorhinolaryngol.* **224:**129–134.

80. Schibeci, A. and Schacht, J., 1977, Action of neomycin on the metabolism of polyphosphoinositides in the guinea pig kidney, *Biochem. Pharmacol.* **26:**1769–1774.

81. Marche, P., Koutouzov, S., and Girard, A., 1983, Impairment of membrane phosphoinositide metabolism by aminoglycoside antibiotics: Streptomycin, amikacin, kanamycin, dibekacin, gentamicin and neomycin, *J. Pharmacol. Exp. Ther.* **227:**415–420.

82. Berridge, M. J., 1984, Inositol triphosphate and diacylglycerol as second messengers, *Biochem. J.* **220:**345–360.

83. Kirschbaum, B. B., 1984, Interactions between renal brush border membranes and polyamines, *J. Pharmacol. Exp. Ther.* **229:**409–416.

84. Josepovitz, C., Pastoriza-Munoz, E., Timmerman, D., Scott, M., Feldman, S., and Kaloyanides, G. J., 1982, Inhibition of gentamicin uptake in rat renal cortex in vivo by aminoglycosides and organic polycations, *J. Pharmacol. Exp. Ther.* **223:**314–321.

85. Brasseur, R., Laurent, G., Raysschaert, J. M. and Tulkens, P., 1984, Interactions of aminoglycoside antibiotics with negatively charged lipid layers: Biochemical and conformational studies, *Biochem. Pharmacol.* **33:**629–637.

86. Weinberg, J. M. and Humes, H. D., 1980, Mechanisms of gentamicin-induced dysfunction of renal cortical mitochondria. I. Effects on mitochondrial respiration, *Arch. Biochem. Biophys.* **205:**222–231.

87. Weinberg, J. M., Harding, P. G., and Humes, H. D., 1980, Mechanisms of gentamicin-induced dysfunction of renal cortical mitochondria. II. Effects on monovalent cation transport, *Arch. Biochem. Biophys.* **205:**232–239.

88. Walker, P. D. and Shah, S. V., 1987, Gentamicin enhanced production of hydrogen peroxide by renal cortical mitochondria, *Am. J. Physiol.* **253:**C495–C499.

89. Walker, P. D. and Shah, S. V., 1988, Evidence suggesting a role for hydroxyl radical in gentamicin-induced acute renal failure in rats, *J. Clin. Invent.* **81:**334–341.

90. Josepovitz, J. C., Pastoriza-Munoz, E., Timmerman, D., Scott, M., Feldman, S., and Kaloyanides, G. J., 1982, Inhibition of gentamicin uptake in rat renal cortex in vivo by aminoglycosides and organic polycations, *J. Pharmacol. Exp. Ther.* **223:**314–321.

91. Humes, H. D., Sastrasinh, M., and Weinberg, J. M., 1984, Calcium is a competitive inhibitor of gentamicin-renal membrane binding interactions and dietary calcium supplementation protects against gentamicin nephrotoxicity, *J. Clin. Invest.* **73:**134–147.

92. Bennett, W. M., Elliott, C. W., Houghton, D. C., Gilbert, D. N., Defehr, J., and McCarron, D. A., 1982, Reduction of experimental gentamicin neophrotoxicity in rats by dietary calcium loading, *Antimicrob. Agents Chemother.* **22:**503–512.

93. Williams, P. D., Hottendorf, G. H., and Bennett, D. B., 1986, Inhibition of renal membrane binding and nephrotoxicity of aminoglycosides, *J. Pharmacol. Exp. Ther.* **237:**919–925.

94. Swanson, D. P., Dick, T. J., Simms, S. M. *et al.*, 1985, Product selection criteria for intravascular ionic contrast media, *Clin. Pharmacol.* **4:**527–538.

95. Grainger, R. G., 1980, Osmolality of intravascular radiological contrast media, *Br. J. Radiol.* **53:**739–746.

96. Dawson, P., 1984, New contrast agents: Chemistry and pharmacology, *Invest. Radiol.* **19**(Suppl.): S298–S300.

97. Golman, K., Olivecrona, H., Gustafson, C., *et al.*, 1980, Excitation and depression of non-anesthetized rabbits following injection of contrast media into the subarachnoid space, *Acta. Radiol.* **362**(Suppl):83–86.

98. Humes, H. D. and Nguyen, V. D., 1987, Acute renal failure and toxic nephropathy, *Contemp. Nephr.* **4:**401–462.

99. Arend, L. J., Bakris, G. L., Burnett, J. C. Jr., *et al.*, 1987, Role for intrarenal adenosine in the renal hemodynamic response to contrast media, *J. Lab. Clin. Med.* **110:**406–411.

100. Lund, H. G., Einzig, S., Rysavy, J., *et al.*, 1984, Effect of prostaglandin inhibition on the renal vascular response to ionic and non-ionic contrast media in the dog, *Acta Radiol. Diag.* **25:**407–510.

101. Katzberg, R. W., Morris, T. W., Lasser, E. C., *et al.*, 1986, Acute systemic and renal hemodynamic effects of meglumine/sodium diatrizoate 75% and iopamidol in euvolemic and dehydrated dogs, *Invest. Radiol.* **21:**793–797.

102. Messana, J. P., Cieslinski, D. A., Nguyen, V. D., and Humes, H. D., 1988, Comparison of the toxicity of the radiocontrast agents, iopamidol and diatrizoate, to rabbit renal proximal tubule cells in vitro, *J. Pharmacol. Exp. Therap.* **244:**1139–1144.

H. DAVID HUMES and JOSEPH M. MESSANA

103. Humes, H. D., Cieslinski, D. A., and Messana, J. M., 1987, Pathogenesis of radiocontrast-induced acute renal failure: Comparative nephrotoxicity of diatrizoate and iopamidol, *Diagn. Imaging* (Suppl.):12–18, May.
104. Lund, G., Eihzig, S., Rysavy, J., *et al.*, 1984, Role of ischemia in contrast-induced renal damage: An experimental study, *Circulation* **69**:783–789.
105. Weinberg, J. M. and Humes, H. D., 1983, Renal tubule cell integrity during mercuric chloride and gentamicin nephrotoxicity, in: *Acute Renal Failure: Correlation between Morphology and Function* (K. Solez and A. Whelton, Eds.), Marcel Dekker, New York, pp. 179–194.
106. Venkatachalam, M. A., 1981, Morphologic factors in acute renal failure, in: *Acute Renal Failure* (B. M. Brenner and J. H. Stein, Eds.), Churchill Livingstone, New York, pp. 79–107.
107. Brezis, M., Rosen, S., Silva, P., and Epstein, F. H., 1984, Selective vulnerability of the medullary thick ascending limb to anoxia in the isolated perfused rat kidney, *J. Clin. Invest.* **73**:182–189.
108. Humes, H. D. and Weinberg, J. M., 1983, Alterations in renal tubular cell metabolism in acute renal failure, *Mineral Electrolyte Metab.* **9**:290–305.
109. Humes, H. D. and Weinberg, J. M., 1983, Cellular energetics in acute renal failure, in: *Acute Renal Failure* (B. M. Brenner and J. M. Lazarus, Eds.), Saunders, Philadelphia, pp. 47–98.
110. Siegel, M., Rice, J., Barnes, J., Osgood, R., and Stein, J., 1983, Protective effect of mini dose ouabain in ischemic renal failure in the dog, *Clin. Res.* **31**:518A.
111. Weinberg, J. M., 1985, Oxygen deprivation–induced injury to isolated rabbit kidney tubules, *J. Clin. Invest.* **76**:1193–1208.
112. Brezis, M., Rosen, S., Silva, P., Spokes, K., and Epstein, F. H., 1984, Polyene toxicity in renal medulla: Injury mediated by transport activity, *Science* **224**:66–68.
113. Gaudio, K. M., Taylor, M. R., Chaudry, I. H., Kashgarian, M., and Siegel, N. J., 1982, Accelerated recovery of single nephron function by the post ischemic infusion of ATP-MGCl$_2$, *Kidney Int.* **22**:13–20.
114. Gaudio, K. M., Ardito, T. A., Reilly, H. F., Kashgarian, M., and Siegel, N. J., 1983, Accelerated cellular recovery after ischemic renal injury, *Am. J. Pathol.* **112**:338–346.
115. Siegel, N. J., Glazier, W. B., Chaudry, I. H., Gaudin, K. M., Lytton, B., Baue, A. E., and Kashgarian, M., 1980, Enhanced recovery from acute renal failure by the postischemic infusion of adenine nucleotides and magnesium chloride in rats, *Kidney Int.* **17**:338–349.
116. Weinberg, J. M. and Humes, H. D., 1986, Increases of cell ATP produced by exogenous adenine nucleotides in isolated rabbit renal tubules, *Am. J. Physiol.* **250**:F720–F733.
117. Venkatachalam, M. A., Patel, Y. J., Kreisberg, J. I., and Weinberg, J. M., 1988, Energy thresholds that determine membrane integrity and injury in a renal epithelial cell line (LLC-PK$_1$), Relationships to phospholipid degradation and unesterified fatty acid accumulation, *J. Clin. Invest.* **31**:745–758.
118. Nguyen, V. D., Cieslinski, D. A., and Humes, H. D., 1988, Importance of adenosine triphosphate in phospholipase A$_2$ induced rabbit renal proximal tubule cell injury, *J. Clin. Invest.* **82**:1098–1105.
119. Weinberg, J. M., 1988, Adenine nucleotide metabolism by isolated kidney tubules during oxygen deprivation, *Biochem. Med. Met. Biol.* **39**: 319–329.
120. Epps, D. E., Palmer, J. W., Schmid, H. H. O., and Pfeiffer, D. R., 1982, Inhibition of permeability-dependent Ca^{2+} release from mitochondria by N-acylethanolamines, a class of lipids synthesized in ischemic heart tissues, *J. Biol. Chem.* **257**:1383–1391.
121. Beatrice, M. C., Palmer, J. W., and Pfeiffer, D. R., 1980, The relationship between mitochondrial membrane permeability, membrane potential, and the retention of Ca^{2+} by mitochondria hydroperoxide, *J. Biol. Chem.* **255**:8663–8671.
122. Beatrice, M. C., Stiers, D. L., and Pfeiffer, D. R., 1982, Increased permeability of mitochondria during Ca^{2+} release induced by t-butyl hydroperoxide or oxalacetate, the effect of ruthenium red, *J. Biol. Chem.* **257**:7161–7170.
123. Chien, K. R., Abrams, J., Serroni, A. *et al.*, 1978, Accelerated phospholipid degradation and

associated membrane dysfunction in irreversible, ischemic liver cell injury, *J. Biol. Chem.* **253:** 4809–4817.

124. Humes, H. D., 1986, Role of calcium in pathogenesis of acute renal failure, *Am. J. Physiol.* **250:** F579–F589.

125. Weinberg, J. M. and Humes, H. D., 1985, Calcium transport and inner mitochondrial membrane damage in renal cortical mitochondria, *Am. J. Physiol.* **248:**F876–F889.

126. Broekemeier, K. M., Schmid, P. C., Schmid, H. H., and Pfeiffer, D. R., 1985, Effects of phospholipase A_2 inhibitors on ruthenium red-induced Ca^{2+} release from mitochondria, *J. Biol. Chem.* **260:**105–113.

127. Okayasu, T., Curtis, M. T., and Farber, J. L., 1985, Structural alterations of the inner mitochondrial membrane in ischemic liver cell injury, *Arch. Biochem. Biophys.* **236:**638–645.

128. Palmer, J. W., Schmid, P. C., Pfeiffer, D. R., and Schmid, H. O., 1981, Lipids and lipolytic enzyme activities of rat heart mitochondria, *Arch. Biochem. Biophys.* **221:**674–682.

129. Malis, C. D. and Bonventre, J. V., 1986, Mechanism of calcium potentiation of oxygen free radical injury to renal mitochondria, *J. Biol. Chem.* **261:** 14201–14208.

130. Braughler, J. M., Duncan, L. A., and Goodman, T. J., 1985, Calcium enhances in vitro free radical-induced damage to brain synaptosomes, mitochondria, and cultured spinal cord neurons, *J. Neurochem.* **45:**1288–1293.

131. Au, A. M., Chan, P. H., and Fishman, R. A., 1985, Stimulation of phospholipase A_2 activity by oxygen-derived free radicals in isolated brain capillaries, *J. Cell Biochem.* **27:**449–453.

132. DiMonte, D., Bellomo, G., Thor, H., Nicotera, P., and Orrenius, S., 1984, Menadione-induced cytotoxicity is associated with protein thiol oxidation and alteration in intracellular Ca^{2+} homeostasis, *Arch. Biochem. Biophys.* **235:**343–350.

133. Weglicki, W. B., Dickens, B. F., and Mak, I. T., 1984, Enhanced lysosomal phospholipid degradation and lysophospholipid production due to free radicals, *Biochem. Biophys. Res. Commun.* **124:**229–235.

134. Sevanian, A., Stein, R. A., and Mead, J. F., 1981, Metabolism of epoxidized phosphatidylcholine by phospholipase A_2 and epoxide hydrolase, *Lipids* **16:**781–789.

135. Humes, H. D. and Weinberg, J. M., 1986, Toxic nephropathies, in: *The Kidney,* 3rd ed. (B. M. Brenner and F. C. Rector, Eds.), Saunders, Philadelphia, pp. 1491–1532.

136. Nohl, H., Jordan, W., and Youngman, R. J., 1986, Quinones in biology: Function in electron transfer and oxygen activation, *Adv. Free Radical Biol. Med.* **2:**211–279.

137. Mak, I. T., Kramer, J. H. and Weglicki, W. B., 1986, Potentiation of free radical-induced lipid peroxidative injury to sarcolemmal membranes by lipid amphiphiles, *J. Biol. Chem.* **261:**1153–1157.

138. Cross, Carroll E., Halliwell, B., Borish, E. T., Pryor, W. A., Ames, B. N., Saul, R. L., McCord, J. M., and Harman, D. 1987, Oxygen radicals and human disease, *Ann. Intern. Med.* **107:**526–545.

139. Baud, L. and Ardaillou, R., 1986, Reactive oxygen species: Production and role in the kidney, *Am. J. Physiol.* **251:**F765–F776.

140. Ward, P. A., Johnson, K. J. and Till, G. O., 1986, Oxygen radicals and microvascular injury of lungs and kidneys, *Acta Physiol. Scand.* **548**(Suppl.):79–85.

141. Ratych, R. E. and Bulkey, G. B., 1986, Free-radical-mediated postischemic reperfusion injury in the kidney, *J. Free Radical Biol. Med.* **2:**311–319.

142. Fridovich, I., 1978, The biology of oxygen radicals. The superoxide radical is an agent of oxygen toxicity: Superoxide dismutases provide an important defense, *Science* **201:**875–880.

143. McCord, J. M. and Fridovich, I., 1978, The biology and pathology of oxygen radicals, *Ann. Intern. Med.* **89:**122–127.

144. Fridovich, I., 1983, Superoxide radical: An endogenous toxicant, *Annu. Rev. Pharmacol. Toxicol.* **23:**239–257.

145. Reed, D. J. and Fariss, M., 1984, Glutathione depletion and susceptibility, *Pharmacol. Rev.* **36**(2):25S–33S.

146. Suttorp, N., Toepfer, W., and Roka, L., 1986, Antioxidant defense mechanisms of endothelial cells: Glutathione redox cycle versus catalase, *Am. J. Physiol.* **251:**C671–C680.

147. Jones, D. P., Eklow, L., Thor, H., and Orrenous, S., 1981, Metabolism of hydrogen peroxide in isolated hepatocytes: Relative contributions of catalase and glutathione peroxidase in decomposition of endogenously generated H_2O_2, *Arch. Biochem. Biophys.* **210**(2):505–516.

148. Eklow, L., Moldeus, P., and Orrenous, S., 1984, Oxidation of glutathione during hydroperoxide metabolism, *Eur. J. Biochem.* **138:**459–463.

149. Freeman, B. A. and Crapo, J. D., 1982, Free radicals and tissue injury, *Lab. Invest.* **47:**412–426.

150. Guarnieri, C., Flamigni, F., and Caldarere, C. M., 1980, Role of oxygen in the cellular damage induced by re-oxygenation of hypoxic heart, *J. Mol. Cell. Cardiol.* **12:**797–808.

151. Liu, J., Simon, L. W., Phillips, J. R., and Robin, E. D., 1977, Superoxide dismutase activity in hypoxic mammalian systems, *J. Appl. Physiol.* **42:**107–110.

152. McCord, J. M., 1985, Oxygen-derived free radicals in postischemic tissue injury, *N. Engl. J. Med.* **312:**159–163.

153. Engerson, T. D., McDelvey, T. G., Rhyne, D. B., Boggio, E. B., Snyder, S. J., and Jones, H. P., 1987, Conversion of xanthine dehydrogenase to oxidase in ischemic rat tissue, *J. Clin. Invest.* **79:** 1564–1570.

154. Nohl, H. and Jordan, W., 1986, The mitochondrial site of superoxide formation, *Biochem. Biophys. Res. Commun.* **138**(2):533–539.

155. Weiss, S. J. and Silvka, A., 1981, Monocyte and granulocyte-mediated tumor cell destruction, *J. Clin. Invest.* **69:**255–262.

156. Klebanoff, S. J., 1980, Oxygen metabolism and the toxic properties of phagocytes, *Ann. Intern. Med.* **93:**480–489.

157. Gibson, D. D., Hawrylko, J., and McCay, P. B., 1985, GSH-dependant inhibition of lipid peroxidation: Properties of a potent cytosolic system which protects cell membranes, *Lipids* **20**(10):704–411.

158. Del Maestro, R. F., 1980, An approach to free radicals in medicine and biology, *Acta Physiol. Scand.* **492:**153–168.

159. Slater, T. F., 1984, Free-radical mechanisms in tissue injury, *Biochem. J.* **222:**1–15.

160. Sevanian, A. and Hochstein, P., 1985, Mechanisms and consequences of lipid peroxidation in biological systems, *Annu. Rev. Nutr.* **5:**365–390.

161. Sevanian, A. and Kim, E., 1985, Phospholipase A_2 dependant release of fatty acids from peroxidized membranes, *J. Free Rad. Biol. Med.* **1:**263–271.

162. Maridonneau, I., Braquet, P., and Garay, R. P., 1983, Na^+ and K^+ transport damage induced by oxygen free radicals in human red cell membranes, *J. Biol. Chem.* **258:**3107–3113.

163. Curtis, M. T., Gilfor, D., and Farber, J. L., 1984, Lipid peroxidation increases the molecular order of microsomal membranes, *Arch. Biochem. Biophys.* **235:**644–649.

164. Bellomo, G., Mirabelli, F., and Orrenius, S., 1983, Critical role of sulfhydryl group(s) in ATP-dependent $Ca++$ sequestration by the plasma membrane fraction from rat liver, *FEBS Lett.* **163:** 136–139.

165. Nicotera, P., Moore, M., Mirabelli, F., Bellomo, G., and Orrenius, S., 1985, Inhibition of hepatocyte plasma membrane Ca^{2+}-ATPase activity by menadione metabolism and its restoration by thiols, *FEBS Lett.* **181:**149–153.

166. Di Monte, D., Bellomo, G., Thor, H., Nicotera, P., and Orrenius, S., 1984, Menadione-induced cytotoxicity is associated with protein thiol oxidation and alteration in intracellular Ca^{2+} homeostasis, *Arch. Biochem. Biophys.* **235:**343–350.

167. Messana, J. M., Cieslinski, D. A., O'Connor, R. P., and Humes, H. D., 1988, The role of glutathione in protection against exogenous oxidant injury to rabbit renal proximal tubules, *Am. J. Physiol.* **255:** F874–F884.

168. Paller, M. S., Hoidal, J. R., and Ferris, T. F., 1984, Oxygen free radicals in ischemic acute renal failure in the rat, *J. Clin. Invest.* **74:**1156–1164.

169. Ouriel, K., Smedira, N. G., and Ricotta, J. J., 1985, Protection of the kidney after temporary ischemia; free radical scavengers, *J. Vasc. Surg.* **2**:49–53.
170. Baker, G. L., Corry, R. J., and Autor, A. P., 1985, Oxygen free radical induced damage in kidneys subjected to warm ischemia and reperfusion, *Ann. Surg.* **202**(5):628–641.
171. Paller, M. S. and Hebbel, R. P., 1986, Ethane production as a measure of lipid peroxidation after renal ischemia, *Am. J. Physiol.* **251**:F839–F843.
172. Paller, M. S., 1986, Hypothroidism protects against free radical damage in ischemic acute renal failure, *Kidney Int.* **29**:1161–1166.
173. Koyama, I., Bulkley, G. B., Williams, G. M., and Im, M. J., 1985, The role of oxygen free radicals in mediating the reperfusion injury or cold-preserved ischemic kidneys, *Transplantation* **40**(6):590–595.
174. Green, C. J., Healing, G., Lunec, J., Fuller, B. J., and Simpkin, S., 1986, Evidence of free-radical-induced damage in rabbit kidneys after simple hypothermic preservation and autotransplantation, *Transplantation* **41**(2):161–165.
175. Green, C. J., Healing, G., Simpkin, S., Fuller, B. J., and Lunec, J., 1986, Reduced susceptibility to lipid peroxidation in cold ischemic rabbit kidneys after addition of desferrioxamine, mannitol, or uric acid to the flush solution, *Cryobiology* **23**:358–365.
176. Bennett, J. F., Bry, W. I., Collins, G. M., and Halasz, N. A., 1987, The effects of oxygen free radicals on the preserved kidney, *Cryobiology* **24**:264–269.
177. Linas, S. L., Whittenburg, D., and Repine, J. E., 1987, O_2 metabolites cause reperfusion injury after short but not prolonged renal ischemia, *Am. J. Physiol.* **253**:F685–F691.
178. Linas, S. L., Shanley, P. F., White, C. W., Parker, N. P., and Repine, J. E., 1987, O_2 metabolite-mediated injury in perfused kidneys is reflected by consumption of DMTU and glutathione, *Am. J. Physiol.* **253**:F692–F701.
179. White, M., Hunt, D., Humes, H. D., and Weinberg, J. M., 1985, Effects of allopurinol on ischemic injury to isolated tubules, *Kidney Int.* **27**:239.
180. Toledo-Pereyra, L. H., Simmons, R. L., Olson, L. C., and Najarian, J. S., 1977, Clinical effect of allopurinol on preserved kidneys: A randomized double-blind study, *Ann. Surg.* **185**:128–131.
181. Chatterjee, S. N. and Berne, T. V., 1976, Protective effect of allopurinol in renal ischemia, *Am. J. Surg.* **131**:658–659.
182. Vasko, K. A., DeWall, R. A., and Riley, A. M., 1972, Effect of allopurinol in renal ischemia, *Surgery* **71**:787–790.
183. Toledo-Pereyra, L. H., Simmons, R. L., and Najarian, J. S., 1974, Effect of allopurinol on the preservation of ischemic kidneys perfused with plasma or plasma substitutes, *Ann. Surg.* **180**:780–782.
184. Jackson, N. M., O'Connor, R. P., and Humes, H. D., 1986, Response of isolated renal proximal tubule segments to hypoxia–reoxygenation or chemically induced oxidative stress, *Toxicologist* **6**:269.
185. Nguyen, V. D., Messana, J. M., Cieslinski, D. A., and Humes, H. D., 1987, Exogenous glutathione supplementation increases cellular glutathione level of renal proximal tubule segments and prevents hypoxia-induced proximal tubule segment injury, *Clin. Res.* **35**:636A.
186. Nguyen, V. D., Messana, J. M., Cieslinski, D. A., and Humes, H. D., 1988, Effect of glutathione depletion on hypoxia-induced injury to rabbit renal proximal tubule segments, *Kidney Int.* **33**:363.

9

The Kidney in Systemic Disease

Cindy L. Corpier and Wadi N. Suki

1. Introduction

A wide variety of systemic diseases have injurious effects on the kidney. As in the previous edition of this volume, we will restrict our review to multiorgan disorders which affect the renal microvasculature and the nephrologic consequences of tumors. Since the last writing of this chapter, a great deal has been learned about the pathogenesis of diabetic nephropathy and the halting of its progression. Drugs and infectious agents have become more evident in their associations with the thrombotic microangiopathies, while there is less to report in the areas of scleroderma and the renal effects of tumors.

2. Disorders of the Renal Microvasculature

The thrombotic microangiopathies (TMA), especially hemolytic uremic syndrome (HUS), diabetes mellitus, and sickle cell disease, will comprise the bulk of this section. The discussion of scleroderma is brief owing to the small number of publications in this area since 1986, and the reader is referred to Volume 4 (pp. 467–469) for more detail.

CINDY L. CORPIER and WADI N. SUKI • Renal Section, Baylor College of Medicine, The Methodist Hospital, Houston, Texas 77030.

2.1. Thrombotic Microangiopathies

Syndromes characterized by microangiopathic hemolytic anemia and micro-vascular thrombosis are referred to as the TMAs, a term originally applied by Symmers in 1952.[1] This designation includes HUS, thrombotic thrombocytopenic purpura (TTP), and postpartum renal failure. The pathologic features of both TTP and HUS have been extensively reviewed recently.[2-4] Renal involvement has been described as occurring in three patterns. In some cases microangiopathic glomerular lesions may predominate, in others the prevalent lesion is that of arterial thrombosis, and finally, combined glomerular and vascular involvement may be seen. A preponderance of vascular lesions is indicative of a more severe process. The specific glomerular abnormality is evidenced by a thickening of the capillary walls due to the subendothelial deposition of a "fluffy material" consisting of strands of fibrin, fragments of platelets, extensions of mesangial cells, trapped endothelial cells, and microfibrils. The mesangium is generally affected by swelling and re-ticulation of the matrix which may evolve to mesangiolysis. Expansion of the mesangium may result in glomerular capillary narrowing. Glomerular thrombosis is usually absent in mild disease and, when present, rarely involves the entire capillary tuft. The thrombi have been shown to consist of platelets and fibrin. Renal outcome in TMA is influenced by the percentage of glomeruli affected. The severity of the renal lesion is highly variable from case to case. Likewise, the distribution of the thrombosis in other organs varies widely.

It has been proposed recently that the standard points of differentiation be-tween TTP and HUS do not clearly separate the syndromes and that they instead may represent alternative expressions of a single entity.[5] Both are characterized by histopathologically identical lesions, a Coombs-negative hemolytic anemia, frag-mentation of red blood cells (RBCs), and thrombocytopenia. The clinical presenta-tion of TTP usually includes neurologic manifestations, fever, and a variable inci-dence of renal dysfunction. Preferential renal involvement without multiorgan features has been the standard definition of HUS. However, renal manifestations have been reported in up to 80% of patients with TTP, and neurologic perturbations may complicate HUS.[6] Therefore, clear separation clinically may not be possible.

Although the pathologic lesion has been well described and the clinical man-ifestations consistent with TMA generally agreed upon, the pathophysiology has been more elusive. TMA occurs in a multitude of diverse settings which seem to share the common mechanism of vascular endothelial damage. Disruption of the endothelial lining eventually leads to thrombus formation in the microvasculature. Remuzzi et al. reviewed the role of prostacyclin (PGI_2) in TMA.[7] PGI_2 is an extremely potent inhibitor of platelet aggregation which antagonizes the effects of thromboxane A2. After release from endothelial cells, PGI_2 is rapidly degraded to the more stable compound 6-keto-$PGF_1\alpha$. Depressed PGI_2-stimulating activity and decreased levels of 6-keto-$PGF_1\alpha$ have been reported in patients with HUS and TTP. This has been demonstrated in both the adult and atypical childhood forms of HUS. Since the expected response to endothelial injury is enhanced production of

PGI_2, two explanations for these results have been put forward. The low levels of PGI_2 production detected may be a consequence of repeated stimulation of the endothelium which outstrips the cells' synthetic capacity. Alternatively, a stimulating factor usually present in normal plasma may be lacking in TMA. The observation that defective stimulation of PGI_2 release by plasma from patients with HUS can be restored by plasma infusion is supportive of this hypothesis.[8] Recent reports in both children and adults of elevated levels of PGI_2 metabolites have conflicted with earlier data.[9,10] Hautekeete et al. reported elevated 6-keto-$PGF_1\alpha$ levels in two adult patients.[10] They suggest that extensive injury to endothelial cells could lead to massive prostacyclin release resulting in elevated levels of the metabolite. Hemolysis of RBCs to which prostacyclin has bound could also be responsible for these findings.

Several compounds have been implicated as the mediators of the endothelial damage. Bacterial endotoxin (verotoxin, Shiga toxin), neuraminidase, and drugs, particularly cyclosporine and mitomycin C, have all been shown to be capable of injuring vascular endothelium. TMA is known to complicate several types of active infections and postvaccination settings. Bacterial, rickettsial, viral, and fungal infections have all been associated (reviewed in Ref. 11). An enteric pathogen not recognized as causative of diarrheal disease until 1982, *Escherichia coli* O157:H7, has been linked to HUS.[12] This organism causes copious, bloody diarrhea which may be accompanied by fever or fecal leukocytes. Enterohemorrhagic *E. coli* (EHEC) is the term for this strain of the organism. A phage-encoded toxin, verotoxin, which is cytotoxic for HeLa and Vero cells, has been identified in patients with hemorrhagic colitis and HUS.[13,14] Verotoxin is thought to be identical to the Shiga toxin produced by *Shigella dysenteriae* 1.

Cases of HUS following enteric infection with *E. coli* O157:H7 and other serotypes led to a prospective study of this association in Seattle, Washington.[15] Fourteen cases were identified in which 12 had diarrhea as part of the prodromal illness. Seven of these patients (58%) had evidence of *E. coli* O157:H7 in their stool. The group concluded that this organism is associated with the majority of cases of HUS in the Pacific Northwest and may have been overlooked in the past as normal flora. A retrospective, epidemiological study in King County, Washington, identified 33 cases of childhood HUS between 1971 and 1980 in which 23 developed bloody diarrhea as part of their prodrome.[16] The presence of enteric pathogens was not commented on in this study.

The apparent importance of *E. coli* O157:H7 in diarrheal illness and HUS has prompted studies directed toward development of a rapid screening tool for this strain. Levine et al. reported their evaluation of a DNA probe prepared from a segment of the EHEC plasmid.[17] This probe was found to be both highly sensitive and specific for *E. coli* O157:H7.

A syndrome sometimes referred to as chemotherapy-related HUS (CR-HUS) has been described in patients treated with antineoplastic agents. The drug most commonly associated is the antibiotic mitomycin C (MMC). One review published in July 1987 tabulated 128 reported cases.[3] An additional nine cases in which MMC was used were identified in the literature through August 1988.[18-21] CR-HUS following treatment with MMC has a reported incidence of 2–10% and occurs in a variety of malignancies. Gastric, colorectal, and breast carcinomas account for the majority of tumors seen in this circumstance. The occurrence of CR-HUS is uncommon when the cumulative dose of MMC is less than 30 mg/m^2 or when fewer than two cycles of therapy have been administered. The onset of symptoms is often within 2 months of the last dose; however, it may occur as late as 9 months after completion of therapy. Other drugs that have been implicated in this syndrome include cisplatin, bleomycin, daunorubicin combined with cytosine arabinoside, and methyl CCNU (reviewed in Refs. 3 and 22).

Development of CR-HUS is usually associated with clinical remission and is much less common in the setting of progressive cancer. In addition to the triad of microangiopathic hemolytic anemia, thrombocytopenia, and renal failure, most patients have systemic hypertension. An unusual characteristic of CR-HUS is the frequent exacerbation of hemolysis following blood transfusions. Pulmonary edema, also a frequent manifestation of CR-HUS, likewise may be precipitated by RBC transfusions. One series documented pulmonary edema in 12 patients who showed no other signs of volume overload.[23] Respiratory symptoms followed RBC transfusion in nine patients and were spontaneous in the remaining three. In another group of 39 patients with CR-HUS, 19 developed pulmonary edema.[24] Accelerated hypertension, left ventricular failure, and volume overload may contribute to the pulmonary insufficiency in these cases; however, other factors appear to be more important. MMC use predisposes patients with CR-HUS to noncardiogenic pulmonary edema, possibly through the mechanism of direct endothelial damage.[24] This is distinct from the pulmonary interstitial toxicity caused by the drug, which behaves similarly to bleomycin-induced lung disease.[18] Activation of intravascular clotting by either tumor products or constituents of RBC transfusions resulting in pulmonary vascular microthrombi could also initiate the deterioration in lung function.[20,23] Cardiac and neurologic abnormalities may be present in conjunction with the other features of CR-HUS and can also be significantly worsened by blood transfusions. Patients treated with bleomycin-containing regimens have exhibited Raynaud's phenomenon as part of their syndrome.[25]

The usual laboratory abnormalities of TMA are present in these patients. Of note, circulating immune complexes (CIC) have been elevated in the majority of cases tested. Renal histology reveals a picture similar or identical to HUS of other causes. At autopsy, microthrombi may be limited to the kidney or widespread, with the brain and lungs being the two most common extrarenal sites of involvement.

The exact pathogenetic mechanisms involved in development of CR-HUS are not clearly understood. Direct endothelial injury by MMC or CICs may be at play. The immune complexes are composed of IgG, complement, and a glycoprotein antigen. Antibodies eluted from these complexes have been shown to react with adenocarcinoma cells but not with normal tissue.[23,26] It has been suggested that reduction of the tumor burden with either chemotherapy or surgical resection results in a state of antigen–antibody "equivalence" favoring the formation of immune complexes. The accumulation of such CICs in blood vessels may damage the endothelial lining, cause platelet aggregation, and promote microvascular thrombosis. Such a scenario would explain the existence of CR-HUS when little or no tumor remains.

The prognosis of CR-HUS tends to be poor, with 75% of patients dying within 4 months of diagnosis.[24] Refusal of dialytic therapy for severe renal failure has been one of the factors responsible for the high mortality. It has been recommended that patients receiving agents associated with this syndrome be monitored for hemolysis and urinary abnormalities such as hematuria or proteinuria.[3] Discontinuation of the responsible drug may prevent further deterioration of renal function and hematologic status. If the diagnosis of CR-HUS does become evident, RBC and platelet transfusions should be given as sparingly as possible, with careful monitoring for pulmonary compromise. There is no specific treatment for CR-HUS. Supportive medical care, including anithypertensive agents, diuretics, and/or dialysis, is usually required. Plasmapheresis and plasma exchange have been used in these patients. CICs are usually decreased by these modalities, with accompanying hematologic improvement; however, renal failure is not commonly reversed. Immunoperfusion, a form of plasma therapy in which autologous plasma is filtered over staphylococcal protein A (SPA) filters and then reinfused into patients, has met with better success. SPA is known to bind both individual and complexed IgG molecules. This property has been put to advantage in a procedure designed to remove CICs from plasma. In 11 patients with CR-HUS who underwent this treatment, stabilization of renal function occurred in six and hematologic improvement was achieved in nine.[27] It remains to be seen if this therapeutic option will prove to be of benefit in larger groups of patients.

Other relationships between malignancies and TMA have been described. HUS as a preleukemic manifestation was suggested by the case of a 4½ year-old boy who developed acute lymphocytic leukemia (ALL).[28] Recovery from biopsy-proven HUS was followed in 8 months by the development of ALL. HUS in the setting of untreated malignancy has been infrequently noted. Two well-documented episodes occurred in a 64-year-old man diagnosed as having metastatic adenocarcinoma of the prostate 8 months after the onset of HUS.[29] Three similar cases were cited. A single episode of HUS in a patient treated for small cell carcinoma of the lung is the first report of this association.[30] This case was atypical in that CICs were not detectable, MMC was not used, and the patient responded to conventional therapy for HUS. Renal outcome was favorable in all three of these reports.

Features of both HUS and Henoch–Schönlein purpura were seen in a patient who presented with Kawasaki syndrome.[31] HUS and Kawasaki syndrome have previously been identified together, but this is an unusual association.

Another important category of TMA is that which occurs in the setting of tissue transplantation. Bone marrow and renal transplantation will be discussed separately. TMA following bone marrow transplantation we found mentioned in the literature three times prior to 1986, involving six patients. Cyclosporine was used as part of the posttransplant regimen in all of them.[32–34] Shulman et al. reported clinical and histologic findings that were consistent with TMA in three bone marrow graft recipients.[33] Two of these cases had also exhibited acute graft-vs.-host disease (GVHD); however, comparison of the pathologic findings in a group with GVHD but not treated with cyclosporine failed to reveal similar features. More recently three individuals who were not treated with cyclosporine developed HUS following bone marrow grafting.[35] All nine of the reported patients died. At least five of them exhibited GVHD and five were found to have cytomegalovirus infections. While the TMA may have played a significant role in the poor prognosis of these patients, other, sometimes multiple, complications of bone marrow transplantation were present in each case.

The presence of TMA in renal allograft recipients may represent either *de novo* or recurrent disease. In the "precyclosporine" era TMA was seen in transplant patients usually as a manifestation of acute allograft rejection (reviewed in Ref. 36). It has become apparent with the advent of cyclosporine that TMA may occur not only as a result of allograft rejection but as a toxic effect of the drug.[37,38] Three of the four cases were reported improved with dosage reduction or conversion to an azathioprine–corticosteroid regimen. Differentiation of cyclosporine-induced TMA from allograft rejection may require renal biopsy since the typical signs of rejection are often not evident in cyclosporine-treated patients.

Recurrence of TMA in both cadaveric and living–related donor renal transplants has been well documented. As early as 1982, recurrent HUS following cadaveric transplantation was thought to be triggered by cyclosporine and an advisement against its use in this situation was made.[39] One review identified four recurrences in 29 patients who received renal allografts for TMA.[36] The group concluded that TMA was not a contraindication for renal transplantation. These findings are in contradistinction to those of the group in Minneapolis.[40] Fourteen patients received 20 allografts, with all but one from living–related donors. Recurrence was definite in seven cases and probable in three others. One patient developed HUS in both living–related and cadaveric donor allografts. The authors recommended that neither cyclosporine nor Minnesota antilymphocyte globulin be used in patients whose original disease was HUS. Two other groups have found much lower rates of recurrence among their patients.[41,42] Workers in Leiden transplanted eight individuals whose original disease was HUS and saw a recurrence in one. Interestingly, use of oral contraceptives may have been the precipitating factor in that case. In the Australia and New Zealand registry, approximately 10% of those transplanted for HUS suffered graft failure due to recurrent disease. It is impossible from these small groups of patients to arrive at definite conclusions about the risk of recurrent TMA in renal allografts. We do know that the condition reappears in both cadaveric and living–related donor transplants as well as in both the presence and absence of cyclosporine therapy. These recurrent episodes usually result in loss of graft function. Decisions regarding immunosuppressive therapy must weigh the relative risks of graft loss from rejection vs. recurrent TMA.

Maintenance dialysis and/or renal transplantation becomes necessary when

TMA progresses to end-stage renal failure. Several modalities have been used in attempt to interrupt progression of the renal lesion. We have briefly discussed therapy in CR-HUS. Plasmapheresis and antiplatelet agents have been advocated by one group based on their experience with four patients, although others have not had similar results.[43] Treatment of TTP has been extensively reviewed.[44] Plasma exchange, albeit in small groups, has a response rate of approximately 80%. This is better than results obtained when patients received whole blood exchange transfusions or plasma infusions alone. The use of vincristine combined with plasmapheresis has been recommended based on one group's follow-up (6–12 months) in four patients with TTP.[45] Since the major risk of plasmapheresis is incurred from the plasma which is administered, the possibility of additional benefit over plasma infusion alone would seem to dictate its use in these cases. If plasmapheresis is unavailable, then plasma infusions should be the first-line therapy in adult TMA. The proposed role of PGI_2 in the pathogenesis of TMA has led to its use in treatment. The results of PGI_2 infusions have been variable and no conclusions on the therapeutic value can be made at this time (studies summarized in Ref. 7).

In contrast to the adult forms, TMA in children is generally not treated with plasma infusions. Rizzoni *et al.* studied 32 children prospectively and found no difference in outcome over a 2-year follow-up period.[46] However, in cases with extensive central nervous system involvement, use of plasma exchange therapy may be indicated. Sheth *et al.* reported the case of a 12-year-old girl who suffered progressive neurologic deterioration in spite of plasma infusion and whole blood exchange.[47] Plasma exchange therapy was associated with overall improvement.

In summary, childhood forms of TMA are associated with a good prognosis, and plasma therapies are probably not warranted except in cases with serious neurologic involvement. Adult TMA usually has a poorer prognosis, and strong consideration should be given to plasma infusion and/or exchange during the acute stages of the illness. The role of prostacyclin infusion in treatment of TMA is not yet established.

2.2. Diabetes Mellitus

The development of clinical proteinuria (the excretion of in excess of 300 mg of protein a day or 200 μg/min) secondary to diabetic nephropathy is considered a poor prognostic sign. This is in part due to the fact that these patients will ultimately develop end-stage renal disease and require dialysis or transplantation. It is estimated that in excess of 25% of all the patients undergoing dialysis in the United States today are diabetic. Just as important, however, proteinuria in the insulin-dependent diabetic is a predictor of increased cardiovascular mortality. In a study from the Steno Memorial Hospital in Denmark, Borch-Johnsen and Kreiner[48] report on 2890 patients with insulin-dependent diabetes screened for proteinuria. Of these, 2642 patients were entered into the study. Proteinuria was present in 722 patients, and in this group 109 deaths were observed during the period of follow-up, whereas the number expected for a nondiabetic group matched for sex and age was only 2.97. In the much larger group without proteinuria, 101 deaths were observed but only 23.3 were expected. Thus, in patients with proteinuria the relative mortality from cardiovascular disease was 37 times that in the general population, whereas in patients without proteinuria it was only 4.2 times that in the general population. In both the proteinuric and nonproteinuric insulin-dependent diabetic patient groups relative mortality from cardiovascular disease in women was 2–2.6 times that of men. Important factors contributing to this accelerated cardiovascular mortality in patients with clinical diabetic nephropathy are the development of hypertension and hypercholesterolemia. This is supported by a study from the University of Manchester[49] in which 22 insulin-dependent diabetics with clinical diabetic nephropathy were matched for sex, age, duration of diabetes, and concentration of hemoglobin A_1 with 22 other insulin-dependent diabetics with normal albumin excretion rate (AER). The patients with proteinuria had three to four times the incidence of ischemic heart disease, peripheral vascular disease, and proliferative retinopathy. These patients had significantly higher systolic and diastolic blood pressures, lower high-density-lipoprotein cholesterol, and a tendency for increased serum cholesterol.

With these grim observations, pointing to the seriousness of developing clinical diabetic nephropathy in the insulin-dependent diabetic, it is somewhat comforting to know that the incidence of this disorder appears to be declining. In another study from the Steno Memorial Hospital in Denmark,[50] 2658 patients diagnosed as type I diabetics between 1933 and 1972 were followed longitudinally. Of patients diagnosed between 1933 and 1942, 40.6% developed persistent proteinuria, whereas of patients diagnosed between 1953 and 1962, 26.9% developed persistent proteinuria, a 30% decrease. However, in all four decades the peak incidence of proteinuria was found after 15–17 years of diabetes duration, the lowest incidence was found in patients developing diabetes after the age of 20, and males showed the highest incidence of proteinuria. Of course, the reasons for the declining incidence of overt diabetic nephropathy are not known, but a number of factors are presumed to have contributed, including the introduction of longer-acting forms of insulin, the production of highly purified insulin preparations, the increased emphasis on blood sugar control, and the intensified and improved methods for home blood sugar monitoring. It is also possible that improved dietary monitoring and emphasis on slimness over the years could have played a role. In this study patients with lower body mass index had a lower incidence of proteinuria.

It is clear from the foregoing that diabetic nephropathy is a grave complication of insulin-dependent diabetes mellitus, but it is also clear that only about one-third of these patients are destined to develop nephropathy. It could be valuable, therefore, if those patients destined to develop clinical diabetic nephropathy could somehow be identified. Summarizing clinical investigations spanning a period of over 15 years, Mogensen[51] recently pointed to elevated urine albumin excretion (UAE) and a high glomerular filtration rate (GFR) as the major predictors of follow-up diabetic nephropathy, hypertension, and a decline in renal function.

2.2.1. Microalbuminuria

Normal adults excrete on average approximately 4.5 μg/min of albumin. This rate of albumin excretion is well below the detection limit of methods used for ordinary office urinalysis. Using assay tools (radioimmunoassay, radioimmunodiffusion) capable of detecting these subclinical rates of albumin excretion, it was found that after a mean follow-up of 10 years patients whose initial AER exceeded 15 μg/min, had an 80% risk of developing clinical proteinuria, while no patient excreting less than 15 μg/min of albumin developed clinical proteinuria.[51] Thus, this level of subclinical albuminuria has been labeled microalbuminuria and, when present in two or more urine samples collected over a period of 6 months, has been considered a sign of incipient diabetic nephropathy. Overt diabetic nephropathy is considered to be present when urinary excretion is greater than 200 μg/min or 300 mg/day in at least two urine samples over a similar period of time. During the phase of incipient diabetic nephropathy, increased GFR is generally present, diabetic retinopathy is more advanced, and the blood pressure is 10–15% higher than that in control subjects.

2.2.2. Hyperfiltration

As indicated earlier, increased GFR has been correlated with progression of diabetic nephropathy. A great deal of investigative effort has been expended, therefore, in attempting to understand the pathogenesis of hyperfiltration and to develop means of normalizing the GFR. However, the GFR is not at all predictable from the serum creatinine.[52] Furthermore, in a study by Norden and co-workers,[52] the endogenous creatinine clearance overestimated GFR as measured by ^{51}Cr EDTA by 0–180%. Thus, only markers of glomerular filtration, such as inulin, iothalamate, and EDTA, can be relied on in studies of GFR in diabetic patients.

Two factors, the blood glucose level and dietary protein intake, appear to play a role in modulating the GFR in the hyperfiltering diabetic patient. In a study by Wiseman and co-workers[53] it was shown that a brief period of euglycemia induced by overnight insulin infusion did not correct the hyperfiltration of a group of hyperfiltrating diabetics. In this group, unlike a group of normal controls or of normal filtering diabetics, a period of sustained glucose-induced hyperglycemia resulted in a significant increase of GFR by almost 12%. This increase in GFR was accompanied by a corresponding, although smaller, increase (5.8%) in renal plasma flow (RPF), resulting in increase in the filtration fraction of 9.2%. It is not clear, however, whether sustained euglycemia might result in correction of hyperfiltration. In a study from Oslo, Norway,[54] continuous subcutaneous insulin infusion (CSII) brought blood glucose and hemoglobin A_1 near the normal range and with that there was a significant decrease in GFR. However, this group of patients had a mean GFR, as measured by ^{51}Cr EDTA, of 119 ± 4 ml/min per 1.73 m^2. Thus, it did not appear that these patients fit into a category of hyperfiltration.

The mechanism of hyperfiltration that accompanies hyperglycemia and diabetes has not been identified. However, increased PGE_2 synthesis appears to play a role. In a study of streptozotocin-induced diabetes in the rat, PGE_2 synthesis in cortical and medullary microsomal fractions was found to be increased.[55] Treatment of the rats with aspirin resulted in a reduction in PGE_2 synthesis and prevented the increase in GFR. Long-term treatment with aspirin prevented the decline in GFR and the thickening of the glomerular basement membrane which is observed in the untreated diabetic rats. These and similar other studies have led investigators to use prostaglandin synthetase inhibitors in clinical diabetic nephropathy. In a study by Hommel et al.,[56] prostaglandin E_2 excretion in the urine of type I insulin-dependent diabetics was found to be increased in those patients with nephropathy when compared to a normoalbuminuric group, and indomethacin in a dose of 150 mg/day significantly reduced urinary PGE_2 excretion, the AER, and fractional clearance of albumin.

These interesting studies notwithstanding, it remains to be determined whether long-term euglycemia and long-term correction of hyperfiltration with prostaglandin synthesis inhibitors will arrest the progression of incipient diabetic nephropathy and prevent the ultimate development of overt clinical diabetic nephropathy and its subsequent progression to end-stage renal disease.

The ingestion of a protein meal has been known to raise the glomerular filtration rate in normal individuals, and a recent study by Brouhard and co-workers[57] shows a similar increase in GFR in patients with diabetes, the increase being of comparable magnitude. This increase in GFR was accompanied by an increase in glucagon, and the administration of somatostatin prevented the increase in GFR and the increase in plasma glucagon in both control subjects and diabetics. The diabetic patients, who had a higher GFR than the healthy volunteers, tended to have higher plasma glucagon and plasma growth hormone levels, although the differences were not significant. Thus, the ingestion of protein by increasing GFR could conceivably have adverse effects in diabetic patients.

In a survey of protein intake in young, type I diabetics compared to normal subjects, Kupin and co-workers[58] found that both groups consumed substantial amounts of protein in their diets, the average being 1.86 g/kg per day in controls and 2.17 g/kg per day in the diabetics. Both groups were then studied on diets containing 3.5 and 1.5 g/kg per day of protein. GFR and RPF decreased markedly and to a similar degree in both groups when protein intake was reduced, although the GFR was significantly greater in the diabetic patients than it was in the controls. Thus, modest reductions in protein intake, to levels that could easily be complied with, resulted in a 16.2% decrease in the GFR of type I diabetics. The effect of protein restriction on incipient diabetic nephropathy was studied by Cohen et al.[59] in a group of insulin-dependent diabetics with AER ranging between 15 and 200 μg/min. When these patients were crossed over from their normal-protein diet (median 92 g/day) to a low-protein diet (median 47 g/day), albumin excretion rate fell from a mean of 23.0 μg/min to 15.4 μg/min. This decrease in albumin excretion rate was accompanied by a significant fall in median GFR and in fractional renal clearance of albumin. Thus, short-term changes in dietary protein can ameliorate the two early predictors of diabetic nephropathy. However, recognizing the difficulty in compliance with dietary restrictions, it will be many years before it can be determined whether reduced protein intake can modify the long-term course of diabetic nephropathy.

In patients with well-established diabetic nephropathy due to insulin-dependent diabetes mellitus and with progressive renal dysfunction, a diet containing 40 g of high-biologic-value protein was found to be associated with salutory changes in renal function.[60] Daily urinary protein excretion rate decreased significantly in these patients from 2.1 g to 0.14 g, accompanied by an increase in the serum albumin level from 3.5 to 4.3 g/dl. Thus, even in patients with advanced diabetic nephropathy, protein restriction appears to be beneficial.

2.2.3. Hypertension

Both hypertension and diabetes mellitus are prevalent in the general population. An increase in blood pressure above control is noted early in insulin-dependent diabetes mellitus, even when diabetic nephropathy is in its incipient stage.[51] However, hypertension becomes an invariable accompaniment of clinically apparent diabetic nephropathy. Nevertheless, diabetics may develop essential hypertension, and the distinction between this form of hypertension and renal hypertension due to diabetic nephropathy is important. In an effort to identify differences, Christensen et al.,[61] in Aarhus, Denmark, investigated patients with incipient nephropathy and patients with overt diabetic nephropathy and compared them to patients with essential hypertension and to healthy controls. When UAE was plotted against blood pressure, a nearly complete separation was observed between the diabetic and nondiabetic hypertensive groups with respect to urinary albumin excretion as a function of systolic blood pressure and mean arterial blood pressure. Although in both groups UAE increased with the severity of blood pressure elevation, at any level of blood pressure UAE in diabetics was as much as 100 times that in nondiabetic essential hypertensives. Conversely, at any level of UAE blood pressure was about 70 mm Hg higher in the nondiabetic essential hypertensive than in the diabetic. Said differently, the levels of urinary albumin excretion seen in patients with early clinical diabetic nephropathy are seen only in patients with severe essential hypertension. Conversely, patients with diabetes mellitus who develop essential hypertension would not be expected to have significant elevation of urinary albumin excretion.

As stated earlier, hypertension and diabetic nephropathy are associated with accelerated macrovascular disease and cardiovascular mortality.[48,49] Intuitively, it seems important to control hypertension in the patient with diabetic nephropathy. In confirmation of this expectation and of earlier studies, Parving and his group,[62] in Denmark, recently published a study on 11 insulin-dependent diabetics with overt diabetic nephropathy followed for almost 10 years. During 32 months of follow-up prior to intervention, the patients were observed to have an increasing mean arterial blood pressure, increasing protein excretion, and a declining GFR, the rate of decline being 0.94 ml/min per month. These patients were then begun on a program of treatment consisting predominantly of metoprolol, hydralazine, and furosemide. The normalization of blood pressure over the ensuing period of 72 months resulted in a decrease in protein excretion and a decrease in the rate of decline of GFR to an initial value of 0.29 ml/min per month, and in the last 2 years of follow-up, to a value of 0.1 ml/min per month. These studies clearly indicate that control of hypertension can effectively postpone the development of renal insufficiency in patients with overt diabetic nephropathy.

Because of its apparent importance to the patient with diabetes mellitus, the treatment of hypertension in the diabetic has recently received a fair amount of attention, as evidenced by a special statement on this subject published by the Working Group on Hypertension in Diabetes.[63] In this report the Working Group appears to be advocating the step-care approach to the treatment of hypertension in diabetics: in other words, an approach in which second and third drugs are added to a first drug until control of hypertension is achieved, all the time using small to moderate doses of the different drugs. The group also appears to advocate the use of diuretics as a first-line treatment. However, Kaplan and his colleagues,[64] from Dallas, have taken issue with this approach and we are sympathetic to their point of view. In the first place, diuretics cause hypokalemia, they worsen blood sugar control, they stimulate the renin–angiotensin system, which may worsen proteinuria, and they cause hypercholesterolemia. Furthermore, the Working Group goes on to state that β-adrenergic receptor-inhibiting agents are frequently indicated in the diabetic hypertensive and can be used safely. However, these agents can also impair glucose tolerance and can aggravate insulin-induced hypoglycemia, obscure the symptoms of hypoglycemia, raise diastolic blood pressure during hypoglycemic attacks, and also cause hyperlipidemia. Kaplan and co-workers[64] point out that the use of α-adrenergic inhibitory agents and of angiotensin converting enzyme inhibitors (CEI) is superior first-line therapy in patients with both diabetes mellitus and hypertension since these agents do not adversely affect the control of diabetes mellitus and have more favorable lipid profiles.

With respect to CEIs, a number of studies in experimental models of renal disease and of diabetic nephropathy have now shown the renal protective effect of this group of agents. In rats made diabetic by the injection of streptozotocin, and kept moderately hyperglycemic with daily insulin injections, systemic hypertension does not develop.[65] These rats, however, display the expected increase in single-nephron GFR, which appears to be due both to high glomerular plasma flow (Q_A) and to elevated mean glomerular capillary pressure (P_{GC}). The use of the CEI enalapril resulted in a small decrease in mean arterial pressure without a significant change in SNGFR or Q_A. However, P_{GC} was reduced to normal levels. With this correction of glomerular hypertension, the increase in urinary albumin excretion seen in the diabetic rats after 14 months of follow-up was completely abolished. Morphologic examination of the kidneys revealed preservation of glomerular structure, whereas glomerular sclerosis was seen in the untreated rats. These intriguing animal studies seem to have their parallel in studies in normotensive diabetic patients studied at the Hospital Saint-Louis in Paris.[66] In this study, 20 patients with incipient diabetic nephropathy due to insulin-dependent diabetes mellitus (UAE of 30–300 mg/24 hr) were randomized to one of two groups, a placebo group and a group receiving 20 mg of enalapril daily. Over the ensuing 6 months, blood pressure fell slightly in the enalapril group, and while GFR rose from 130 ml/min per 1.73 m^2 to 141 ml/min per 1.73 m^2, AER declined from 124 mg/24 hr to 37 mg/24 hr, whereas in the placebo group AER increased from 81 mg/24 hr to 183 mg/24 hr. It appears, therefore, that treatment with CEIs, even before systemic hypertension had set in but at a time when microalbuminuria was evident, may result in an improvement in the AER, an early predictor of future development of overt diabetic nephropathy. Whether, if such treatment is sustained, the development of diabetic nephropathy will be forestalled or prevented remains to be determined in future studies.

2.2.4. Superimposed Renal Disease

In addition to essential hypertension, patients with diabetes mellitus may also develop superimposed renal parenchymal disease due to causes other than their diabetic state. Although there have been a number of reports of superimposed nondiabetic renal disease, the frequency of this coincidence has not been studied. In a study by Hommel and co-workers,[67] 1024 type 1 diabetic patients were investigated of whom 184 (18%) were found to have persistent proteinuria. Microscopic hematuria, defined as three or more erythrocytes per high-power field in two or more sterile urine specimens, was found in 23 of these type 1 diabetic patients with persistent proteinuria (12.5%). There were no differences in blood pressure, the duration of diabetes, the serum creatinine concentration, or the prevalence of retinopathy between the two groups. Kidney biopsy was performed in 13 of the 23 patients with microscopic hematuria, and while diabetic glomerulosclerosis was present in all 13 patients, nine patients were found to have a nondiabetic superimposed renal disease consisting of mesangioproliferative glomerulonephritis in five, membranous glomerulonephritis in three, and sarcoidosis in one. It was concluded that microscopic hematuria is an important clue to the presence of superimposed renal parenchymal disease in type 1 diabetic patients with diabetic nephropathy and well-preserved kidney function.

2.2.5. Renal Replacement Therapy

When diabetic nephropathy culminates in renal failure, patients have the option either of undergoing peritoneal or hemodialysis or of receiving a renal transplant. Although dialysis is lifesaving, survival of diabetic patients is inferior to that of nondiabetic patients treated with this modality. Renal transplantation, however, appears to be an outstanding option for the diabetic with end-stage renal disease. The experience in kidney transplantation in diabetic patients at the University of Minnesota was recently summarized by Sutherland and co-workers.[68] In the period between July 1, 1979, and December 31, 1984, 384 diabetics received renal allografts, 49% of these being from cadaveric donors, 33% from HLA nonidentical related donors, and 18% from HLA identical siblings. The recipients of grafts from donors other than HLA identical siblings were splenectomized, and all patients received five or more blood transfusions prior to transplantation. It is most encouraging that graft survival rates for diabetic vs. nondiabetic recipients were similar in all donor categories. Patient survival rates were also the same for diabetic and nondiabetic recipients of kidneys from related donors. Only in recipients of cadaveric kidneys was patient survival lower for diabetics than for nondiabetic recipients, the figures being 79% patient survival for the diabetic cadaveric graft recipients vs. 90% for the corresponding nondiabetic group. In a subgroup of 139 diabetics receiving grafts from HLA mismatched donors, treatment with azathioprine and cyclosporine was compared. In these diabetic patients cadaver graft survival rates were higher in the cyclosporine-treated than in the azathioprine-treated groups. Thus, even though the results of transplantation in diabetic patients have been outstanding, they promise to improve further among recipients of cadaveric grafts in the cyclosporine era. Unfortunately, however, normalization of the chemical milieu by kidney transplantation does not seem to alter the course of the vascular complications of diabetic recipients.

A study of insulin-dependent diabetics receiving cadaveric renal transplants at the Hennepin County Medical Center in Minneapolis, Minnesota, showed a higher rate of vascular disease after transplantation in diabetic recipients, both in those with and in those without vascular disease prior to transplantation.[69] Furthermore, there was an amputation rate in diabetic transplant recipients of 18%. Of the vascular diseases studied in this report, coronary artery disease, manifested by angina, myocardial infarction, or both, was a very important component. Obviously, it would be very important to be able to identify patients with preexisting coronary disease because of the 67% recurrence rate in these patients after transplantation. One method for screening these patients prior to transplantation is the noninvasive exercise thallium imaging method. This approach appears to be a very useful tool, according to a study by Felsher and co-workers.[70] In this study, the presence of a normal image and an exercise heart rate greater than 120 beats/min was highly discriminating in identifying a subgroup of patients that over the period of follow-up was free of cardiovascular events. Such an approach may be used, therefore, in screening diabetic renal transplant candidates prior to transplantation in order for therapeutic measures to be undertaken in those found to have abnormalities.

2.3. Sickle Cell Hemoglobinopathy

Renal and urologic abnormalities are common in patients affected by sickle cell hemoglobinopathies (SCH). Sickle cell trait occurs in approximately 8% of the black American population.[71] Sickle cell disease, defined as homozygosity for two abnormal genes, is present in about 1% of the black population.[72] Together with those affected by sickle cell anemia (S-S) and SCH in populations other than black, a substantial number of individuals are at risk for complications.

The urologic manifestations of SCH include hematuria, papillary necrosis, urinary tract infection, and priapism. A pediatric population consisting of 321 patients with SCH followed between 1970 and 1984 at Children's Hospital in Philadelphia was reviewed.[71] Gross hematuria occurred in three patients and all had papillary necrosis documented by excretory urography (intravenous pyelography; IVP). Microhematuria was incidentally noted in 16%. Urinary tract infections (UTI) affected 10% of the patients and were recurrent in one-third. *Escherichia coli* was the most common pathogen and was present in greater than 50% of the cases. Three of ten patients with recurrent UTIs who underwent IVPs showed changes indicative of reflux nephropathy. These findings suggest that children with SCH and UTIs should be screened radiographically for urinary tract abnormalities. Priapism which responded to medical therapy occurred in 8 of 155 male patients in the study. An additional two were affected and required surgical intervention. Risk of impotence in these children appears to be quite low when they are treated with hydration and hypertransfusion.

Most episodes of gross hematuria resolve spontaneously, with no need for surgery. Renal autotransplantation was reported in one patient who exhibited recurrent bleeding over a 7-month period.[73] Her postoperative course was punctuated by gross hematuria on only two occasions over a 38-month period. The mechanism responsible for this improvement is unclear. It has been suggested that correction of some abnormality in local hemodynamics effected by relocation of the kidney in the iliac fossa may be responsible. As a treatment for otherwise difficult-to-control bleeding, this procedure has the advantage when compared to nephrectomy of maintaining the patient with two functional kidneys.

The incidence and prognosis of sickle glomerulopathy (SG) was examined retrospectively in an adult population.[74] SG, a glomerular lesion that somewhat resembles membranoproliferative glomerulonephritis, is associated with hyperchloremic, hyperkalemic renal tubular acidosis (type IV) and the nephrotic syndrome. The renal histology consists of mesangial expansion and glomerular basement membrane (GBM) duplication without electron-dense deposits. Twelve patients with protein excretion in excess of 2 g/24 hr were identified from a group of 240 adults with sickle cell anemia. Nine of them had SG by renal biopsy. The cause of SG is speculative. The authors hypothesize that chronic activity of the mesangium causes its proliferation and extension along the endothelial aspect of the GBM. Formation of new GBM material on the inner side would then create the double-contour pattern seen histologically.

The prognosis of SG in the group studied was poor. Four patients were dead within 2 years of follow-up and another three progressed to end-stage renal failure. This represents a very unfavorable comparison with the remainder of those affected by sickle cell anemia.

The results of a national study on the natural history of renal allografts in SCH indicate that transplantation is a therapeutic option in these patients.[72] Data collected from 110 centers identified 45 transplants in 40 patients, 11 of which were from living-related donors (LRD). Patient mortality within the first year was 12%. Graft survival was 82% in the LRD group and 62% in the cadaveric donor group.

These data indicate that both patient and graft survival rates compare favorably with those observed in the population without SCH. Less encouraging results have been reported by the Birmingham, Alabama, group.[75] Six individuals with sickle cell anemia and two with sickle cell disease were transplanted in that center between 1968 and 1986. One-year graft survival in these patients was only 25%. Sickling resulted in the loss of four allografts, all within 5 months of transplantation. These workers concluded that transplantation offered no advantage over dialysis in SCH. Progressive diminution in allograft function attributed to repeated sickle cell crises was reported in one other patient.[76]

2.4. Scleroderma

In the previous volume of *Contemporary Nephrology* the subsets of scleroderma (or systemic sclerosis) were described. Estimates of renal involvement in systemic sclerosis have been variable, depending on the criteria used. Scleroderma renal crisis, a syndrome characterized by the sudden onset of malignant hypertension, rapidly progressive renal failure, and elevated plasma renin activity (PRA), occurs in about 5–15% of patients in the series reported.[77] Treatment with the angiotensin-converting enzyme (ACE) inhibitors has been associated with successful management of hypertension. However, both positive and negative responses of the renal disease have been seen.[78–80] Enalapril, the second ACE inhibitor released for clinical use, also has been found to be effective in scleroderma renal crisis.[81] Treatment over a 1-month period in one patient resulted in decreased levels of aldosterone, increased PRA, and improved renal function. Another group has indicated that preliminary data show captopril and enalapril to be equally useful in this disorder.[77] It is likely, therefore, that ACE inhibition rather than some other effect of captopril is the important factor.

The life-threatening nature of scleroderma renal crisis requires prompt management of renal failure and hypertension. Systemic sclerosis, however, can manifest a rapidly progressive course in the skin and viscera other than the kidneys. There have now been several anecdotal reports of regression of diffuse systemic sclerosis following treatment with cyclosporine.[82–84] In one such report a flare of the disease was associated with discontinuation of the drug for 2½ weeks.[82] Reinstitution of cyclosporine was followed by gradual improvement. Further study of this mode of therapy appears warranted.

3. Renal Consequences of Tumors

Solid and hematologic tumors of many types can affect renal function. One of the most common tumors that leads to impairment of renal function is multiple myeloma. Traditionally renal insufficiency has been associated with a poor overall prognosis. Factors related to prognosis have been retrospectively reviewed in three different studies.[85–87] Two agreed that the histologic finding best correlated with poor renal outcome was tubular interstitial damage.[85,86] In the two studies that addressed mortality, both found survival to parallel return of renal function.[85,87] The period of time to recovery was frequently quite prolonged. Dehydration, infections, and hypercalcemia have often been detected at the time that renal failure is initially recognized. It also appears that the use of nonsteroidal antiinflammatory drugs may be important, especially if combined with dehydration.[85] Naproxen use was reported to precipitate acute renal failure in two patients eventually found to have multiple myeloma.[88]

Other hematologic malignancies as well may exhibit important renal manifestations. Acute tumor lysis syndrome was seen in a patient treated for prolymphocytic leukemia.[89] This fatal complication was unexpected because of the low response rate to therapy which is usual in this disease. Oncogenous osteomalacia due to light-chain nephropathy was well documented in two individuals, one each with myeloma and chronic lymphocytic leukemia.[90] Both were found to have complete healing of the bone lesions following treatment with phosphorus repletion.

References

1. Symmers, W. S. T. C., 1952, Thrombotic microangiopathic haemolyic anaemia (thrombotic microangiopathy), *Br. Med. J.* **2:**897.
2. Churg, J. and Strauss, L., 1985, Renal involvement in thrombotic microangiopathies, *Semin. Nephrol.* **5:**46.
3. Murgo, A. J., 1987, Thrombotic microangiopathy in the cancer patient including those induced by chemotherapeutic agents, *Semin. Hematol.* **24:**161.
4. Kwaan, H. C., 1987, Clinicopathologic features of thrombotic thrombocytopenic purpura, *Semin. Hematol.* **24:**71.
5. Remuzzi, G., 1987, HUS and TTP: Variable expression of a single entity, *Kidney Int.* **32:**292.
6. Eknoyan, G. and Riggs, S. A., 1986, Renal involvement in patients with thrombotic thrombocytopenic purpura, *Am. J. Nephrol.* **6:**117.
7. Remuzzi, G., Zoja, C., and Rossi, E., 1987, Prostacyclin in thrombotic microangiopathy, *Semin. Hematol.* **24:**110.
8. Remuzzi, G., Misiani, R., Marchesi, D., Livio, M., Mecca, G., Gaetano, G., and Donati, M. B., 1979, Treatment of the hemolytic uremic syndrome with plasma, *Clin. Nephrol.* **12:**279.
9. Stuart, M. J., Spitzer, R. E., Walenga, R. W., and Boone, S., 1985, Prostanoids in hemolytic uremic syndrome, *J. Pediatr.* **106:**936.
10. Hautekeete, M. L., Nagler, J. M., Cuykens, J. J., Parizel, G., Laekeman, G. M., and Herman, A. G., 1986, 6-Keto-PGF$_1$ α levels and prostacyclin therapy in 2 adult patients with hemolytic uremic syndrome, *Clin. Nephrol.* **26:**157.
11. Kwaan, H. C., 1987, Miscellaneous secondary thrombotic microangiopathy, *Semin. Hematol.* **24:** 141.
12. Riley, L. W., Remis, R. S., Helgerson, S. D., McGee, H. B., Wells, J. G., Davis, B. R., Hebert, R. J., Olcott, E. S., Johnson, L. M., Hargrett, N. T., Blake, P. A., and Cohen, M. L., 1983, Hemorrhagic colitis associated with a rare *Escherichia coli* serotype, *N. Engl. J. Med.* **308:**681.
13. Karmali, M. A., Petric, M., Steele, B. T., and Lim, C., 1983, Sporadic cases of haemolytic-uremic syndrome associated with faecal cytotoxin-producing *Escherichia coli* in stools, *Lancet* **1:**619.
14. O'Brien, A. D., Newland, J. W., Miller, S. F., Holmes, R. K., Smith, H. W., and Formal, S. B.,

1984, Shiga-like toxin converting phages from *Escherichia coli* strains that cause hemorrhagic colitis or infantile diarrhea, *Science* **226**:694.

15. Neill, M. A., Tarr, P. I., Clausen, C. R., Christie, D. L., and Hickman, R. O., 1987, *E. coli* O157:H7 as the predominant pathogen associated with the hemolytic uremic syndrome: A prospective study in the Pacific Northwest, *Pediatrics* **80**:37.

16. Tarr, P. I. and Hickman, R. O., 1987, Hemolytic uremic syndrome epidemiology: A population-based study in King County, Washington, 1971 to 1980, *Pediatrics* **80**:41.

17. Levine, M. M., Xu, J., Kaper, J. B., Lior, H., Prado, V., Tall, B., Nataro, J., Karch, H., and Wachsmuth, K., 1987, A DNA probe to identify enterohemorrhagic *Escherichia coli* of O157:H7 and other serotypes that cause hemorrhagic colitis and hemolytic uremic syndrome, *J. Infect. Dis.* **156**:175.

18. Verweij, J., van der Burg, M. E. L., and Pinedo, H. M., 1987, Mitomycin C-induced hemolytic uremic syndrome. Six case reports and review of the literature on renal, pulmonary and cardiac side effects of the drug, *Radiol. Oncol.* **8**:33.

19. Mergenthaler, H. G., Binsack, T., and Wilmanns, W., 1988, Carcinoma-associated hemolytic-uremic syndrome in a patient receiving 5-fluorouracil-adriamycin-mitomycin C combination chemotherapy, *Oncology* **45**:11.

20. Jain, S. and Seymour, A. E., 1987, Mitomycin C associated hemolytic uremic syndrome, *Pathology* **19**:58.

21. D'Elia, J. A., Aslani, M. D., Schermer, S., Cloud, L., Bothe, A., and Dzik, W., 1987, Hemolytic-uremic syndrome and acute renal failure in metastatic adenocarcinoma treated with mitomycin: Case report and literature review, *Renal Failure* **10**:107.

22. Fillastre, J. P., Viotte, G., Morin, J. P., and Moulin, B., 1988, Nephrotoxicity of antitumoral agents, *Adv. Nephrol.* **17**:175.

23. Cantrell, J. E., Phillips, T. M., and Schein, P. S., 1985, Carcinoma-associated hemolytic uremic syndrome: A complication of mitomycin-C therapy, *J. Clin. Oncol.* **3**:723.

24. Sheldon, R. and Slaughter, O., 1986, A syndrome of microangiopathic hemolytic anemia, renal impairment, and pulmonary edema in chemotherapy-treated patients with adenocarcinoma, *Cancer* **58**:1428.

25. Jackson, A. M., Rose, B. D., Graff, L. G., Jacobs, J. B., Schwartz, J. H., Strauss, G. M., Yang, J. P. S., Rudnick, M. R., Eltenbein, I. B., and Narins, R. G., 1984, Thrombotic microangiopathy and renal failure associated with antineoplastic chemotherapy, *Ann. Intern. Med.* **101**:41.

26. Zimmerman, S. E., Smith, F. P., Phillips, T. M., Coffey, R. J., and Schein, P. S., 1982, Gastric carcinoma and thrombotic thrombocytopenic purpura: Association with plasma immune complex concentrations, *Br. Med. J.* **284**:1432.

27. Korec, S., Schein, P. S., Smith, F. P., Neefe, J. R., Woolley, P. V., Goldberg, R. M., and Phillips, T. M., 1986, Treatment of cancer-associated hemolytic uremic syndrome with staphyloccal protein A immunoperfusion, *J. Clin. Oncol.* **4**:210.

28. Salcedo, J. R. and Fusner, J., 1986, Hemolytic uremic syndrome followed by acute lymphocytic leukemia, *Int. J. Pediatr. Nephrol.* **7**:169.

29. Sennesael, J. J., Vanden Houte, K. M., Spapen, H. D., de Bruyne, R. M. G., and Verbeelen, D. L., 1987, Recurrent hemolytic uremic syndrome and metasatic malignancy, *Am. J. Nephrol.* **7**:60.

30. Avvento, L., Gordon, S., Silberberg, J. M., Zarrabi, M. H., and Zucker, S., 1988, Hemolytic uremic syndrome in a patient with small cell lung cancer, *Am. J. Hematol.* **27**:221.

31. Heldrick, F. J., Jodorkovsky, R. A., Lake, A. M., and Parnes, C. A., 1987, Kawasaki syndrome: HUS and HSP complicating its course and management, *Maryland Medical Journal* **36**:764.

32. Powles, R. L., Clink, H. M., Spence, D., Morgenstern, G., Watson, J. G., Selby, P. J., Woods, M., Barrett, A., *et al.*, 1980, Cyclosporin A to prevent graft-versus-host disease in man after allogeneic bone-marrow transplantation, *Lancet* **1**:327.

33. Shulman, H., Striker, G., Deeg, H. J., Kennedy, M., Storb, R., and Thomas, E. D., 1981, Nephrotoxicity of cyclosporin A after allogeneic marrow transplantation, *N. Engl. J. Med.* **305**:1392.

34. Atkinson, K., Biggs, J. C., Hayes, J., Ralston, M., Dodds, A. J., Concannon, A. J., and Naidoo, D., 1983, Cyclosporin A associated nephrotoxicity in the first 100 days after allogeneic bone marrow transplantation: three distinct syndromes, *Br. J. Haematol.* **54**:59.

35. Marshall, R. J. and Sweny, P., 1986, Haemolytic-ureamic syndrome in recipients of bone marrow transplants not treated with cyclosporin A, *Histology* **10**:953.

36. Bonsib, S. M., Ercolani, L., Ngheim, D., and Hamilton, H. E., 1985, Recurrent thrombomicroangiopathy in a renal allograft, *Am. J. Med.* **79**:520.

37. Van Buren, D., Van Buren, C. T., Flechner, S. M., Maddox, A. M., Verani, R., and Kahan, B. D., 1985, De novo hemolytic uremic syndrome in renal transplant recipients immunosuppressed with cyclosporine, *Surgery* **98**:54.

38. Verpooten, G. A., Paulus, G. J., Roels, F., and DeBroe, M. E., 1987, De novo occurrence of hemolytic–uremic syndrome in a cyclosporine-treated renal allograft patient, *Transpl. Proc.* **19**: 2943.

39. Leithner, C., Sinzinger, H., Pohanka, E., Schwarz, M., Kretschmer, G., and Syre, G., 1982, Recurrence of haemolytic uraemic syndrome triggered by cyclosporin A after renal transplantation, *Lancet* **1**:1470.

40. Hebert, D., Sibley, R. K., and Mauer, S. M., 1986, Recurrence of hemolytic uremic syndrome in renal transplant recipients, *Kidney Int.* **30**:S51.

41. Berg-Wolf, M. G., Kootte, A. M., Weening, J. J., and Paul, L. C., 1988, Recurrent hemolytic uremic syndrome in a renal transplant recipient and review of the Leiden experience, *Transplantation* **45**:248.

42. Mathew, T. H., 1988, Recurrence of disease following renal transplantation, *Am. J. Kidney Dis.* **12**: 85.

43. Chow, S., Roscoe, J., and Cattran, D. C., 1986, Plasmapheresis and antiplatelet agents in the treatment of the hemolytic uremic syndrome secondary to mitomycin, *Am. J. Kidney Dis.* **12**:407.

44. Shepard, K. V. and Bukowski, R. M., 1987, The treatment of thrombotic thrombocytopenic purpura with exchange transfusions, plasma infusions, and plasma exchange, *Semin. Hematol.* **24**: 178.

45. Sennett, M. L. and Conrad, M. E., 1986, Treatment of thrombotic throbocytopenic purpura, *Arch. Intern. Med.* **146**:266.

46. Rizzoni, G., Claris-Appiani, A., Edefonti, A., Facchin, P., Franchini, F., Gusmano, R., Imbasciati, E., Pavanello, L., Perfumo, F., and Remuzzi, G., 1988, Plasma infusion for hemolytic-uremic syndrome in children: Results of a multicenter controlled trial, *J. Pediatr.* **112**:284.

47. Sheth, K. J., Leichter, H. E., Gill, J. C., and Baumgardt, A., 1987, Reversal of central nervous system involvement in hemolytic uremic syndrome by use of plasma exchanges, *Clin. Pediatr.* **26**: 651.

48. Borch-Johnsen, K. and Kreiner, S., 1987, Proteinuria: value as predictor of cardiovascular morality in insulin dependent diabetes mellitus, *Br. Med. J.* **294**:1651–1654.

49. Winocour, P. H., Durrington, P. N., Ishola, M., Anderson, D. C., and Cohen, H., 1987, Influence of proteinuria on vascular disease, blood pressure, and lipoproteins in insulin dependent diabetes mellitus, *Br. Med. J.* **294**:1648–1651.

50. Kofoed-Enevoldsen, A., Borch-Johnsen, K., Kreiner, S., Nerup, J., and Deckert, T., 1987, Declining incidence of persistent proteinuria in type I (insulin-dependent) diabetic patients in Denmark, *Diabetes* **36**:205–209.

51. Mogensen, C. E., 1987, Microalbuminuria as a predictor of clinical diabetic nephropathy, *Kidney Int.* **31**:673–689.

52. Norden, G., Bjorck, S., Graneras, G., and Nyberg, G., 1987, Estimation of renal function in diabetic nephropathy. Comparison of five methods, *Nephron* **47**:36–42.

53. Wiseman, M. J., Mangili, R., Alberetto, M., Keen, H., and Viberti, G., 1987, Glomerular response mechanisms to glycemic changes in insulin-dependent diabetics, *Kidney Int.* **31**:1012–1018.

54. Dahl-Jorgensen, K., Brinchmann-Hansenn, O., Hansenn, K. F., Ganes, T., Kierulf, P., Smeland,

E., Sandvik, L., and Aagenaes, O., 1986, Effect of near normoglycaemia for two years on progression of early diabetic retinopathy, nephropathy, and neuropathy: The Oslo study, *Br. Med. J.* **293:** 1195–1199.

55. Moel, D. I., Safirstein, R. L., McEvoy, R. C., and Hsueh, W., 1987, Effect of aspirin on experimental diabetic nephropathy, *J. Lab. Clin. Med.* **110:**300–307.

56. Hommel, E., Mathiesen, E., Arnold-Larsen, S., Edsberg, B., Olsen, U. B., and Parving, H-H., 1987, Effect of indomethacin on kidney function in type I (insulin-dependent) diabetic patients with nephropathy, *Diabetologia* **30:**78–81.

57. Brouhard, B. H., LaGrone, L. F., Richards, G. E., and Travis, L. B., 1987, Somatostatin limits rise in glomerular filtration rate after a protein meal, *J. Pediatr.* **110:**729–734.

58. Kupin, W. L., Cortes, P., Dumler, F., Feldkamp, C. S., Kilates, M. C., and Levin, N. W., 1987, Effect on renal function of change from high to moderate protein intake in type I diabetic patients, *Diabetes* **36:**73–79.

59. Cohen, D., Dodds, R., and Viberti, G., 1987, Effect of protein restriction in insulin dependent diabetics at risk of nephropathy, *Br. Med. J.* **294:**795–798.

60. Evanoff, G. V., Thompson, C. S., Brown, J., and Weinman, E. J., 1987, The effect of dietary protein restriction on the progression of diabetic nephropathy. A 12-month follow-up, *Arch. Intern. Med.* **147:**492–495.

61. Christensen, C. K., Krusell, L. R., and Mogensen, C. E., 1987, Increased blood pressure in diabetics: essential hypertension or diabetic nephropathy? *Scand. J. Clin. Lab. Invest.* **47:**363–370.

62. Parving, H-H., Anderson, A. R., Smidt, U. M., Hommel, E., Mathiesen, E. R., and Svendsen, P. A., 1987, Effect of antihypertensive treatment on kidney function in diabetic nephropathy, *Br. Med. J.* **294:**1443–1447.

63. Working Group on Hypertension in Diabetes, 1987, Statement on hypertension in diabetes mellitus. Final report, *Arch. Intern. Med.* **147:**830–842.

64. Kaplan, N. M., Rosenstock, J., and Raskin, P., 1987, A differing view of treatment of hypertension in patients with diabetes mellitus, *Arch. Intern. Med.* **147:**1160–1162.

65. Anderson, S. and Brenner, B. M., 1987, Therapeutic implications of coverting-enzyme inhibitors in renal disease, *Am. J. Kidney Dis.* **10**(Suppl. 1):81–87.

66. Marre, M., LeBlanc, H., Suarez, L., Guvenne, T.-T., Menard, J., and Passa, P., 1987, Converting enzyme inhibition and kidney function in normotensive diabetic patients with persistent microalbuminuria, *Br. Med. J.* **294:**1448–1452.

67. Hommel, E., Carstensen, H., Skott, P., Larsen, S., and Parving, H-H., 1987, Prevalence and causes of microscopic haematuria in type I (insulin-dependent) diabetic patients with persistent proteinuria, *Diabetologia* **30:**627–630.

68. Sutherland, D. E. R., Fryd, D. S., Payne, W. D., Asher, N., Simmons, R. L., and Najarian, J. S., 1987, Kidney transplantation in diabetic patients, *Transpl. Proc.* **19**(Suppl. 2):90–94.

69. Rao, K. V. and Andersen, R. C., 1987, The impact of diabetes on vascular complications following cadaver renal transplantation, *Transplantation* **43:**193–197.

70. Felsher, J., Meissner, M. D., Hakki, A-H., Heo, J., Kane-Marsch, S., and Iskandrian, A. S., 1987, Exercise thallium imaging in patients with diabetes mellitus. Prognostic implications, *Arch. Intern. Med.* **147:**313–317.

71. Tarry, W. F., Duckett, J. W., and Snyder, H. M., 1987, Urological complications of sickle cell disease in a pediatric population, *J. Urol.* **138:**592.

72. Chatterjee, S. N., 1987, National study in natural history of renal allografts in sickle cell disease or trait: a second report, *Transpl. Proc.* **19:**33.

73. Qunibi, W. Y., 1988, Renal autotransplantation for severe sickle cell hematuria, *Lancet* **8579:**236.

74. Bakir, A. A., Hathiwala, S. C., Ainis, H., Hryhorczuk, D. O., Rhee, H. L., Levey, P. S., and Dunea, G., 1987, Prognosis of the nephrotic syndrome in sickle glomerulopathy, *Am. J. Nephrol.* **7:** 110.

75. Barber, W. H., Delerhol, M. H., Julian, B. A., Curtis, J. J., Luke, R. G., Alexander, R. W., and

Dietheim, A. G., 1987, Renal transplantation in sickle cell anemia and sickle disease, *Clin. Trans.* 1:169.

76. Miner, D. J., Jorkasky, D. K., Perloff, L. J., Grossman, R. A., and Tomaszewski, J. E., 1987, Recurrent sickle cell nephropathy in a transplanted kidney, *Am. J. Kidney Dis.* **10**:306.

77. Shapiro, A. P. and Medsger, T. A., 1988, Renal involvement in systemic sclerosis, in: *Diseases of the Kidney*, Volume II (R. W. Schrier and G. W. Gottschalk, eds.), Little, Brown, Boston, p. 2273.

78. Lopez-Ovejano, J. A., Saal, S. D., D'Angelo, W. A., Cheigh, J. S., Stenzel, K. H., and Laragh, J. H., 1979. Reversal of vascular and renal crises of scleroderma by oral angiotensin-converting-enzyme blockade, *N. Engl. J. Med.* **300**:1417.

79. Thurm, R. H. and Alexander, J. C., 1984, Captopril in the treatment of scleroderma renal crisis, *Arch. Intern. Med.* **144**:733.

80. Waeber, B., Schaller, M-D., Wauters, J-P., and Brunner, H. R., 1984, Deterioration of renal function in hypertensive patients with scleroderma despite blood pressure normalization with captopril, *Klin. Wochenschr.* **62**:728.

81. Milsom, S. R. and Nicholls, M. G., 1986, Successful treatment of scleroderma renal crisis with enalapril, *Br. Med. J.* **62**:1059.

82. Yocum, D. E. and Wilder, R. L., 1987, Cyclosporin A in progressive systemic sclerosis, *Am. J. Med.* **83**:369.

83. Appelboom, T. and Itzkowitch, D., 1987, Cyclosporine in successful control of rapidly progressive scleroderma, *Am. J. Med.* **82**:866.

84. Zachariae, H. and Zachariae, E., 1987, Cyclosporin A in systemic sclerosis, *Br. J. Dermatol.* **116**:741.

85. Rota, S., Mougenot, B., Baudouin, B., De Meyer-Bras-seur, M., LeMaitre, V., Michel, C., Mignon, F., Rondeau, E., Vanhille, P., Verroust, P., and Ronco, P., 1987, Multiple myeloma and severe renal failure: A clinicopathologic study of outcome and prognosis in 34 patients, *Medicine* **66**:126.

86. Pasquali, S., Zuccelli, P., Casanova, S., Cagnoli, L., Confalonieri, R., Pozzi, C., Banfi, G., Lupo, A., and Bertani, T., 1987, Renal histological lesions and clinical syndromes in multiple myeloma, *Clin. Nephrol.* **27**:222.

87. Pozzi, C., Pasquali, S., Donini, U., Casanova, S., Banfi, G., Tiraboschi, G., Furci, L., Porri, M. T., Ravelli, M., Lupo, A., Schena, F. P., Brunati, C., Imbasciati, E., and Locatelli, F., 1987, Prognostic factors and effectiveness of treatment in acute renal failure due to multiple myeloma: a review of 50 cases, *Clin. Nephrol.* **28**:1.

88. Wu, M. J., Kumar, K. S., Kulkarni, G., and Kaiser, H., 1987, Multiple myeloma in naproxen-induced acute renal failure, *N. Engl. J. Med.* **317**:170.

89. Gomez, G. A. and Han, T., 1987, Acute tumor lysis syndrome in prolymphocytic leukemia, *Arch. Intern. Med.* **147**:375.

90. Rao, D. S., Parfitt, A. M., Villanueva, A. R., Dorman, P. J., and Kleerekoper, M., 1987, Hypophosphatemic osteomalacia and adult fanconi syndrome due to light-chain nephropathy, *Am. J. Med.* **82**:333.

10

Congenital Disorders of the Kidneys and Tumors
Alport's Syndrome and Electrolyte and Metabolic Disorders in Apudomas

Julio E. Benabe, Luis Baez, and Manuel Martinez-Maldonado

1. Alport's Syndrome

In 1902, Guthrie[1] described the unusual occurrence of renal disease in 12 members of a family. In 1927, Alport observed the association of deafness with renal failure in the same family.[2] Over the next few decades, the finding of several other families in whom progressive hereditary nephritis coexisted with deafness clearly suggested that this association was indeed a distinct form of hereditary nephritis.[3-8] Williamson named the entity Alport's syndrome in 1961.[9] More recent reports have expanded the classic dyad of aural and renal defects to include other abnormalities, including ocular defects, thrombocytopathia, hypoparathyroidism, and others.[10-21] Renal disease, however, is the hallmark of Alport's hereditary nephritis.

JULIO E. BENABE • Renal Section, Medical Service, Veterans Administration Hospital, University of Puerto Rico School of Medicine, San Juan, Puerto Rico 00936. LUIS BAEZ • Hematology Section, Medical Service, Veterans Administration Hospital, University of Puerto Rico School of Medicine, San Juan, Puerto Rico 00936. MANUEL MARTINEZ-MALDONADO • Medical Service, Veterans Administration Hospital, University of Puerto Rico School of Medicine, San Juan, Puerto Rico 00936.

1.1. Clinical Features

Alport's hereditary nephritis is a familial disorder characterized by a progressive course. Hematuria in childhood is typical, yet an adult type has also been recognized. In the latter, macroscopic hematuria is not common and renal impairment may be absent for years.[22] Once renal failure appears, however, its progression is an inexorable as in the juvenile form. Episodes of gross hematuria in children often may occur after an upper respiratory tract infection.[12] Proteinuria may be a common finding but may be absent or intermittent in female patients or in male patients in the early stage of the disease.[23-25] Very heavy or increasing proteinuria implies a worse prognosis.[12,26-28] Both the juvenile and the adult type of the syndrome are characterized by the inevitable development of renal failure in affected males, as well as in some females. Alport was the first to recognize that the disease carried a worse prognosis in males than in females.[2,29] More recently, Rumpelt has shown that the clinical course was more severe in males, and this finding correlated with a higher rate of basement membrane alterations.[30] Basement membrane showed splitting (61%) and thinning (6%) in males; the figures were 16% and 21%, respectively, in females. The splitting lesion is more prominent as males age, but this is not so in females. Thus, this study suggests that the thinning lesion of the glomerular basement membrane may be of minor importance.

Grünfeld[28] reviewed 36 cases of hereditary nephritis in women with persistent urinary abnormalities. Of the 36, renal failure developed in nine at age 35 years or less; five developed renal failure at 45 years or more. The remaining 22 patients had normal renal function, and their ages ranged from 19 to 48 years. A comparison of the female patients older than 30 years who developed renal failure with those who did not permitted identification of some of the indicators of the evolution of renal disease to end-stage disease. These included gross hematuria in childhood, neural hearing loss, a family history of Alport's syndrome, and the presence of diffuse thickening and splitting of the glomerular basement membrane.

Hearing and ocular defects have been the most frequently associated nonrenal abnormalities. Farboody and co-workers[31] found a 60% incidence of hearing loss in their study of 23 new kindreds. In most of the cases there was loss of high-frequency hearing. Gleeson has reported a uniformly slow rate of progression of the hearing loss in 11 patients with Alport's syndrome.[32] Tone decay was negligible, which together with a high speech discrimination is consistent with end-organ defect. Gleeson also confirmed the functional integrity of the retrocochlear pathways as far as the inferior colliculus, suggesting that the primary hearing defect in these patients laid in the cochlea.[32] Histologic examination did not reveal any consistent pathologic changes.[33-35] The most common finding was a decrease in spiroganglion cells of the basal cochlear turn and spongivesicular changes involving the spiral ganglia with atrophy of the organ of Corti.[33-35] Temporal bones fixed within 2 hr of death disclosed that the stria vascularis was the most severely involved structure: Thickening and lamellation of its capillary basement membrane similar to that seen in the glomerular lesion was found.[36]

It has been recognized that hearing loss augurs a poor prognosis in both males and females; in the latter group hearing loss is less frequent and renal failure less severe than in the former.[12-28] As a rule, patients of any sex without deafness have less severe renal disease.[12,26,37] On the other hand, deafness may be present and not accompanied by progression to renal failure.[38,39] The presence of renal disease and deafness, even if familial, is not diagnostic of Alport's syndrome. Uniformly, hematuria has been present, but the diagnosis rests on the findings on renal biopsy.

Ocular defects are not as common as hearing abnormalities, but carry a more significant diagnostic weight. The triad of nephritis, deafness, and ocular changes may be the most important clinical feature for the diagnosis.[40] Spherophakia has been reported occasionally.[31,41] More frequent and specific is anterior lenticonus.[42,43] Lenticonus is more common in males and is usually, although not invariably, bilateral. When present it is very difficult to see the fundus clearly because of severe refractive error. Macular or perimacular lesions are quite characteristic and consist of bright whitish or yellowish dense granulations located in the perimacular regions of both eyes and involving the more superficial layer of the retina just beneath the internal limiting membrane.[21,44] Moreover, patients with perimacular changes exhibit renal failure considerably earlier than those without. Habib and co-workers[41] have also shown that 77% of patients with perimacular changes started dialysis before 30 years of age, as opposed to 13% of patient without perimacular changes. These findings suggest that ocular lesions, both lenticonus and perimacular changes, are features of prognostic significance; their presence and the presence of deafness are reliable indicators of a poor prognosis.

1.2. Pathology and Pathogenesis

The basis lesion of Alport's syndrome has been demonstrated by ultrastructural studies to consist of glomerular basement membrane thickening with splitting and splintering of the lamina densa.[12,25,31,41,45] Yoshikawa et al.[46] described the glomerular basal lamina as being irregularly thickened, and the lamina densa to show replication with a "basket weave" pattern enclosing electron-lucent lacunae frequently containing small, dense particles. They concluded that a "basket weave" pattern is confined to hereditary nephritis. On light microscopy, sections stained with methenamine silver show focally thickened glomerular basement membrane in early cases.[12,41] Subsequently, segmental or global glomerular sclerosis and changes seen in chronic interstitial nephritis (periglomerular fibrosis, tubular atrophy, and interstitial fibrosis with foam cells) can be seen but these changes are of no diagnostic value. The glomerular ultrastructure with widespread lamellation of the glomerular basement membrane is highly characteristic of Alport's syndrome. Nevertheless, it is not specific and may be seen only focally, as well as with other nephropathies[31,46-49] Early in the course diffuse or focal thinning of the glomerular basement membrane (GBM) similar to that in benign familial hematuria may be seen.[12,49,50] Immunofluorescence is usually negative or shows only minor focal staining.[12,51]

The abnormal structure of the basement membrane has led to speculations on the pathogenesis of the disease. Spear in 1973[52] proposed that in Alport's syndrome the abnormality may reside in a structural gene at a locus governing the composition of basement membrane in the glomerulus, inner ear, and lens capsule. Studies examining the composition of the GBM in Alport's syndrome have shown that, in comparison with age-and-sex-matched control kidneys, the basement membranes from Alport's patients showed a slight increase in proline and glycine, slight decreases in half cystein and hydroxyproline, without changes in the hydroxylysine content or the carbohydrate composition.[53] Habib and co-workers[41] found a decrease in hydroxyproline content as the most characteristic modification in the amino acid composition of the GBM in Alport's syndrome. Tina et al.[54] as well as Veltischev and co-workers[55] have shown increased urinary excretion of hydroxylysine glycosides in Alport's syndrome. However, the significance of these findings is controversial since Schroder et al.[56] did not find any change in urine excretion of this compound.

Other evidence of altered GBM composition is derived from the studies by McCoy et al.[57] and Olson et al.[58] These investigators demonstrated the absence of GBM antigens in hereditary nephritis, related to the nephritogenic antigen commonly observed in Goodpasture's syndrome. Jenis et al.[59] have shown that absence of anti-GBM staining correlated with the severity of GBM splitting identified by electron microscopy. In a recent study Kashtan and co-workers[60] probed epidermal basement membranes from members of kindreds with Alport-type familial nephritis for the presence of antigens reactive with Goodpasture sera (GPS). They found absence of a 28-kilodalton-molecular-weight monomer and a 24-kilodalton monomer of the noncollagenous globular domain of type IV collagen consistent with the hypothesis of an abnormality of a basement membrane constituent lying in type IV collagen. More recently, Kleppel and co-workers[61] demonstrated the absence of 28-kilodalton noncollagenous monomers of type IV collagen in GBM from Alport's familial nephritis. It has also been shown that lack of Goodpasture antigen reactivity is uniformly associated with the absence of serum amyloid P component, a known constituent of normal GBM.[62] Amyloid P component has also been shown to be absent in the GBM of Alport-type hereditary nephritis.

The use of monoclonal antibodies against GBM can identify patients with Alport's syndrome. All patients without evidence of hereditary nephritis had strong binding of antibodies against GBM in one study. In contrast, 12 of 13 patients with strong evidence of hereditary nephritis showed no binding or greatly reduced binding.[63]

Thus, the available data are consistent with the hypothesis that a genetic defect that determines the GBM composition is most likely the cause of Alport's syndrome. The available evidence suggests that the mode of inheritance is heterogeneous. Some families have shown autosomal dominant inheritance, while in others an X-linked dominant inheritance of either juvenile or adult type has been demonstrated.[64–68]

2. Electrolyte and Metabolic Disorders in Apudomas

Apudomas are well-differentiated neoplasms exhibiting indolent growth patterns and associated with long-term survival even when metastases are present. They can produce and secrete biogenic amines and polypeptide hormones that can result in complex syndromes with occasionally fatal metabolic and electrolyte complications.[69,70] The concept of apudomas was introduced by Pearse based on the common cytochemical characteristics of amine precursor uptake and decarboxylation (APUD) of these cells.[71] These tumors are normally found in the carotid body, adrenal medulla, thyroid, melanocytes, sympathetic system, and enteric and pancreatic islets, and the embryogenesis and ultrastructure characteristics suggest that they arise from the primitive neuroectoderm.[72] There is, however, experimental evidence to suggest that at least the pancreatic islet cells do not originate from the neural crest.[69]

Many APUD tumors occur in familial syndromes of multiple endocrine neoplasias. These syndromes affect family members in an autosomal dominant fashion with a high degree of penetrance. Multiple endocrine neoplasia (MEN) syndromes can be classified into three well-described patterns of endocrine gland involvement: (1) Wermer's syndrome (MEN I) is characterized by the presence of parathyroid hyperplasia, pancreatic islet cell tumors, and pituitary adenomas; (2) Sipple's syndrome (MEN II) includes medullary carcinoma of thyroid, parathyroid hyperplasia, and pheochromocytomas; (3) multiple mucosal neuroma syndrome (MEN III) includes medullary carcinoma of thyroid, bilateral pheochromocytomas, and multiple mucosal neuromas.[73–76] Overlapping of syndromes occurs in a sporadic fashion, as in the case of the association of pancreatic islet cell tumors and pheochromocytomas.[77]

Also, some syndromes have a high incidence of other neoplasia, such as MEN I and intestinal carcinoids and lipomas. A sizable number of these tumors also occur sporadically without any evidence of a hereditable or familial pattern.

2.1. Pheochromocytomas

Pheochromocytomas are APUD tumors that originate from chromaffin cells of the sympathetic nervous system. These tumors produce and secrete excessive amounts of catecholamines (epinephrine/norepinephrine). They are located in the adrenal in 90% of cases. Diagnosis is dependent on demonstration of high levels of free norepinephrine or its major metabolite, 3,4-dihydroxyphenylglycol (DHPG), in urine.[78] In addition, clinical manifestations of hypertension, headaches, palpitations, and diaphoresis are strongly suggestive of the disease. A recent study has shown that gas chromatography–mass spectrophotometric analysis for free norepinephrine in 24-hr urine samples had a 100% sensitivity and 98% specificity among 1192 urine samples. By contrast, there was 82% sensitivity and 95% specificity among 358 plasma samples. Measurements of plasma DHPG may sometimes

Table I. APUD Tumors

Syndrome	Cell of origin	Hormone	Clinical findings	Electrolyte disorders	Remarks
Pheochromocytoma	Sympatho chromaffin cell	Epinephrine/ norepinephrine	40% paroxysmal hypertension, headaches, palpitations, diaphoresis	Rarely hypercalcemia	10% extraadrenal, 10% malignant, 70% bilateral in familial cases
Medullary CA of thyroid	C cell (parafollicular)	Calcitonin	Thyroid mass, cervical adenopathy, watery diarrhea	Mild volume contraction	20% have MEN II
Carcinoid	Enterochromaffin cell	Serotonin, histamine, brady-kanin	58% flushing and diarrhea, 10% asthma, 12% asymptomatic, 37% cardiopathy	Hypokalemia, metabolic acidosis (if severe diarrhea)	90% appendix, small intestine, rectum; median survival with unresectable disease is 5 years
Insulinoma	B-islet cell	Insulin	Fasting hypoglycemia, neuroglycopenic signs	Hypercalcemia (MEN I)	10% are malignant, 90% are benign adenomas
Glucagonoma	A-islet cell	Glucagon	Dermatitis, diabetes mellitus, weight loss, anemia	Hypoaminoacidemia	High incidence of thromboembolisms, 70% are malignant tumors (necrolytic migratory erythema)
VIPoma	A-, B-, D-islet cells	VIP, PHI, prostaglandins	Secretory diarrhea, hypochlorhydria, flushing (20%), hyperglycemia (30%)	Volume contraction hypokalemia (100%), metabolic acidosis hypercalcemia (50%)	60% liver metastasis at diagnosis, pheochromocytoma, ganglioneuromas, small cell CA associated with high VIP
Gastrinomas	D-islet cells	Gastrin	Recurrent, intractable peptic ulcers, diarrhea (30%)	Hypercalcemia (25%)	MEN I in 25%, 90% pancreatic, 80% multifocal
Somatostatinoma	D-islet cell D (duodenal)	Somatostatin	Diabetes, hypoglycemia, gallbladder disease, diarrhea/steatorrhea, hypochlorydia, weight loss	Volume contraction hypocalcemia	60% pancreatic in origin, other found in duodenum
P Pomas	D-islet cells	Pancreatic polypeptide	Abdominal pain, hepatomegaly, watery diarrhea	Hypokalemia	PP levels increased in MEN I syndrome
Neurotensinomas	A–D-islet cell	Neurotensin, VIP	Water diarrhea, edema, hypotension, flushing, diabetes, cyanosis	Hypercalcemia, metabolic acidosis	Difficult to separate from VIPoma

prove useful in reducing the rate of false positive results.[78] Electrolyte disorders are usually not a presenting abnormality in patients with pheochromocytoma. In rare cases, these tumors can produce ectopic ACTH causing hypokalemia, metabolic alkalosis, and Cushing's syndrome.[79] Hypercalcemia can be seen in patients with familial pheochromocytoma as part of the hyperparathyroidism seen in MEN type II.[80]

In some cases of nonfamilial pheochromocytomas concomitant hypercalcemia can be present in the absence of parathyroid neoplasia and can be corrected by surgical removal of the tumor.[81,82] Various mechanisms have been suggested to explain the hypercalcemia in nonfamilial pheochomocytomas: (1) ectopic parathyroid hormone (PTH) production by adrenal tumor, (2) PTH-like hormone secreted by the tumor that stimulates adenylate cyclase, and (3) catecholamine activation of osteoclasts leading to bone resorption.[83] Studies done on tumor extracts from a patient with hypercalcemia-associated pheochromocytoma demonstrated the presence of bone-resorbing activity in a fetal rat bone assay. The extract caused stimulation of renal cortical adenylate cyclase similar to PTH, but the bone-resorbing activity was not abolished by preincubation with PTH antisera. Extracts from normocalcemic phechromocytoma failed to show this activity.[83]

2.2. Medullary Carcinoma of the Thyroid

During embryogenesis, the ultimobrachial body is incorporated into the lateral lobes of the thyroid and gives rise to the parafollicular or C cells (calcitonin). These cells are derived from the neural crest, strain with silver nitrate (argyrophilic), and are able to uptake and decarboxylate amine precursors. They secrete calcitonin, a 32-amino-acid polypeptide.[84]

The major physiologic action of calcitonin in humans is that of lowering serum calcium by reducing bone resorption. Calcitonin also inhibits PTH effects on bone, decreases alkaline phosphatase and pyrophosphatase activities, and inhibits hydroxyproline production. *In vitro* studies have shown that calcitonin directly inhibits osteoclast function.[85] The effect of calcitonin on bone resorption diminishes upon prolonged exposure. This "escape phenomenon" probably occurs as a result of down-regulation of receptors.

Medullary carcinoma of thyroid arise as a neoplastic transformation of parafollicular C cells. They account for 8% of all thyroid carcinomas. In 70–80% the tumor occurs in a sporadic, nonfamilial fashion. In 20–30% they occur as part of the MEN types II and III or rarely as familial, poorly characterized non-MEN syndromes. Most of the sporadic tumors tend to be unilateral and unifocal whereas familial tumors are commonly bilateral and multifocal.

In a study of large series of patients with nonfamilial medullary carcinoma of thyroid seen at M. D. Anderson Hospital, the most common presenting manifestation was that of a palpable thyroid nodule (94% of cases).[86] Diarrhea was a prominent feature in 29% of patients. In contrast, in patients with tumor and the MEN II syndrome, diagnosis was suspected in 50% cases, when family members were tested for elevated basal or stimulated levels of immunoreactive calcitonin. Basal levels of calcitonin can fall within the normal range of 30–40% of cases, but provocative tests with pentagastrin and/or calcium infusions lead to abnormally high circulating levels in almost all patients with medullary cancer of thyroid.[87] Other malignancies such as lung and breast cancer can cause high levels of immunoreactive calcitonin, yet hypocalcemia does not occur.

Total thyroidectomy is the only curative treatment for medullary cancer of thyroid. In cases of familial tumors, much care must be taken to diagnose and treat underlying pheochromocytomas prior to attempts at thyroid surgery in order to avoid life-threatening hypertensive crisis.[88]

Early diagnosis and treatment in patients with MEN II is associated with a 90% cure rate. The prognosis is poorer in patients with sporadic tumors or those with MEN type III; the death rate due to progressive tumor is close to 50%.

2.3. Carcinoid Tumors

In 1907, Oberndorfer described small intestinal tumors as "kazenoid" (carcinoid) because of their histologic resemblance to carcinomas, yet they followed a more benign course.[89] The syndrome of flushing, diarrhea, bronchoconstriction, and cardiac disease was recognized by Thorson et al. and attributed to serotonin secretion by these tumors.[90]

The mayority of carcinoid tumors are found in the gastrointestinal tract and the lungs, although they have been reported to occur in the thymus, prostate, skin, and other organs.[91] In the gastrointestinal tract they arise from enterochromaffin or K (Kultchinsky) cells of the mucosal crypts. Cytologically similar cells are found in proximal bronchi and trachea. These cells are part of the APUD system and are able to take amine precursors (aromatic amino acids) such as tryptophan and produce decarboxylation.

The syndrome is a consequence of the hormones released by the neoplastic cells. The diarrhea is most likely caused by serotonin. The use of antiserotonin agents such as cyproheptadine or methylsergide will control the bowel movements and ameliorate the diarrheic bouts. This controls the potential electrolyte disorders that may be seen in this syndrome, particularly hypokalemia and volume contraction.[92]

The attacks of flushing occur mainly in the head and neck area and upper trunk. They are short lived (1–2 min) and become generalized in very rare cases, when the vasodilatation can be severe enough to cause hypotension and syncope. Bronchoconstriction, when it occurs, usually follows an attack of flushing.

Many humoral mediators are implicated in the carcinoid flushing, including histamine, bradykinin, prostaglandins, and substances P and K (tachykinins). Histamine appears to be the predominant mediator of the flushing attacks in patients with gastric carcinoids since they can be abolished by the use of combined H_1 and H_2 blocking agents.[93]

Measurement of the levels of serotonin and its metabolite (5-HIAA) in the urine and the serotonin levels in plasma and platelet granules permits assessment of the activity of the tumors.

Small primary tumors in the appendix and rectum are cured with surgery in more than 90% of cases. The presence of liver metastasis makes the disease incurable. Tumor debulking surgery is indicated in some cases to afford palliation of symptoms. Interferons and somatostatin analogs are useful palliative intervention for the incurable patient, particularly in stopping the diarrheic and flushing episodes. Chemotherapeutic agents used with limited success in symptomatic patients include adryamicin, DTIC, streptozotocin, and 5-FU.[94,95]

2.4. Pancreatic Islet Cell Tumors

Islet cell tumors are APUDomas that originate from endocrine cells of the pancreas. They share many common features, such as similar histopathology, multiple hormone productions, and metastasis to regional lymph nodes and liver. The clinical symptoms and signs produced depend on the predominant hormones and polypeptides secreted by tumor cells.

2.4.1. Vipoma

One of the most dramatic syndromes of electrolyte and water disturbance is that caused by a pancreatic islet cell tumor that secretes a hormone known as vasoactive intestinal polypeptide (VIP). Patients present with severe secretory watery diarrhea (pancreatic cholera) leading to life-threatening hypokalemia, metabolic acidosis, and volume contraction.[96] Stool volume is usually greater than 3 liters/24 hr and diarrhea persists despite fasting. Potassium losses in the stools can reach levels greater than 400 meq/24 hr. Diarrheic fluid is isotonic with plasma and stool pH is greater than 7.5 owing to bicarbonate secretion. In addition, hyperglycemia and hypercalcemia can accompany this syndrome. Measurement of gastric fluid will demonstrate hypochlorhydria.

Although this tumor frequently produces and secretes other hormones and peptides, most of the clinical findings can be explained by tumor secretion of VIP.[97] *In vitro* experiments have demonstrated that VIP causes chloride secretion when applied to the serosal surface of intestinal mucosa.[98-100] Also, intravenous infusions of VIP given to healthy volunteers can produce the syndrome.[101] VIP abolishes water and sodium absorption and causes active chloride secretion (against electrochemical gradient) in the small bowel and bicarbonate secretion in the colon.[102] VIP effects in the intestinal mucosa are thought to occur by stimulation of the adenylate cyclase/cyclic AMP system, but measurements of cyclic nucleotides in tissue obtained from jejunal biopsies in vipoma patients have failed to document a rise in cyclic AMP.[103] Volunteers given high doses of VIP can experience episodes of flushing, vasodilatation as evidenced by occasional fall in blood pressure, and a decrease in stimulated gastric acid output. This evidence indicates that VIP mediates many of the findings of the clinical syndrome.

Intestinal water and electrolyte handling may be modified by other peptides secreted by VIP tumor cells; for example, peptide histidine methionine, which can be found in high levels in plasma in these patients, can cause modest diarrhea.[102]

Hypercalcemia can occur in up to 50% of patients with watery diarrhea syndrome.[96] In rare cases the hypercalcemia can be explained on the basis of MEN I which includes parathyroid adenomas, but in most cases PTH levels are normal. *In vitro* studies have shown that VIP can cause bone resorption via a cyclic AMP–dependent mechanism, so it may directly contribute to the hypercalcemia.[104]

The diagnosis of a VIP-secreting tumor can be established in a patient with severe watery diarrhea, metabolic acidosis, hypokalemia, flushing, a normal 24-hr urine for 5-HIAA, and an elevated (usually three or four times the normal level, depending on the assay) VIP level in plasma. In 50% of cases, metastases to regional lymph nodes and liver are present.[96]

In some cases, tumor debulking (surgery) or cytotoxic chemotherapy can offer some palliation of symptoms. Tumor growth will continue, and tumor debulking (surgery), cytotoxic chemotherapy, and embolization of hepatic metastasis are of limited benefit in most cases. Palliation of symptoms can be offered with various substances, particularly somatostatin, that decrease the secretion of VIP by the tumor. Also, drugs that inhibit target organ effects, such as opiates and loperamide, may be useful.[96,102]

While most other APUD tumors will not regularly produce prominent electrolyte disorders as part of their initial clinical findings, in some well-documented cases, these tumor cells can produce and secrete other peptide hormones (ACTH, serotonin, VIP, PTH, prostaglandin, kallikrein) that can cause serious electrolyte (potassium, calcium, sodium, magnesium) and water disorders.[96,102]

2.4.2. Gastrinoma

In 1955, Zollinger and Ellison described a syndrome of recurrent peptic ulcer disease and pancreatic tumors.[105] It was later recognized that the syndrome was produced by an islet cell tumor of the pancreas that secreted a gastric secretagogue (gastrin) responsible for the gastric hyperacidity and the recurrent ulcerogenic diathesis.

It is well recognized now that in 60% of patients with gastrin-secreting islet cell tumors (gastrinomas), other endocrine neoplasia of pituitary and parathyroids glands coexists as part of the MEN I syndrome.[106] Almost 100% of gastrinoma/MEN I patients have evidence of hyperparathyroidism.[107]

In a recent study of 75 consecutive patients with Zollinger–Ellison (Z–E) syndrome, the presence of concomitant Cushing syndrome was noted.[108] Five percent of patients with the sporadic form of Z–E syndrome had severe symptoms due to ectopic production of ACTH by the tumor. Nineteen percent of patients with Z–E syndrome and MEN I syndrome had Cushing syndrome due to pituitary production of ACTH.

Most patients with gastrinoma syndrome present with peptic ulcer disease signs, symptoms, or complications.[109] In 30% of cases a major complaint is severe, intractable diarrhea. The diarrhea is usually secretory in nature, but rarely will lead to prominent electrolyte or water imbalances, in contrast to other islet cell tumors (VIP-secreting tumors). The diarrhea is caused by large amounts of hydrochloric acid reaching the small bowel, with inhibition of water and sodium absorption. High gastrin levels will also induce chloride and water secretion. A fall in the pH of duodenal and jejunal contents, steatorrhea, and malabsorption can ensue as a result of inactivation of pancreatic lipase.[110]

Acid intestinal contents can also impair vitamin B_{12}/intrinsic factor absorption in distal ileum, leading to megaloblastosis and worsening diarrhea.[110] The diagnosis can be established in the patient with ulcerogenic diathesis and high basal and stimulated levels of immunoreactive gastrin in the presence of gastric hyperacidity. Other conditions of hypergastrinemia, such as pernicious anemia, atrophic gastritis, antral G-cell hyperplasia, pyloric stenosis, short bowel syndrome, and chronic renal failure, must be ruled out.[109] In 50–85% of cases, a primary tumor can be found in the pancreas. In 10–20% of cases, the primary tumor is not found or can arise from the duodenal or stomach mucosa. In patients with MEN I syndrome, the tumors are slow growing and can appear years after the diagnosis of gastrinoma has been made on clinical grounds.

Owing to the multifocal nature of the pancreatic tumor and to the presence of liver and lymph node metastasis, surgical cure occurs in less than 20% of patients.[111] Yet, good palliation of symptoms can be accomplished with the use of H_2 blockers, such as cimetidine and ranitidine.

In a recent study of patients with islet cell tumors and liver metastasis, good palliation of symptoms was obtained with sequential hepatic artery embolization.[112] Chemotherapeutic agents such as 5-FU or streptozotozin are of limited value in this disease.

2.4.3. Glucagonomas

In 1966 McGavran et al.[113] described the first well-documented case of an A_2-cell carcinoma of the pancreas secreting glucagon and causing a typical rash and mild diabetes mellitus. Since then, multiple clinical types of glucagonomas have been described: (1) glucagonoma with a typical glucagonoma clinical syndrome, (2) solitary glucagonomas with or without diabetes, (3) multiple concurrent islet cell tumors (glucagonomas, insulinomas, gastrinomas), (4) multiple glucagonomas with MEN type I, and (5) solitary microglucagonomas of the elderly.[114,115]

The most typical manifestation of the glucagonoma syndrome is the presence of a necrolytic migratory erythematous rash.[116] Initially, it presents with papules and macules with superficial scaling, progressing to blistering, crusting, and hyperpigmentation. The etiology of the rash is unknown, but is most probably related to zinc and amino acid deficiency typically found in patients with the full-blown syndrome. The rash initially responds to zinc treatment, but may remit despite supplementation. The rash also parellels the development of profound hypoaminoacidemia (especially of citrulline, proline, ornithine, tyrosine, glycine, threonine, and alanine) and can be corrected by amino acid replacement.[117,118] The changes in amino acid concentrations are due to glucagon-induced gluconeogenesis and not to amino aciduria, and they can be reproduced in normal, healthy volunteers by exogenous glucagon administration. Other manifestations of the glucagonoma syndrome include (1) diabetes mellitus, (2) normocytic normochromic anemia, (3) weight loss, (4) thromboembolic phenomena (30% of cases), and (5) painful glossitis, stomatitis, and angular cheilosis.

Diagnosis can usually be established by detecting high plasma levels of glucagon in patients with the characteristic symptoms and signs. The malignant nature of this tumor is apparent by the local–regional and distant metastasis (to liver) documented in 60% of cases. Exploratory laparotomy with removal of primary tumor and debulking of metastatic lesions is the only curative approach.[119]

The use of a somatostatin analog (Sandoz, SMS 201-995) can reduce glucagon production by the tumor, and palliation is thus obtained. In some cases, worsening of glucose intolerance and weight loss can occur with somatostatin treatment owing to a decrease in other pancreatic hormones, especially insulin.[120]

2.4.4. Insulinomas

Insulinomas are rare tumors of beta-islet cells of pancreas. The incidence is less than one per million people per year. In 5% of cases the tumor is part of the MEN I syndrome. In 60 consecutive cases described by Service *et al.* from the Mayo Clinic, 78% of the tumors were found to be benign solitary adenomas of pancreas; in only 8% were the tumors malignant and exhibiting metastasis.[121]

Patients present with signs and symptoms of hypoglycemia secondary to insulin secretion by the tumor. Most of the presenting clinical features of patients with insulinomas can be attributed to the effects of hypoglycemia on the brain or to its effect of releasing catecholamines. Confusion, abnormal behavior, amnesia, and even unconsciousness occur in 50–80% of cases. Combinations of diplopia, blurred vision, sweating, palpitation, and weakness are noted in 85% of cases. Approximately 20% of patients are initially misdiagnosed as having a primary neurologic or psychiatric condition.[119]

Surgical excision of the tumor is curative in a high percentage of cases. In patients with advanced tumors and metastases, debulking surgery can provide palliative relief of symptoms. Diazoxide, a nondiuretic benzothiadiazine, can be used to ameliorate symptoms in inoperable patients.[122] This drug, initially synthesized as a hypotensive agent, can cause hyperglycemia by inhibiting insulin release directly and by stimulating glycogenolysis. Cytotoxic treatments with 5-FU and streptozotozin have been of limited benefit. The benefits of somatostatin analogs in the treatment of islet cell tumors await confirmatory studies for insulinomas.[123]

2.4.5. Somatostatinoma

Somatostatin was discovered in 1968, during a search for a hypothalamic growth hormone inhibitory factor.[124] Hellman and Lernmark found somatostatin in extracts of pancreatic islet A cells.[125] This tetradecapeptide belongs to a family of peptides with inhibitory function on a variety of endocrine glands. It inhibits the release of neurohormones (GH,TSH, prolactin, ACTH) from the pituitary. It blocks the release of various gastroenteropancreatic hormones (gastrin, cholecystokinin, pancreozymin, secretin, motilin, insulin, glucagon, and VIP).[126] It also inhibits the release of renin from the juxtaglomerular apparatus. In fact, infusions of somatostatin to volunteers produce hyporeninemia. The mechanism of this action seems to be mediated by beta antagonism.[127] Further studies have shown that somatostatin can practically inhibit all gastrointestinal and pancreatic endocrine and exocrine functions. It also inhibits gastric acid release (basal and stimulated), gallbladder contraction, and intestinal absorption. The native protein and the long-acting synthetic analog (sandozstatin) are also affective in blocking the release of hormones from various endocrine tumors (vipomas, glucagonomas, insulinomas, carcinoids).

In a recent article, Vinik *et al.* reviewed the clinical features of the somatostatinoma syndrome.[128] Twenty-seven cases were of pancreatic origin and 21 cases originated in the duodenum and jejunum. In 78% of cases of pancreatic tumor, nonketotic diabetes mellitus was a common presenting feature, but occurred in only 14% of primary intestinal tumors. Hypoglycemic attacks did not occur when the primary tumor was in the intestine, but occurred in 30% of patients with pancreatic tumors. An explanation for this is not apparent. Weight loss is frequently present. Contributing factors are hypochloridia, diarrhea, and steatorrhea, which are common complaints in 90% of patients with pancreatic tumors. Of interest is the coexistance of neurofibromas, café au lait spots, and pheochromocytomas in 25% of intestinal tumors.

Somatostatinomas are commonly malignant tumors and metastases are found in 70% of cases. Surgery (tumor debulking) is indicated in all patients in an attempt to cure or palliate symptoms.[128]

2.4.6. Pancreatic Polypeptide Cell Tumors

Pancreatic polypeptide hormone was isolated and characterized by Kimmel *et al.* in 1975.[129] This peptide is produced by D_1 cells which are widely scattered throughout the pancreas and its ducts. No specific physiologic function for this hormone has been recognized, although there is some evidence that it might work by inhibiting gallbladder contraction and some pancreatic enzyme secretion.

Pancreatic endocrine tumors are frequently composed of multiple cell types. In one series, 55% of tumors were found to contain mixed cell types by immunocytochemistry and radioimmunochemistry of tumor cells.[130] In 30% of tumors, pancreatic polypeptide cells were found, and this was most striking in VIP-producing tumors. In some cases, pancreatic polypeptide cell hyperplasia coexisted with functioning islet cell tumors, and cells were not part of the malignant process.

Pancreatic polypeptide cell tumors have been considered "silent" tumors, but in a review of 21 cases by Vinik et al.[128], 50% of patients with these tumors had weight loss and 30% had watery diarrhea as presenting complaints. Also, 30% of cases had other endocrine neoplasia as part of the MEN I syndrome. In patients with elevation of pancreatic polypeptide hormone and a pancreatic mass, exploratory laparotomy and tumor resection is indicated. Chemotherapy and somatostatin can prove useful for palliation of patients with unresectable disease.

2.4.7. Neurotensinoma

Neurotensin was initially isolated from bovine hypothalamus by Carraway and Leeman.[131] A 13-amino-acid polypeptide, it can cause hypotension, hyperglycemia, vasodilation, and cyanosis. Most cases of neurotension-secreting tumors also produce VIP and present with the watery diarrhea, hypokalemia, acidosis syndrome. In these cases, it becomes difficult to evaluate the role of neurotensin in the clinical presentations.[132]

References

1. Guthrie, L. G., 1902, Idiopathic or congenital hereditary and family hematuria, Lancet 1:1243–1246.
2. Alport, A. C., 1927, Hereditary familial congenital hemorrhagic nephritis, Br. Med. J. 101:504–506.
3. Sturtz, G. S. and Burke, E. C., 1956, Hereditary hematuria, nephropathy and deafness; preliminary report, N. Engl. J. Med., 254:1123–1126.
4. Sohar, E., 1956, Renal disease, inner ear deafness, and ocular changes; a new heredofamilial syndrome, AMA Arch. Intern. Med. 97:627–630.
5. Goldbloom, R. B., 1957, Hereditary renal disease associated with nerve deafness and ocular lesions, Pediatrics 20:241–247.
6. Nieth, H., 1959, A contribution to the syndrome of hereditary hematuria, nephropathy and deafness, Verh. Deutsch. Ges. Inn. Med. 65:664–667.
7. Klotz, R. E., 1959, Congenital hereditary kidney disease and hearing loss: A case history. AMA Arch. Otolaryngol. 69:560–565.
8. Russell, E. P. and Smith, J. J., 1959, Hereditary hematuria, AMA J. Dis. Child. 98:401–409.
9. Williamson, D. A. J., 1961, Alport's syndrome of hereditary nephritis with deafness, Lancet 2:1321–1323.
10. Eckstein, J. D., Filip, D. J., and Watts, J. C., 1975, Hereditary thrombocytopenia, deafness, and renal disease, Ann. Intern. med. 82:639–645.
11. Epstein, C. J., Sahud, M. A., Piel, C. F., Goodman, J. R., Bernfield, M. R., Kusner, J. H., and Ablin, A. R., 1972, Hereditary macrothrombocytopathia, nephritis and deafness. Am. J. Med. 52:299–310.
12. Gubler, M. C., Levy, M., Broyer, M., Naizot, C., González, G., Perrin, D., and Habib, R.,

1981, Alport's syndrome: A report of 58 cases and a review of the literature, *Am. J. Med.* **70**:493–505.

13. Peterson, L. C., Rao, K. V., Crosson, J. T., and White, J. G., 1985, Fechtner syndrome—A variant of Alport's syndrome with leukocyte inclusions and macrothrombocytopenia, *Blood* **65**:397–406.

14. Barakat, A. Y., D'Albora, J. B., Martin, M. M., and Jose, P., 1977, Familial nephrosis, nerve deafness, and hypoparathyroidism, *J. Pediatr.* **91**:61–64.

15. Passwell, J. H., David, R., Boichis, H., and Herzfeld, S., 1981, Hereditary nephritis with associated defects in proximal renal tubular function, *J. Pediatr.* **98**:85–87.

16. Marin, O. S. M. and Tyler, H. R., 1961, Hereditary interstitial nephritis associated with polyneuropathy, *Neurology* **11**:999–1005.

17. Wallace, I. R. and Jones, J. H., 1960, Familial glomerulonephritis and aminoaciduria, *Lancet* **1**:941–943.

18. Goyer, R. A., Reinords,, J., Burke, J., and Burkholder, P., 1968, Hereditary renal disease with neurosensory hearing loss, prolinuria and ichthyosis, *Am. J. Med. Sci.* **256**:166–179.

19. Brivet, F., Girot, R., Barbanel, C.; Gazengel, C., Maier, M., and Crosnier, J., 1981, Hereditary nephritis associated with May–Hegglin anomaly, *Nephron* **29**:59–62.

20. Hansen, M. S., Behnke, O., Pedersen, N. T., and Bidebaek, A., 1978, Magathrombocytopenia associated with glomerulonephritis, deafness and aortic cystic medianecrosis, *Scand. J. Haematol.* **21**:197–199.

21. Perrin, D., Jungers, P., Grunfeld, J. P., Delons, S., Noel, L. H., and Zenatti, C., 1979, Perimacular changes in Alport's syndrome, *Clin. Nephrol.* **13**:163–167.

22. O'Neill, W. M., Atkin, C. L., and Bloomer, H. A., 1978, Hereditary nephritis: A re-examination of its clinical and genetic features, *Ann. Intern. Med.* **88**:176–182.

23. Kaufman, D. B., McIntosh, R. M., Smith, F. G., and Vernier, R. L., 1970, Diffuse familial nephropathy: A clinico pathological study, *J. Pediatr.* **77**:37–41.

24. Ferguson, A. C. and Rance, C. P., 1972, Hereditary nephropathy with nerve deafness (Alport's syndrome), *Am. J. Dis. Child.* **124**:84–86.

25. Hinglais, N., Grunfeld, J. P., and Bois, E. P., 1972, Characteristic ultrastructural lesions of the glomerular basement membrane in progressive hereditary nephritis (Alport's syndrome), *Lab. Invest.* **27**:473–487.

26. Grunfeld, J. P., Noel, L. H., Hafez, S., *et al.*, 1985, Renal prognosis in women with hereditary nephritis, *Clin. Nephrol.* **23**:267–273.

27. Grunfeld, J. P., Bois, E. P., and Hinglais, N., 1973, Progressive and nonprogressive hereditary chronic nephritis, *Kidney Int.* **4**:216–228.

28. Grünfeld, J. P., 1985, The clinical spectrum of hereditary nephritis, *Kidney Int.* **27**:83–92.

29. Schneider, R. G., 1963, Congenital hereditary nephritis with nerve deafness, *NY J. Med.* Sept. 15:2644–2648.

30. Rumpelt, H. J., 1979, Hereditary nephropathy (Alport's syndrome): Correlation of clinical data with glomerular basement membrane alterations, *Clin. Nephrol.* **13**:203–207.

31. Farboody, G. H., Valenzuela, R., McCormack, L. J., Kallen, R., and Osborne, 1D. G., 1979, Chronic hereditary nephritis: A clinicopathologic study of 23 new kindreds and review of the literature, *Chronic Hered. Nephritis* **10**:655–668.

32. Gleeson, M. J., 1984, Alport's syndrome: Audiological manifestations and implications, *J. Laryngol. Otol.* **98**:449–465.

33. Rinlemann, W. F., 1976, Auditory manifestations of Alport's disease syndrome, *Trans. Am. Acad. Ophthalmol. Otol.* **82**:375–378.

34. Odkvist, L. M., Kylen, P., and Lundberg, M., 1976, Two families with Alport's syndrome, *Acta Otolaryngol.* **82**:234–239.

35. Myers, G. J. and Tyler, H. R., 1972, The etiology of deafness in Alport's syndrome, *Arch. Otolaryngol.* **96**:333–340.

36. Arnold, W., 1980, Uberlegungen zur Pathogenese des cochleo-renalen Syndroms. *Acta. Otolaryngol.* (Stockh.) **89:**330–336.
37. Cassady, G., Brown, K., Cohen, M., and DeMaria, W., 1965, Hereditary renal dysfunction and deafness, *Pediatrics* **35:**967–979.
38. Chazan, J. A., Zacks, J., Cohen, J. J., and Garella, S., 1971, Hereditary nephritis. Clinical spectrum and mode of inheritance in five new kindreds, *Am. J. Med.* **50:**764–771.
39. Purriel, P., Drets, M., Pascale, E., Sánchez-Cestau, R., Borrás, A., Ferreira, W. A., De Lucca, A., and Fernández, L., 1970, Familial hereditary nephropathy (Alport's syndrome), *Am. J. Med.* **49:**753–773.
40. Sohar, E., 1956, Renal disease, inner ear deafness, and ocular changes, *Arch. Intern. Med.* **97:** 627–630.
41. Habib, R., Gubler, M., Hinglais, N., Noel, L., Droz, D., Levy, M., Mahieu, P., Foidart, J., Perrin, D., Bois, E., and Grunfeld, J., 1982, Alport's syndrome: Experience at Hopital Necker, *Kidney Int.* **21:**S20–S28.
42. Perrin, D., 1964, Le syndrome d'Alport, *Ann. Ocul.* **197:**329–346.
43. Arnott, E. J., Crawford, M. D. A., and Toghill, P. J., 1966, Anterior lenticonus and Alport's syndrome, *Br. J. Ophthalmol.* **50:**390–403.
44. Polak, B. C. P. and Hogewind, B. L., 1977, Macular lesions in Alport's syndrome, *Am. J. Ophthalmol.* **84:**532–535.
45. Spear, G. S. and Slusser, R. J., 1972, Alport's syndrome: Emphasizing electron microscopic studies of the glomerulus, *Am. J. Pathol.* **69:**213–219.
46. Yoshikawa, N., Cameron, A. H., and White, R. H. R., 1981, The glomerular basal lamina in hereditary nephritis, *J. Pathol.* **135:**199–209.
47. Kohaut, E. C., Singer, D. B., Nevels, B. K., and Hill, L. L., 1976, The specificity of split renal membranes in hereditary nephritis, *Arch. Pathol. Lab. Med.* **100:**475–479.
48. Hill, G. S., Jenis, E. H., and Goodloe, S., 1974, The nonspecificity of the ultrastucture lesion in hereditary nephritis: With additional observations on benign familial hematuria, *Lab. Invest.* **31:** 516–532.
49. Yum, M., and Bergstein, J. M., 1983, Basement membrane nephropathy: A new classification for Alport's syndrome and asumptomatic hematuria based on ultrastructural findings, *Hum. Pathol.* **14:**996–1003.
50. Piel, C. F., Biava, C. G., and Goodman, J., 1982, Glomerular basement membrane attenuation in familial nephritis and "benign" hematuria, *J. Pediatr.* **101:**358–365.
51. Spear, G. S., 1984, Hereditary nephritis (Alport's syndrome), *Clin. Nephrol.* **21:**3–6.
52. Spear, G. S., 1973, Alport's syndrome: A consideration of pathogenesis, *Clin. Nephrol.* **1:**336–338.
53. DiBona, G. F., 1983, Alport's syndrome: A genetic defect in biochemical composition of basement membrane of glomerulus, lens, and inner ear? *J. Lab. Clin. Med.* **101:**817–820.
54. Tina, L. U., Lou, M. F., Dizio, D., and Calcagno, P. L., 1979, Alteration of collagen metabolism in hereditary nephritis, *Pediatr. Res.* **13:**774–776.
55. Veltischev, Y., Ignatova, M., Ananenko, A., Klembovsky, A., Daihin, E., Brydun, A., and Degtyareva, E., 1983, Hereditary nephritis and hypoplastic dysplastic nephropathy: Hydroxylysine glycoside excretion and the glomular basement membrane, *Int. J. Pediatr. Nephrol.* **4:**149–154.
56. Schroder, C. H., Monnens, L. A. H., Lith-Zanders, H. M. A., Trijbels, J. M. F., Veerkamp, J. H., and Langeveld, J. P. M., 1986, Urinary excretion hydroxylysine and its glycosides in Alport's syndrome and several other glomerulopathies, *Nephron* **44:**103–107.
57. McCoy, R. C., Johnson, K., Stone, W., and Wilson, C., 1982, Absence of nephritogenic GMB antigen(s) in some patients with hereditary nephritis, *Kidney Int.* **21:**642–452.
58. Olson, D. L., and Anand, S. K., Landing, B. H., Heuser, E., Grushkin, C. M., and Lieberman, E., 1980, Diagnosis of hereditary nephritis by failure of glomeruli to bind anti-glomerular basement membrane antibodies. *Pediatrics* **96:**697–699.

59. Jenis, E. H., Valeski, J. E., and Calcagno, P. L., 1981, Variability of anti-GBM binding in hereditary nephritis, *Clin. Nephrol.* **15**:11–14.
60. Kashtan, C., Fish, A., Kleppel, M., Yoshioka, K., and Michael, A., 1986, Nephritogenic antigen determinants in epidermal and renal basement membranes of kindreds with Alport-type familial nephritis, *J. Clin. Invest.* **78**:1035–1044.
61. Kleppel, M., Kashtan, C., Butkowski, R., Fish, A. and Michael, A., 1987, Alport familial nephritis, *J. Clin. Invest.* **80**:263–266.
62. Melvin, T., Kim, Y., and Michael, A., 1968, Amyloid P component is not present in the glomerular basement membrane in Alport-type hereditary nephritis, *Am. J. Pathol.* **125**:460–464.
63. Savage, C., Kershaw, M., Pusey, C., Barratt, T., Reed, A., Pincott, J., Dillon, M., and Lockwood, C., 1986, Use of a monoclonal antibody in differential diagnosis of children with haematuria and hereditary nephritis, *Lancet* **1**:1459–1461.
64. Hasstedt, S., Atkin, C., and San Juan, A., 1986, Genetic heterogeneity among kindreds with Alport syndrome, *Am. J. Hum. Genet.* **38**:940–953.
65. Evans, S. H., Erickson, R., Kelsch, R., and Peirce, J., 1980, Apparently changing patterns of inheritance in Alport's hereditary nephritis: Genetic heterogeneity versus altered diagnostic criteria, *Clin Genet.* **17**:285–292.
66. Hasstedt, S. and Atkin, C., 1983, X-linked inheritance of Alport syndrome: Family P revisited, *Am. J. Hum. Genet.* **35**:1241–1251.
67. Atkin, C. L., Gregory, M. C., and Border, W. A., 1988, Alport syndrome, in: *Diseases of the Kidney*, 4th ed. (R. W. Schrier and C. W. Gottschalk, eds.), Little, Brown, Boston, pp. 617–641.
68. Feingold, J., Bois, E., Chompret, A., Broyer, M., Gubler, M., and Grunfeld, J., 1985, Genetic heterogeneity of Alport syndrome, *Kidney Int.* **27**:672–677.
69. Mazzaferri, E. L. and O'Dorisio, T. M., 1987, Endocrine tumors: Special problems in diagnostic and management, *Semin. Oncol.* **14**(3):237–246.
70. Moertel, C. G., 1987, An odyssey in the land of small tumors, *J. Clin. Oncol.* **5**(10):1503–1522.
71. Pearse, A. G. E., 1968, Common cytochemical and ultrastructural characteristics of cells producing polypeptide hormones, *Proc. R. Soc. Lond.* **170**:71–80.
72. Pearse, A. G. E., 1980, The APUD concept and hormone production, *Clin. Endocrinol. Metab.* **9**: 211–222.
73. Wermer, P., 1954, Genetic aspects of adenomatosis of endocrine glands, *Am. J. Med.* **16**:363–371.
74. Sipple, J. H., 1961, The association of pheochromocytoma with carcinoma of the thyroid gland, *Am. J. Med.* **31**:163–166.
75. Williams, E. D. and Pollock, D. J., 1966, Multiple mucosal neuromata with endocrine tumors: A syndrome allied to Von Recklinghousin's disease, *J. Pathol. Bacteriol.* **91**:71–88.
76. Leskin, M., 1985, Multiple endocrine neoplasia, in: *Williams Endocrinology*, 7th ed. (J. Wilson and D. Foster, eds.), Saunders, Philadelphia, pp. 1274–1289.
77. Carney, J. A., Go, V. L. M., and Gordon, H., 1980, Familiar pheochromocytomas and islet cell tumors of the pancreas, *Am. J. Med.* **68**:515–521.
78. Duncan, M. W., Compton, P., Lazauus, L., and Smythe, G. A., 1988, Measurements of norepinephrine and 3,4-Dehydroxyphenylglycol in urine and plasma for the diagnosis of pheochromocytoma, *N. Engl. J. Med.* **319**:136–142.
79. Forman, B. H., Marban, E., and Kayne, R., 1979, Ectopic ACTH syndrome due to pheochromocytoma, *Yale J. Biol. Med.* **52**:181.
80. Lips, K. J. M., Veer, J. S., and Struyvenberg, A., 1981, Bilateral occurrence of pheochromocytoma in patients with MEN type II, *Am. J. Med.* **70**:1051–1059.
81. Gray, R. S. and Gillon, J., 1976, Normotensive pheochromocytoma with hypercalcemia: Correction after adrenalectomy, *Br. J. Med.* **1**:378.
82. Heath, H. and Edis, A. J., 1979, Pheochromocytoma associated with hypercalcemia and ectopic secretion of calcitonin, *Ann. Intern. Med.* **91**:208–210.

83. Stewart, A. F., Hoecker, J. L., Mallet, L. E., Segre, G. V., Amatruda, T. T., and Visnery, A., 1985, Hypercalcemia in pheochromocytoma, *Ann. Intern. Med.* **102:**776–779.
84. Tashjian, A. H., Wolfe, H. J., and Voelkel, E. F., 1974, Human calcitonin, *Am. J. Med.* **56:**840–849.
85. Holtrop, M. E., Raisz, L. G., and Simmons, H. A., 1974, The effects of parathyroid hormone, colchicine and calcitonin on the ultrastructure and activity of osteoclast in organ culture, *J. Cell. Biol.* **60:**346–355.
86. Saad, M. F., Ordonez, N. G., Rashid, R. K., Guido, J. J., Hill, C. S., Hickey, R. C., and Samaan, N. A., 1984, Medullary carcinoma of thyroid: A study of the clinical and prognostic factors in 161 patients, *Medicine* **63**(6):319–342.
87. Samaan, N. A., Castillo, S., and Schultz, P. N., 1980, Serum calcitonin after pentagastrin in patients with broncogenic and breast cancer, *J. Clin. Endocrinol. Metab.* **51:**237–241.
88. Sizemore, G. W., 1987, Medullary carcinoma of thyroid, *Semin. Oncol.* **14**(3):306–314.
89. Oberndorfer, S., 1970, Uber die klienen dumdarn-carcinome, *Verh. Dtsch. Patholges.* **11:**113–116.
90. Thorson, G., Bjork, G., and Bjorkmann, G., 1954, Malignant carcinoid of the small intestine with metastasis to the liver, vascular heart disease, peripheral vasomotor symptoms, bronchoconstriction and an unusual type of cyanosis, *Am. Heart J.* **47:**795–817.
91. Feldman, J. M., 1987, Carcinoid tumors and syndrome, *Semin. Oncol.* **14**(3):237–246.
92. Oates, J. A., 1986, The carcinoid syndrome, *N. Engl. J. Med.* **315**(11):702–704.
93. Roberts, L. S., Marney, S. R., and Oates, J. A., 1979, Blockade of the flush associated with gastric carcinoids by combined H_1 and receptor antagonist, *N. Engl. J. Med.* **300:**236–238.
94. Kvols, L. K., Moertel, C. G., O'Connell, M. J., Schutt, A. J., Rubin, J., and Hann, R. G., 1986, The treatment of the malignant carcinoid syndrome, *N. Engl. J. Med.* **315:**663–666.
95. Creutzfeld, T. W. and Stockmann, F., 1987, Carcinoids and carcinoid syndrome, *Am. J. Med.* **82:**4–16.
96. Mekhjian, H. S. and O'Dovisio, T. M., 1987, Vipoma syndrome, *Semin. Oncol.* **14:**3, 282–291.
97. Modlin, I. M., Bloom, S. R., and Mitchell, S. J., 1978, Experimental evidence for vasoactive intestinal peptide as the cause of the watery diarrhea syndrome, *Gastroenterology* **75:**1051–1055.
98. Schwartz, C. J., Kimberg, D. V., Sheevin, H. W., Field, M., and Said, S. I., 1974, Vasoactive intestinal peptide stimulation of adenylate cyclase and active electrolyte secretion of intestinal mucosa, *J. Clin. Invest.* **54:**536–544.
99. Eklund, S., Brunsson, I., Jodal, M., and Lundgren, O., 1987, Evidence against cAMP mediating VIP induced intestinal secretion, *Acta Physiol. Scand.* **129**(1):115–125.
100. Krejs, G. J., Barkley, R. M., Read, N. W., and Fordtran, J. S., 1978, Intestinal secretion induced by VIP. A comparison with cholera toxin, *J. Clin. Invest.* **61:**1337–1345.
101. Kane, M. G., O'Dorisio, T. M., and Krejs, G. J., 1983, Production of secretory diarrhea by intravenous infusion of vasoactive intestinal peptide, *N. Engl. J. Med.* **309:**1482.
102. Krejs, G. J., 1987, Vipoma syndrome, *Am. J. Med.* **82**(58):37–48.
103. Schwartz, S. E., Fitzgerald, M. A., and Levine, R. A., 1975, Normal jejunal cyclic nucleotide in a patient with secretory diarrhea, *Arch. Intern. Med.* **138:**1403.
104. Hohmann, E. ., Levine, L., and Tashijian, A. H., 1983, Vasoactive intestinal peptide stimulates bone resorption via a cyclic adenosine 3'-5'-monophosphate-dependent mechanism, *Endocrinology* **112:**1233–1239.
105. Zollinger, R. M. and Ellison, E. H., 1955, Primary peptic ulcerations of the jejunum associated with islet cell tumor of the pancreas, *Am. Surg.* **142:**709–728.
106. Lamer, C. B., Stadil, F., and Van Tougeren, J. H., 1978, Prevalence of endocrine abnormalities in patients with Z–E syndrome, *Am. J. Med.* **64:**607–612.
107. Betts, J. B., O'Malley, B. P., and Rosenthal, F. D., 1980, Hyperparathyroidsm: a prerequisite for the Zollinger–Ellison syndrome in MEN I, *Q. J. Med.* **49:**69–76.
108. Maton, P. N., Gardner, J. D., and Jensen, R. T., 1986, Cushing syndrome in patients with the Zollinger–Ellison syndrome, *N. Engl. J. Med.* **315:**1–5.

109 Zollinger, R. M., 1987, Gastrinoma: The Zollinger–Ellison syndrome, *Semin. Oncol.* **14**(3):247–252.

110. Shimoda, S., Sounders, D. R., and Rubin, C., 1968, The Zollinger–Ellison syndrome with steatorrea: Mechanisms of fat and B_{12} malabsorption. *Gastroenterology* **55**:705–710.

111. Ellison, E. C., Carey, L. C., Sparks, J., O'Dorisio, T. M., Merkhjian, H. S., Fromkes, J. J., Caldwell, J. H., and Thomas, F. B., 1987, Early surgical treatment of gastrinomas, *Am. J. Med.* **82**:17–22.

112. Ajani, J. A., Carrasco, H., Charsan Gavej, C., Samaan, N. A., Levin, B., and Wallace, S., 1988, Islet cell tumors metastatic to the liver: Effective palliation by hepatic artery embolization, *Ann. Intern. Med.* **108**:340–344.

113. McGavarn, H. H., Unger, R. H., and Recant, L., 1966, A glucagon-secreting alpha-cell carcinoma of the pancreas, *N. Engl. J. Med.* **274**:1408–1413.

114. Ruttman, E., Kloppel, G., Bommer, G., Kiehn, M., and Heitz, P. V., 1980, Pancreatic glucagonoma with or without syndrome, *Virch. Arch. Pathol. Anat. Histol.* **388**:51–67.

115. Warner, T. F., Block, M., Hafez, R., Mack, E., Lloyd, R. V., and Bloom, S. R., 1983, Celucagonomas: Ultrastructure and immunocytochemistry. *Cancer* **51**:1090–1096.

116. Bloom, S. R. and Polak, J. M., 1987, Glucagonoma syndrome, *Am. J. Med.* **82**:25–35.

117. Norton, J. A., Kahn, C. R., and Schiebinger, R., 1979, Amino acid deficency and the skin rash associated with glucagonoma syndrome, *Ann. Intern. Med.* **91**:213–215.

118. Boden, G., Razvani, I., and Owens, O. E., 1984, Effects of glucagon on plasma amino acids, *J. Clin. Invest.* **73**:785–793.

119. Guenther, B., 1987, Insulinoma and glucagonoma. *Semin. Oncol.* **14**:253–262.

120. Boden, G., Ryan, I. G., and Eisenschmid, B. L., 1986, Treatment of inoperable glucagonoma with long acting somatostatin analogue SMS 201–995, *N. Engl. J. Med.* **314**:1686–1689.

121. Service, F. J., Dale, A. J. D., Elveback, L. R., and Jiang, N. S., 1976, Insulinoma clinical and diagnostic features of 60 consecutive cases, *Mayo Clin. Proc.* **51**:417–149.

122. Yabo, R., Viktora, J., and Stagnet, M., 1965, Studies concerning the hypoglycemic effects of diazoxide and its mode of action, *Diabetes* **14**:591–594.

123. Osei, H. and O'Dorisio, T., 1985, Malignant insulinoma: Effects of somatostatin analogue, *Ann. Intern. Med.* **103**:223–225.

124. Krulich, L., Dhaviwal, A. P., and McCann, S. M., 1968, Stimulatory and inhibitory effects of purified hypothalamic extracts on growth hormone release, *Endocrinology* **83**:783–790.

125. Hellman, B. and Lernmark, A., 1969, Inhibition of *in vitro* insulin secretion by an extract of pancreatic A_1 cells, *Endocrinology* **84**:1484–1487.

126. Krejs, G., Orci, L., Conlon, J. M., and Ravazzola, M., 1979, Somatostatin syndrome, *N. Engl. J. Med.* **301**:285–292.

127. Rosenthal, J., Escobar, F., and Raptis, S., 1977, Prevention by somatostatin of rise in blood pressure and plasma renin mediated by beta-receptor stimulation, *Clin. Endocrinol.* **6**:455–462.

128. Vinik, A. I., Strodel, W. E., Eckhauser, F. E., Moattaui, A. R., and Lloyd, R., 1987, Somatostatinomas, P-Pomas, neurotensinomas, *Semin. Oncol.* **14**:263–281.

129. Kimmel, J. R., Hayden, L. J., and Pollock, H. G., 1975, Isolation and characterization of a new pancreatic polypeptide hormone, *J. Biol. Chem.* **250**:9369–9376.

130. Larsson, L., Schwartz, T., Lundquist, G., Chance, . E., Sundler, F., Rehfeld, J. F., Grimelius, L., and Fabrenburg, J., 1976, Occurrence of human pancreatic polypeptide in pancreatic endocrine tumors, *Am. J. Pathol.* **85**:675–684.

131. Carraway, R. and Leeman, S. E., 1973, The isolation of a new hypotensive peptide, neurotensin, firm bovine hypothalamus, *J. Biol. Chem.* **248**:6854–6861.

132. Bloom, S. R., Lee, Y. C., and Lacroute, J. M., 1983, Two patients with pancreatic apudomas secreting neurotension and VIP, *GUT* **24**:448–452.

11

The Uremic Syndrome

Stephen Brennan and Garabed Eknoyan

1. Introduction

The symptom complex that constitutes the uremic syndrome has long been recognized. Its earliest, most eloquent and succinct description probably was given by Aretaeus of Cappadocia in his *The Causes and Indications of Acute and Chronic Diseases* sometime during the first century of our era.[1] In Chapter III, titled "On the Affections about the Kidneys," he states:

> Certain persons pass bloody urine periodically. . . . they are very pale, inert, sluggish, without appetite, without digestion; and if discharge [of urine] has taken place, they are languid and relaxed in their limbs, but light and agile in their head. But if the periodical evacuation [of urine] does not take place, they are afflicted with headache; their eyes become dull, dim and rolling: hence many become epileptic; others are swollen, misty, dropsical; and others again are affected with melancholy and paralysis.

While the centuries have added little more to this vivid description of the clinical consequences of renal failure, the underlying mechanisms, of which Aretaeus had no notion whatsoever, continue to be methodically explored and gradually unraveled. The results of these efforts since the publication of Volume 4 of this series are summarized in this chapter.

2. Uremic Toxins

Since dialysis reverses some of the abnormalities associated with renal failure, the uremic syndrome may be the consequence of accumulation of noxious sub-

STEPHEN BRENNAN and GARABED EKNOYAN • Renal Section, Department of Medicine, Baylor College of Medicine Houston, Texas 77030.

stances in the blood and tissues. Despite intensive search, no single definite uremic toxin has been identified. Of the different factors that have been incriminated, only in the case of parathyroid hormone (PTH) has convincing evidence been offered for a role in the pathogenesis of uremia. The fact remains that PTH alone cannot account for most of the manifestations of uremia. Actually, PTH appears most likely to play a permissive and synergistic role in addition to whatever other toxins (or deficiencies) may exist.[2] As each organ system is considered in this review, the potential pathogenetic role of various incriminated toxins, including PTH, will be discussed.

The so-called "middle molecules" have been proposed as major toxins. A sophisticated array of scientific technology has been utilized in the search for these middle-molecular-weight toxins, and several abnormal peaks identified chromatographically in the plasma and dialysate of uremic patients have been implicated.[3] However, none of these substances has yet been adequately characterized or shown to bear a consistent relationship to the objective measures of the abnormalities that characterize the uremic syndrome. Furthermore, one study has demonstrated that neither hemodialysis nor peritoneal dialysis alters the plasma concentration of middle molecules or any subfraction of thereof.[4]

Attention has also been focused on trace elements. Aluminum overload is associated with distinct neurologic and bone abnormalities in uremic patients,[5] but this condition is a result of the treatment of uremia, rather than its cause. Zinc deficiency may be responsible for disorders of gustatory, endocrine, and immune function in uremia[6] and will be discussed in greater detail in the appropriate sections of this chapter. Selenium deficiency has been reported in dialysis patients compared to normal controls and has also been associated with accelerated atherogenesis, congestive cardiomyopathy, and predisposition to neoplasia.[7,8] However, neither hemodialysis nor peritoneal dialysis acutely alters selenium levels. The selenium deficiency may be nutritional in origin.[8]

Many polypeptides,[3] organic acids,[9] guanidino compounds,[10] and other amines[11] have been noted to be present in abnormal quantities in uremic subjects. Their precise role in the etiology of the uremic state, if any, remains to be ascertained.

3. Progression of Renal Dysfunction

In the broadest sense, there are two principal goals to the dietary management of uremia. The first is to assist in maintaining homeostasis (by restricting sodium, potassium, phosphate, and fluid), to correct nutritional deficiencies (with vitamin supplements), and to relieve uremic symptoms (by protein restriction). Recently, attention has focused on an additional role for dietary management of the progression of renal failure. It is not clear how protein restriction prevents the inexorable downhill course of renal failure, but mounting experimental and clinical evidence suggests that nutritional modifications, other than protein restriction, may favorably affect the outcome of renal disease.

Several studies have now documented that protein restriction is accompanied by a decrease in intraglomerular capillary pressure (P_{GC})[12,13] and glomerular filtration rate (GFR), in both uremic and normal individuals.[14] Humoral changes, including alterations in renin–angiotensin[15] and glomerular prostaglandin production,[16] have been noted to occur in response to protein depletion. These findings make it possible to anticipate the adjunctive use of a pharmacologic approach in combination with less restrictive dietary measures to forestall the requirement for dialysis in patients with renal failure.

3.1. Protein Restriction

There is considerable evidence, in both humans and animals, that protein restriction exerts a protective effect on the course of progressive renal failure. The results of prospective cooperative studies on the role of diet in progressive uremia are eagerly awaited. The data accumulated thus far are certainly encouraging. High-calorie, low-protein food products which are palatable are available, albeit at a cost that is some 2- to 10-fold higher than conventional foods.[17]

A principal concern in studies of protein restriction is the possibility of malnutrition and negative nitrogen balance. In a study of six patients treated with diets containing about 0.6 g/kg body weight of protein but of variable caloric intake (15, 25, 35, or 45 kcal/kg body weight daily), the likelihood of negative nitrogen balance and the rate of urea generation were correlated inversely with the caloric content of the diet.[18] In an experimental model of chronic renal failure induced in rats by ¾ nephrectomy comparable stabilization of GFR was noted in animals fed an isocaloric diet containing either 6% or 14% protein when compared to 22%-protein diets. However, the group ingesting 6% protein sustained significant growth retardation.[19]

The dietary supplementation of extremely low-protein diets with essential amino acids and their keto analogs has been reported to prevent the negative nitrogen balance associated with severe protein restriction. However, in a study of 12 patients (serum creatinine 6.8–16.3 mg/dl) on very low nitrogen (0.04 g N/kg per day) diets supplemented with essential amino acids and keto acids, negative nitrogen balance (as assessed by body weight, midarm muscle circumference, and other anthropometric measurements) was sustained despite an intake of 50 kcal/kg body weight daily.[20] On the other hand, in a follow-up study of 15 patients with moderate renal failure (mean creatinine clearance 18.3 ml/min) eating a diet containing 0.55 g/kg body weight protein for 14.9 months, no evidence of malnutrition on either biochemical or anthropometric studies was noted despite slower progression of renal failure as compared to a control group on an ad lib diet.[21] Thus, the optimal level of protein ingestion which will halt progression of renal failure without causing malnutrition has yet to be determined.

In addition to the beneficial effects of a low-protein diet on renal clearance, improvements in the histologic stigmata of progressive renal disease and glomerular permselectivity characteristics have been documented in animal studies. Measurements of the fractional clearance of albumin and IgG have demonstrated a rapid decrease in proteinuria toward normal following initiation of low-protein diets in rats[12] and human subject.[15]

3.2. Phosphate Restriction

For the most part, the phosphorus content of a diet closely parallels its protein content; thus, protein restriction obligates a degree of phosphorus restriction as well. There is now convincing evidence that the beneficial effects of protein and phosphate restriction on progression are additive. Rats subjected to 5/6 nephrectomy, receiving diets of identical caloric and protein composition, had significantly slower progression of renal failure and better control of serum phosphorus when consuming a low-phosphate diet.[22] A salutory effect of phosphate restriction on proteinuria, renal function, and morphology has been demonstrated in experimental models of diabetes mellitus, glomerulonephritis, and renal ablation.[23]

3.3. Uremic Manifestations

An additional benefit derived from protein restriction is the amelioration of some of the biochemical and metabolic derangements associated with uremia. Protein restriction with keto-analog supplementation decreased parathyroid hormone levels and serum phosphate concentration in 10 hemodialysis patients compared to eight control dialysis patients on their usual diets.[24]

Another benefit of dietary modification in uremia is improvement of linear growth in children. Three children with moderate uremia (creatinine clearance 20–25 ml/min per 1.73 m^2) received nocturnal nasogastric caloric supplements amounting to 50 kcal/kg body weight each night. Over a period of 11–16 months, linear growth improved from < 5% to 95% of standard growth scores while serum creatinine remained stable.[25]

Protein restriction does not appear to exert a significant effect on the abnormalities of lipid transport characteristic of the uremic state. On the other hand, a diet low in protein and phosphate was shown to decrease insulin resistance and improve the carbohydrate tolerance of uremic children, an effect that could not be attributed to improvements in secondary hyperparathyroidism.[26] Other dietary alterations may have an effect on the course of progressive renal failure. Nephrectomized rats fed a diet high in polyunsaturated fatty acids had less biochemical and morphologic stigmata of progression than a control group fed beef tallow.[27] Carbohydrate restriction in general, and glucose restriction in particular, was associated with less rapid deterioration of renal function in a rat model of chronic renal failure.[28]

3.4. Acquired Cystic Disease

A consequence of long-term uremia which is recognized with increasing frequency is the acquisition of cystic lesions in the kidneys,[29] which have the potential of becoming infected, rupturing with consequent bleeding beneath the renal capsule or into the perirenal space,[30] or undergoing malignant degeneration.[31-33] In a study of 100 patients receiving either hemodialysis or peritoneal dialysis, 63 patients had sonographic evidence of acquired cystic kidney disease.[29] This was mainly correlated with duration of dialysis and was independent of the modality of dialysis. Although an unexpected rise in hematocrit may be a sign of acquired cysts, it is by no means a universal finding. Most reported malignancies were discovered incidentally, although abnormal cytology of the urinary sediment has been an indicator of such a change.[31] Occasional cases of metastatic disease have been reported.

3.5. Hypertension and Progression of Uremia

Altered intraglomerular hemodynamic derangements have been shown to be associated with progressive uremia. Treatments of systemic or intraglomerular hypertension may be able to correct some of these abnormalities and slow the deterioration of renal function if hemodynamic events are the chief culprits. Results along these lines have been somewhat conflicting. In a group of 17 patients with moderate to severe chronic renal insufficiency (creatinine clearance 12–66 ml/min), followed at monthly intervals without a change in diet, the progression of renal failure was significantly slowed compared to the 2-year period prior to the initiation of improved blood pressure control.[34] In another retrospective review of 40 patients with diabetes mellitus it was noted that the rate of increase in serum creatinine was 0.036 mg/dl per month if the mean arterial pressure was <115 mm Hg, as compared to a rate of 0.3 mg/dl per month in those who had a mean arterial pressure >125 mm Hg.[35] Hypertension was also synergistic with other nephrotoxins in accelerating uremia in diabetics. A study employing multivariate analysis has shown that age and mean blood pressure appear to be independently inversely correlated with GFR.[36]

Although human studies imply that any form of blood pressure control is beneficial in arresting progression, it is clear from animal studies that not all antihypertensive regimens are equally effective. Angiotensin converting enzyme inhibition (CEI) treatment in rats subjected to subtotal nephrectomy led to a decrease in glomerulosclerosis and plasma creatinine concentration compared to no treatment.[37] Another study compared the effects of CEI or calcium channel blockade to no treatment in the rat remnant kidney model. Even though similar reductions in blood pressure were accomplished, only CEI was associated with significant improvement in renal histology and progression.[38] A favorable outcome with CEI (but not identical control of blood pressure with other agents) has also been demonstrated in diabetic animal models, even if begun well after the onset of renal injury.[39] On the other hand, the effect of antihypertensive drugs may not be entirely mediated via hemodynamic properties. The use of verapamil in subtotally nephrectomized rats was associated with protection against renal dysfunction, pathologic injury, and nephrocalcinosis as well as improved survival, despite no change in blood pressure.[40] By the same token, correction of the hyperlipidemia of renal failure has been shown experimentally to retard the course of experimental renal failure and development of glomerulosclerosis, independent of any change in glomerular capillary pressure.[41]

4. The Skin

With the widespread availability of dialysis, the major uremic skin abnormalities (i.e., uremic frost and poor wound healing) have become much less common. However, a constellation of new dermal abnormalities has arisen to take their place. The vast majority of dialysis patients have some cutaneous problem. Skin biopsies performed on 63 uremic patients (53 of whom were on maintenance hemodialysis) revealed an increase in thickness of the basement membrane and mast cell infiltration as the principal histologic abnormalities.[42] The microscopic changes were directly correlated with the duration of dialysis, raising the possible role of a cutaneous reaction to some component of the dialysis equipment. Reversal of these changes occurred in 72–100% of patients following a successful renal transplant.[43,44] Skin thinning in uremia has been shown to be the primary reason for poor wound healing in these individuals.[45]

The major symptomatic complaint of patients with advanced renal failure, even before the initiation of dialysis, is pruritus. Several lines of evidence suggest that secondary hyperparathyroidism may be the principal culprit. Several studies continue to document the high calcium content of uremic skin[46] and the frequently dramatic relief of pruritus following subtotal parathyroidectomy. However, PTH cannot be the sole reason for pruritus, since correlation between plasma PTH levels and symptoms is poor. Some studies have postulated increased skin content of divalent anions (e.g., phosphate or sulfate),[47] vitamin A, or dermal mast cell degranulation and consequent histamine release[42] as factors contributing to the pruritus of uremia. Treatment of pruritus consists of good skin hygiene and use of diphenhydramine or hydroxyzine. Patients failing these measures can obtain some relief with ultraviolet radiation.

The transepidermal elimination of abnormal skin structural elements, termed reactive perforating collagenosis,[48] is seen with much greater frequency in uremic subjects than in the general population. Dialysis removes plasma porphyrins only poorly,[49] and the coexistence of a bullous dermatosis which closely resembles porphyria cutanea tarda with elevated porphyrins has led to the description of so-called "pseudoporphyria." True porphyria cutanea tarda is rarely seen in dialysis patients.[50] Diagnostic radiology tests are occasionally associated with unusual skin reactions in renal failure. A case of severe dermoepidermal necrosis with necrotizing vasculitis and skin iodide vegetations following an intravenous pyelogram has been reported.[51] One patient with severe calcinosis cutis who underwent a nuclear technetium 99m scan had diffuse dermal uptake of the isotope, possibly from adsorption of technetium onto dermal deposits of hydroxyapatite.[52]

5. The Muscles and Joints

5.1. Muscles

After skin problems, the most distressing symptoms encountered in end-stage renal disease are muscle pain, weakness, and cramps. Typically, patients notice proximal muscle weakness which may be disabling. Myopathy may be the dominant finding in progressive renal insufficiency. This is dramatically illustrated in the case report of a patient who had progressive muscle weakness for 3 years before the diagnosis of renal failure was made, in whom the institution of dialysis led to significant improvement of the muscular symptoms.[53] Renal failure is associated with elevated levels of plasma and urine myoglobin,[54] due to diminished renal elimination of myoglobin rather than increased myolysis. Fatal rhabdomyolysis has been reported in a dialysis patient following an upper respiratory infection.[55]

Metabolic abnormalities of muscle are receiving greater recognition as factors contributory to uremic myopathy. Several studies have now shown an increased rate of muscle catabolism, due to either increased degradation or decreased synthesis of muscle or both.[56] These abnormalities are related at least partly to postreceptor abnormalities in insulin-mediated myocyte carbohydrate metabolism.[57−59] Sodium-dependent amino acid uptake into muscle cells is impaired in acute uremia,[60] but sodium-independent amino acid uptake is unaffected.[61] Intramyocytic levels of high-energy phosphates, total adenine nucleotides, and metabolic substrates are depressed in uremia.[62−64]

Although convincing evidence for a role of parathyroid hormone in the myopathy exists, there is no direct effect of PTH on muscle cell glucose uptake, protein metabolism, or amino acid transport.[65] Intracellular acidosis has been proposed as the signal for changes in muscle metabolism, since intracellular pH and bicarbonate concentration have been shown to be low in uremic patients when compared to normal controls.[64,66] Furthermore, some of the metabolic abnormalities in muscle can be reversed following the administration of bicarbonate.[66]

Exercise training can greatly improve abnormal muscle catabolism[58,59] in addition to cardiovascular fitness.[67] This will be discussed in greater detail in Section 8.1. The discovery of low levels of carnitine and various carnitine acyl esters[68,69] has raised enthusiasm about the possible use of carnitine supplements as treatment for uremic myopathy. Unfortunately, although carnitine levels improve following drug administration, symptomatic response has been disappointing.[70]

5.2. Joints and Juxtaarticular Structures

Carpal tunnel syndrome (CTS) is being encountered with increasing frequency in patients with end-stage renal disease. The lesions tend to progress more rapidly in uremic subjects on dialysis than subjects without renal failure, leading to its earlier identification and institution of therapeutic measures in dialysis patients.[71] CTS in uremia is most often due to the synovial deposition of an abnormal amyloid protein very similar or identical to beta-2 microglobulin (B_2-M),[72,73] a low-molecular-weight protein (11,800) daltons) which is normally catabolized and excreted by the kidney. B_2-M accumulates in dialysis patients.[74] It is unclear whether B_2-M is deposited in other organs as well.[75,76] Synovial fluid amyloid concentration correlates well with the presence of synovial amyloid deposits.[77] The degree of amyloid deposition in synovial structures is best correlated with duration of uremia and of dialysis.[78] Hemodialysis with standard cuprophane membranes does not remove B_2-M.[74]

Destructive arthropathies also occur in renal failure and have several potential etiologies. In addition to amyloid-related disease, crystalline arthritis[79–81] and infections[82] are frequent offenders. A report of 73 dialysis patients from France noted a destructive arthropathy in 29 subjects.[83] Many of these joint changes may be related to secondary hyperparathyroidism or aluminum toxicity. Joints most frequently affected include the knees, hips, shoulders, and a surprisingly high incidence of hand and/or wrist involvement.[80,83,84] When crystals are found in joint effusions, they are most commonly calcium salts of hydroxyapatite, pyrophosphate, or oxalate.[79,83,85,86] A relatively low white cell count in the effusion is not unusual and may partly explain the generally poor response to nonsteroidal antiinflammatory agents.[80]

Spontaneous tendon rupture continues to be encountered occasionally in azotemic patients.[87,88] The neuropathic arthropathy of Charcot is remarkable for its infrequency in dialysis subjects, in whom the incidence of peripheral neuropathy is high.

6. The Gastrointestinal System

Since the advent of maintenance dialysis, such gastrointestinal (GI) manifestations of uremia as uremic colitis and hemorrhage have greatly decreased in frequency. Nevertheless, a host of new ailments has appeared, which affect a great majority of patients with end-stage renal disease.

6.1. Oral Cavity

Abnormalities in the oral cavity are frequently encountered in advanced uremia. Dysgeusia and diminished taste acuity frequently occur. Taste threshold is inversely related to glomerular filtration over a range of creatinine clearances from 5 to 75 ml/min. Taste abnormalities appear to be largely responsive to zinc supplementation.[6] A population of pediatric dialysis patients has been shown to have normal taste perception and thresholds at a time when zinc levels were normal.[89] Recovery of normal taste follows successful renal transplantation.

The hard tissues of the mouth are also affected. Dental caries are decreased in frequency in dialysis patients owing to the relatively alkaline ambient pH resulting from high levels of urea in saliva. Mobility of teeth in their sockets, possibly related to osteomalacia of the bony structures of the jaw or deposition of aluminum-containing crystals in the periodontium, is a major cause of tooth loss.[90] Close cooperation with a dentist familiar with these patients is essential, especially in patients awaiting transplantation.[91]

6.2. Esophagus

Esophagitis is the most common lesion affecting the esophagus in uremia, accounting for 17% of cases of upper GI hemorrhage in dialysis patients. Esophageal motility is also occasionally disturbed, perhaps as a result of uremic autonomic neuropathy. Esophageal dysmotility may account for some of the increased frequency of vomiting seen in this population.

6.3. Stomach and Duodenum

In an autopsy series of 94 patients with GFR < 10 ml/min, gastric disorders were found commonly.[92] The highest incidence of upper GI tract pathology (58%) was present in patients who had never been dialyzed or who had been dialyzed for less than 1 month. The prevalence of gastric lesions was inversely related to duration of dialysis. In patients who had been dialyzed for longer than 1 month the prevalence was only 31%. The most common lesions were gastritis, gastric ulcers, and peptic ulcers. Despite the decrease in anatomic abnormalities noted after the initiation of dialysis in this autopsy study, clinically evident gastric problems were more frequent in the dialyzed group. Additional support for this observation comes from a longitudinal endoscopic study, in which clinically relevant gastritis, duodenitis, or ulcers were noted more frequently after the initiation of dialysis or transplantation.[93]

Angiodysplasias of the stomach and duodenum are the most common causes of upper GI bleeding in end-stage renal disease.[92] These lesions also occur with an increased frequency in the colon. It has been suggested that the ratio of blood urea nitrogen (BUN)/creatinine has a very high diagnostic specificity in distinguishing upper vs. lower GI source of bleeding independent of the level of residual renal function.[94] Upper endoscopy is unlikely to unearth an occult source of bleeding in patients with an unexplained fall in hematocrit but no other evidence to suggest GI blood loss.[95]

Gastric acid secretion is depressed in uremic patients prior to the initiation of dialysis and improves after either dialysis or transplantation.[96] However, serum gastrin levels are high in uremia, and it is suggested that gastric acid secretion is depressed owing to an abnormally low sensitivity to gastrin-induced acidification. Some authors have found no correlation between gastric histology and acid secretion,[96] while others have noted an increase in antral gastrin cell density in end-stage renal disease.[97] Gastric emptying of solids and liquids is well preserved in uremia. Anorexia and early satiety have been postulated to be due in part to central nervous system opiate abnormalities, but a study in rats showed that administration of opioids increased food intake only in the control group, and not in uremic animals.[98]

Duodenal polyps are more common in uremia than in normal subjects.[93] These polyps arise from hyperplasia of Brunner's glands in patients with a low resting gastric pH and elevated levels of pepsinogen II. Duodenal calcium absorption is impaired in experimental uremia, probably owing to abnormalities of vitamin D metabolism.[99]

6.4. Intestines

Intestinal necrosis and ischemic enteritis are occasionally seen in uremic patients. The mortality in colonic infarction is quite high (75%) in dialysis subjects.[100] Risk factors for the development of infarction include frequent hypotensive episodes while on dialysis and large weight losses due to emesis, diarrhea, or ultrafiltration.[100] Uremia *per se* increases the severity of experimental ischemic colitis.[101] Unexplained colonic perforation continues to be seen in the occasional dialysis patient.[102] Intestinal necrosis due to sorbitol enemas containing the potassium binding resin sodium polystyrene has been reported clinically and documented experimentally.[103] Interestingly, in the experimental studies sorbitol was suggested as the offending agent. One dialysis unit has reported a cluster of five cases of pseudomembraneous enterocolitis due to *Clostridium difficile* enterotoxin–producing bacteria.[104] Perirectal or perineal abcess can be more difficult to diagnose in dialysis patients than in otherwise healthy patients.[105]

Studies in an experimental model of renal failure in rats revealed an adaptive increase in fecal potassium excretion. This was considered to be secondary to increased colonic Na,K-ATPase activity. Human studies have been unable to document an increase in Na,K-ATPase activity, although net rectal potassium secretion increases about 2.5-fold in end-stage renal disease.[106,107] Active potassium secretion, transepithelial potential, net sodium and water absorption, and plasma aldosterone levels are all unchanged[106,108,109]; thus the mechanism of increased rectal potassium secretion remains unclear.

6.5. Liver and Biliary Tree

Chronic hepatitis, defined as persistent elevation of SGOT for at least 1 year, has been reported in 3.4% of dialysis patients. Of these, 50% are patients who are hepatitis B surface antigen positive.[110] It has been suggested that hepatitis B virus DNA assays may have more sensitivity than conventional serologic testing in the diagnosis of hepatitis, particularly in uremic individuals who are on maintenance dialysis.[111]

Hepatic parenchymal cell function is abnormal in uremia. The activity of the enzyme pyruvate kinase is depressed in experimental chronic renal failure.[112,113]

Hepatic production of urea and ammonia is increased in uremia, but no change in glucose production is present.[114] Instead, accumulation of intermediates of carbohydrate metabolism (lactate, pyruvate, and glutamate) is noted. The ability of pholorhizin to reproduce these biochemical abnormalities suggests a role of relative insulinopenia or an elevated glucagon:insulin ratio in mediating the liver metabolic abnormalities.[114] In contrast to the abnormalities of hepatic parenchymal cell function, hepatic Kupffer cell and endothelial cell function appear to be normal in uremia, at least as assessed indirectly by serum beta-*N*-acetyl hexosaminidase levels.[115]

The biliary tract is generally normal in uremia. Levels of serum alkaline phosphatase are frequently elevated, but this is generally secondary to metabolic bone disease. The intestinal isoenzyme of alkaline phosphatase may also be the source of elevated levels in some patients.[116] It is of interest in this regard that renal and intestinal alkaline phosphatase are indistinguishable with currently available assay methods. The gallbladder is of normal thickness in uremia, despite the presence of hypoalbuminemia which tends to cause edema of the gallbladder wall.[117] A curious finding is the occasional visualization of the gallbladder during scintigraphy with technetium 99m–labeled red cells to localize GI bleeding. It is felt that this represents the perferential excretion of labelled heme in the biliary tree in uremia.[118] Cholangiocellular carcinoma occurs with slightly increased frequency in patients with end-stage renal disease.[119]

A combination of dialysis, ultrafiltration, and peritoneovenous shunting has been successfully utilized in the management of uremic patients with cirrhotic or nephrogenic ascites.[120]

6.6. Pancreas

Pancreatic lesions are common in dialysis patients. An autopsy study of 78 dialysis patients revealed the presence of an anatomic abnormality in the pancreas in 60%.[121] The most common finding was pancreatitis in 28% of patients; other lesions included fibrosis, hemosiderin deposits, calcification, cystic changes, and amyloidosis. In another postmortem review, amyloid deposition in the islets of Langerhans was seen in 6 of 10 dialysis patients, as compared to 1 of 15 nonuremic controls.[122]

Acute pancreatitis occurs in dialysis patients with an estimated 10-year incidence of 2.3%.[123] The mortality of acute pancreatitis in dialysis patients is about 20–30%.[123,124] The diagnosis can be somewhat difficult to establish, particularly in patients on peritoneal dialysis.[125] The presence of abdominal pain, fever, nausea and vomiting, hyperamylasemia, and peritoneal fluid leukocytosis may be due to either peritonitis or pancreatitis. A review of 43 stable hemodialysis patients found that 81% had an elevated serum amylase level.[126] Serum amylase levels greater than three times the upper limit of normal or the presence of amylase in the peritoneal fluid was consistent with a diagnosis of pancreatitis.

7. The Pulmonary System

The most common pulmonary problem in dialysis patients is pulmonary edema. This condition may present a variety of radiographic guises[127] and consequently may not be easy to diagnose. Subclinical volume overload in the pulmonary circulation cannot easily be excluded as a cause of abnormal pulmonary function tests. Volume overload of the extracellular fluid space and left ventricular failure are the most common causes of pulmonary edema, but abnormal pulmonary capillary permeability may play a contributory role in some circumstances. Acute increases in left atrial pressure by balloon distention lead to greater increases in transcapillary protein transudation in the lungs of acutely nephrectomized animals compared to sham-operated controls.[128] In humans with uremia, pulmonary epithelial permeability has been shown to be increased and can be improved with dialysis.[129] Another study has shown, however, that uremic patients have less leaky pulmonary capillaries than those of patients with adult respiratory distress syndrome or cardiogenic edema and are, in fact, unchanged compared to normal controls.[130]

Pulmonary calcification is another fairly frequent finding in uremia, being noted in 20% of patients in a postmortem study and in 22% of pediatric patients studied with nuclear scanning[131] The process may be exacerbated in some patients after transplantation.[132] Respiratory failure in these patients may be severe or even lethal. Some authors have suggested a role for secondary hyperparathyroidism in the pathogenesis of the disorder,[132] while others have concluded that aluminum deposition and duration of dialysis are major factors.[131] Bone-seeking isotopes (e.g., technetium 99m diphosphonate), but not gallium 67, are useful diagnostically in identifying or detecting the presence of pulmonary calcification.[133]

Obstructive sleep apnea may develop or be worsened by uremia. In one obese male patient, intensive dialysis was able to completely reverse the process.[134] It is conceivable that insomnia in dialysis patients may be partly related to sleep apnea or nocturnal hemoglobin desaturation, since abnormal sleep patterns are common in both dialysis and sleep apnea patients.

Hypoxia, both in arterial blood and at the cellular level, is a constant finding during hemodialysis.[135] In patients receiving acetate as the principal dialysate buffer, diffusive losses of carbon dioxide into dialysate, with the consequent reduction in PCO_2, is a major factor leading to hypoventilation and subsequent hypoxia. Active investigation into the role of complement-mediated leukocyte sequestration in pulmonary capillaries is ongoing. Complement activation primarily via the alternative pathway, as measured by effluent blood levels of C3a and C5a,[136] can be regularly found within 30 min of the onset of hemodialysis with the first use of a new cuprophane dialyzer and is associated with symptomatic shortness of breath and leukopenia. A relatively selective decrease in polymorphonuclear leukocytes has been documented in one study. There is significant variability in the magnitude of complement activation between individuals and from one type of dialyzer membrane to the next.[137−139] Saturation of complement activating sites on dialysis membranes has been suggested by studies of dialyzer reuse.[140,141] Furthermore, a progressive decrease in binding of C5a to neutrophils has been shown after exposure to dialysis membranes *in vitro*.[140]

Pleural effusions may develop in dialysis patients, as a result of either increased fluid entry from subpleural capillaries or defective lymphatic drainage of pleural fluid. A syndrome of uremic pleuritis which is an often hemorrhagic, necrotizing, and consists of a fibrinous sterile exudate has been described.[142] Although spontaneous remissions and recurrences are sometimes seen in such patients, decortication may be required. In one patient, uremic pleuritis was noted incidentally during the course of a radionuclide renogram.[143]

Airway resistance is unchanged during the hemodialysis procedure.[144] No clinically significant changes in pulmonary function tests are noted during continuous ambulatory peritoneal dialysis.[145]

8. The Cardiovascular System

Abnormalities of the cardiac, vascular, and hemodynamic function are common in patients with renal failure. The superimposition of rapid and often major changes in volume, electrolyte, and solute composition of the extracellular fluid induced during dialysis presents an added challenge which unmasks these abnormalities and contributes to much of the untoward symptomatology attributed to the dialytic procedure.

8.1. Heart

Myocardial performance is frequently affected early in clinical and experimental uremia. The presence or absence of cardiac disease is an important predictor of the ultimate prognosis of patients with end-stage renal disease. An autopsy study found that cardiac disease was a much more likely cause of death in dialysis patients than in age-and-sex-matched controls, and that deaths from congestive heart failure were particularly likely.[146] The reasons for the excess of cardiovascular disease in uremia are many, and include hypertension, volume overload, anemia, and hyperlipidemias in addition to the myocardial depressant effects of endogenous uremic toxins.

Asymptomatic patients at various levels of renal insufficiency usually display elevations in left ventricular (LV) end-diastolic volume both at rest and during exertion.[147] In such patients, LV stroke work does not increase normally following exercise. Coupled with the anemia and hypertension of renal failure, this will invariably result in increased cardiac work that accounts for many of the symptoms and structural abnormalities of these patients. The response to physical exercise is abnormal in uremia, with a decrease in oxygen consumption[148] and cardiovascular capacity[149] demonstrable in the majority of patients. This occurs even in the presence of normal catecholamine levels, although the cardiac response to beta agonists is depressed[150] (probably due to deficient activity of cardiac adenylate cyclase), and the cardiac binding of alpha-1 adrenergic agents is also depressed.[151] Of special clinical relevance is the fact that the presence of poor exercise tolerance is a marker for rehabilitation potential in these patients; the likelihood of remaining employed 1 year after starting dialysis has been directly correlated with baseline exercise tolerance. Exercise training has been repeatedly shown to improve the physical work capacity and maximal oxygen consumption of these patients, as well as their lipid abnormalities, glucose tolerance, and blood pressure control,[152,153] and possibly their hematocrit and depressive symptoms as well.[152]

In general, the immediate effects of hemodialysis (HD) and peritoneal dialysis (PD) on cardiac performance are comparable. Following dialysis, LV systolic volume and end-diastolic volume decrease and the velocity of circumferential shortening fraction increases.[154] Stroke volume and cardiac output generally are unchanged or decrease, while LV ejection fraction may increase. One study has shown that the best cardiovascular response to either PD or HD is seen in patients with the poorest left ventricular function before therapy.[154] The effects of changes in extracellular fluid volume are insufficient to explain the observed effects on myocardial performance, since different effects are noted when comparing dialysis, ultrafiltration, and hemofiltration with comparable degrees of volume loss.[155] Changes in serum electrolyte composition that occur during dialysis may be responsible for some of the improvement in contractility. In particular, the dialysis-induced increase in ionized calcium has been convincingly shown to improve LV function. Additionally, two patients on continuous ambulatory peritoneal dialysis (CAPD) have been described who developed a dilated cardiomyopathy following parathyroidectomy, one of whom improved following administration of calcium.[156] The presence of 2 liters of dialysate in the peritoneal cavity does not affect hemodynamics while patients are recumbent. On the other hand, the presence of peritoneal dialysate attenuates the normal orthostatic decrease in systolic blood pressure and increase in heart rate when patients are upright.[157]

The etiology of the depressed myocardial function is unclear. PTH has been implicated as a potential depressant of myocardial cell contractility. Conflicting results have been obtained with parathyroidectomy. A study of experimental uremia induced by 7/8 nephrectomy in rats showed that parathyroidectomy ameliorated many of the cardiac metabolic changes associated with uremia, such as decreased myocardial oxygen consumption, depressed ATP content, and increased calcium content, but cardiac index was not improved.[158] It has been shown in humans that the degree of diastolic dilation of the LV was inversely related to the level of circulating PTH.[147] A possible morphologic basis for the poor cardiac function of uremic subjects has come to light with the discovery of structural abnormalities of the myocardial basement membrane and the abnormal distribution of anionic binding sites on the sarcolemmal membranes.[159] A constant biochemical finding in uremic individuals has been the presence of increased calcium content of the myocardium. A study of experimental uremia in rats has shown that administration of verapamil is able to prevent the development of cardiac histologic abnormalities.[160] Reports of patients with severe myocardial calcification have appeared in the literature,[161] and a role of oxalate in the deposition of calcium deposits has been proposed.[162] The precise pathophysiologic role of these findings awaits further clarification.

Because of the development of symptomatic congestive heart failure, many uremic patients receive digitalis chronically. Attempting to maintain therapeutic drug levels in these patients can be very difficult. Digoxin but not digitoxin undergoes substantial renal elimination,[163] and neither drug is appreciably removed by dialysis. An endogenous substance with digoxinlike immunoreactivity (DLI) can be identified in the majority of dialysis patients not on cardiac glycosides,[164] and the plasma level of DLI can vary depending on the assay employed. These substances are rarely detected in patients with normal renal function and do not bear a consistent relationship to the degree of renal function impairment. In general, the levels of DLI do not exceed 0.23 ng/ml in individuals who are not on digitalis preparations, but values as high as 2.9 ng/ml have been found.[164–166] Given the narrow therapeutic window of the cardiac glycosides, the possibility of prescribing an inadequate dose of digoxin to uremic patients, solely on the basis of their drug level, is very real. On the other hand, substances that exhibit DLI have also been shown to inhibit Na,K-ATPase[165] and thus may well exert a pharmacologic effect. The clinical relevance of DLI remains under active investigation.

Patients with end-stage renal disease have many of the risk factors associated with atherosclerosis, including hyperlipidemia, hypertension, diabetes mellitus, and hyperuricemia. Despite the presence of multiple risks, it is not at all clear that uremia *per se* either causes a greater mortality from coronary artery disease or leads to accelerated atherogenesis. Myocardial infarction is the cause of death in 13% of dialysis patients, and significant coronary artery disease is seen in 60% of patients coming to autopsy, figures comparable to those seen in nonuremic controls.[146] One study suggests that ischemic heart disease is no more progressive in renal failure than it is in persons with normal renal function.[167] The diagnosis of myocardial infarction should not present a problem clinically; although 8% of dialysis subjects have a modestly elevated MB creatine kinase activity, enzyme levels in acute myocardial infarction are on the average eight fold higher than the highest levels seen in uremic controls (153 IU/liter vs. 20 IU/liter). However, one study suggests that elevated baseline levels of MB creatine kinase in otherwise stable dialysis patients are a highly significant predictor for the subsequent development of cardiac disease.[168] Cardiac surgery presents no extraordinary risk to the uremic patient.[169,170] Cardiovascular morbidity and mortality are similar to those in nonuremic controls undergoing the same procedure,[169] and symptomatic relief of anginal complaints can be expected in over 90% of patients following aortocoronary bypass grafting.[170] However, there may be an increased risk in uremic patients who are diabetic. In a study of 60 diabetic patients preparing for renal transplantation, thallium treadmill stress testing was performed, followed by coronary angiography in those with abnormal thallium results. Only seven patients had normal thallium treadmill tests, and the remainder underwent coronary angiography; 23 of the 53 catheterized patients were found to have significant stenoses, with a perioperative mortality of 43.5% following renal transplant in this subgroup. No perioperative cardiovascular morbidity or mortality was noted in the group with normal coronary arteries.[171] These patients did not undergo routine coronary revascularization prior to transplant.

Valvular abnormalities are common in end-stage renal disease patients. On careful scrutiny, abnormalities can be discerned in all four cardiac valves. Calcification of the aortic valve was noted in 28% of long-term dialysis patients (mean duration of dialysis 7.5 years) and was directly correlated to duration of end-stage renal disease.[172] Clinically important aortic stenosis was seen in 6/174 dialysis patients (a highly significant increase in incidence compared to nonuremics). Only one of the six patients with aortic stenosis had a bicuspid aortic valve.[173] Mitral annular calcification is even more common, being noted in 36% of 87 long-term dialysis subjects. One of these 31 patients developed mitral stenosis as a consequence.[172] Pulmonic valve insufficiency is a well-recognized cause of diastolic murmurs in dialysis patients. It is caused by pulmonary hypertension and is improved or corrected by either dialysis or transplantation.

8.2. Atrial Natriuretic Peptides

Whereas endocrinelike granules in atrial myocytes were first described 30 years ago, the potent vasorelaxant, diuretic, and natriuretic properties of atrial extracts were discovered only within the past decade.[174] Atrial natriuretic peptide (ANP) is a polypeptide hormone of 28 amino acids which is released from the atria in response to various stimuli, including atrial distention and tachycardia. The role of other stimuli such as hormonal or neural factors in mediating the release of ANP is disputed. One of the principal physiologic roles that has been proposed for ANP is in the regulation of extracellular fluid volume status. Plasma levels of ANP increase in acutely saline loaded animals and humans and decline in volume depletion. The function or expression of other volume regulatory and vasoconstrictive hormones (e.g., renin, angiotensin II, aldosterone, and vasopressin) is modified by physiologic levels of ANP.

Plasma levels of ANP are elevated in chronic renal failure and end-stage renal disease.[175,176] The usual predialysis concentration of ANP is two- to eightfold higher than in normal controls and decreases promptly with dialysis.[175–180] In healthy subjects, ANP in plasma is present as a single immunoreactive moiety (i.e., the 28-amino-acid intact hormone),[174,181] and most studies in uremics have also found only the intact hormone in the circulation.[175,178,182] With the development of increasingly sensitive assays, however, other biologically active forms have also been identified.[181,183] Amino terminal fragments of pro-ANP consisting of amino acids 1–30 and 31–67 are detected in the circulation of uremic patients and have been shown to exert both natriuretic and vasorelaxant effects.[183] At least one study has detected a second peak of ANP immunoreactivity in uremics which is not present in controls.[181] By obtaining a large volume of pooled ultrafiltrate from dialysis patients (1000 liters), it has been discovered that very little ANP crosses the dialyzer membrane; that which does cross is exclusively the intact active hormone.[182]

The elevated fractional excretion of sodium (FE_{Na}) and single-nephron glomerular filtration rate which characterize renal failure have now been postulated to be due, at least in part, to the effects of ANP, released in response to the chronic mild volume overload characteristic of renal insufficiency. Rats subjected to a 5/6 nephrectomy respond to infusions of ANP with a decrease in systolic blood pressure of 20% coupled with an increase in GFR of 24% and an increase in FE_{Na} to 9–15%, raising the possibility of a therapeutic role for ANP in the treatment of advanced uremia.[184,185] Many studies have suggested that the etiology of elevations in plasma ANP in uremic patients is volume expansion. Several lines of evidence support this conclusion. In patients with chronic renal failure, either HD, ultrafiltration, or hemofiltration is associated with a rapid decrease in ANP levels,[177,179,180] whereas no change in ANP is seen following isovolemic ultrafiltration.[186] While plasma levels of ANP do not correlate with the plasma creatinine concentration,[175,176] a good correlation is noted with predialysis weight, intradialytic weight loss, and hematocrit.[179,181,187,188] One group of patients with chronic renal failure had a 22% decrease in ANP levels following isolated ultrafiltration and a supranormal response (ANP levels 150% of preultrafiltration baseline) to infusion of a volume of isotonic saline equal to that lost during ultrafiltration.[189] In another study, ANP levels in patients with chronic uremia correlated best with blood pressure[175]; however, in this study, the ANP levels of patients without cardiomegaly were no different from those of controls. It is possible that ANP is important primarily in regulating acute changes in extracellular fluid volume rather than chronic ones, since there was no detectable difference in ANP levels of rats in the steady state studied on different dietary sodium intake or during mineralocorticoid escape.[190] Because of its sensitivity to changes in volume status, and because of the frequent difficulty in determining the clinical state of hydration in uremic patients, serial determinations of ANP may prove to be clinically useful in the assessment of dialysis dry weights and as a means to quantify the adequacy of extracellular fluid volume during dialysis.

8.3. Pericardium

The widespread use of dialysis has greatly diminished the incidence of clinically apparent pericarditis, although pericardial disease continues to be found and is considered a cause of cardiac mortality in autopsy series of dialysis patients.[146] The availability of diagnostic echocardiography has brought new insights into the problem of pericarditis in uremic subjects. One study of 1058 HD patients, followed for an average of 13.7 years, identified 161 episodes of pericarditis in 136 patients.[191] Patient survival in this group was 89.7%, despite the fact that 57 patients sustained cardiac tamponade or pretamponade. Hemodynamic compromise was less likely in effusions that developed within the first 2 weeks after initiation of dialysis.

The primary treatment of dialysis-related pericarditis is intensive dialysis for 10–14 days. For patients with recurrent or intractable effusions despite a trial of intensive dialysis, or for patients with acute hemodynamic compromise (i.e., tamponade), surgical intervention (often combined with intrapericardial instillation of nonabsorbable steroids) has been quite effective in producing long-lasting remissions from pericarditis.[191–194] Although PD may be less effective than HD in the treatment of uremic pericardial effusions, in one study the incidence of pericarditis in patients undergoing PD was only 5%, as compared to a 25% incidence in HD patients.[154]

Although volume overload plays an important role in the etiology of uremic pericardial effusions, the exact pathophysiology of pericarditis in these individuals remains uncertain. Occasionally, drug-induced pericarditis can occur, and may even be fatal.[195] Reports of clustering of some cases of pericarditis have led to the suggestion of a viral infectious etiology,[196] and the possibility of infectious pericarditis should not be overlooked in these immune-compromised individuals exposed to a host of invasive procedures.

8.4. Hyperlipidemia

Abnormal lipid metabolism has been implicated as a factor responsible in part for the increased risk of vascular occlusive disease in uremic patients. Compared to normal controls, renal failure is associated with elevations in serum levels of triglycerides (TG), low-density-lipoprotein (LDL) and very-low-density-lipoprotein (VLDL) cholesterol, and low concentrations of high-density lipoprotein (HDL) cholesterol.[197–199] Decreases in the activity of the lipid catabolic enzymes lipoprotein lipase and lecithin:cholesterol acetyltransferase have also been noted.[199,200] These findings suggest that the lipid abnormalities found in uremia may be secondary to decreased degradation rather than overproduction of lipoproteins. This may, in turn, be due to a state of relative insulin deficiency in uremia. In a study of nephrectomized rats, uremic animals were found to be hypoinsulinemic in addition to having low levels of lipoprotein lipase and high VLDL levels.[200] These lipid abnormalities were reversed by chronic insulin infusion. Other hormonal influences on lipid homeostasis have also been investigated. Thyroid hormone deficiency has been associated with increased levels of an abnormal prebeta VLDL and increased risk of coronary artery disease and cerebrovascular events.[201] However, uremic rats treated with triiodothyronine had no difference in lipid levels compared to placebo-treated uremic animals.[202] A correlation has been noted between the levels of alkaline phosphatase and serum triglycerides (TG) in long-term dialysis patients, suggesting a pathogenetic role for PTH; indeed, parathyroidectomy led to a decrease in the TG levels of these patients.[203]

HDL subfractions are altered in the uremic state.[204] In particular, a decrease in HDL_2 cholesterol levels has been found in patients with varying degrees of chronic renal failure, and an inverse correlation noted between the concentration of serum creatinine and HDL_2 cholesterol. Other abnormalities in the fractionation of lipoproteins include the demonstration of so-called double prebeta hyperlipopro-teinemia in the plasma of uremic subjects[198] and qualitative changes in the ap-olipoproteins.[197,205] A defect in the transport of cholesterol from HDL to VLDL and LDL has also been described,[206] but its possible contribution to accelerated atherosclerosis is unknown.

The evidence that correction of dyslipidemias in chronic renal failure will reduce ischemic cardiac events is equivocal. Nevertheless, experimental evidence does support the notion that lipid abnormalities may cause vascular disease in uremics. Thus, it seems prudent to attempt to lower lipids in uremia. Certainly, adherence to an appropriate diet and regular exercise schedule, cessation of smok-ing, and attempts to maintain ideal body weight are desirable. All these measures require a high degree of commitment and motivation from the patient. It has been suggested that the dialysate buffer composition (acetate vs. bicarbonate) and glucose concentration, frequency of dialysis, or mode of therapy (HD vs. CAPD) can contribute to the incidence of lipid abnormalities.[196,206,207] Certainly, drugs associated with hyperlipidemias (e.g., beta blockers and androgens) should be avoided if possible. Lipid-lowering agents have been shown to be effective in lowering plasma lipid levels in uremic patients; however, the toxicity of these compounds makes their general recommendation impossible.[208,209]

8.5. Vasculature

The vascular tree of uremic patients is subjected to a variety of insults, both hemodynamic and metabolic. As a result, there is accelerated development of vascular degenerative lesions which lead ultimately to ischemic cardiac, cere-brovascular, and peripheral vascular disease. Hypertension is present in over 75% of patients with renal failure and is a major contributor to vascular disease in this population. Volume overload is certainly the major factor in the pathogenesis of hypertension of uremia, and ultrafiltration is of benefit in the majority of hyperten-sive dialysis patients, but volume overload is by no means the only problem.

Plasma renin activity (i.e., the rate of conversion of renin substrate to an-giotensin I after addition of renin to plasma) is increased in uremic patients.[210,211] Angiotensin converting enzyme (ACE) levels are high in dialysis patients, provid-ing a rationale for the use of ACE inhibitors in the treatment of dialysis-associated hypertension. On the other hand, several studies have documented a decreased pressor response to angiotensin II in dialysis patients.[211,212] It may be that continu-ous exposure to high circulating levels of endogenous angiotensin II leads to down-regulation of receptor density as a cause of decreased vascular reactivity to an-giotensin II.

The sympathetic nervous system also plays a role in the hypertension of uremia. Circulating levels of free norepinephrine and dopamine and conjugated epinephrine are elevated in renal failure.[213] It also appears that the negative feed-back of circulating norepinephrine on the activity of the sympathetic nervous system is depressed in uremics. The pressor response of uremics to exogenous norepinephrine is reduced.[211,214] PTH appears to play a permissive role in the pressor response to catecholamines in uremia. Uremic rats treated with norepinephrine have a blunted hypertensive response which can be restored to normal following either parathyroidectomy or inhibition of prostaglandin synthesis with indomethacin.[214,215] Bromocriptine was shown to decrease blood pressure and norepinephrine in a report of nine hypertensive dialysis patients,[216] indicating a possible role for prolactin in sympathetic control in some patients.

The calcium content of vascular structures is increased in clinical and experimental renal failure. One study of 143 patients with end-stage renal disease examined with plain radiographs of the extremities demonstrated arterial calcification in all, which was severe in 58 patients.[217] This had a marked tendency to progress in 57% of the subjects, whereas regression occurred in only 13%. Decreasing dialysate calcium concentration from 3.5 to 2.5 meq/liter was associated with a minor decrease in blood pressure (4.6 mm Hg).[218] In animal models, dietary calcium restriction has been shown to markedly decrease the vascular morphologic changes associated with long-term uremia.[219] Administration of calcium to uremic rats results in a hypertensive response which is attenuated by prior parathyroidectomy.[215] A possible method for the study of vascular reactivity to calcium and other stimuli in resistance vessels in humans has recently been described. Essentially, the reactivity of vessels obtained by biopsy of subcutaneous adipose tissue is measured after exposure to various vasoactive substances.[220]

It has been suggested that circulating inhibitors of Na,K-ATPase may be important mediators of hypertension in uremia. Several studies have demonstrated a correlation between Na,K-ATPase inhibition and hypertension in uremic and nonuremic subjects.[221–223] However, other studies have shown no correlation to blood pressure[124] and suggest that the inhibitory activity and blood pressure are more likely related to the state of sodium balance and volume overload as independent epiphenomena.

Identification of the operative mechanism in the causation of hypertension in uremic patients is of more than academic interest, since the control of hypertension is of major importance in the rate of progression of chronic renal failure. Individually tailored treatment of these patients will hopefully delay the need for end-stage therapy and reduce morbidity and mortality from cardiovascular disease once dialysis is undertaken.

Subclavian vein stenosis, due to prior temporary vascular access, is occasionally unmasked following placement of a permanent dialysis vascular access on the same side.[225,226]

9. The Hematopoietic System

9.1. Red Blood Cells

One of the most frequent abnormalities in uremic patients, as well as the source of numerous symptoms, is a severe hypoproliferative anemia. The pathogenesis of the anemia is multifactorial and results from erythropoietin deficiency, circulating inhibitors of erythropoietin activity, and metabolic abnormalities resulting in short-ened red cell survival. A frequently underestimated factor in the anemia of chronic renal disease is the role of blood loss due to the frequent and sometimes unnecessary diagnostic phlebotomy. This has been estimated to amount to about 1130 ml/year in a group of stable hemodialysis patients.[227]

9.1.1. Erythropoietin Deficiency

The principal site of erythropoietin (Epo) production is the kidney. The cell(s) responsible for the production of Epo remain unknown, although cortical tubular cells have been implicated. A deficiency in Epo production is the predominant cause of the anemia of most patients with chronic renal failure.[228] Epo may be quantified by either bioassay or radioimmunoassay (RIA). Correlation between the two methods is generally good and may facilitate the study of hormone kinetics and inhibitors due to the simplicity of the RIA.

Patients with renal failure have lower levels of Epo at any hemoglobin level than patients with iron deficiency anemia of comparable degree.[229] There are, however, some uremic patients with elevated levels of Epo by the RIA method who are severely anemic. This has been attributed to the presence of inhibitors of Epo which suppress the bone marrow or the detection of biologically inactive, but immunoreactive forms of the hormone. Despite the relatively depressed levels of circulating Epo in the plasma, the little that is present retains its ability to stimulate erythropoiesis, albeit at a reduced level. Dialysis patients who experience a spon-taneous hemorrhage have been noted to sustain an increase in their Epo levels and to undergo reticulocytosis; conversely, these same patients had a decrease in Epo levels and diminished reticulocyte production after transfusion.[230]

Perhaps the most effective argument in favor of Epo deficiency as the patho-genetic mechanism involved in the anemia of uremia has been the observation of human subjects treated with recombinant human Epo. In early trials of patients treated with this drug, a striking dose-dependent increase in the hematocrit was invariably noted.[231-234] Following administration of Epo, there was an increase in the reticulocyte count followed shortly thereafter by an increase in the hematocrit. Achieving a hemoglobin concentration of 10 g/dl has been reported in several studies. The use of Epo is not without potentially serious side effects, however. These include exacerbation of hypertension, particularly in patients with poorly controlled blood pressure at the onset of therapy. Hypertensive encephalopathy has been recorded in patients receiving Epo.[231,234] An increased predilection to vascular thrombosis of the dialysis access route,[231,234] as well as in the systemic circulation (presumably on the basis of increased viscosity of the blood[232]), is also a potential concern. Increases in serum concentrations of creatinine and potassium have been seen in most patients.[233] This is probably related to either poorer dietary compliance or less efficient dialysis, since an increase in the hematocrit will necessitate a lower plasma flow rate through the dialyzer at the same blood flow rate. Nevertheless, the therapeutic promise of synthetic Epo is so great that its commercial availability is eagerly awaited.

Epo levels increase soon after renal transplantation and decrease during acute rejection episodes.[235] Low levels of circulating Epo can be detected in anatomically anephric patients, implying an extrarenal source of production in some patients.[236,237] One such source may be the liver, although its exact role in erythropoiesis needs further elucidation.

9.1.2. Inhibition of Erythropoiesis

Despite the clear-cut role of Epo cited in the previous section and the reported absence of Epo inhibition in some studies,[228] both *in vitro* and *in vivo* evidence continues to accrue for the presence of inhibitors of erythropoiesis in uremic serum. A ferrokinetic study of six hemodialysis patients, before and after switching to CAPD, demonstrated an increase in red cell volume in all six and increased red cell survival in three, despite undetectable changes in the Epo levels.[238] These results suggest the more efficient removal of an Epo inhibitor (or a direct marrow toxin) via peritoneal dialysis. Monocytes and macrophages from uremic subjects inhibit the *in vitro* proliferation of erythrocytic precursors, possibly via elaboration of PGE_2 or decreased levels of interleukin 1.[239] Heme synthesis in red blood cell precursors has been found to be decreased in hemodialysis patients despite normal number of erythroblasts and normal response of those erythroblasts to Epo *in vitro,* suggesting the presence of an *in vivo* inhibitor.[240] It has been suggested that PTH,[241] angiotensin II,[242] plasma glycosidases,[243,244] and an unidentified "middle molecule"[245] may be the specific repressive factor of erythropoiesis. On the other hand, the *in vivo* significance of these *in vitro* inhibitors has been questioned, since contrary to earlier studies, uremic serum was shown to lack specificity in terms of bone marrow suppression.[246]

Abnormalities of trace metal homeostasis have been implicated in the pathogenesis of uremic anemia. Correction of an existing copper deficiency was reported to be effective in one patient with pancytopenia and chronic renal failure.[247] Zinc deficiency has been incriminated as another possible offender in the abnormality of heme synthesis which is characterized by decreased activity of delta-aminolevulinic acid dehydrase.[248] There has been growing concern about the possible role of aluminum intoxication in the pathogenesis of a severe microcytic anemia which is generally accompanied by near-total absence of peripheral sideroblasts.[249] Aluminum enters red blood cells from the plasma with ease, and the intracellular levels of aluminum in erythrocytes are nearly identical to those in plasma or serum.[250] Patients with uremia are predisposed to GI hemorrhage, as discussed in an earlier section, and are by no means immune from the potential development of iron deficiency. This is especially true in patients given deferoxamine for the treatment of aluminum intoxication,[249] in whom negative iron balance may be an unwanted side effect. Ferritin levels in general parallel marrow ion stores in uremia, but may be misleading particularly in patients with the so-called hemochromatosis alleles (HLA A3, B7, or B14).[251]

Androgens are useful in the treatment of anemia in dialysis patients. There is some evidence that anabolic steroids act by increasing red cell survival in uremia.[252] Deficiency of folic acid may be a factor in some dialysis patients with anemia, since this vitamin is dialyzable.

9.1.3. Altered Metabolism and Shortened Lifespan

Red cell survival is decreased in uremia. This is due at least partly to the increased osmotic fragility of the red cells, making them more susceptible to early removal by the reticuloendothelial system. It has been suggested that PTH contributes to this defect,[253] possibly via stimulation of a membrane Ca-ATPase.[254] Increased red blood cell (RBC) deformability in uremia, noted in the presence of PTH, is calcium dependent, inhibited by the calcium channel blocking drug verapamil, and reproduced in the absence of PTH by the calcium ionophore A23187.[255] The abnormal osmotic fragility of uremic RBCs is primarily a property of older cells.[253]

The loss of sialic acid from red cell membranes decreases RBC survival, and speculation about the possible role of enzymes that remove sialic acid from red cells and Epo continues.[243] As yet, there is no direct evidence that cleavage of sialic acid from cell membranes or Epo has a major role in the anemia of renal failure.

The regulation of ion transporters in erythrocyte membranes has been the subject of intense study, since the ionic permeability of RBCs correlates directly with the hematocrit.[256] Potassium content of red cells is decreased in azotemic patients,[256,257] and red cell calcium and sodium are increased.[256,258] For the most part, red cell Na,K-ATPase activity has been found to be decreased,[259] although some investigators have found unchanged[260] or increased[256] Na–K pump activity. Similarly, no consensus has been reached on the activity of RBC Na–Li countertransport or Na–K–Cl cotransport in uremia.[260–262] The effect of dialysis on erythrocyte content and transport of electrolytes is similarly uncertain, perhaps because of the confounding influence of dialysate composition and degree of weight loss during dialysis. However, the intracellular sodium level in RBCs of dialysis patients is usually low, although some investigators have found normal or even increased sodium concentrations in some subsets of patients.

In patients with severe renal failure, whether dialyzed or not, there is an increase in RBC content of adenosine triphosphate (ATP) and 2,3-diphospho-glycerate (DPG).[257,263,264] The pH of uremic red cells is decreased[263] and improves following dialysis with either acetate or bicarbonate as the source of base. The correction of cellular ATP levels is less complete, but is independent of the dialysate base used.[263] Guanosine triphosphate (GTP) levels are also commonly elevated during uremia. Both ATP and GTP levels in erythrocytes are normalized after renal transplantation.[264]

9.2. Hemostasis

Although other abnormalities of the coagulation cascade exist, the most important factor predisposing uremic patients to abnormal bleeding is platelet dysfunction. A slight decrease in absolute platelet count has been documented, but megakaryocytes are normal in number in the bone marrow of uremic individuals.[265] Thrombopoiesis is also diminished. However, these quantitative defects in platelet count are thought to be relatively minor in comparison to the qualitative abnormalities in platelet aggregation.

Some methods of examining platelet function (e.g., thromboelastography) suggest an *in vitro* hypercoagulability in uremia.[266] This is almost certainly an *in vitro* artifact, however, due to the common coexistence of anemia and hyperfibrinogenemia in patients with renal failure. Platelet aggregation to most stimuli, including ADP, collagen, ristocetin, epinephrine, and arachidonate, is impaired.[267] Theories abound to explain the hemostatic abnormalities in uremic patients. It has been shown that fibrinogen binding to uremic platelets, an early step in platelet aggregation, is decreased despite a normal number of fibrinogen receptors on uremic platelets. However, this defective fibrinogen binding can be corrected by the addition of arachidonic acid.[268] Thus, defective production or release of arachidonic acid in uremia may interfere with normal platelet function. Defects in platelet cyclooxygenase do not appear to be a significant cause of thrombocytopathy in uremia.[269] Oxalic acid, which is known to be elevated in the plasma of renal failure patients, inhibits platelet aggregation induced by ADP.[270]

A developmental defect in platelets has been suggested by studies examining megakaryocyte DNA content. There is an inverse correlation between the levels of BUN or creatinine and the DNA content of megakaryocytes in uremia, which suggests lower ploidy of uremic platelet precursors.[271] Since higher ploidy is generally associated with the ultimate production of more reactive platelets, a postulated uremic inhibition of DNA replication could lead to less reactive platelet formation. The abnormal platelet function is largely a property implicit to the platelets themselves and much less so to a serum factor, since normal platelets in uremic serum have normal aggregation, and uremic platelets in normal serum have decreased aggregation. However, adherence of normal platelets to subendothelium is decreased in the presence of uremic serum.[267]

Evidence both for and against a role for PTH in mediating platelet abnormalities has been advanced. The bulk of the evidence at present suggests only a limited, if any, role for PTH in the pathogenesis of uremic bleeding. One study found no correlation between chemical or clinical evidence of hyperparathyroidism and platelet abnormalities, and therapy of hyperparathyroidism with $1,25-(OH)_2$-vitamin D had no effect of platelet aggregation.[272] The presence of a circulating inhibitor of platelet aggregation has been suggested by the observation of improved platelet function in some patients following transfer from hemodialysis to peritoneal dialysis. However, this finding may be explained as an effect of hypoalbuminemia, which is more common in PD patients and also improves platelet aggregation.[273]

Of therapeutic interest is the effect of desmopressin (1-deamino-8-D-arginine vasopressin) in the treatment of the bleeding diathesis of uremia. Desmopressin acutely, but transiently decreases the bleeding time in uremia and has had dramatic success in the control of clinical uremic bleeding.[274-276] Also of interest is the use of conjugated estrogens in uremic bleeding. In one trial, estrogens had their maximum effect in 5–7 days but improved bleeding times for up to 14 days.[277] There was no effect on von Willebrand factor concentration or structure, or on platelet aggregation; the mechanism of action of estrogens in uremic bleeding remains to be exactly defined, but seems to be due to a vascular wall effect of estrogens in contrast to that of desmopressin on von Willebrand factor.

9.3. Leukocytes

The neutropenia that occurs during dialysis has already been discussed in Section 7. The chemotactic response of neutrophils and neutrophilic C5a receptors is decreased in dialysis patients. The oxidative metabolism of neutrophils and monocytes is decreased in response to chemotactic, but not to nonchemotactic, stimuli.[278] Uremic serum may stimulate oxidative metabolism in leukocytes under some circumstances,[279,280] but the significance of this finding is uncertain. Uremic serum appears to decrease the number of leukocyte clones in culture without affecting their maturation.[281] White cell ATP levels and adenylate cyclase function are abnormal in both children and adults with uremia.[282] Pyruvate kinase activity is also low in uremic adults.[282] Phagocytosis by peritoneal macrophages and neutrophils is decreased in renal failure.[11,283] Hemodialysis has the ability to acutely improve neutrophil chemotaxis.[284]

10. The Immune System

Abnormalities in immune function are extremely common in renal failure patients and can be recognized clinically by impaired reactivity of skin to delayed-type hypersensitivity testing, increased susceptibility to opportunistic bacterial and fungal infections, an increased incidence of neoplasia, and increased allograft survival in the uremic host.[119,285–290] The mechanisms that impair immunity in uremia are not clearly defined, but abnormalities of both cellular and humoral immunity have been identified.

10.1. Cell-Mediated Immunity

Abnormalities in total lymphocyte number and specific subpopulations are a universal finding in uremia.[291–295] Total lymphocyte count and T-lymphocyte number are decreased. T4+ cells (helper-inducer) are frequently, but not universally, decreased, and T8+ cells (suppressor) are usually, but not invariably, increased. This leads to a decrease in the T4/T8 ratio, which is considered to underlie many of the immune derangements of uremia. A rat model of chronic uremia demonstrated involution of the thymus 20 weeks after 5/6 nephrectomy, followed 2 weeks thereafter by increase in skin graft survival, decreased reactivity of mixed lymphocyte cultures, impaired resistance to tumor induction, and a marked decrease in the number of killer T cells.[293] B-cell functions have been less extensively studied, but T-cell-dependent B-cell proliferation is diminished in uremia, as is the T-cell-independent B-cell response to *Staphylococcus aureus*.[296] *In vitro* B-cell colony growth is inhibited by uremic adherent macrophages.[297] The mechanisms causing these abnormalities in cellular immunity are under active investigation.

Much interest in the immune regulation in renal failure has centered on lymphokines, e.g., interleukins (IL) or interferons. In patients on maintenance dialysis, IL-1, which is identical to endogenous pyrogen, has been isolated from the dialyzer in large amounts if standard, nonsterile dialysate is used, but not if sterile pyrogen-free saline is used.[298] This may be responsible for the sixfold increase in the incidence of fever in uremic patients while on hemodialysis.[299] Il-1, normally undetectable, was present in six of seven uremic patients predialysis, increased during hemodialysis, and was associated with an increment in temperature.[300] IL-1 production may be decreased in macrophages from patients whose peritoneal dialysis is complicated with frequent episodes of peritonitis.[301] IL-2 production has been found to be decreased in most, but not all, studies of uremic individuals.[302–304] The number of cells with IL-2 receptors is usually, but not invariably, found to be depressed as well.[294] The decreased response of uremic lymphocytes to concanavalin A, phytohemagglutinin, or pokeweed mitogen can be restored toward normal with exogenous IL-2.[304] Increases in the production of gamma interferon and PGE_2 have also been implicated in immune suppression of uremia.[301,303]

An attempt has been made to identify putative circulating inhibitors of lymphocyte function. The improved T-cell function in a subgroup of patients on CAPD has been attributed to the removal of an inhibitor.[292] Uremic serum was able to diminish blast transformation of normal lymphocytes exposed to mitogens, by a mechanism distinct from cyclic AMP.[305] Uremic serum was further able to induce a population of supressor cells by a mechanism distinct from induction due to concanavalin A.[306] A pentapeptide identified in uremic sera has been shown to have powerful immunomodulatory properties in *in vitro* assays at concentrations equal to that detected in the circulation.[307] Noncytotoxic Fc gamma receptor blocking antilymphocyte antibodies of the IgG class are present in many multiple-transfused uremic patients.[308] Vitamin E levels in mononuclear cells are low in uremia, and vitamin E supplementation is associated with a decrease in T8+ cells.[309]

Transfusions of blood have a major immunosuppressive effect in uremia.[310] The mechanism of this effect is thought to be largely due to induction of T8+ clones. In fact, the major reason for suppressed cutaneous immunity in anergic dialysis patients is considered to be transfusion related.[311]

Cell-mediated immunity is generally improved following either hemodialysis or peritoneal dialysis. CAPD improves skin responses of cellular immunity,[312] and hemodialysis acutely increases T3+ and T4+ cells while simultaneously decreasing T8+ and Ia+ cells, thus improving the T4/T8 ratio.[313] An important exception is that peritoneal dialysis seems to impair cellular immunity of resident peritoneal macrophages, at least in some patients.[314] This is expressed as a decrease in phagocytosis and phagocyte viability. The major factor responsible for this might be the low pH of commercially available dialysate solutions.[315] At one time, it was felt that cytotoxic therapy may be of benefit in uremia by selectively eliminating suppressor clones; this has not been borne out experimentally.[316]

10.2. Humoral Immunity

Humoral immunity is substantially less affected than cellular immunity in uremic patients. The erythrocyte sedimentation rate is elevated in 93% of hemodialysis patients and is above 100 mm/hr in about 20% of them.[317] The ESR correlates with the patient's age, degree of anemia, and hypocalcemia. Total gamma globulins are not depressed in renal failure, although polymorphisms at the DNA level in the Ig gene region have been described.[318] Endotoxin levels are frequently elevated, but bear a poor relationship to symptomatic "endotoxemia."[319] The serum of uremic patients contains a factor that inhibits the antimicrobial effect of sublethal doses of the cephalosporin antibiotic cefuroxime,[320] and this can be corrected toward normal with hemodialysis. Protein C activity in plasma is markedly decreased in uremia owing to the presence of an inhibitor.[321]

Vaccination is often recommended for uremic subjects, but suboptimal antibody responses are frequently encountered. Most uremic subjects require two injections of influenza vaccine in order to develop an adequate response.[322] Lack of efficacy of flu vaccine has been associated with high RBC Mg^{2+} content. Patients who receive hepatitis B vaccine prior to the initiation of dialysis have a better antibody response than those already on dialysis. Furthermore, the plasma-derived vaccine appears to be more immunogenic than the recombinant vaccine in dialysis patients.[323] Hemodialysis patients have a much weaker antibody response and lose their antibody titers to pneumococcal vaccinations much faster than either renal transplant recipients or controls.[324] On a more positive note, varicella vaccine was able to induce antibodies in 20 of 23 initially seronegative children on dialysis, and booster doses increased the antibody titers in 41 of 47 seropositive children.[325]

The acquired immunodeficiency syndrome (AIDS) is a public health concern of enormous magnitude.[326] AIDS is associated with a number of renal syndromes and is appearing at increasing frequency among chronic dialysis patients. In dialysis patients, the incidence of seropositivity for the infectious agent (HTLV-III or HIV) confirmed by Western blot or lymphocyte culture is in the range of 1–5% at this time.[327,328] The incidence of nosocomial transmission appears acceptably low provided isolation measures similar to those employed for hepatitis B surface antigen–positive patients are used.[328]

11. The Nervous System

Neurologic complications are an inevitable feature in dialysis patients and frequently form the basis of the presenting complaints in terminal uremia. On the other hand, neurologic findings may be extremely subtle and detectable only with sensitive electrophysiologic testing. Clinically significant abnormalities occur in the central nervous system, peripheral nerves, and autonomic nervous system and may be a principal component of the presenting symptom complex.

11.1. Central Nervous System

Anatomic abnormalities are demonstrable by computerized tomography (CT) of the brain in the majority of patients with end-stage renal disease. A group of 69 hemodialysis patients studied by CT revealed cortical atrophy in 56.5%, ventricular atrophy in 15.9%, low-density areas consistent with ischemia in 10.1%, and calcification in 4.5%.[329] The frequency of these findings correlated with the duration of uremia. Dialysis does not have an acute effect on the density of intracranial structures or size of the ventricular system.[330] The incidence of cerebral hemorrhage is about fivefold higher in dialysis patients than in the general population, but bland cerebral infarcts may be decreased compared to the general population.[331] One reason for the increase in hemorrhagic strokes, with a decrease in ischemic disease, might be an effect of heparin. This notion is supported by a report of a patient with osteogenesis imperfecta who sustained a spontaneous subdural hematoma during hemodialysis.[332]

Electroencephalographic abnormalities are common in uremia. Nine children on hemodialysis were noted to have a decrease in beta and alpha activity prior to dialysis, findings consistent with decreased vigilance. After dialysis, alpha and beta activity was improved.[333] In another study, electroencephalographic (EEG) improvements were found to occur in pediatric patients treated with high sodium (148–150 mmol/liter) concentrations in the dialysate.[334] Changes in adult EEG patterns with dialysis are extremely subtle, if indeed they occur at all.[330]

Extremely sensitive electrophysiologic testing usually reveals some abnormalities. Visual-evoked potential responses were abnormal, even in the absence of clinical findings, in a group of dialysis patients.[335] Auditory brain stem–evoked potentials were found to be abnormal in 24% of 38 stable chronic dialysis patients and improved after each dialysis treatment.[336] The endocochlear potential was found to be decreased in a study of experimental renal failure in rats.[337] Abnormal visual-evoked potentials may be reversed after renal transplantation.[338] Uremic optic neuropathy, which may respond favorably to corticosteroids, has been described.[339] A reversible uremic auditory neuropathy has also been reported.[340]

There has been a resurgence of interest in the potential role of endogenous opioids (enkephalins, endorphins) in the pathogenesis of uremic central nervous system (CNS) findings. Plasma met-enkephalin levels are elevated in hemodialysis patients and decrease slightly following dialysis.[341] Plasma leu-enkephalin levels are depressed in dialysis patients and are unchanged during the dialysis treatment. However, administration of naloxone is unable to either prevent or effectively treat dialysis induced hypotension,[342] nor does it correct the excessive secretion of prolactin commonly seen in dialysis patients[343] (see Section 12). Opioids presumably have no role in the anorexia of uremia.[98] Thus, from the available evidence, endogenous opioids do not appear to make a major contribution to most CNS symptoms or signs in uremia.

Numerous metabolic abnormalities occur in the brain of uremic animals and humans. A role has been postulated for the abnormal handling of glutamine, glycine, and the branched-chain and aromatic amino acids in the pathophysiology of uremic encephalopathy.[344] The function of synaptic junctions in the brain is abnormal in uremia, revealing increased sodium permeability, decreased Na,K-ATPase activity, and normal water and urea permeability.[345] Most studies have found an increase in calcium content of the brain in uremia, and the improvement in auditory evoked potentials induced by dialysis is probably related to changes in serum calcium.[336] However, the importance of calcium has been challenged in kinetic studies of ^{45}Ca uptake and distribution.[346] The function or synthesis of the neurotransmitters dopamine, serotonin, and gamma-aminobutyric acid may be impaired in renal failure.[344]

Of the many substances in uremia that have been proposed as "the" neurotoxin, the greatest support has been for parathyroid hormone.[2] It is clear, however, that the role of PTH is mainly permissive, as both the biochemical and clinical findings of uremic encephalopathy can occur in parathyroidectomized subjects. Aminolevulinic acid (ALA) levels are elevated both in uremic subjects and in those with acute intermittent porphyria; however, there is no evidence that ALA is directly neurotoxic in either condition.[347] Since there is no apparent correlation between CNS findings and involvement of peripheral nerves, the same toxin is unlikely to be involved in both conditions.[347]

It is important to consider some possible iatrogenic causes of neurologic deterioration in patients with renal failure. The now well-known syndrome of dialysis dementia has been attributed to aluminum intoxication from contaminated water supplies.[5] Awareness of the problem has led to a marked decrease in the incidence of dialysis dementia. Phosphate-binding aluminum hydroxide gels have been implicated in the development of a subacute encephalopathy which was rapidly reversed with deferoxamine therapy.[348] Many drugs, including commonly used antihypertensive agents, have significant CNS depressive side effects. Reversible parkinsonism has been reported in two dialysis patients receiving metaclopropamide as an antiemetic.[349]

Anesthetic agents, including narcotics and spinal anesthetics, may have changes in their biologic effects in uremic subjects. For the most part, mechanisms of action remain to be determined, but simple changes in binding or metabolism do not appear to be adequate to explain the functional differences noted in patients with advanced renal failure.[350]

11.2. Peripheral Nervous System

A peripheral sensorimotor neuropathy is common in renal failure. The lower limbs are more commonly affected than the upper.[351] Diffuse involvement along the length of the affected nerves is the rule.[352] At least 50% of renal failure patients present with clinically evident peripheral neuropathy,[353] and the proportion of patients with abnormal nerve conduction velocities (or the even more sensitive sensory-evoked potentials) is higher still.[354] Patients with end-stage renal disease on the basis of diabetes millitus tend to have the worst degree of peripheral neuropathy. Ulnar nerve involvement is more common in uremic than diabetic peripheral neuropathy.[351]

The response of uremic polyneuropathy to various treatment modalities has been mixed. Generally speaking, the neuropathy tends to stabilize or improve slightly, either clinically or electrophysiologically, with either hemodialysis or peritoneal dialysis.[353,355] One study has suggested that cuprophan dialysis membranes are associated with worse clinical neuropathy than polyacrylonitrile membranes.[356] Renal transplantation usually results in substantial clinical improvement of the peripheral neuropathy. A manifestation of peripheral neuropathy known as the "restless-leg" syndrome may be amenable to treatment with levodopa.[357] Uremic patients are commonly hyperuricemic and may be prone to develop acute gout, necessitating treatment with colchicine. There are reports of patients with renal failure who developed acute colchicine neuropathy.[358]

11.3. Autonomic Nervous System

Derangements of autonomic function are common in renal failure. A study of 67 uremic patients, both prior to and following the initiation of dialysis, found parasympathetic abnormalities in 65% and sympathetic dysfunction in an additional 24%.[359] Dialysis seems to stabilize or improve autonomic neuropathy.[360,361] Autonomic function has been reported as either unchanged or improved following renal transplantation.[362,363]

Abnormalities of sympathetic function are mainly expressed as disorders of circulating catecholamine levels and altered end-organ responsiveness. Catecholamine levels are increased in renal failure,[364,365] although at least some of the increase can be attributed to methodologic considerations and the presence of sulfoconjugated catecholamines.[366] Beta-adrenergic function is altered in uremia. Inhibitors of agonist binding to beta-adrenoreceptors have been described.[367,368] However, beta-2-receptor density is increased in renal failure.[368] Sympathetically mediated extrarenal potassium disposal is impaired in uremia.[369] There is no strong evidence for a dominant role of PTH in either parasympathetic or sympathetic dysfunction in renal insufficiency.[367,370]

11.4. Neurobehavioral Disorders

Depression is commonly encountered in dialysis patients. As many as 30–50% of adult dialysis patients may have symptoms of a major depressive disorder.[371–373] Other frequent findings in uremic patients include anxiety, personality disorders, and mania.[374–376] Since some aspects of the patients' psychological state are closely related to functional recovery,[372] it is important to provide as much social and emotional support as possible. It has been suggested that depression may be overdiagnosed in end-stage renal disease, and that many "depressive" symptoms are in fact due to uremia.[377] Although it seems intuitively obvious that a good support structure (group therapy, intact family unit, and so forth) should be associated with at least as good survival as occurs in its absence, both improvements and declines in patient survival have been correlated with good psychologic and family support.[378–380] Depression commonly worsens with increasing duration of dialysis, although correction of chemical abnormalities by dialysis is associated with an increase in intelligence quotient and cognitive skills in children.[381]

Other family members can often be devastated when a child, parent, or sibling has advanced uremia requiring dialysis.[382,383] Transplantation does not cure the ailing psyche, but instead presents a new set of problems and a new series of emotional ills.

12. The Endocrine System

Endocrine abnormalities develop early in renal failure and increase in severity during the course of progression to end-stage renal disease. Several factors contribute to the pathogenesis of endocrine abnormalities in renal failure. With the onset of reduction in renal function, the capacity of the kidneys as a principal route of excretion and biodegradation of hormones and their substrates becomes compromised. As renal failure progresses, the uremic environment *per se* begins to exert a detrimental effect on endocrine function as hormone synthesis, feedback systems, and end-organ responsiveness become jeopardized. Additionally, poor nutrition and medical treatment will influence the type and magnitude of endocrine abnormalities that occur in chronic renal failure.[384,385]

A role for opioids in the altered function of endocrine organs in renal failure has also been postulated.[386] Elevated plasma levels of some,[387] but not all,[388] circulating opioids have been found in patients with chronic renal failure. An effect of opioids in normal endocrine function has been demonstrated on the basis of structural, stimulation, and inhibition studies.[389–391] The studies in patients with renal failure are based on the use of naloxone, a high-affinity blocker of all three types of opioid receptors: mu, delta, and kappa. Blockade of opioid receptors significantly improved glucose tolerance and glucose-induced secretion in uremic patients and blunted the response of calcium-induced calcitonin secretion and suppression of PTH. These results were taken to indicate the existence of hyperendorphism in end-stage renal failure.[386]

The presumption that the endocrine abnormalities of renal failure abate after successful transplantation appears to be true only in two-thirds of such cases. In a retrospective analysis of 275 transplanted cases, a variety of endocrine abnormalities (hyperparathyroidism, sexual dysfunction, growth retardation, hyperinsulinism) persisted in 71 patients, independent of the adequacy of function of the transplanted kidney.[392]

12.1. Carbohydrate Metabolism

The principal defect in the compromised carbohydrate metabolism of uremic patients is resistance to insulin. The cellular basis of insulin resistance is due mainly to impairment of the postreceptor responsiveness to insulin. In an experimental model of acute uremia, studies of insulin-mediated metabolism of epitrochlearis muscle revealed no change in insulin sensitivity, but a decreased responsiveness to insulin of glucose uptake, glycogen synthesis, and glucose oxidation.[393] The decreased glycogen synthesis, which at maximal insulin concentrations was 54% less than normal, was attributed to a 23% decrease in the total activity of muscle glycogen synthetase and the percentage of enzyme present in the activated form in uremic animals. Glycogen phosphorylase activity was unchanged. Muscle protein degradation was increased in both the absence and presence of insulin.[393]

In addition to the postreceptor binding defect, another reason for the abnormal carbohydrate metabolism appears to be the presence in uremic plasma of dialyzable substances which reversibly inhibit insulin binding, leading to altered insulin sensitivity. In a study of 20 uremic patients before and after dialysis, predialysis binding of radioactive insulin to erythrocytes was 50% lower than in normal subjects.[394] Dialysis treatment resulted in a rapid increase in binding of about 55%. Serial studies in two patients showed a steady time-dependent increase in insulin binding of about 24% per hour. After an intravenous glucose load, the plasma insulin–glucose ratio decreased in parallel with the increase in binding of insulin assayed after dialysis.[394]

Postmortem studies of end stage renal disease (ESRD) patients treated with long-term hemodialysis have revealed a considerable increase in the prevalence of pancreatic pathology.[121] Of special relevance to the carbohydrate intolerance is the demonstration of hyaline replacement of the islets of Langerhans in 6 of 10 autopsied cases reported from Japan.[122] Electron microscopy revealed the presence of amyloid fibrils in the deposits. Clinically, glucose was present in the urine of one of the three patients studied premortem and a moderate elevation of the glucose level in two other cases.[122] Whether these lesions, which apparently develop in the course of dialytic management, result in impaired insulin secretion and thereby constitute an added contributory factor to the glucose intolerance of uremia remains to be ascertained.

The abnormalities in insulin sensitivity and insulin-mediated glucose metabolism notwithstanding, the insulin-mediated potassium uptake and potassium-mediated release of insulin are well preserved and, in fact, are markedly increased in renal failure. In a remnant kidney model of experimental renal failure in dogs, the peak increments of insulin response to potassium chloride infusion (2 meq/kg per hr) was increased (140 ± 16 μU/ml in uremia vs. 39 ± 3 μg/ml in controls).[395] Analysis of potassium distribution revealed a marked decrease in potassium transfer from the extracellular to the intracellular compartment of uremic dogs. This acute sensitivity of pancreatic beta cells for insulin release in response to potassium is clearly important to the extrarenal maintenance of potassium balance in renal failure.

Hyperglucagonemia, due to impaired degradation of the peptide by the diseased kidney, is a characteristic feature of the uremic state.[385] It has been shown that the canine and rat hepatocyte convert glucagon to a metabolite lacking the amino-terminal residues of the hormone.[396] These fragments accumulate in chronic renal failure, and studies of glucagon metabolism by carboxy-terminal radioimmunoassay could lead to underestimation of glucagon extraction by the liver.

12.2. Thyroid Gland

Because of disturbances in thyroid hormone kinetics and binding, tests of thyroid gland function are abnormal in about one-third to one-half of patients with chronic renal failure even though thyroid function is normal in the majority of patients.[385] Evidence continues to accrue for the now well-established pattern of these changes, which consists of decreased binding of thyroxine (T_4) to protein, with consequent low total and less commonly low free T_4 levels; impaired conversion of T_4 to triiodothyronine (T_3), which has been attributed to the impaired activity of renal 5'-deiodinase; normal response to exogenous thyroid-stimulating hormone (TSH); and a slow or subnormal response of TSH to thyrotropin-releasing hormone (TRH).[397–400] Kinetic, transfer, and distribution studies of thyroxine are not different from normal in patients with chronic renal failure.[401] The basic mechanism for the low total T_4 level is inhibition of binding to proteins, despite normal levels of thyroid-binding globulin (TBG).[402] Competition with free fatty acids for protein binding sites has been proposed as one mechanism responsible for the abnormality of TBG-bound T_4.[400,403] Also, there may be a decrease in the TBG level in some patients on chronic hemodialysis.[404]

The abnormalities of T_4 and T_3 notwithstanding, no deficiency of thyroid hormone seems to exist at the cellular level. In a rat model of uremia, chronic supplementation of T_3 for 5 weeks induced no significant change in body weight gain; serum insulin, glucose, glycerol, nonesterified fatty acids, total glycerides, total cholesterol, or total choline phospholipids; or triglyceride production and degradation rates.[405] On the other hand, a blunted peripheral tissue responsiveness to exogenous T_3 administration to patients in chronic renal failure has been demonstrated, as determined from measurements of basal oxygen uptake and peripheral blood mononuclear leukocyte ouabain binding.[406] By the same token, a stimulatory effect of erythropoiesis has been demonstrated in an experimental model of anemic uremic rats given relatively high doses of T_3 (50 μg/kg per day) for 10 days.[407] This has led to the suggestion of the potential therapeutic use of T_3 for the anemia of renal failure. However, the low T_3 levels frequently found in patients with renal failure may confer a protective effect by minimizing the protein catabolism of these patients. Nitrogen balance studies in seven patients, during T_3 supplementation and its suppression by sodium ipodate, revealed a significant negative correlation between T_3 concentration and nitrogen balance ($r = -0.63$, $p < 0.005$).[408] The putative protection of low T_3 levels against protein breakdown is supported by another cross-sectional study of 19 patients on hemodialysis and of 11 patients on continuous ambulatory peritoneal dialysis.[409] In hemodialysis patients T_4 and T_3 levels were significantly decreased, whereas in peritoneal dialysis patients they were normal. In hemodialysis patients, a significant correlation was found between

T_3 and serum proteins, whereas in peritoneal dialysis patients, a positive correlation was found between T_3 and triceps skinfold thickness. The overload of carbohydrate presented during peritoneal dialysis was postulated to have normalized the thyroid hormones in patients on peritoneal dialysis.[409]

Diagnostic difficulties are encountered when hypothyroidism occurs in patients with chronic renal failure.[410] Several of the typical features of renal failure are similar to those of hypothyroidism and are accompanied by the usually low T_4 and T_3 levels. In addition, the TSH may be slightly elevated or at the upper limit of normal, principally because of the reduced clearance of TSH fragments in renal failure.[411] Furthermore, the TSH response to TRH is usually blunted in uremia due to poor nutritional status and excess endogenous dopamine levels.[412] Thus, the demonstration of the appropriate TSH response to TRH must be observed for the correct diagnosis of hypothyroidism in uremic patients. A blunted response of TSH to TRH does not exclude the diagnosis of borderline hypothyroidism. In such instances the test should be repeated periodically to substantiate clear evidence of hypothyroidism.

There seems to be a correlation between the abnormalities of thyroid function tests and the glucose intolerance of renal failure. In a study of 60 patients on dialysis, the serum T_3 level and T_3/T_4 molar ratio were significantly lower and the reverse T_3 (RT_3) higher in those with glucose intolerance. In fact, serum RT_3 showed a diagnostic specificity of 94.2% and a sensitivity of 100% for the presence of an abnormal oral glucose tolerance test.[413]

12.3. Gonads

Primary failure of normal gonadal function and that of its hypothalamic–hypophyseal regulatory mechanism develop early in the course of renal failure, worsen with progressive deterioration of renal failure, and ultimately come to account for much of the sexual complaints of ESRD patients.

12.3.1. Male

In a study of testicular function in experimental uremia induced by 5/6 nephrectomy in mature male rats, the levels of testosterone (T) and androstenedione (A) in serum and testicular interstisial fluid were significantly depressed as early as 1 week after the induction of renal failure.[414] An increment in the follicle-stimulating hormone (FSH) level did not occur until 4 weeks after nephrectomy, whereas the levels of luteinizing hormone (LH) remained within the normal range throughout the 4-week period of this study. Primary Leydig cell dysfunction also occurs and fails to respond to chorionic gonadotropin administration despite correction of the testosterone levels following gonadotropin therapy.[415]

In patients with chronic renal failure the characteristic hormonal abnormalities that ultimately develop are low levels of A, T, and dihydrotestosterone (DHT), with normal levels of testosterone-binding globulin; whereas the levels of FSH, LH, and prolactin (PRL) are elevated.[416-419] Part of the defect in uremic hypogonadism is due to aberrant hypothalamic pulsatile responsiveness, while that of hypophyseal responsiveness remains normal.[416-418] The hormonal derangements do not improve following institution of hemodialysis, and actually may be magnified by it.[417,420] A partial improvement in T levels is noted following a low-protein diet supplemented with essential amino acids and ketoanalogs.[420,421] In a study comparing 18 patients on dietary restriction to eight patients on hemodialysis, the changes in gonadal function showed a direct relation to the serum PTH levels, leading to the suggestion of a contributory role of secondary hyperparathyroidism to uremic hypogonadism.[420]

The very high levels of PRL that occur in some patients further contribute to the suppression of gonadal function. The abnormal levels of PRL, which is under dopaminergic control, seem to be aggravated by the elevated levels of dopamine in ESRD patients.[422] Its lowering with dopaminergic antagonists can improve the levels of circulating T and can improve sexual function in some patients.[423,424] In contrast to humans, responses to dopaminergic agonists and antagonists, either *in vivo* or *in vitro*, are not impaired with experimental renal failure studied at 8 weeks, indicating that hyperprolactinemia occurs on a nondopaminergic basis relatively early in the course of renal failure in the rat.[425] A principal reason for the hyperprolactinemia in uremic males is its reduced clearance, which correlates positively with the level of renal function.[426] The elevated circulating levels of PRL are due to increases in little PRL without major changes in the big and big–big forms of PRL.[426] Of interest is the observation that salmon calcitonin, at a subhypocalcemic dose (10 MRC units over 30 min), significantly suppresses PRL selection by 40% in patients with reduced renal function (GFR 35 ml/min).[427] Correction of hyperprolactinemic hypogonadism may be important for the prevention of osteoporosis associated with such states.[42U]

12.3.2. Female

The gonadal hormonal abnormalities noted in females are similar to those noted in males. The serum levels of PRL, LH, and FSH are increased, while those of estrogen, estradiol, and progesterone are low, and the pulsatile release of gonadotropins is compromised.[416,424,429] The elevated PRL levels appear to contribute to the dysfunctional uterine bleeding and metrorrhagia of uremic women. In a study of nine uremic women, lowering of PRL with bromocriptine therapy reduced the menorrhagia in four and the metrorrhagia in three women.[424]

12.4. Adrenal Glands

Although the half-life of cortisol is increased in renal failure, the daily pattern of plasma cortisol secretion is not different from normal.[430] However, the degree of suppression after dexamethasone is significantly lower in uremic subjects, possibly because of the prolonged cortisol half-life in renal failure. None of a group of seven uremic subjects had suppressed plasma cortisol after 1 mg dexamethasone orally the night before. After 48-hr suppression, they did suppress. Thus, normal suppression of plasma cortisol can be achieved in uremia, if the duration of dexamethasone administration is prolonged sufficiently to compensate for the prolongation of cortisol half-life. The volume of distribution, clearance, and half-life of dexamethasone are normal. However, its intestinal absorption may be decreased. Thus, in patients who do not suppress after oral dexamethasone, it is essential to measure plasma dexamethasone levels or use the intravenous dexamethasone suppression test.[430] The half-life of prednisone is increased in renal failure. An adaptive increase in hepatic clearance of prednisone has been shown in 5/6 nephrectomized rats.[431] While the plasma concentration of free dopamine and norepinephrine levels are high in most patients with renal failure, that of epinephrine is not different from controls. In a study of 35 patients, the conjugated level of these catecholamines was also altered. The sulfoconjugated levels of all three catecholamines were increased; glucuroconjugated dopamine and norepinephrine were unchanged, while the level of epinephrine was increased.[432] The physiologic significance of these changes in conjugated catecholamines remain to be defined.

The increased plasma aldosterone levels in renal failure are necessary for the maintenance of normal potassium homeostasis. In a study of 16 patients with renal failure, there was significant correlation between aldosterone excretion and fractional excretion of potassium ($r = 0.53$).[433] Despite the elevated basal levels of aldosterone, the diseased kidney continues to respond with normal increments in the renal excretion of potassium following the administration of exogenous aldosterone.[434] Furthermore, in an experimental model of renal failure in dogs, the increased basal secretion of aldosterone increased appropriately when the potassium load was acutely increased by higher dietary intake (from 60 to 200 meq/day) or by the intravenous infusion of potassium (2 meq/kg over 1 hr).[395] Angiotensin II appears necessary for an adequate aldosterone response to potassium stimulation. Inhibition of converting enzyme results in a significant reduction in the basal aldosterone secretion and a consequent increase in the plasma potassium concentration from 3.9 ± 0.2 meq/liter to 5.4 ± 0.4 meq/liter.[433] It seems then that, independent of basal elevated aldosterone levels, the hyperkalemia noted in some patients with chronic renal failure is in part due to a relative degree of hypoaldosteronism, for the prevailing hyperkalemia, and can be aggravated by converting enzyme inhibitors. The pathogenesis of this acquired relative hypoaldosteronism does not seem to be due to dopaminergic inhibition of aldosterone[435] and remains to be clarified.

The plasma levels of active renin and trypsin-activated inactive renin are decreased in renal failure.[436] The plasma renin activity and angiotensin II levels are increased, reflecting increased converting enzyme activity.[437] The hyperdipsia noted in some patients with chronic renal failure on hemodialysis appears to be mediated by this increased production of angiotensin II and may be ameliorated after the administration of an angiotensin converting enzyme inhibitor.[437]

12.5. Growth Factors

Methodologic problems continue to plague the determination of somatomedin levels in renal failure, making it difficult to interpret the conflicting results reported in the literature.[438-440] By the same token, the response of growth hormone to growth hormone–releasing hormone is variable, but tends to be increased.[441] The importance of this issue is particularly relevant to children with renal failure whose growth is retarded. Treatment with recombinant growth hormones seems to be promising in the partial resolution of this problem.[442]

12.6. Parathyroid Glands and Renal Osteodystrophy

Secondary hyperparathyroidism is a well-established early complication of renal failure. Phosphate retention, diminished synthesis of $1,25\text{-}(OH)_2\text{-}D3$, and abnormal set-point for calcium-regulated PTH release all participate in the state of compensatory hypersecretion of PTH that characterizes patients with renal failure. The normal interrelationship of these three factors in regulating serum calcium and serving as calcium-independent feedback regulators of each other is disturbed in renal failure and thereby magnifies the abnormalities of each of the others. Decreased degradation of PTH by the diseased kidney further contributes to the elevated levels of PTH encountered in patients with renal failure, particularly that of the C-terminal fragments of PTH whose excretion depends on the kidney.[443]

Although hypocalcemia is the main factor that ultimately accounts for the genesis of secondary hyperparathyroidism of renal failure, it may not be essential for its development. In a study of experimental renal failure in dogs, in which hypocalcemia was prevented by feeding a high-calcium diet, PTH levels increased from 64 ± 7.7 to 118 ± 21 pg/ml, and serum $1,25\text{-}(OH)_2\text{-}D3$ decreased from 25.4 ± 3.8 to 12.2 ± 3.6 pg/ml.[444] On the other hand, prevention of the decrease in $1,25\text{-}(OH)_2\text{-}D3$ by its exogenous administration, at a dosage that did not alter serum ionized calcium (75–100 mg twice daily), prevented the increase in PTH. Thus, low levels of $1,25\text{-}(OH)_2\text{-}D3$, independent of changes in serum calcium, appear to contribute to the altered regulation of PTH secretion in renal insufficiency.[444]

PTH and $1,25\text{-}(OH)_2\text{-}D3$ act together to regulate calcium homeostasis. That PTH is trophic to $1,25\text{-}(OH)_2\text{-}D3$ synthesis has long been known. There is also increasing evidence that $1,25\text{-}(OH)_2\text{-}D3$ has a direct counterregulatory effect on the parathyroid gland, which is rich in stereospecific, high-affinity receptors for $1,25\text{-}(OH)_2\text{-}D3$. In a study of hyperplastic parathyroid glands obtained from seven patients with chronic renal failure, the binding of radiolabeled $1,25\text{-}(OH)_2\text{-}D3$ was significantly lower than that of the parathyroid glands obtained from transplanted patients and adenomas removed from patients with primary hyperparathyroidism.[445] This reduced binding by parathyroid cells of 1,25-$(OH)_2$-D3 in renal failure coupled with the low serum levels of 1,25-$(OH)_2$-D3 in kidney disease would compromise the counterregulatory effect of 1,25-$(OH)_2$-D3 on PTH secretion. The resultant increased release of PTH at any given level of calcium would then account for the increased set-point for calcium suppression of PTH release. In order to compensate for this increased need for PTH the parathyroid gland responds by hypertrophy and proliferation. The result is the progressive development of diffuse hyperplasia of the parathyroid glands during the course of progressive renal failure and early period of maintenance dialysis. The evolution to nodular hyperplasia seems to occur in patients maintained on dialysis for over 4 years.[446]

The salutary effect of exogenous supplementation with vitamin D_3 or its metabolites continues to be documented by different centers worldwide.[447-451] Replacement therapy is particularly important in advanced renal failure, since unlike early or moderate renal failure (GFR 30–50 ml/min), phosphate reduction alone may no longer be effective to increase the endogenous production of 1,25-$(OH)_2$-De.[452-454] Substantial degradation of 1,25-$(OH)_2$-D3 occurs in the intestine, and in some cases, where oral replacement therapy is not effective, intravenous administration may be necessary.[455] Experimental evidence indicates that pharmacologic doses of 1,25-$(OH)_2$-D3 and a low-calcium diet enhance the GI absorption and tissue loads of aluminum.[456] Therefore, patients supplemented with 1,25-$(OH)_2$-D3 who are exposed to aluminum may be at greater risk of aluminum-associated bone disease. To circumvent this dire eventuality, the use of alternative phosphate binders, such as calcium carbonate, has been recommended.[457] The development of yet another complication of exogenous vitamin D therapy, hypercalcemia, should be carefully monitored in such patients.

Circulating osteocalcin, which normally reflects the rate of bone formation, is elevated in renal failure. However, multiple immunoreactive forms of osteocalcin appear to accumulate in uremia. In a study of 18 patients on maintenance dialysis it was shown that in contrast to the single sharp peak of osteocalcin present in normal serum, in pooled sera from patients with high osteoclastic resorptive surfaces identified by histomorphometry there were five additional immunoreactive peaks, while three additional peaks were detected in sera from patients with lower osteoclastic surfaces.[458]

With the successful prevention of hyperparathyroid bone disease parathyroidectomy is rarely necessary in patients with ESRD. It must be kept in mind, however, that once clinical evidence of hyperparathyroid bone disease develops, the response to vitamin D_3 supplementation, as assessed by bone histomorphometry, is less complete in patients treated with parathyroidectomy followed by vitamin D_3 supplementation, despite similar biochemical and radiographic responses, compared to patients without clinical parathyroid disease.[459] Still, subtotal parathyroidectomy with autotransplantation can benefit patients with clearly established severe progressive hyperparathyroidism causing clinical bone disease associated with hypercalcemia and high levels of PTH. Features such as soft tissue calcification, pruritus, vessel wall calcification, and peripheral ischemia respond less favorably or predictably.[460–463] The pharmacologic inhibition of PTH is a substitute for surgery. The initial promise of the usefulness of H_2-receptor antagonists continues to be refuted.[464] The role of a new hypocalcemic agent, WR-2721, with strong inhibitory activity of PTH secretion, is certainly promising,[465] but remains to be demonstrated clinically.

Brown tumors, though much less common in secondary than in primary hyperparathyroidism, do occur in patient on maintenance dialysis. They must be entertained in the differential diagnosis of severe localized bone pain. Their unusual localization, such as in the orbital bones or vertebrae, results in unexpected visual abnormalities and paraplegia.[466,467]

Of therapeutic interest is the effect of calcium channel blockers on PTH. In uremic male Wistar rats, injection of verapamil increased the already elevated levels of PTH by 62% in rats with moderate renal failure, a value significantly greater than the 21% increase noted in the control rats.[468] The implication of prolonged treatment of patients with progressive renal failure with calcium channel blockers may not be devoid of detrimental effects.

References

1. Adams, F., 1986, The extant works of Aretaeus, the Cappodocian. Sydenham Society, Wertheimer and Co., London.
2. Klahr, S. and Slatopolsky, E., 1986, Toxicity of parathyroid hormone in uremia, *Annu. Rev. Med.* **37**:71–78.
3. Kaplan, B., Gotfried, M., and Ravid, M., 1986, Amino acid containing compounds in uremic serum—Search for middle molecules by high performance liquid chromatography, *Clin. Nephrol.* **26**:66–71.
4. Valek, A., Spustova, V., Lopot, F., Erben, J., and Dzurik, R., 1986, Can plasma concentration of middle molecules contribute to assessment of adequate dialysis treatment? *Artif. Organs* **10**:37–44.
5. Mayor, G. H., and Burnatowska-Hledin, M., 1986, The metabolism of aluminum and aluminum-related encephalopathy, *Semin. Nephrol.* **6**(4 Suppl. 1):1–4.
6. Muirhead, N., Kertesz, A., Flanagan, P. R., Hodsman, A. B., Hollomby, D. J., and Valberg, L. S., 1986, Zinc metabolism in patients on maintenance and hemodialysis, *Am. J. Nephrol.* **6**:422–426.
7. Foote, J. W., Hinks, L. J., and Lloyd, B., 1987, Reduced plasma and white blood cell selenium levels in hemodialysis patients, *Clin. Chim. Acta* **164**:323–328.
8. Dworkin, B., Weseley, S., Rosenthal, W. S., Schwartz, E. M., and Weiss L., 1987, Diminished blood selenium levels in renal failure patients on dialysis: Correlations with nutritional status, *Am. J. Med. Sci.* **293**:6–12.
9. Shaykh, M., Bazilinski, N., McCaul, D. S., Ahmed, S., Dubin, A., Musiala, T., and Dunea, G., 1985, Fluorescent substances in uremic and normal serum, *Clin. Chem.* **31**:1988–1992.
10. DeDeyn, P., Marescau, B., Lornoy, W., Becaus, I., Van Leuven, I., Van Gorp, L., and Lowenthal, A., 1987, Serum guanidino compound levels and the influence of a single hemodialysis in uremic patients undergoing maintenance hemodialysis, *Nephron* **45**:291–295.
11. Farinelli, A., Fiocchi, O., Stabellini, G., Stabellini, N., Marangoni, C., and Spisani, S., 1987, Effect on leukocyte locomotion and superoxide production by uremic toxins and polyamines, *Int. J. Artif. Organs* **10**:37–40.
12. Nath, K. A., Kren, S. M., and Hostetter, T. H., 1986, Dietary protein restriction in established renal injury in the rat. Selective role of glomerular capillary pressure in progressive glomerular dysfunction, *J. Clin. Invest.* **78**:1199–1205.

13. Zeller, K. R., 1987, Effects of dietary protein and phosphorus restriction on the progression of chronic renal failure, *Am. J. Med. Sci.* **294:**328–340.

14. Levine, M. M., Kirschenbaum, M. A., Chaudhari, A., Wong, M. W., and Bricker, N. S., 1986, Effect of protein on glomerular filtration rate and prostanoid synthesis in normal and uremic rats, *Am. J. Physiol.* **251:**F635–F641.

15. Rosenberg, M. E., Swanson, J. E., Thomas, B. L., and Hostetter, T. H., 1987, Glomerular and hormonal responses to dietary protein intake in human renal disease, *Am. J. Physiol.* **253:**F1083–F1090.

16. Ito, Y., Barcelli, U., Yamashita, W., Weiss, M., Deddens, J., and Pollack, V. E., 1987, A low protein-high linoleate diet increases glomerular PGE_2 and protects renal function in rats with reduced renal mass, *Prostaglandins Leukotrienes Med.* **28:**277–284.

17. Van Duyn, M. A., 1987, Acceptability of selected low protein products for use in a potential diet therapy for chronic renal failure, *J. Am. Diet. Assoc.* **87:**909–914.

18. Kopple, J. D., Monteon, F. J., and Shaib, J. K., 1986, Effect of energy intake on nitrogen metabolism in nondialyzed patients with chronic renal failure, *Kidney Int.* **29:**734–742.

19. Friedman, A. L., and Pityer, R., 1986, Beneficial effect of moderate protein restriction on growth, renal function and survival in young rats with chronic renal failure, *J. Nutr.* **116:** 2466–2477.

20. Lucas, P. A., Meadows, J. H., Roberts, D. E., and Coles, G. A., 1986, The risks and benefits of a low protein-essential amino acid-keto acid diet, *Kidney Int.* **29:**995–1003.

21. Acchiardo, S. R., Moore, L. W., and Cockrell, S., 1986, Does low protein diet halt the progression of renal insufficiency? *Clin. Nephrol.* **25:**289–294.

22. Lumlertgul, D., Burke, T. J., Gillum, D. M., Alfrey, A. C., Harris, D. C., Hammond, W. S., and Schrier, R. W., 1986, Phosphate depletion arrests progression of chronic renal failure independent of protein intake, *Kidney Int.* **29:**658–666.

23. Alfrey, A. C., 1988, Effect of dietary phosphate restriction on renal function and deterioration, *Am. J. Clin. Nutr.* **47:**531–536.

24. Lindenau, K., Kokot, F., and Frohling, P. T., 1986, Suppression of parathyroid hormone by therapy with a mixture of ketoanalogues/amino acids in hemodialysis patients, *Nephron* **43:** 84–86.

25. Strife, C. F., Quinlan, M., Mears, K., Davey, M. L., and Clardy, C., 1986, Improved growth of three uremic children by nocturnal nasogastric feedings, *Am. J. Dis. Childhood* **140:**438–443.

26. Mak, R. H., Turner, C., Thompson, T., Haycock, G., and Chantler, C., 1986, The effect of a low protein diet on glucose metabolism in children with uremia, *J. Clin. Endocrinol. Metab.* **63:**985–989.

27. Barcelli, U. O., Miyata, J., Ito, Y., Gallon, L., Laskarszewski, P., Weiss, M., Hitzemann, P., and Pollak, V. E., 1986, Beneficial effects of polyunsaturated fatty acids in partially nephrectomized rats, *Prostaglandins* **32:**211–219.

28. Kleinbenecht, C., Laouari, D., Hinglais, N., Habib, R., Dodu, C., Lacour, B., and Broyer, M., 1986, Role of amount and nature of carbohydrates in the course of experimental renal failure, *Kidney Int.* **30:**687–693.

29. Thompson, B. J., Jenkins, D. A., Allan, P. L., Elton, R. A., and Winney, R. J., 1986, Acquired cystic disease of the kidney in patients with end-stage chronic renal failure: A study of prevalence and aetiology, *Nephrol. Dial. Transplant.* **1:**38–48.

30. Levine, E., Grantham, J. J., and MacDougall, M. L., 1987, Spontaneous subcapsular and perinephric hemorrhage in end-stage kidney disease: Clinical and CT findings, *Am. J. Radiol.* **148:** 755–758.

31. Numez, D., Yrizarry, J. M., Nadij, M., Beerman, R., and Morillo, G., 1986, Renal cell carcinoma complicating long-term dialysis: Computed tomography-guided aspiration cytology, *J. Comput. Tomogr.* **10:**51–53.

32. Bretan, P. N., Busch, M. P., Hricak, H., and Williams, R. D., 1986, Chronic renal failure: A significant risk factor in the development of acquired renal cysts and renal cell carcinoma. Case reports and review of the literature, *Cancer* **57:**1871–1879.

33. Hughson, M. D., Buchwald, D., and Fox, M., 1986, Renal neoplasia and acquired cystic kidney disease in patients receiving long-term dialysis, *Arch. Pathol. Lab. Med.* **110**:592–601.

34. Bergstrom, J., Alvestrand, A., Bucht, H., and Gutierrez, A., 1986, Progression of chronic renal failure in man is retarded with more frequent clinical follow-ups and better blood pressure control, *Clin. Nephrol.* **25**:1–6.

35. Aubia, J., Hojman, L., Chine, M., Lloveras, J., Masramon, J., Llorach, I., Cuevas, X., and Puig, J. M., 1987, Hypertension and nephrotoxicity in the rate of decline in kidney function in diabetic nephropathy, *Clin. Nephrol.* **27**:15–20.

36. Lindeman, R. D., Tobin, J. D., and Shock, N. W., 1987, Hypertension and the kidney, *Nephron* **47**(Suppl. 1):62–67.

37. Jackson, B., Whitty, M., Debrevi, L., and Cubela, R., 1987, Preservation of renal structure and function in the rat remnant kidney model of chronic renal failure by enalapril treatment, *Pathology* **19**:38–42.

38. Jackson, B., Debrevi, L., Cubela, R., Whitty, M., and Johnston, C. I., 1986, Preservation of kidney function in the rat remnant kidney model of chronic renal failure by blood pressure reduction, *Clin. Exp. Pharmacol. Physiol.* **13**:319–323.

39. Anderson, S., and Brenner, B. M., 1987, Therapeutic implications of converting-enzyme inhibitors in renal disease, *Am. J. Kidney Dis.* **10**(Suppl. 1):81–87.

40. Harris, D. C., Hammond, W. S., Burke, T. J., and Schrier, R. W., 1987, Verapamil protects against progression of experimental chronic renal failure, *Kidney Int.* **31**:41–46.

41. O'Donnell, M. P., Kasiske, B. L., Cleary, M. P., and Keane, W. F., 1985, Effects of genetic obesity on renal structure and function in the Zucker rat, *J. Lab. Clin. Med.* **106**:605–610.

42. Ichimaru, K., and Horie, A., 1987, Microangiopathic changes of subepidermal capillaries in end-stage renal failure, *Nephron* **46**:144–149.

43. Altmeyer, P., Kachel, H. G., Schafer, G., and Fossbinder, W., 1986, Normalization of uremic skin changes following kidney transplantation, *Hautarzt* **37**:217–221.

44. Bencini, P. L., Montagnino, G., Sala, F., DeVecchi, A., Crosti, C., and Tarantino, A., 1986, Cutaneous lesions in 67 cyclosporine-treated renal transplant recipients, *Dermatologica* **172**:24–30.

45. Yue, D. K., McLennan, S., Marsh, M., Mai, Y. W., Spaliviero, J., Delbridge, L., Reeve, T., and Turtle, J. R., 1987, Effects of experimental diabetes, uremia, and malnutrition on wound healing, *Diabetes* **36**:295–299.

46. Marumo, F., Nakamura, M., Sato, N., Shimada, H., Tsukamoto, S., and Iwanami, S., 1985, Deranged Ca, Al, and Mg content in the tissues of patients with chronic renal failure, as measured by non-destructive neutron activation analysis, *Int. J. Artif. Organs* **8**:319–324.

47. Cole, D. E., and Boucher, M. J., 1986, Increased sweat sulfate concentration in chronic renal failure, *Nephron* **44**:92–95.

48. Yuzuk, S., Trau, H., Stempler, D., Sofer, E., Levy, A., and Schewach-Millet, M., 1985, Reactive perforating collagenosis, *Int. J. Dermatol.* **24**:584–586.

49. Anderson, C. D., Rossi, E., and Garcia-Webb, P., 1987, Porphyrin studies in chronic renal failure patients on maintenance hemodialysis, *Photodermatology* **4**:14–22.

50. McColl, K. E., Simpson, K., Laiwah, A. Y., Thompson, G. G., McDougall, A., and Moore, M. R., 1986, Hemodialysis-related porphyria cutanea tarda—Treatment failure with charcoal hemoperfusion, *Photodermatology* **3**:169–173.

51. Lauret, P., Godin, M., and Bravard, P., 1985, Vegetating iodides after an intravenous pyelogram, *Dermatologica* **171**:468–469.

52. Larsen, M. J., Adcock, K. A., and Satterlee, W. G., 1985, Dermal uptake of technetium-99m MDP in calcinisis cutis, *Clin. Nucl. Med.* **10**:780–782.

53. Berretta, J. S., Holbrook, C. T., and Haller, J. S., 1986, Chronic renal failure presenting as proximal muscle weakness in a child, *J. Child. Neurol.* **1**:50–52.

54. Feinfeld, D. A., Briscoe, A. M., Nurse, H. M., Hotchkiss, J. L., and Thompson, G. E., 1986, Myoglobinuria in chronic renal failure, *Am. J. Kidney Dis.* **8**:111–114.

55. Muto, S., and Tabei, K., Asano, Y., and Hosoda, S., 1987, A case of rhabdomyolysis in chronic renal failure, *Jpn. J. Med.* **26:**76–80.

56. Li, J. B., and Wassner, S. J., 1986, Protein synthesis and degradation in skeletal muscle of chronically uremic rats, *Kidney Int.* **29:**1136–1143.

57. May, R. C., Clark, A. S., Goheer, M. A., and Mitch, W. E., 1985, Specific defects in insulin-mediated muscle metabolism in acute uremia, *Kidney Int.* **28:**490–497.

58. Davis, T. A., Klahr, S., and Karl, I. E., 1987, Glucose metabolism in muscle of sedentary and exercised rats with azotemia, *Am. J. Physiol.* **252:**F138–F145.

59. Davis, T. A., Klahr, S., and Karl, I. E., 1987, Insulin-stimulated protein metabolism in chronic azotemia and exercise, *Am. J. Physiol.* **253:**F164–F169.

60. Maroni, B. J., Karapanos, G., and Mitch, W. E., 1986, System A amino acid transport in incubated muscle: effects of insulin and acute uremia, *Am. J. Physiol.* **251:**F74–F80.

61. Maroni, B. J., Karapanos, G., and Mitch, W. E., 1986, System ASC and sodium independent neutral amino acid transport in muscle of uremic rats, *Am. J. Physiol.* **251:**F81–F86.

62. Krog, M., Ejerblad, S., and Agren, A., 1986, Enzyme activities and adenine nucleotide content in aorta, heart muscle and skeletal muscle from uremic rats, *Br. J. Exp. Pathol.* **67:**431–438.

63. Del Canale, S., Fiaccadori, E., Ronda, N., Soderlund, K., Antonucci, C., and Guariglia, A., 1986, Muscle energy metabolism in uremia, *Metabolism* **35:**981–983.

64. Del Canale, S., Fiaccadori, E., Coffrini, E., Vitali, P., Ronda, N., Antonucci, C., Arduini, U., and Guariglia, A., 1986, Uremic acidosis and intracellular buffering, *Scand. J. Urol. Nephrol.* **20:** 301–306.

65. Wassner, S. J., and Li, J. B., 1987, Lack of an acute effect of parathyroid hormone within skeletal muscle, *Int. J. Pediatr. Nephrol.* **8:**15–20.

66. May, R. C., Kelly, R. A., and Mitch, W. E., 1987, Mechanisms for defects in muscle protein metabolism in rats with chronic uremia. Influence of metabolic acidosis, *J. Clin. Invest.* **79:**1099–1103.

67. Painter, P., Messer-Rehak, D., Hanson, P., Zimmerman, S. W., and Glass, N. R., 1986, Exercise capacity in hemodialysis, CAPD, and renal transplant patients, *Nephron* **42:**47–51.

68. Warner, C., Forstner-Wanner, S., Schaeffer, G., Schollmeyer, P., and Horl, W. H., 1986, Serum free carnitine, carnitine esters and lipids in patients on peritoneal dialysis and hemodialysis, *Am. J. Nephrol.* **6:**206–211.

69. Rodriguez-Segada, S., Alonso de la Pena, C., Paz, J. M., Novoa, D., Arcocha, V., Romero, R., and Del Rio, R., 1986, Carnitine deficiency in haemodialysed patients, *Clin. Chim. Acta* **159:**249–256.

70. Rocchi, L., Feola, I., Calvani, M., D'Iddio, S., Alfarone, C., and Frascarelli, M., 1986, Effects of carnitine administration in patients with chronic renal failure undergoing periodic dialysis, evaluated by computerized electromyography, *Drugs Exp. Clin. Res.* **12:**707–711.

71. Fontanesi, G., Giancecchi, F., Tartaglia, I., Rotini, R., and Borgatti, P. P., 1986, Carpal tunnel syndrome. Comparative study between normal and dialyzed patients, *Ital. J. Orthop. Traumatol.* **12:**207–215.

72. Gorevic, P. D., Casey, T. T., Stone, W. J., DiRaimondo, C. R., Prelli, F. C., and Frangione, B., 1985, Beta-2 microglobulin is an amyloidogenic protein in man, *J. Clin. Invest.* **76:**2425–2429.

73. Gejyo, F., Odani, S., Yamada, T., Honma, N., Saito, H., Suzuki, Y., Nakagawa, Y., Kobayashi, H., Maruyama, Y., and Hirasawa, Y., 1986, Beta-2 microglobulin: A new form of amyloid protein associated with chronic hemodialysis, *Kidney Int.* **30:**385–390.

74. Blumberg, A., and Burgi, W., 1987, Behavior of beta 2-microglobulin in patients with chronic renal failure undergoing hemodialysis, hemodiafiltration, and continuous ambulatory peritoneal dialysis (CAPD), *Clin. Nephrol.* **27:**245–249.

75. Noel, L. H., Zingraff, J., Bardin, T., Atienza, C., Kuntz, D., and Drueke, T., 1087, Tissue distribution of dialysis amyloidosis, *Clin. Nephrol.* **27:**175–178.

76. Munoz-Gomez, J., Gomez-Perez, R., Llopart-Buisan, E., and Sole-Arques, M., 1987, Clinical

picture of the amyloid arthropathy in patients with chronic renal failure maintained on haemodialysis using cellulose membranes, *Ann. Rheum. Dis.* **46:**573–579.

77. Munoz-Gomez, J., Gomez-Perez, R., Sole-Arques, M., and Llopart-Buisan, E., 1987, Synovial fluid examination for the diagnosis of synovial amyloidosis in patients with chronic renal failure undergoing hemodialysis, *Ann. Rheum. Dis.* **46:**324–326.

78. Linke, R. P., Hampl, H., Bartel-Schwarze, S., and Eulitz, E., 1987, Beta-2 microglobulin, different fragments and polymers thereof in synovial amyloid in long term hemodialysis, *Biol. Chem. Hoppe Seyler* **368:**137–144.

79. Yano, E., Takeuchi, A., and Yoshioka, M., 1985, Hydroxyapatite associated arthritis in a patient undergoing chronic hemodialysis, *Int. J. Tissue React.* **7:**527–534.

80. Reginato, A. J., Ferreiro Seoane, J. L., Barbazan Alvarez, C., Mitja Piferrer, J., Vidal Meijon, L., Pascual Turon, R., Vasconez, F., Rivera, E. R., Clayburne, G., and Rothfuss, S., 1986, Arthropathy and cutaneous calcinosis in hemodialysis oxalosis, *Arthritis Rheum.* **29:**1376–1396.

81. Kaplan, P., Resnick, D., Murphey, M., Heck, L., Phalen, J., Egan, D., and Rutsky, E., 1987, Destructive noninfectious spondyloarthropathy in hemodialysis patients: A report of four cases, *Radiology* **162:**241–247.

82. Spencer, J. D., 1986, Bone and joint infections in a renal unit, *J. Bone Joint Surg.* **68:**489–493.

83. Benhamou, C. L., Rouchon, J. P., Geslin, N., Pierre, D., Viala, J. F., and Barthez, J. P., 1987, Arthropathies of the limbs in dialyzed renal failure patients, *Presse Med.* **16:**119–122.

84. Naidich, J. B., Karmel, M. I., Mossey, R. T., Bluestone, P. A., and Stein, H. L., 1987, Osteoarthropathy of the hand and wrist in patients undergoing longterm hemodialysis, *Radiology* **164:**205–209.

85. Chou, C. T., Wasserstein, A., Schumacher, H. R., and Fernandez, P., 1985, Musculoskeletal manifestations in hemodialysis patients, *J. Rheumatol.* **12:**1149–1153.

86. Schumacher, H. R., Reginato, A. J., and Pullman, S., 1987, Synovial fluid oxalate deposition complicating rheumatoid arthritis with amyloidosis and renal failure. Demonstration of intracellular oxalate crystals, *J. Rheumatol.* **14:**361–366.

87. Burgess, R. C., and Guise, E. R., 1985, Infrapatellar tendon ruptures, *Orthopedics* **8:**362–364.

88. Novoa, D., Romero, R., and Forteza, J., 1987, Spontaneous bilateral rupture of the quadriceps tendon in uremia and kidney transplantation, *Clin. Nephrol.* **27:**48 (Letter).

89. Shapera, M. R., Moel, D. I., Kamath, S. K., Olson, R., and Beauchamp, G. K., 1986, Taste perception of children with chronic renal failure, *J. Am. Diet. Assoc.* **86:**1359–1362.

90. Boyce, B. F., Prime, S. S., Halls, D., Johnston, E., Critchlow, H., MacDonald, D. G., and Junor, B. J., 1986, Does osteomalacia contribute to development of oral complications of oxalosis? *Oral Surg. Oral Med. Oral Pathol.* **61:**272–277.

91. Eigner, T. L., Jastak, J. T., and Bennett, W. M., 1986, Achieving oral health in patients with renal failure and renal transplants, *J. Am. Dent. Assoc.* **113:**612–616.

92. Chacati, A., and Godon, J. P., 1987, Effect of haemodialysis on upper gastrointestinal tract pathology in patients with chronic renal failure, *Nephrol. Dial. Transplant.* **1:**233–237.

93. Ala-Kaila, K., 1987, Upper gastrointestinal findings in chronic renal failure, *Scand. J. Gastroenterol.* **22:**372–376.

94. Snook, J. A., Holdstock, G. E., and Bamforth, J., 1986, Value of a simple biochemical ratio in distinguishing upper and lower sites of gastrointestinal hemorrhage, *Lancet* **1:**1064–1065.

95. Gupta, S., Walker, D. L., Keshavarzian, A., and Hodgson, H. J., 1987, Upper endoscopy for occult bleeding in renal failure, *J. Clin. Gastroenterol.* **9:**43–45.

96. Ala-Kaila, K., Pasternack, A., Kataja, M., Keyrilainen, O., and Sipponen, P., 1987, Sensitivity of gastric acid secretion in patients with chronic renal failure, *Scand. J. Gastroenterol.* **22:**1123–1129.

97. El Ghonaimy, E., Barsoum, R., Soliman, M., El Fikky, A., Rashwan, S., El Rouby, O., Haddad, S., El Khashab, O., Abou Zeid, M., and Hassaballah, N., 1985, Serum gastrin in chronic renal failure: Morphological and physiological correlations, *Nephron* **39:**86–94.

98. Levine, A. S., Morley, J. E., and Raij, L., 1986, Opiates and the anorexia of uremia, *Physiol. Behav.* **37:**835–838.

99. Goligorsky, M. S., Chaimovitz, Shany, S., Rapoport, J., Sharony, Y., and Haichenco, J., 1986, Verapamil improves defective duodenal calcium absorption in experimental chronic renal failure, *Mineral Electrolyte Metab.* **12:**363–370.

100. Diamond, S. M., Emmett, M., and Henrich, W. L., 1986, Bowel infarction as a cause of death in dialysis patients, *JAMA* **256:**2545–2547.

101. Gomella, L. G., Flanigan, R. C., Hagihara, P. F., Lucas, B. A., and McRoberts, J. W., 1986, The influence of uremia and immunosuppression on an animal model for ischemic colitis, *Dis. Colon Rectum* **29:**724–727.

102. Alexander, P., Schuman, E., and Vetto, R. M., 1986, Perforation of the colon in the immunocompromised patient, *Am. J. Surg.* **151:**557–561.

103. Lillemoe, K. D., Romolo, J. D., Hamilton, S. R., Pennington, L. R., Burdick, J. F., and Williams, G. M., 1987, Intestinal necrosis due to sodium polystyrene (Kayexalate) in sorbitol enemas: Clinical and experimental for the hypothesis, *Surgery* **101:**267–272.

104. Leung, A. C., Orange, G., McLay, A., and Henderson, I. S., 1985, *Clostridium difficile*—associated colitis in uremic patients, *Clin. Nephrol.* **24:**242–248.

105. Stone, W. J., and Alford, R. H., 1986, Perirectal and perineal infections in end-stage renal disease patients, *Uremia Invest.* **9:**53–62.

106. Panese, S., Martin, R. S., Virginillo, M., Litardo, M., Siga, E., Arrizurieta, E., and Hayslett, J. P., 1987, Mechanism of enhanced transcellular potassium secretion in man with chronic renal failure, *Kidney Int.* **31:**1377–1382.

107. Martin, R. S., Panese, S., Virginillo, M., Gimenez, M., Litardo, M., Arrizurieta, E., and Hayslett, J. P., 1986, Increased secretion of potassium in the rectum of humans with chronic renal failure, *Am. J. Kidney Dis.* **8:**105–110.

108. Sandle, G. I., Gaiger, E., Tapster, S., and Goodship, T. H., 1987, Evidence for large intestinal control of potassium homeostasis in uraemic patients undergoing long-term dialysis, *Clin. Sci.* **73:**247–252.

109. Sandle, G. I., Gaiger, E., Tapster, S., and Goodship, T. H., 1986, Enhanced rectal potassium secretion in chronic renal insufficient: Evidence for large intestinal potassium adaptation in man, *Clin. Sci.* **71:**393–401.

110. Parfrey, P. S., Farge, D., Forbes, R. D., Dandavino, R., Kenick, S., and Guttman, R. D., 1985, Chronic hepatitis in end-stage renal disease: Comparison of HBsAg-negative and HBsAg positive patients, *Kidney Int.* **28:**959–967.

111. Pao, C. C., Yang, W. L., Huang, C. C., Hsu, J. L., Lin, S. S., Ken, R., Chao, Y., Sun, C. F., Liaw, Y. F., and Lin, J. Y., 1987, Hepatitis type B virus DNA in patients receiving hemodialysis: Correlation with other HBV serological markers, *Nephron* **46:**155–160.

112. Imai, E., Yamauchi, A., Noguchi, T., Tanaka, T., Fujii, M., Mikami, H., Fukuhara, Y., Ando, A., Orita, Y., and Kamada, T., 1987, Effects of chronic renal failure on the regulation of pyruvate kinase, *Metabolism* **36:**601–606.

113. Caro, J. F., Sinha, M. K., and Dohm, G. L., 1987, Effect of chronic uremia on fructose 2,6-biphosphate glycolytic and gluceoneogenic enzymes in the rat liver, *Biochem. Biophys. Res. Commun.* **144:**352–358.

114. Klim, R. A., Albajar, M., Hems, R., and Williamson, D. H., 1986, Effects of chronic uremia on the formation of glucose and urea plus ammonia from L-alanine, L-glutamine and L-serine in isolated rat hepatocytes, *Clin. Sci.* **70:**627–634.

115. Scapa, E., Neuman, M., Weissgarten, S., Modai, D., and Eschar, J., 1986, Serum beta-*N*-acetyl hexosaminidase levels in chronic renal failure, *Enzyme* **36:**207–211.

116. Alpers, D. H., DeSchryver-Kecskemeti, K., Goodwin, C. L., Tindira, C. A., Harter, H., and Slatopolsky, E., 1988, Intestinal alkaline phosphatase in patients with chronic renal failure, *Gastroenterology* **94:**62–67.

117. Kaftori, J. K., Pery, M., Green, J., and Gaitini, D., 1987, Thickness of the gallbladder wall

inpatients with hypoalbuminemia: A sonographic study of patients on peritoneal dialysis, *Am. J. Radiol.* **148:**1117–1118.

118. Brill, D. R., 1985, Gallbladder visualization during technetium-99m-labelled red cell scintigraphy for gastrointestinal bleeding, *J. Nucl. Med.* **26:**1408–1411.
119. Kantor, A. F., Hoover, R. N., Kinlen, L. J., McMullan, M. R., and Fraumenti, J. F., 1987, Cancer in patients receiving long-term dialysis treatment, *Am. J. Epidemiol.* **126:**370–376.
120. Hobar, P. C., Turner, W. W., and Valentine, R. J., 1987, Successful use of the Denver peritoneovenous shunt in patients with nephrogenic ascites, *Surgery* **101:**161–164.
121. Vaziri, N. D., Dure-Smith, B., Miller, R., and Mirahmadi, M., 1987, Pancreatic pathology in chronic dialysis patients—An autopsy study of 78 cases, *Nephron* **46:**347–349.
122. Suda, K., and Ariwa, R., 1987, The islets of Langerhans in uremic patients receiving chronic hemodialysis, *Nephron* **46:**134–136.
123. Rutsky, E. A., Robards, M., Van Dyke, J. A., and Rostand, S. G., 1986, Acute pancreatitis in patients with end-stage renal disease without transplantation, *Arch. Intern. Med.* **146:**1741–1745.
124. Van Dyke, J. A., Rutsky, E. A., and Stanley, R. J., 1986, Acute pancreatitis associated with end-stage renal disease, *Radiology* **160:**403–405.
125. Caruana, R. J., Wolfman, N. T., Karstaedt, N., and Wilson, D. J., 1986, Pancreatitis: An important cause of abdominal symptoms in patients on peritoneal dialysis, *Am. J. Kidney Dis.* **7:** 135–140.
126. Royse, V. L., Jensen, D. M., and Corwin, H. L., 1987, Pancreatic enzymes in chronic renal failure, *Arch. Intern. Med.* **147:**537–539.
127. Kohen, J. A., Opsahl, J. A., and Kjellstrand, C. M., 1986, Deceptive patterns of uremic pulmonary edema, *Am. J. Kidney Dis.* **7:**456–460.
128. Peterson, B. T., Brooks, J. A., and Hyde, R. W., 1986, Lung fluid balance during acute renal failure in sheep, *J. Appl. Physiol.* **60:**1333–1340.
129. Belcher, N. G., and Rees, Pj, 1986, Changes in pulmonary clearance of technetium labelled DTPA during haemodialysis, *Thorax* **41:**381–385.
130. Rocker, G. M., Morgan, A. G., Pearson, D., Basran, G. S., and Shale, D. J., 1987, Pulmonary vascular permeability to transferrin in the pulmonary oedema of renal failure, *Thorax* **42:**620–623.
131. Drachman, R., Baillet, G., Gagnadoux, M. F., de Vernejoul, P., and Broyer, M., 1986, Pulmonary calcifications in children on dialysis, *Nephron* **44:**46–50.
132. Milliner, D. S., Lieberman, E., and Landing, B. H., 1986, Pulmonary calcinosis after renal transplantation in pediatric patients, *Am. J. Kidney Dis.* **7:**495–501.
133. Lecklitner, M. L., and Foster, R. W., 1985, Absence of gallium-67 avidity in diffuse pulmonary calcification, *Clin. Nucl. Med.* **10:**632–634.
134. Fein, A. M., Niederman, M. S., Ibriano, L., and Rosen, H., 1987, Reversal of sleep apnea in uremia by dialysis, *Arch. Intern. Med.* **147:**1355–1356.
135. Knudsen, F., and Thorgaard Andersen, P., 1985, Cellular hypoxia during hemodialysis. Demonstration of intradialytic release of purine and pyrimidine metabolites, *Blood Purif.* **3:**179–183.
136. Knudsen, F., Nielsen, A. H., Pedersen, J. O., and Jersild, C., 1985, On the kinetics of complement activation, leucopenia, and granulocyte-elastase release induced by hemodialysis, *Scand. J. Clin. Lab. Invest.* **45:**759–766.
137. Horl, W. H., Steinhauer, H. B., and Schollmeyer, P., 1985, Plasma levels of granulocyte elastase during hemodialysis: Effects of different dialyzer membranes, *Kidney Int.* **28:**791–796.
138. Schohn, D. C., Jahn, H. A., Eber, M., and Hauptmann, G., 1986, Biocompatibility and hemodynamic studies during polycarbonate versus cuprophane membrane dialysis, *Blood Purif.* **4:**102–111.
139. Danielson, B. G., Hallgren, R., and Venge, P., 1986, Patient reactions and granulocyte degranulation during hemodialysis with cuprophane and polycarbonate membranes. A double-blind study, *Blood Purif.* **4:**147–150.
140. Lewis, S. L., Van Epps, D. E., and Chenoweth, D. E., 1987, Leukocyte C5a receptor modulation during hemodialysis, *Kidney Int.* **31:**112–120.

141. Suzuki, Y., Uchida, J., Tsuji, H., Kuzuhara, K., Hara, S., Nihei, H., Ogura, Y., Otsubo, O., and Mimura, N., 1987, Acute changes in C3a and C5a in an anaphylactoid reaction in hemodialysis patients, *Tohoku J. Exp. Med.* **152**:35–45.

142. Maher, J. F., 1987, Uremic pleuritis, *Am. J. Kidney Dis.* **10**:19–22.

143. Abdel-Dayem, H. M., Nawaz, M. K., Suhaili, A. R., and Kouris, K., 1986, Uremic pleural effusion detected on radionuclide renogram *Clin. Nucl. Med.* **11**:196–197.

144. Willroth, P. O., and Tredt, H. J., 1986, Airway resistance in dialysis patients, *Z. Gesamte Inn. Med.* **41**:48–50.

145. Beasley, C. R., Ripley, J. M., Smith, D. A., and Neale, T. J., 1986, Pulmonary function in chronic renal failure patients managed by continuous ambulatory peritoneal dialysis, *NZ Med. J.* **99**:313–315.

146. Clyne, N., Lins, L. E., and Pehrsson, S. K., 1986, Occurrence and significance of heart disease in uraemia. An autopsy study, *Scand. J. Urol. Nephrol.* **20**:307–311.

147. London, G. M., Fabiani, F., Marchais, S. J., de Vernejoul, M. C., Guerin, A. P., Safar, M. E., Metivier, F., and Llach, F., 1987, Uremic cardiomyopathy: An inadequate left ventricular hypertrophy, *Kidney Int.* **31**:973–980.

148. Beasley, C. R., Smith, D. A., and Neale, T. J., 1986, Exercise capacity in chronic renal failure patients managed by continuous ambulatory peritoneal dialysis, *Aust NZ J. Med.* **16**:5–10.

149. Kettner-Melsheimer, A., Weiss, M., and Huber, W., 1987, Physical work capacity in chronic renal disease, *Int. J. Artif. Organs* **10**:3–8.

150. Mann, J. F., Jakobs, K. H., Riedel, J., and Ritz, E., 1986, Reduced chronotropic responsiveness of the heart in experimental uremia, *Am. J. Physiol.* **250**:H846–H852.

151. Meggs, L. G., Ben-Ari, J., Gammon, D., Choudhury, M., and Goodman, A. I., 1986, Effect of chronic uremia on the cardiovascular alpha 1 receptor, *Life Sci.* **39**:169–179.

152. Goldberg, A. P., Geltman, E. M., Gavin, J. R., Carney, R. M., Hagberg, J. M., Delmez, J. A., Naumovich, A., Oldfield, M. H., and Harter, H. R., 1986, Exercise training reduces coronary risk and effectively rehabilitates hemodialysis patients, *Nephron* **42**:311–316.

153. Painter, P. L., Nelson-Worel, J. N., Hill, M. M., Thornbery, D. R., Shelp, W. R., Harrington, W. R., and Weinstein, A. B., 1986, Effects of exercise training during hemodialysis, *Nephron* **43**: 87–92.

154. Alpert, M. A., Van Stone, J., Twardowski, Z. J., Ruder, M. A., Whiting, R. B., Kelly, D. L., and Madsen, B. R., 1986, Comparative cardiac effects of hemodialysis and continuous ambulatory peritoneal dialysis, *Clin. Cardiol.* **9**:52–60.

155. Henderson, L. W., 1986, Heterogeneity of the cardiovascular response to hemofiltration, *Kidney Int.* **29**:901–907.

156. Feldman, A. M., Fivush, B., Zahkor, K. G., Ouyang, P., and Baughman, K. L., 1988, Congestive cardiomyopathy in patients on continuous ambulatory peritoneal dialysis, *Am. J. Kidney Dis.* **11**:76–79.

157. Kong, C. H., Raval, U., and Thompson, F. D., 1986, Effect of 2 liters of intraperitoneal dialysate on the cardiovascular system, *Clin. Nephrol.* **26**:134–139.

158. el-Belbessi, S., Brautbar, N., Anderson, K., Campese, V. M., and Massry, S. G., 1986, Effect of chronic renal failure on heart. Role of secondary hyperparathyroidism, *Am. J. Nephrol.* **6**:369–375.

159. Lee, Y. S., 1986, Alterations of ultrastructure and anionic molecular organization in the basement membranes of chronic uremic myocardium, *Am. J. Nephrol.* **6**:435–442.

160. Zahavi, I., Chagnac, A., Djaldetti, M., Katz, M., and Levi, J., 1985, Effect of verapamil on uremic myocardial disease in the rat, *J. Submicrosc. Cytol.* **17**:637–644.

161. de Moraes, C. R., 1986, Calcification of the heart: A rare manifestation of chronic renal failure, *Pediatr. Radiol.* **16**:422–424.

162. Zazgornik, J., Balcke, P., Rokitansky, A., Schmidt, P., Kopsa, H., Minar, E., and Graninger, W., 1987, Excessive myocardial calcinosis in a chronic hemodialyzed patient, *Klin. Wochenschr.* **65**:97–100.

163. Rambausek, M., and Ritz, E., 1985, Digitalis in chronic renal insufficiency, *Blood Purif.* **3:**4–14.

164. Witherspoon, L., Schuler, S., Alyea, K., Figueroa, J., and Neely, H., 1986, Digoxin-like substance in term pregnancy, newborns, and renal failure, *J. Nucl. Med.* **27:**1418–1422.

165. Vasdev, S., Johnson, E., Longerich, L., Prabhakaran, V. M., and Gault, M. H., 1987, Plasma endogenous digitalis-like factors in healthy individuals and in dialysis-dependent and kidney transplant patients, *Clin. Nephrol.* **27:**169–174.

166. Gault, H., Vasdev, S., Vlasses, P., Longerich, L., and Dawe, M., 1986, Interpretation of serum digoxin values in renal failure, *Clin. Pharmacol. Ther.* **39:**530–536.

167. Castro, L., Hofling, B., Hassler, R., Hillebrand, G., Land, W., Kreuzer, E., Kemkes, B., Gurland, H. J., and Erdmann, E., 1985, Progression of coronary and valvular heart disease in patients on dialysis, *Trans. Am. Soc. Artif. Intern. Organs* **31:**647–650.

168. Medeiros, L. J., Schotte, D., and Gerson, B., 1987, Reliability and significance of increased creatine kinase MB isoenzyme in the serum of uremic patients, *Am. J. Clin. Pathol.* **87:**103–108.

169. Zamora, J. L., Burdine, J. T., Karlberg, H., Shenaq, S. M., and Noon, G. P., 1986, Cardiac surgery in patients with end-stage renal disease, *Ann. Thorac. Surg.* **42:**113–117.

170. Marshall, W. G., Rossi, N. P., Meng, R. L., and Wedige-Stecher, T., 1986, Coronary artery bypass grafting in dialysis patients, *Ann. Thorac. Surg.* **42**(6 Suppl.):S12–S15.

171. Philipson, J. P., Carpenter, B. J., Itzkoff, J., Hakala, T. R., Rosenthal, J. T., Taylor, R. J., and Puschett, J. B., 1986, Evaluation of cardiovascular risk for renal transplantation in diabetic patients, *Am. J. Med.* **81:**630–634.

172. Maher, E. R., Young, G., Smyth-Walsh, B., Pugh, S., and Curtis, J. R., 1987, Aortic and mitral valve calcification in patients with end-stage renal disease, *Lancet* **2:**875–877.

173. Maher, E. R., Pazianas, M., and Curtis, J. R., 1987, Calcific aortic stenosis: A complication of chronic uraemia, *Nephron* **47:**119–122.

174. Atlas, S. A., and Laragh, J. H., 1986, Atrial natriuretic peptide: a new factor in hormonal control of blood pressure and electrolyte homeostasis, *Annu. Rev. Med.* **37:**397–414.

175. Yamamoto, Y., Higa, T., Kitamura, K., Tanaka, K., Kanagawa, K., Matsuo, H., 1987, Plasma concentration of human atrial natriuretic polypeptide in patients with impaired renal function, *Clin. Nephrol.* **27:**84–86.

176. Hasegawa, K., Matsushita, Y., Inoue, T., Morii, H., Ishibashi, M., and Yamaji, T., 1986, Plasma levels of atrial natriuretic peptide in patients with chronic renal failure, *J. Clin. Endocrinol. Metab.* **63:**819–822.

177. Wilkins, M. R., Wood, J. A., Adu, D., Lote, C. J., Kendall, M. J., and Michael, J., 1986, Change in plasma immunoreactive atrial natriuretic peptide during sequential ultrafiltration and haemodialysis, *Clin. Sci.* **71:**157–160.

178. Espiner, E. A., Nicholls, M. G., Yandle, T. G., Crozier, I. G., Cuneo, R. C., McCormick, D., and Ikram, H., 1986, Studies on the secretion, metabolism and action of atrial natriuretic peptide in man, *J. Hypertens.* (Suppl.) **4:**S85–S91.

179. Larochelle, P., Beroniade, V., Gutkowska, J., Cusson, J. R., Lecrivain, A., du Soich, P., Cantin, M., and Genest, J., 1987, Influence of hemodialysis on the plasma levels of the atrial natriuretic factor in chronic renal failure, *Clin. Invest. Med.* **10:**350–354.

180. Zoccali, C., Ciccarelli, M., Mallamaci, F., Delpino, D., Salnitro, F., Parlongo, S., and Maggiore, Q., 1986, Effect of ultrafiltration on plasma concentrations of atrial natriuretic peptide in haemodialysis patients, *Nephrol. Dial. Transplant.* **1:**188–191.

181. Ogawa, K., Smith, A. I., Hodsman, G. P., Jackson, B., Woodcock, E. A., and Johnston, C. I., 1987, Plasma atrial natriuretic peptide: Concentrations and circulating forms in normal men and patients with chronic renal failure, *Clin. Exp. Pharmacol. Physiol.* **14:**95–102.

182. Forssman, K., Hock, D., Herbst, F., Schulz-Knappe, P., Talartschik, J., Scheler, F., and Forssman, W. G., 1986, Isolation and structural analysis of the circulating human cardiodilatin (alpha ANP), *Klin. Wochenschr.* **64:**1276–1280.

183. Winters, C. J., Sallman, A. L., Meadows, J., Rico, D. M., and Vesely, D. L., 1988, Two new

hormones: Prohormone atrila natriuretic peptides 1-30 and 31-67 circulate in man, *Biochem. Biophys. Res. Commun.* **150**:231–236.

184. Cole, B. R., Schwartz, D., Manning, P. T., Katsube, N. C., and Needleman, P., 1986, Atriopeptins: circulating volume regulatory hormones with potential therapeutic role in chronic renal failure, *J. Hypertens.* **4**(Suppl.):S13–S16.

185. Cole, B. R., Kuhnline, M. A., and Needleman, P., 1985, Atriopeptin III. A potent natriuretic, diuretic, and hypotensive agent in rats with chronic renal failure, *J. Clin. Invest.* **76**:2413–2415.

186. Eisenhauer, T., Talartschik, J., and Scheler, F., 1986, Detection of fluid overload by plasma concentration of human atrial natriuretic peptide (h-ANP) in patients with renal failure, *Klin. Wochenschr.* **64**(Suppl. 6):68–72.

187. Fyhrquist, F., Tikkanen, I., Totterman, K. J., Hynynen, M., Tikkanen, T., and Anderson, S., 1987, Plasma atrial natriuretic peptide in health and disease, *Eur. Heart J.* **8**(Suppl. B):117–122.

188. Tulassay, T., Rascher, W., Ganten, D., Scharer, K., and Lang, R. E., 1986, Atrial natriuretic paptide and volume changes in children, *Clin. Exp. Hypertens.* **8**:695–701.

189. Walker, R. G., Swainson, C. P., Yandle, T. G., Nicholls, M. G., and Espiner, E. A., 1986, Exaggerated responsiveness of immunoreactive atrial natriuretic peptide to saline infusion in chronic renal failure, *Clin. Sci.* **72**:19–24.

190. Luft, F. C., Sterzel, R. B., Lang, R. E., Trabold, E. M., Veelken, R., Ruskoaho, H., Gao, Y., Ganten, D., and Unger, T., 1986, Atrial natriuretic factor determinations and chronic sodium homeostasis, *Kidney Int.* **29**:1004–1010.

191. Rutsky, E. A., and Rostand, S. G., 1987, Treatment of uremic pericarditis and pericardial effusion, *Am. J. Kidney Dis.* **10**:2–8.

192. Jungbluth, H., Keusch, G., Russi, E., Porr, O., Baumann, P. C., and Binswanger, U., 1986, Management of cardiac tamponade in uremic pericarditis, *Schweiz. Med. Wochenschr.* **116**:49–54.

193. Daugirdas, J. T., Leehy, D. J., Popli, S., McCray, G. M., Gandhi, V. C., Pifarre, R., and Ing, T. S., 1986, Subxiphoid pericardiostomy for hemodialysis-associated pericardial effusion, *Arch. Intern. Med.* **146**:1113–1115.

194. Kristal, B., Shasha, S. M., Mahmoud, H., and Stamler, B., 1986, Management of uremic pericarditis, *Isr. J. Med. Sci.* **22**:442–444.

195. Krehlik, J. M., Hindson, D. A., Crowley, J. J., and Knight, L. L., 1985, Minoxidil-associated pericarditis and fatal cardiac tamponade, *West. J. Med.* **143**:527–529.

196. Joffe, P., and Johannessen, A. C., 1987, Uraemic pericarditis, an epidemic disease? *Dan. Med. Bull.* **34**:117–118.

197. Sniderman, A., Cianflone, K., Kwiterovich, P. O., Hutchinson, T., Barre, P., and Prichard, S., 1987, Hyperapobetalipoproteinemia: the major dyslipoproteinemia in patients with chronic renal failure treated with chronic ambulatory peritoneal dialysis, *Atherosclerosis* **65**:257–264.

198. Zacchello, G., Pagnan, A., Sidran, M. P., Ziron, L., Braggion, M., Pavanello, L., and Facchin, P., 1987, Further definition of the lipid–lipoprotein abnormalities in children with various degrees of chronic renal insufficiency, *Pediatr. Res.* **21**:462–465.

199. Mendez, A., Perez, G. O., Goldberg, R. B., and Hsia, S. L., 1987, Lipid and lipoprotein levels in undialyzed patients with chronic renal failure, *Am. J. Med. Sci.* **293**:164–170.

200. Roullet, J. B., Lacour, B., Yuert, J. P., and Drueke, T., 1986, Correction by insulin of disturbed TG-rich LP metabolism in rats with chronic renal failure, *Am. J. Physiol.* **250**:E373–E376.

201. Pagnan, A., Zanetti, G., Braggion, M., Ziron, L., Lusiani, L., Visona, A., Castellani, V., and Ronsisvalle, G., 1985, The double pre-beta very low density lipoprotein lipoproteinemia (DPBL): A new dyslipoproteinemic state, *Diabet. Metab.* **11**:343–349.

202. Lacour, B., Roullet, J. B., Ricordel, Y., and Drueke, T., 1987, Chronic triiodothyronine supplementation does not improve the lipoprotein disorders of mildly uremic rats, *Nephron* **45**:129–134.

203. Nishizawa, Y., Miki, T., Okui, Y., Matsushita, Y., Inoue, T., and Morii, H., 1986, Deranged metabolism of lipids in patients with chronic renal failure: Possible role of secondary hyperparathyroidism, *Jpn. J. Med.* **25**:40–45.

204. Rubies-Prat, J., Espinel, E., Joven, J., Ras, M. R., and Pira, L., 1987, High-density lipoprotein cholesterol subfractions in chronic uremia, *Am. J. Kidney Dis.* **9**:60–65.
205. Laszlo, A., Nemeth, M., Joo, I., Kiss, E., Havass, Z., and Szenohradszki, P., 1986, Changes of serum lipids and lipoproteins during haemodialysis treatment in dialysed chronic uraemic patients, *Int. Urol. Nephrol.* **18**:463–470.
206. Dieplinger, H., Schoenfeld, P. Y., and Fielding, C. J., 1986, Plasma cholesterol metabolism in end-stage renal disease. Difference between treatment by hemodialysis or peritoneal dialysis, *J. Clin. Invest.* **77**:1071–1083.
207. Yamamoto, T., and Yamakawa,, M., 1987, Effect of acetate administration on rats with chronic uremia, *Artif. Organs* **11**:208–213.
208. Pasternack, A., Vanttinen, T., Solakivi, C., Kuusi, T., and Korte, T., 1987, Normalization of lipoprotein lipase and hepatic lipase by gemfibrozil results in correction of lipoprotein abnormalities in chronic renal failure, *Clin. Nephrol.* **27**:163–168.
209. Grutzmacher, P., Scheuermann, E. H., Siede, W., Lang, P. D., Abshagen, U., Radtke, H. W., Baldamus, C. A., and Schoeppe, W., 1986, Lipid lowering treatment with benzafibrate in patients on chronic haemodialysis: Pharmacokinetics and effects, *Klin. Wochenschr.* **64**:910–916.
210. Boer, P., Koomans, H. A., and Dorhout Mees, E. J., 1987, Renin and blood volume in chronic renal failure: A comparison with essential hypertension, *Nephron* **45**:7–15.
211. Schohn, D., Weidmann, P., Jahn, H., and Beretta-Piccoli, C., 1985, Norepinephrine-related mechanism in hypertension accompanying renal failure, *Kidney Int.* **28**:814–822.
212. Sorensen, S. S., Danielsen, H., Jespersen, B., and Pedersen, E. B., 1986, Hypotension in end-stage renal disease: Effect of postural change, exercise and angiotensin II infusion on blood pressure and plasma concentrations of angiotensin II, aldosterone and arginine vasopressin in hypotensive patients with chronic renal failure treated by dialysis, *Clin. Nephrol.* **26**:288–296.
213. Cuche, J. L., Jondeau, G., Ruget, G., Selz, F., Piga, J. C., and Harboun, C., 1986, Effects of an intravenous infusion of noradrenaline on plasma concentration of free and sulfoconjugated catecholamines in anesthetized dogs, *Pharmacology* **32**:90–100.
214. Watson, A. J., Stout, R. L., and Whelton, A., 1987, Parathyroidectomy increases peripheral vascular responsiveness to exogenous noradrenaline in the uraemic rat, *Nephrol. Dial. Transplant* **2**:83–85.
215. Iseki, K., Massry, S. G., and Campese, V. M., 1986, Effects of hypercalcemia and parathyroid hormone on blood pressure in normal and renal failure rats, *Am. J. Physiol.* **250**:F924–F929.
216. Degli Esposti, E., Sturani, A., Santoro, A., Zuccala, A., Chiarini, C., and Zucchelli, P., 1985, Effect of bromocriptine treatment on prolactin, noradrenaline and blood pressure in hypertensive haemodialysis patients, *Clin. Sci.* **69**:51–56.
217. Meema, H. E., and Oreopoulos, D. G., 1986, Morphology, progression, and regression of arterial and periarterial calcifications in patients with end-stage renal disease, *Radiology* **158**:671–677.
218. Sherman, R. A., Bialy, G. B., Gazinski, B., Bernholc, A. S., and Eisinger, R. P., 1986, The effect of dialysate calcium levels on blood pressure during hemodialysis, *Am. J. Kidney Dis.* **8**:244–247.
219. Tvedegaard E., 1987, Arterial disease in chronic renal failure—An experimental study in the rabbit, *Acta Pathol. Microbiol. Immunol. Scand.* **290**(Suppl.):1–28.
220. Aalkjaer, C., Pedersen, E. B., Danielsen, H., Fjeldborg, O., Jespersen, B., Kjaer, T., Sorensen, S. S., and Mulvany, M. J., 1986, Morphological and functional characteristics of isolated resistance vessels in advanced uraemia, *Clin. Sci.* **71**:657–663.
221. Devynck, M. A., Pernollet, M. G., and Meyer, P., 1987, Endogenous digitalis-like factors in essential and experimental hypertension, *Int. J. Radiol. Appl. Instrum.* **14**:341–352.
222. Kariya, K., Sano, H., Yamanishi, J., Saito, K., Furuta, Y., and Fukuzaki, H., 1986, A circulating Na$^+$-K$^+$ATPase inhibitor, erythrocyte sodium transport and hypertension in patients with chronic renal failure, *Clin. Exp. Hypertens.* **8**:167–183.
223. Deray, G., Pernollet, M. G., Devynck, M. A., Zingraff, J., Touam, A., Rosenfeld, J., and

Meyer, P., 1986, Plasma digitalislike activity in essential hypertension or end-stage renal disease, *Hypertension* **8**:632–638.

224. Kelly, R. A., O'Hara, D. S., Canessa, M. L., Mitch, W. E., and Smith, T. W., 1985, Characterization of digitalis-like factors in human plasma. Interaction with NaK-ATPase and cross-reactivity with cardiac glycoside specific antibodies, *J. Biol. Chem.* **260**:11396–11405.

225. McNally, P. G., Brown, C. B., Moorhead, P. J., and Raftery, A. T., 1987, Unmasking of subclavian vein obstruction following arteriovenous fistulae for haemodialysis. A problem following subclavian line dialysis? *Nephrol. Dial. Transplant.* **1**:258–260.

226. Currier, C. B., Widder, S., Ali, A., Kuusisto, E., and Sidawy, A., 1986, Surgical management of subclavian and axillary vein thrombosis in patients with a functioning arteriovenous fistula, *Surgery* **100**:25–28.

227. Vaziri, N. D., and Lester, K., 1979, Use of microanalytic laboratory methods to reduce blood loss in dialysis patients, *J. Dial.* **3**:367–374.

228. Pavlovic-Kentera, V., Clemons, G. K., Djukanovic, L., and Biljanovic-Paunovic, L., 1987, Erythropoietin and anemia in chronic renal failure, *Exp. Hematol.* **15**:785–789.

229. Urabe, A., Saito, T., Fukamachi, H., Kubota, M., and Takaku, F., 1987, Serum erythropoietin titers in the anemia of chronic renal failure and other hematological states, *Int. J. Cell Cloning* **5**: 202–208.

230. Walle, A. J., Wong, G. Y., Clemons, G. K., Garcia, J. F., and Niedermayer, W., 1987, Erythropoietin–hematocrit feedback circuit in the anemia of end-stage remal disease, *Kidney Int.* **31**:1205–1209.

231. Casati, S., Passerini, P., Campise, M. R., Graziani, G., Cesana, B., Perisic, M., and Ponticelli, C., 1987, Benefits and risks of protracted treatment with human recombinant erythropoietin in patients having haemodialysis, *Br. Med. J.* **295**:1017–1020.

232. Raine, A. E., 1988, Hypertension, blood viscosity, and cardiovascular morbidity in renal failure: Implications of erythropoietin therapy, *Lancet* **1**:97–100.

233. Eschbach, J. W., Egrie, J. C., Downing, M. R., Browne, J. K., and Adamson, J. W., 1987, Correction of the anemia of end-stage renal disease with recombinant human erythropoietin. Results of a combined phase I and II clinical trial, *N. Engl. J. Med.* **316**:73–78.

234. Winearls, C. G., Oliver, D. O., Pippard, M. J., Reid, C., Downing, M. R., and Cotes, P. M., 1986, Effect of human erythropoietin derived from recombinany DNA on the anemia of patients maintained by chronic haemodialysis, *Lancet* **2**:1175–1178.

235. Rejman, A. S., Grimes, A. J., Cotes, P. M., Mansell, M. A., and Joekes, A. M., 1985, Correction of anaemia following renal transplantation: Serial changes in serum immunoreactive erythropoietin, absolute reticulocyte count, and red cell creatine levels, *Br. J. Haematol.* **61**:421–431.

236. Muto, S., Asano, Y., Hosoda, S., Shionoya, S., Miura, Y., Urabe, A., and Takaku, F., 1987, Polycythemia of end-stage renal failure: No inhibition of erythropoiesis by uremic serum and markedly increased serum erythropoietin level, *Nephron* **46**:34–36.

237. Naets, J. P., Garcia, J. F., Tousaaint, C., Buset, M., and Waks, D., 1986, Radioimmunoassay of erythropoietin in chronic uraemia or anephric patients, *Scand. J. Haematol.* **37**:390–394.

238. Coles, G. A., and Cavill, I., 1986, Erythropoiesis in the anemia of chronic renal failure: The response to CAPD, *Nephrol. Dial. Transplant.* **1**:170–174.

239. Lamperi, S., and Carozzi, S., 1987, Monocyte–macrophage mediated suppression of erythropoiesis in renal anaemia, *Nephrol. Dial. Transplant.* **2**:86–92.

240. Fukushima, Y., Fukuda, M., Yoshida, K., Yamaguchi, A., Nakamtot, Y., Miura, A. B., Harada, T., and Tsuchida, S., 1986, Serum erythropoietin levels and inhibitors of erythropoiesis in patients with chronic renal failure. *Tohuku J. Exp. Med.* **150**:1–15.

241. Pierratos, A., Toor, P., Ayiomamitis, A., Oreoupoulos, D., and Keating, A., 1986, Immunoreactive parathyroid hormone and *in vitro* inhibition of erythropoiesis by uremic serum in patients on continuous ambulatory peritoneal dialysis, *Am. J. Nephrol.* **6**:465–468.

242. Hirakata, H., Onoyama, K., Horik, K., and Fujishima, M., 1986, Participation on the renin–angiotensin system in the captopril-induced worsening of anemia in chronic hemodialysis patients, *Clin. Nephrol.* **26:**27–32.

243. Shannon, J. S., and Lapin, T. R., 1986, Theanaemia of chronic renal failure: A potentially treatable catabolic phenomenon? *Med. Hypotheses* **20:**29–36.

244. Shannon, J. S., Lappin, T. R., Elder, G. E., Roberts, G. M., McGeown, M. G., and Bridges, J. M., 1985, Increased plasma glycosidase and protease activity in uremia: possible role in the aetiology of the anaemia of chronic renal failure, *Clin. Chim. Acta* **153:**203–207.

245. Saito, A., Suzuki, I., Chung, T. G., Okamoto, T., and Hotta, T., 1986, Separation of an inhibitor of erythropoiesis in "middle molecules" form hemodialysis patients with chronic renal failure, *Clin. Chem.* **32:**1938–1941.

246. Delwiche, F., Segal, G. M., Eschbach, J. W., and Adamson, J. W., 1986, Mematopoietic inhibitors in chronic renal failure: Lack of in vitro specificity, *Kidney Int.* **29:**641–648.

247. Ruocco, L., Baldi, A., Cecconi, N., Marini, A., Azzara, A., Ambrogi, F., and Grassi, B., 1986, Severe pancytopenia due to copper deficiency, *Acta Haematol.* **76:**224–226.

248. Yalouris, A. G., Lyberatos, C., Chalevalakis, G., Theodosiadou, E., Billis, A., and Raptis, S., 1986, Some parameters of haem synthesis in dialyzed and non-dialyzed uraemic patients, *Scand. J. Haematol.* **37:**404–410.

249. Swartz, R., Dombrouski, J., Burnatowska-Hledin, M., and Mayor, G., 1987, Microcytic anemia in dialysis patients: Reversible marker of aluminum toxicity, *Am. J. Kidney Dis.* **9:**217–223.

250. van der Voet, G. B., and deWolff, F. A., 1985, Distribution of aluminum between plasma and erythrocytes, *Hum. Toxicol.* **4:**643–648.

251. Quereda, C., Tervel, J. L., Lamas, S., Marcen, R., Matesanz, R., and Ortuno, J., 1987, HLA antigens and serum ferritin in hemodialysis patients, *Nephron* **45:**104–110.

252. Solomon, L. R., and Hendler, E. D., 1987, Androgen therapy in haemodialysis patients. II. Effects on red cell metabolism, *Br. J. Haematol.* **65:**223–230.

253. Malachi, T., Bigin, E., Gafter, U., and Levi, J., 1986, Parathyroid hormone effect on the fragility of human young and old red blood cells in uremia, *Nephron* **42:**52–57

254. Levi, J., Malachi, T., Djaldetti, M., and Bogin, E., 1987, Biochemical changes associated with the osmotic fragility of young and mature erythrocytes caused by parathyroid hormone in relation to the uremic state, *Clin. Biochem.* **20:**121–125.

255. Bogin, E., Earon, Y., and Blum, M., 1986, Effect of parathyroid hormone and uremia on erythrocyte deformability, *Clin. Chim. Acta* **161:**293–299.

256. Thomas, T. H., Mason, C., and Illingworth, K. M., 1986, Changing effects on erythrocyte sodium and potassium during the development of chronic renal failure with anaemia in rats, *Clin. Sci.* **71:**639–646.

257. Jablonska-Skwiecinska, E., Staniszewska, K., and Kowalska, H., 1987, The red cell sodium, potassium, inorganic phosphate, ATP and 2,3 DPG concentrations in chronic renal failure, *Folia Haematol.* **114:**493–495.

258. Barton, I. K., Mansell, M. A., and Grimes, A. J., 1987, Red-cell calcium in patients with renal failure, *Nephron* **47:**123–124.

259. Born, N. A., Aronson, J. K., Hallis, K. F., and Grahame-Smith, D. G., 1986, Cation transport abnormalities *in vivo* in untreated essential hypertension, *Clin. Sci.* **70:**611–616.

260. Corry, D. B., Tuck, M. L., Brickman, A. S., Yanagawa, N., and Lee, D. B., 1986, Sodium transport in red blood cells from dialyzed uremic patients, *Kidney Int.* **29:**1197–1202.

261. DeSanto, N. G., Trevisan, M., DeColle, S., DiMuro, M., DeChiara, F., Latte, M., Franzese, A., Iacono, R., Capasso, G., and Capodicasa, G., 1987, Intraerythrocytic cation metabolism in children with uremia undergoing hemodialysis, *J. Lab. Clin. Med.* **110:**231–236.

262. Trevisan, M., DeSanto, N., Laurenzi, M., DiMuro, M., DeChiara, F., Latte, M., Franzese, A., Aicone, R., Capodicasa, G., and Giordano, C., 1986, Intracellular ion metabolism in erythrocytes and uraemia: The effects of different dialysis treatments, *Clin. Sci.* **71:**545–552.

263. Monti, J. P., Gallice, P., Baas, M., Murisasco, A., and Crevat, A., 1987, Modifications of intra-erythrocytic homeostasis in uremic patients, as studied with 31P nuclear magnetic resonance, *Clin. Chem.* **33:**76–80.

264. Rejman, A. S., Mansell, M. A., Grimes, A. J., and Joekes, A. M., 1985, Rapid correction of red-cell nucleotide abnormalities following successful renal transplantation, *Br. J. Haematol.* **61:**433–443.

265. Gafter, U., Bessler, H., Malachi, T., Zevin, D., Djaldetti, M., and Levi, J., 1987, Platelet count and thrombopoietic activity in patients with chronic renal failure, *Nephron* **45:**207–210.

266. Holloway, D. S., Vagher, J. P., Caprini, J. A., Simon, N. M., and Mockros, L. F., 1987, Thromboelastography of blood from subjects with chronic renal failure, *Thromb. Res.* **45:**817–825.

267. Castillo, R., Lozano, T., Escolar, G., Revert, L., Lopez, J., and Ordinas, A., 1986, Defective platelet adhesion on vessel subendothelium in uremic patients, *Blood* **68:**337–342.

268. DeMinno, G., Cerbone, A., Usberti, M., Cianciaruso, B., Cortese, A., Forace, M. J., Martinez, J., and Murphy, S., 1986, Platelet dysfunction in uremia. II. Correction by arachidonic acid of the impaired exposure of fibrinogen receptors by adenosine diphosphate or collagen, *J. Lab. Clin. Med.* **108:**246–252.

269. Bloom, A., Greaves, M., Preston, F. E., and Brown, C. B., 1986, Evidence against a platelet cyclooxygenase defect in uraemic subjects on chronic haemodialysis, *Br. J. Haematol.* **62:**143–149.

270. Camici, M., Evangelista, L., and Raspolli-Galletti, M., 1986, The effect of oxalic acid on the aggregability of human platelet rich plasma, *Prostaglandins Leukotrienes Med.* **21:**107–110.

271. Winklemann, M., Dorr, U., Pfitzer, P., and Schneider, W., 1986, Is lower ploidy of magakaryocytes another reason for uremic thrombocytopathy? *Klin. Wochenschr.* **64:**540–544.

272. Docci, D., Turci, F., Delvecchio, C., Gollini, C., Baldrati, L., and Pistocchi, E., 1986, Lack of evidence for the role of secondary hyperparathyroidism in the pathogenesis of uremic thrombocytopathy, *Nephron* **43:**28–32.

273. Sloand, E. M., Bern, M. M., and Kaldany, A., 1986, Effect on platelet function of hypo-albuminemia in peritoneal dialysis, *Thromb. Res.* **44:**419–425.

274. Juhl, A. and Jorgensen, F., 1987, DDAVP and life threatening diffuse gastric bleeding in uraemia, *Acta Chir. Scand.* **153:**75–77.

275. Mannucci, P. M., 1986, Desmopressin (DDAVP) for treatment of disorders of hemostasis, *Prog. Hemost. Thromb.* **8:**19–45.

276. Brown, O. E., 1986, Use of desmopressin in children with coagulation disorders, *Int. J. Pediatr. Otorhinolaryngol.* **11:**301–305.

277. Livio, M., Mannucci, P. M., Vigano, G., Mingardi, G., Lombardi, R., Mecca, G., and Remuzzi, G., 1986, Conjugated estrogens for the management of bleeding associated with renal failure, *N. Engl. J. Med.* **315:**731–735.

278. Lewis, S. L., and VanEpps, D. E., 1987, Neutrophil and monocyte alterations in chronic dialysis patients, *Am. J. Kidney Dis.* **9:**381–395.

279. Eckardt, K. U., Eckardt, H., Harber, M. J., and Asscher, A. W., 1986, Analysis of poly-morphonuclear respiratory burst activity in uremic patients using whole-blood chemiluminescence, *Nephron* **43:**274–278.

280. Rhee, M. S., McGoldrick, M. D., and Meuwissen, H. J., 1986, Serum factor from patients with chronic renal failure enhances polymorphonuclear leukocyte oxidative metabolism, *Nephron* **42:**6–13.

281. Schunck, H., Schutt, M., and Langen, P., 1987, The colony-to-cluster ratio in agar cultures of bone marrow. I. Constancy under standardized conditions and alterations in tumour-bearing mice and by various inhibitors added *in vitro, Biomed. Biochim. Acta* **46:**581–586.

282. Metcoff, J., 1986, Malnutrition at the cellular level in uremia: A new frontier for research, *J. Am. Coll. Nutr.* **5:**229–241.

283. Athlin, L., and Domellof, L., 1986, The phagocytic process of human peritoneal macrophages in cancer or uremia, *Acta Pathol. Microbiol. Immunol. Scand.* **94**:63–68.

284. Pedersen, J. O., Knudsen, F., Nielsen, A. H., and Grunnet, N., 1987, The ability of uremic serum to induce neutrophil chemotaxis in relation to hemodialysis, *Blood Purif.* **5**:24–28.

285. Baker, G. L., Oddis, C. V., and Medsger, T. A., 1987, *Pasteurella multocida* polyarticular septic arthritis, *J. Rheumatol.* **14**:355–357.

286. Tapson, J. S., Mansy, H., Freeman, R., and Wilkinson, R., 1986, The high morbidity of CAPD fungal peritonitis—Description of 10 cases and review of treatment strategies, *Q. J. Med.* **61**: 1047–1053.

287. Soubrane, C., Jacobs, C., Jacquillat, C., Dubois, M., Poupon, M. F., Judde, J. G., Maral, J., Beaufils, H., and Jaudon, M. C., 1986, Influence of the uremic state on the development of malignancy. An experimental study in the rat, *Am. J. Nephrol.* **6**:363–368.

288. Neale, T. J., Muir, J. C., Mills, H., Horne, J. G., and Jones, M. R., 1987, Candida albicans vertebral osteomyelitis in chronic renal failure, *Postgrad. Med. J.* **63**:695–698.

289. Eisenberg, E. S., Leviton, I., and Soeiro, R., 1986, Fungal peritonitis in patients receiving peritoneal dialysis: Experience with 11 patients and review of the literature, *Rev. Infect. Dis.* **8**: 309–321.

290. LaRocca, M. T., Mortensen, J. E., and Robinson, A., 1986, Mycobacterium fortuitum peritonitis in a patient undergoing chronic peritoneal dialysis, *Diagn. Microbiol. Infect. Dis.* **4**:161–164.

291. Gluhovschi, G., Golea, O., Schiller, A., Arcan, P., Dragen, I., Nasem, A. K., and Barbu, N., 1987, Urinary infections in patients with chronic renal failure on hemodialysis, *Med. Interne* **25**: 195–203.

292. Shohat, B., Boner, G., Waller, A., and Rosenfeld, J. B., 1986, Cell-mediated immunity in uremic patients prior to and after 6 months' treatment with continuous ambulatory peritoneal dialysis, *Isr. J. Med. Sci.* **22**:551–555.

293. Raskova, J., Czerwinski, D. K., Shea, S. M., and Raska, K., 1986, Cellular immunity and lymphocyte populations in developing uremia in the rat, *J. Exp. Pathol.* **2**:229–245.

294. Raskova, J., Ghobrial, I., Shea, S. M., Ebert, E. C., Eisinger, R. P., and Raska, K., 1986, T cells in patients undergoing chronic hemodialysis: mitogenic response, suppressor activity, and interleukin-2 production and generation, *Diagn. Immunol.* **4**:209–216.

295. Kurz, P., Kohler, H., Meuer, S., Hutteroth, T., and Meyer zum Buschenfelde, K. H., 1986, Impaired cellular immune responses in chronic renal failure: Evidence for a T-cell defect, *Kidney Int.* **29**:1209–1214.

296. Raskova, J., Ghobrial, I., Czerwinski, D. K., Shea, S. M., Eisinger, R. P., and Raska, K., 1987, B-cell activation and immunoregulation in end-stage renal disease patients receiving hemodialysis, *Arch. Intern. Med.* **147**:89–93.

297. Tsakolos, N. D., Theoharides, T. C., Hendler, E. D., Goffinet, J., Dwyer, J. M., Whisler, R. L., and Askenase, P. W., 1986, Immune defects in chronic renal impairment: Evidence for defective regulation of lymphocyte response by macrophages from patients with chronic renal impairment on hemodialysis, *Clin. Exp. Immunol.* **63**:218–227.

298. Port, F. K., VanDeKerkhove, K. M., Kunkel, S. L., and Kluger, M. J., 1987, The role of dialysate in the stimulation of interleukin-1 production during clinical hemodialysis, *Am. J. Kidney Dis.* **10**:118–122.

299. Schaefer, K., von Herrath, D., Hufler, M., and Pauls, A. 1986, The occurence of fever during hemodialysis and hemofiltration. A comparative study, *Int. J. Artif. Organs* **9**:247–250.

300. Lonneman, G., Bingel, M., Koch, K. M., Shaldon, S., and Dinarello, C. A., 1987, Plasma interleukin-1 activity in humans undergoing hemodialysis with regenerated cellulosic membranes, *Lymphokine Res.* **6**:63–70.

301. Lamperi, S., and Carozzi, S., 1986, Suppressor resident peritoneal macrophages and peritonitis incidence in continuous ambulatory peritoneal dialysis, *Nephron* **44**:219–225.

302. Langhoff, E., Hofmann, B., Odum, N., Ladefoged, J., Platz, P., Ryder, L. P., and Svejgaard, A.,

1987, Kinetic analysis of interleukin-2 (IL-2) production and expression of IL-2 receptors by uraemic and normal lymphocytes, *Scand. J. Immunol.* **25:**29–36.

303. Yousefi, S., Vaziri, N. D., Carandang, G., and Cesario, T., 1987, Evaluation of the in vitro production of interferon gamma and other lymphokines in uremic patients, *Proc. Soc. Exp. Biol. Med.* **184:**179–185.

304. Langhoff, E., Ladefoged, J., and Odum, N., 1986, Effect of interleukin-2 and methylprednisolone on *in vitro* transformation of uremic lymphocytes, *Int. Arch. Allergy Appl. Immunol.* **81:**5–11.

305. Modai, D., Weissgarten, J., Cohen, N., Averbukh, Z., Golik, A., Peller, S., Tieder, M., Shaked, U., and Kaufman, S., 1986, The effects of uremic serum and 3'–5' cyclic AMP on blastogenesis of normal lymphocytes, *Thymus* **8:**307–311.

306. Weissgarten, J., Modai, D., Cohen, N., Averbukh, Z., Shaked, U., Tieder, M., Peller, S., and Kaufman, S., 1986, Induction of suppressor cells in normal lymphocytes by uremic serum, *Int. Arch. Allergy Appl. Immunol.* **81:**180–183.

307. Niese, D., Gilsdorf, K., Hiester, E., Dressen, P., Michels, S., and Dengler, H. J., 1986, Immunomodulating properties of the uremic pentapeptide H-asp-leu-trp-glu-lys-OH *in vitro, Klin. Wochenschr.* **64:**642–647.

308. Forwell, M., Gray, K. G., MacSween, R. N., Peel, M. G., Madhok, R., Forbes, C. D., Harvey, J. A., Roberts, J., Ferrell, L., and Sandilands, G. P., 1986, Immunosuppression following alloantigen exposure: A role for lymphocyte Fc gamma-receptor blocking antibodies, *J. Clin. Lab. Immunol.* **19:**53–57.

309. Taccone-Gallucci, M., Giardini, O., Ausiello, C., Piazza, A., Spagnoli, G. C., Bandino, D., Lubrano, R., Taggi, F., Evangelista, B., and Monoco, P., 1986, Vitamin E supplementation in hemodialysis patients: Effects on peripheral blood mononuclear cells lipid peroxidation and immune response, *Clin. Nephrol.* **25:**81–86.

310. Nanishi, F., Inenaga, T., Onoyama, K., Oh, Y., Oochi, N., and Fujishima, M., 1986, Immune alterations in hemodialyzed patients. I. Effect of blood transfusion on T-lymphocyte subpopulations in hemodialyzed patients, *J. Clin. Lab. Immunol.* **19:**167–174.

311. Schot, J. D., and Schuurman, R. K., 1986, Blood transfusion suppresses cutaneous cell mediated immunity, *Clin. Exp. Immunol.* **65:**336–344.

312. Young, G. A., Young, J. B., Young, S. M., Hobson, S. M., Hildreth, B., Brownjohn, A. M., and Parsons, F. M., 1986, Nutrition and delayed hypersensitivity during continuous ambulatory peritoneal dialysis in relation to peritonitis, *Nephron* **43:**177–186.

313. Chida, Y., Sakurai, S., and Yoshiyama, N., 1986, The effect of hemodialysis on lymphocyte subsets during dialysis, *Clin. Nephrol.* **25:**159–164.

314. Alobaidi, H. M., Coles, G. A., Davies, M., and Lloyd, D., 1986, Host defence in continuous ambulatory peritoneal dialysis: The effect of the dialysate on phagocytic function, *Nephrol. Dial. Transplant.* **1:**16–21.

315. Gallimore, B., Gagnon, R. F., and Stevenson, M. M., 1986, Cytotoxicity of commercial peritoneal dialysis solutions towards peritoneal cells of chronically uremic mice, *Nephron* **43:**283–289.

316. Gagnon, R. F., and Lu, D. S., 1985, Mechanism of depressed immunity in chronic renal failure: Effect of cyclophosphamide pretreatment on delayed-type hypersensitivity skin reaction, *J. Clin. Lab. Immunol.* **18:**135–140.

317. Barthon, J., Graves, J., Jens, P., Hamrick, R., and Mayes, M., 1987, The erythrocyte sedimentation rate in end-stage renal failure, *Am. J. Kidney Dis.* **10:**34–40.

318. Demaine, A. G., Taube, D. H., Vaughan, R. W., Kerr, L. A., and Welsh, K. I., 1986, Immunoglobulin heavy chain switch region restriction fragment length polymorphisms are associated with renal disease, *Clin. Exp. Immunol.* **66:**406–413.

319. Nisbeth, U., Hallgren, R., Eriksson, O., and Danielson, B. G., 1987, Endotoxemia in chronic renal failure, *Nephron* **45:**93–97.

320. Munelli Bertazzoni, E., and Panzetta, G., 1986, Antibacterial interaction of cefuroxime and serum from uraemic patients, *J. Antimicrob. Chemother.* **18:**365–373.

321. Sorensen, P. J., Nielsen, A. H., Knudsen, F., and Dyerberg, J., 1987, Defective protein C in uraemia, *Blood Purif.* **5**:29–32.

322. Abdulmassih, Z., Duverlie, G., Morinieree, P., Atik, A., Hannoun, C., Henrotte, J. G., Daniel, P., and Fournier, A., 1987, Response to influenza vaccine in uremic patients: Relation to erythrocyte magnesium and the value of a second injection, *Nephrologie* **8**:23–26.

323. Seaworth, B., Drucker, J., Starling, J., Drucker, R., Stevens, C., and Hamilton, J., 1988, Hepatitis B vaccines in patients with chronic renal failure before dialysis, *J. Infect. Dis.* **157**:332–337.

324. Nikoskelainen, J., Koskela, M., Forsstrom, J., Kasenen, A., and Leinonen, M., 1985, Persistence of antibodies to pneumococcal vaccine in patients with chronic renal failure, *Kidney Int.* **28**:672–677.

325. Broyer, M., and Boudailliez, B., 1985, Varicalla vaccine in children with chronic renal insufficiency, *Postgrad. Med. J.* **61**(Suppl. 4):103–106.

326. Rao, T. K., Friedman, E. A., and Nicastri, A. D., 1987, The types of renal disease in the acquired immunodeficiency syndrome, *N. Engl. J. Med.* **316**:1062–1068.

327. Schaefer, K., Asmus, G., Hufler, M., and von Herrath, D., 1986, HTLV-III antibodies in hemodialysis patients—A consequence of blood transfusions? *Klin. Wochenschr.* **64**:621–622.

328. Goldman, M., Liesnard, C., Vanherweghem, J. L., Dolle, N., Toussaint, C., Sprecher, S., Cogniaux, J., and Thiry, L., 1986, Markers of HTLV-III in patients with end stage renal failure treated by haemodialysis, *Br. Med. J.* **293**:161–162.

329. Cusmano, F., and Savazzi, G. M., 1986, Cerebral computed tomography in uremic and hemodialyzed patients, *J. Comput. Assist. Tomogr.* **10**:567–570.

330. Basile, C., Miller, J. D., Koles, Z. J., Grace, M., and Ulan, R. A., 1987, The effects of dialysis on brain water and EEG in stable chronic uremia, *Am. J. Kidney Dis.* **9**:462–469.

331. Onoyama, K., Kumagai, H., Miishima, T., Tsuruda, H., Tomooka, S., Motomura, K., and Fujishima, M., 1986, Incidence of strokes and its prognosis in patients on maintenance hemodialysis, *Jpn. Heart J.* **27**:685–691.

332. Sayre, M. R., Roberge, R. J., and Evans, T. C., 1987, Nontraumatic subdural hematoma in a patient with osteogenesis imperfecta and renal failure, *Am. J. Emerg. Med.* **5**:298–301.

333. Balzar, E., Saletu, B., Khoss, A., and Wagner, U., 1986, Quantitative EEG: Investigation in children with end stage renal disease before and after hemodialysis, *Clin. Electroencephalogr.* **17**:195–202.

334. Brocard, O., Andre, J. L., and Pierson, M., 1986, Electroencephalographic changes in children dialyzed according to various protocols, *Nephrologie* **7**:181–184.

335. Gambaro, P., Bottacchi, E., Camerlingo, M., D'Allesandro, G., Nebiolo, P. E., Aloatti, S., Marchesan, R., and Mamoli, A., 1987, Central and peripheral involvement in hemodialyzed subjects: Neuro-physiological and nephrological relationships, *Ital. J. Neurol. Sci.* **8**:31–34.

336. Pratt, H., Brodsky, G., Goldsher, M., Ben-david, Y., Harari, R., Podoshin, L., Eliachar, I., Grushka, E., Better, O., and Garty, J., 1986, Auditory brain-stem evoked potentials in patients undergoing hemodialysis, *Electroencephalogr. Clin. Neurophysiol.* **63**:18–24.

337. Urquiza, R., and Morell, M., 1985, The endocochlear potential in experimental renal insufficiency, *Rev. Esp. Fisiol.* **41**:407–410.

338. Brown, J. J., Sufit, R. L., and Sollinger, H. W., 1987, Visual evoked potential changes following renal transplantation, *Electroencephalogr. Clin. Neurophysiol.* **66**:101–107.

339. Knox, D. L., Hanneken, A. M., Hollows, F. C., Miller, N. R., Schick, H. L., and Gonzalez, W. L., 1988, Uremic optic neuropathy, *Arch. Ophthalmol.* **106**:50–54.

340. Anteunis, L. J., and Mooy, J. M., 1987, Hearing loss in a uremic patient: Indicators of involvement of the VIIIth nerve, *J. Laryngol. Otol.* **101**:492–496.

341. Zoccali, C., Ciccarelli, M., Mallamaci, F., Maggiore, Q., Lotti, M., and Zucchelli, G. C., 1987, Plasma met-enkephalin and leu-enkephalin in chronic renal failure, *Nephrol. Dial. Transplant.* **1**:219–222.

342. Sturani, A., Degli Esposti, E., Chiarini, C., Spongano, M., Santoro, A., Zucchelli, P., 1985, Failure of naloxone in reversal hemodialysis-induced hypotension, *Blood Purif.* **3:**184–186.

343. Smith, R., Grossman, A., Gimson, A. E., Besser, G. M., and Rees, L. H., 1985, Effect of liver and renal dysfunction on circulating methionine–enkephalin immunoreactivity, *Neurosci. Lett.* **60:** 301–305.

344. Biasioli, S., D'Andrea, G., Feriani, M., Chiaramonte, S., Fabris, A., Ronco, C., and La Greca, G., 1986, Uremic encephalopathy: An updating, *Clin. Nephrol.* **25:**57–63.

345. Verkman, A. S., and Fraser, C. L., 1986, Water and nonelectrolyte permeability in brain synaptosomes isolated from normal and uremic rabbits, *Am. J. Physiol.* **250:**R306–R312.

346. Adler, A. J., and Berlyne, G. M., 1985, Uptake and distribution of ^{45}Ca in the brain of chronically uremic rats, *Nephron* **41:**354–358.

347. Gorchein, A., and Webber, R., 1987, Delta-aminolevulinic acid in plasma, cerebrospinal fluid, saliva, and erythrocytes: Studies in normal, uraemic, and porphyric subjects, *Clin. Sci.* **72:**103–112.

348. Sprague, S. M., Corwin, H. L., Wilson, R. S., Mayor, G. H., and Tanner, C. M., 1986, Encephalopathy in chronic renal failure responsive to deferoxamine therapy. Another manifestation of aluminum neurotoxicity, *Arch. Intern. Med.* **146:**2063–2064.

349. Sirota, R. A., Kimmel, P. L., Trichtinger, M. D., Diamond, B. F., Stein, H. D., and Yudis, M., 1986, Metaclopropamide-induced parkinsonism in hemodialysis patients. Report of two cases, *Arch. Intern. Med.* **146:**2070–2071.

350. Orko, R., Pitkanen, M., and Rosenberg, P. H., 1986, Subarachnoid anesthesia with 0.75% bupivicaine in patients with chronic renal failure, *Br. J. Anaesth.* **58:**605–609.

351. Fierro, B., Modica, A., D'Arpa, A., Santangelo, R., and Raimondo, D., 1987, Analysis of F-wave in metabolic neuropathies: A comparative in uremic and diabetic patients, *Acta Neurol. Scand.* **75:**179–185.

352. Fierro, B., Modica, A., D'Arpa, A., Santangelo, R., and Raimondo, D., 1986, F-wave study in patients with chronic renal failure on regular haemodialysis, *J. Neurol. Sci.* **74:**271–277.

353. Thomas, P. K., 1978, Screening for peripheral neuropathy in patients treated by chronic hemodialysis, *Muscle Nerve* **1:**396–399.

354. Vogel, P., 1986, Significance of sensory evoked potentials in the diagnosis of polyneuropathy, *Fortschr. Neurol. Psychiatr.* **54:**305–317.

355. Tegner, R., and Lindholm, B., 1985, Uremic polyneuropathy: Different effects of hemodialysis and continuous ambulatory peritoneal dialysis, *Acta Med. Scand.* **218:**409–416.

356. Violante, F., Lorenzi, S., and Fusello, M., 1985, Uremic neuropathy: Clinical and neurophysiological investigation of dialysis patients using different chemical membranes, *Eur. Neurol.* **24:**398–404.

357. Sandyk, R., Bernick, C., Lee, S. M., Stern, L. Z., Iacono, R. P., and Bamford, C. R., 1987, L-Dopa in uremic patients with the restless leg syndrome, *Int. J. Neurosci.* **35:** 233–235.

358. Kuncl, R. W., Duncan, G., Watson, D., Alderson, K., Rogawski, M. A., and Peper, M., 1987, Colchicine myopathy and neuropathy, *N. Engl. J. Med.* **316:**1562–1568.

359. Malik, S., Winney, R. J., and Ewing, D. J., 1986, Chronic renal failure and cardiovascular autonomic function, *Nephron* **43:**191–195.

360. Axelrod, S., Lishner, M., Oz, O., Bernheim, J., and Ravid, M., 1987, Spectral analysis of fluctuations in heart rate: An objective evaluation of autonomic vervous control in chronic renal failure, *Nephron* **45:**202–206.

361. Zaccali, C., Ciccarelli, M., Mallamaci, F., and Maggiore, Q., 1986, Parasympathetic function in haemodialysis patients, *Nephron* **44:** 351–354.

362. Mallamaci, F., Zoccali, C., Ciccarelli, M., and Briggs, J. D., 1986, Autonomic function in uremic patients treated by hemodialysis or CAPD and in transplant patients, *Clin. Nephrol.* **25:**175–180.

363. Solders, G., Persson, A., and Wilczek, H., 1986, Autonomic system dysfunction and polyneuropathy in nondiabetic uremia. A one-year follow-up study after renal transplantation, *Transplantation* **41:**616–619.

364. Romain, Y., Demassieux, S., D'Angelo, G., Gyger, M., and Carriere, S., 1986, Is the platelet phenolsulfotransferase involved in the sulfoconjugation of plasma catecholamines? *Can. J. Physiol. Pharmacol.* **64:**1197–1201.

365. Cuche, J. L., Prinseau, J., Selz, F., Ruget, G., and Baglin, A., 1986, Plasma free, sulfo- and glucuro-conjugated catecholamines in uremic patients, *Kidney Int.* **30:**566–572.

366. Shah, S. D., Clutter, W. E., and Cryer, P. E., 1985, External and internal standards in the single-isotope derivative (radioenzymatic) measurement of plasma norepinephrine and epinephrine, *J. Lab. Clin. Med.* **106:**624–629.

367. Bree, F., Souchet, T., Baatard, R., Fontenaille, C., Lhoste, F., and Tillement, J. P., 1987, Inhibition of (−) [125I]-iodocyanopindolol binding to rat lung beta adrenoreceptors by uremic plasma ultrafiltrates, *Biochem. Pharmacol.* **36:**3121–3125.

368. Souchet, T., Bree, F., Baatard, R., Fontenaille, C., D'Athis, P., Tillement, J. P., Kiechel, J. R., and Lhoste, F., 1986, Impaired regulation of betaa 2-adrenoreceptor density in mononuclear cells during chronic renal failure, *Biochem. Pharmacol.* **35:**2513–2519.

369. Stemmer, C. L., Perez, G. O., and Oster, J. R., 1987, Impairment of beta 2-adrenoreceptor-stimulated potassium uptake in end-stage renal disease, *J. Clin. Pharmacol.* **27:** 628–631.

370. Vita, G., Savica, V., Calabro, R., Padovano, I., Manna, L., Toscano, A., Rotondo, S., and Bellinghieri, G., 1986, Uremic vagal neuropathy: Has parathyroid hormone a pathogenetic role? *Funct. Neurol.* **1:**253–259.

371. Kameko, S., Sato, T., Hirayama, N., Eba, H., Takahashi, N., Suzuki, T., and Funyu, T., 1986, Psychiatric complications of chronic hemodialysis—Importance of psychological and social care, *Jpn. J. Psychiatry Neurol.* **40:**559–570.

372. Rodin, G., and Voshart, K., 1987, Depressive symptoms and functional impairment in the medically ill, *Gen. Hosp. Psychiatry* **9:**251–258.

373. Hong, B. A., Smith, M. D., Robson, A. M., and Wetzel, R. D., 1987, Depressive symptomatology and treatment in patients with end stage renal disease, *Psychol. Med.* **17:**185–190.

374. Glass, C. A., Fielding, D. M., Evans, C., and Ashcroft, J. B., 1987, Factors related to sexual functioning in male patients undergoing hemodialysisand with kidney transplants, *Arch. Sex Behav.* **16:**189–207.

375. Locsey, L., Balogh, L., and Toth, E., 1987, Psychological effects of chronic haemodialysis, *Int. Urol. Nephrol.* **19:**91–100.

376. el-Mallakh, R. S., Schrader, S. A., and Widger, E., 1987, Mania as a presentation of end-stage renal disease, *J. Nerv. Ment. Dis.* **175:**243–245.

377. Devins, G. M., Binik, Y. M., Mandin, H., Burgess, E. D., Taub, K., Letourneau, P. K., Buckle, S., and Low, G. L., 1986–87, Denial as a defense against depression in end-stage renal disease: An empirical test, *Int. J. Psychiatr. Med.* **16:**151–162.

378. Siegal, B. R., Calsyn, R. J., and Cuddihee, R. M., 1987, The relationship of social support to psychological adjustment in end-stage renal disease patients, *J. Chronic Dis.* **40:**337–344.

379. Reiss, D., Gonzalez, S., and Kramer, N., 1986, Family process, chronic illness, and death. On the weakness of strong bonds, *Arch. Gen. Psychiatry.* **43:**795–804.

380. Friend, R., Singletary, Y., Mendell, N. R., and Nurse, H., 1986, Group participation and survival among patients with end-stage renal disease, *Am. J. Public Health* **76:**670–672.

381. Jackson, M., Warrington, E. K., Roe, C. J., and Baker, L. R., 1987, Cognitive function in hemodialysis patients, *Clin. Nephrol.* **27:**26–30.

382. LePontois, J., Moel, D. I., and Cohn, R. A., 1987, Family adjustment to pediatric ambulatory dialysis, *Am. J. Orthopsychiatry* **57:**78–83.

383. Fielding, D., Moore, B., Dewey, M., Ashley, P., McKendrick, T., and Pinkerton, P., 1985, Children with end-stage renal failure: Psychological effects on patients, siblings and parents, *J. Psychosom. Res.* **29:**457–465.

384. Eknoyan, G., 1987, The uremic syndrome. *Contemp. Nephrol.* **4:**513–584.

385. Emmanouel, D. S., Lindheimer, M. D., and Katz, A. I., 1985, Endocrine function, in: *The*

Systemic Consequences of Renal Failure (G. Eknoyan and J. P., Knochel, eds.), Grune & Stratton, Orlando, FL, pp. 177–232.

386. Grzeszczak, W., Kokot, F., and Dulawa, J., 1987, Effects of naloxone administration on endocrine abnormalities in chronic renal failure, *Am. J. Nephrol.* **7:**93–100.

387. Zoccali, C., Ciccarelli, M., Mallamaci, F., Maffiore, Q., Lotti, M., and Zuccheli, G. C., 1987, Plasma met-enkaphalin and leu-enkephalin in chronic renal failure, *Nephrol. Dial. Transpl.* **1:** 219–222.

388. Elias, A. N., Vaziri, N. D., and Maksy, M., 1986, Plasma beta-endorphin and beta-lipotropin in patients with end-stage renal disease. Effects of hemodialysis, *Nephron* **43:**173–176.

389. Pfeiffer, A., and Herz, A., 1984, Endocrine actions of opionids, *Horm. Metab. Res.* **16:**386–397.

390. Bostwick, D. G., Null, W. E., Holmes, D., Weber, E., Barchas, J. D., and Bensch, K. G., 1987, Expression of opioid peptides in tumors, *N. Engl. J. Med.* **317:**1439–1443.

391. Yen, S. S. C., Quigley, M. E., Reid, R. L., Ropert, J. F., and Cotel, N. S., 1985, Neuroendocrinology of opioid peptides and their role in the control of gonadotropin and prolactin secretion, *Am. J. Obstet. Gynecol.* **152:**485–493.

392. Bonomini, V., Campieri, C., Feletti, C., Orsoni, G., and Cangelista A., 1985, Hormonal abnormalities in renal transplantation, *Contrib. Nephrol.* **48:**56–69, 1985.

393. May, R. C., Clark, A. S., Goheer, M. A., and Mitch, W. E., 1985, Specific defects in insulin mediated muscle metabolism in acute uremia, *Kidney Int.* **28:**490–497.

394. Milutinovic, S., Brayer, D., Molnar, V., Stefovic, A., Jankovic, N., Skrabalo, Z., and Rocic, B., 1985, Changes in insulin binding during hemodialysis in uremic patients, *Nephron* **41:**307–313.

395. Tuck, M. L., Davidson, M. B., Asp, N., and Schultze, R. G., 1986, Augmented aldosterone and insulin responses to potassium infusion in dogs with renal failure, *Kidney Int.* **30:**883–890.

396. Hagopian, W. A., and Tager, H. S., 1987, Hepatic glucagon metabolism. Correlation of hormone processing by isolated canine hepatocytes with glucagon metabolism in man and in the dog, *J. Clin. Invest.* **79:**409–417.

397. DeSanto, N. G., Fine, R. N., Carella, C., Leumann, E., Amato, G., Fine, S., Nuzzi, F., Capasso, G., Capodicasa, G., and Lama, G., 1985, Thyroid function in uremic children, *Kidney Int.* **17** (Suppl.):S166–S169.

398. Hardy, M. J., Ragbeer, S. S., and Nascimento, L., 1988, Pituitary–thyroid function in chronic renal failure assessed by a highly sensitive thyrotropin assay, *J. Clin. Endocrinol. Metab.* **66:**233–236.

399. Kohei, S., Inoue, T., and Iino, S., 1986, Serum free thyroid hormones and response of TSH to TRH on nonthyroidal illnesses, *Nippon Naibunpi Gakkai Zasshi* **20:**1231–1243.

400. Liewendahl, K., Tikanoja, S., Mahonen, H., Helenius, T., Valimaki, M., and Tallgren, L. G., 1987, Concentrations of iodothyroinines in serum of patients with chronic renal failure and other nonthyroidal illnesses: Role of free fatty acids, *Clin. Chem.* **33:**1382–1386.

401. Kaptein, E. M., Kaptein, J. S., Chang, E. I., Egodage, P. M., Nicoloff, J. T., and Massry, 1987, Thyroxine transfer and distribution in critical nonthyroidal illnesses, chronic renal failure, and chronic ethanol abuse, *J. Clin. Endocrinol. Metab.* **65:**606–616.

402. Keane, P. M., Walker, W. H., Thornton, G., and Rodbard, D., 1986, Studies of thyroxine binding to plasma proteins in health and disease, *Clin. Biochem.* **19:**52–57.

403. Bregengard, C., Kirkegaard, C., Faber, J., Poulsen, S., Siersbaek-Nielsen, K., and Friis, T., 1987, The influence of free fatty acids on the free fraction of thyroid hormones in the serum as estimated by ultrafiltration, *Acta Endocrinol. (Copenh.)* **116:**102–107.

404. Hegedus, L., Feldt-Rasmussen, U., Andersen, J. R., Poulsen, L. R., and Hansen, J. M., 1987, Serum thyroglobulin in chronic renal failure—Effects of haemodialysis, *Scand. J. Clin. Lab. Invest.* **47:**35–40, 1987.

405. Lacour, B., Roullet, J. B., Ricordel, Y., and Drueke, T., 1987, Chronic triiodothyronine supplementation does not improve the lipoprotein disorders of mildly uremic rats, *Nephron* **45:**129–134.

406. Lim, V. S., Flanigan, M. J., Zavala, D. C., and Freeman, R. M., 1987, Blunted peripheral tissue responsiveness to thyroid hormone in uremic patients, *Kidney Int.* **31:**808–814.

407. Malgor, L. A., Barrios, L., de Albarenque, M. E., Berges, E., de Markowsky, E. E., Montiel, E., and Mussin, S. M., 1986, Erythropoietic effects of renal failure in rats: Comparative studies with testosterone and erythropoietin, *Exp. Hematol.* **14**:250–256.

408. Lim, V. S., Flanigan, M. J., Zavala, D. C., and Freeman, R. M., 1985, Protective adaptation of low serum triiodothyronine in patients with chronic renal failure, *Kidney Int.* **28**:541–549.

409. Verger, M. F., Verger, C., Hatt-Magnien, D., and Perrone, F., 1987, Relationship between thyroid hormones and nutrition in chronic renal failure, *Nephron* **45**:211–215.

410. Rao, M. D., Bay, W. H., George, J. M., and Herbert, L. A., 1986, Primary hypothyroidism in chronic renal failure, *Clin. Nephrol.* **25**:11–14.

411. Ridgway, E. C., Weintraub, B. D., and Maloof, F., 1976, Metabolic clearance and production rates of human thyrotropin, *J. Clin. Invest.* **43**:338–346.

412. Elias, A. N., Vaziri, N. D., Pandian, M. R., Iyer, K., and Ansari, M. A., 1987, Dopamine and TSH secretion in uremic male rats, *Horm. Res.* **27**:102–108.

413. De Marchi, S., Cecchin, E., Villalta, D., and Tesio, F., 1987, Serum reverse T_3 assay for predicting glucose intolerance in uremic patients on dialysis therapy, *Clin. Nephrol.* **27**:189–198.

414. Nazian, S. J., and Dietz, J. R., 1987, Reproductive changes during the early stages of chronic renal insufficiency in the male rat, *Biol. Reprod.* **37**:105–111.

415. Tsitouras, P. D., Kowatch, M. A., Briefel, G. R., Kalbfleisch, J. H., Harman, S. M., and Blackman, M. R., 1985, *In vivo* pretreatment with human chorionic gonadotropin fails to reverse the dysfunction of isolated Leydig cells from chronically uremic rats, *Biol. Reprod.* **33**:781–789.

416. Rodger, R. S., Morrison, L., Dewar, J. H., Wilkinson, R., Ward, M. K., and Kerr, D. N., 1985, Loss of pulsatile luteinizing hormone secretion in men with chronic renal failure, *Br. Med. J. (Clin. Res.)* **291**:1598–1600.

417. Mendoza, C., Carreras, A., Ruiz, E., Ortega, E., Hervas, J., and Osorio, C., 1985, Hypothalamo-hypophyseo-gonadal axis in individuals with chronic renal insufficiency subjected to hemodialysis, *Rev. Esp. Fisiol.* **41**:443–446.

418. van Coevorden, A., Stolear, J. C., Dhaene, M., van Jerweghem, J. L., and Mockel, J., 1986, Effect of chronic oral testosterone undecanoate administration on the pituitary–testicular axes of hemodialyzed male patients, *Clin. Nephrol.* **26**:48–54.

419. Ramirez, G., Butcher, D., Brueggemeyer, C. D., and Ganguly, A., 1987, Testicular defect: the primary abnormality in gonadal dysfunction of uremia, *South. Med. J.* **80**:798–801.

420. Barsotti, G., Ciardella, F., Morelli, E., Fioretti, P., Melis, G., Paoletti, A., Niosi, F., Caprioli, R., Fosso, A., and Carbone, C., 1985, Restoration of blood levels of testosterone in male uremics following a low protein diet supplemented with essential amino acids and ketoanalogues, *Contrib. Nephrol.* **49**:63–69.

421. Fioretti, P., Melis, G. B., Ciardella, F., Barsotti, G., Orlandi, M. C., Paoletti, A. M., and Giovannetti, S., 1986, Parathyroid function and pituitary–gonadal axis in male uremics: effects of dietary treatment and of maintenance hemodialysis, *Clin. Nephrol.* **25**:155–158.

422. Elias, A. N., Vaziri, N. D., and Maksy, M., 1985, Plasma norepinephrine, epinephrine, and dopamine levels in end-stage renal disease, *Arch. Intern. Med.* **145**:1013–1015.

423. Ermolenko, V. M., Kukhtevich, A. V., Dedov, I. I., Bunatian, A. F., Melnichenko, G. A., and Gitel, E. P., 1986, Parlodel treatment of uremic hypogonadism in men, *Nephron* **42**:19–22.

424. Kukhtevich, A. V., Ermolenko, V. M., Dedov, I. I., Melnichenko, G. A., and Gitel, E. P., 1985, Treatment of uremic hypogonadism with parlodel, *Ter. Arkh.* **57**:39–41.

425. Torres-Noriega, J., and Frohman, L. A., 1986, Hyperprolactinemia associated with chronic renal failure in the rat, *Horm. Metab. Res.* **18**:241–243.

426. Rodriguez-Puyol, D., Martin-Oar, J. E., Cachofiero, M. V., del Pino, D., Lopez-Novoa, J. M., and Hernando, L., 1986, Molecular heterogeneity of circulating prolactin in chronic uremic men and renal transplant recipients, *J. Clin. Endocrinol. Metab.* **62**:352–356.

427. Pun, K. K., Varghese, Z., and Moorhead, J. F., 1987, Reduction of serum prolactin after salmon calcitonin infusion in patients with impaired renal function, *Acta Endocrinol. (Copenh.)* **115**:243–246.

428. Greenspan, S. L., Neer, R. M., Ridgway, E. C., and Klibanski, A., 1986, osteoporosis in men with hyperprolactinemic hypogonadism, *Ann. Intern. Med.* **104**:777–782.

429. Rodger, R. S., Dewar, J. H., Turner, S. J., Watson, M. J., and Ward, M. K., 1986, Anterior pituitary dysfunction in patients with chronic renal failure treated by hemodialysis or continuous ambulatory peritoneal dialysis, *Nephron* **43**:169–172.

430. Workman, R. J., Vaughn, W. K., and Stone, W. J., 1986, Dexamethasone suppression testing in chronic renal failure: Pharmacokinetics of dexamethasone and demonstration of a normal hypothalamic–pituitary–adrenal axis, *J. Clin. Endocrinol. Metab.* **63**:741–746.

431. Egfjord, W., Langhoff, E., Daugaard, H., and Olgaard, K., 1987, Increased clearance rate of prednisone in the isolated perfused liver of uremic rats, *Nephron* **45**:53–58.

432. Prinseau, J., Ruget, G., Selz, F., Baglin, A., Fritel, D., and Cuche, J. L., 1986, Plasma catecholamines, free and conjugated in the hemodialyzed chronic renal failure patient, *Arch. Mal. Coeur* **79**:835–839.

433. Zanella, M. T., Mattei, E., Jr., Draibe, S. A., Kater, C. E., and Ajzen, H., 1985, Inadequate aldosterone response to hyperkalemia during angiotensin converting enzyme inhibition in chronic renal failure, *Clin. Pharmacol. Ther.* **38**:613–617.

434. Hene, R. J., Koomans, H. A., Boer, P., Dorhout Mees, E. J., 1987, Effect of high-dose aldosterone infusions on renal electrolytr excretion in patients with renal insufficiency, *Am. J. Nephrol.* **7**:33–37.

435. Krishna, G. G., Chusid, P., and Hoeldtke, R. D., 1987, Effect of dopaminergic blockade on plasma aldosterone in acquired hypoaldosteronism, *Nephron* **47**:184–189.

436. Lifshits, N. L., Ermolenko, V. M., Tatsievskii, V. A., and Klepikov, P. V., 1985, Inactive renin in patients with chronic and terminal renal insufficiency, *Ter. Arkh.* **57**:106–109.

437. Yamamoto, T., Shimizu, M., Morioka, M., Kitano, M., Wakabayashi, H., and Aizawa, N., 1986, Role of angiotensin II in the pathogenesis of hyperdipsia in chronic renal failure, *JAMA* **256**:604–608.

438. Shoelson, S. E., Polonsky, K. S., Nakabayashi, T., Jaspan, J. B., and Tager, H. S., 1986, Circulating forms of somatostatinlike immunoreactivity in human plasma, *Am. J. Physiol.* **250**:E428–E434.

439. Powell, D. R., Rosenfeld, R. G., Sperry, J. B., Baker, B. K., and Hintz, R. L., 1987, Serum concentrations of insulin-like growth factor (IGF)-1, IGF-2, and unsaturated somatomedin carrier proteins in children with chronic renal failure, *Am. J. Kidney Dis.* **10**:287–292.

440. Powell, D. R., Rosenfeld, R. G., Baker, B. K., Liu, F., and Hintz, R. L., 1986, Serum somatomedin levels in adults with chronic renal failure: the importance of measuring insulin-like growth factor I (IGF-I) and IGF-II in acid-chromatographed uremic serum, *J. Clin. Endocrinol. Metab.* **63**:1186–1192.

441. Bessarione, D., Perfumo, F., Giusti, M., Ginevri, F., Mazzocchi, G., Gusmano, R., and Giordano, G., 1987, Growth hormone response to growth hormone-releasing hormone in normal and uraemic children. Comparison with hypoglycaemia following insulin administration, *Acta Endocrinol. (Copenh.)* **114**:5–11.

442. Rochiccioli, P., Pienkowski, C., Bouissou, F., Sablayrolles, B., and Barthe, P., 1986, Partial somatotropin deficiency in a case of chronic renal insufficiency with renal transplantation. Efficacy of treatment with human growth hormone, *Arch. Fr. Pediatr.* **43**:51–53.

443. Breslau, N. A., 1987, Update on secondary forms of hyperparathyroidism, *Am. J. Med. Sci.* **294**:120–131.

444. Lopez-Hilker, S., Galceran, T., Chan, Y. L., Rapp, N., Martin, K. J., and Slatopolsky, E., 1986, Hypocalcemia may not be essential for the development of secondary hyperparathyroidism of chronic renal failure, *J. Clin. Invest.* **78**:1097–1102.

445. Korkor, A. B., 1987, Reduced binding of [^{3}H]-1,25-dihydroxyvimatin D3 in the parathyroid glands of patients with renal failure, *N. Engl. J. Med.* **316**:1573–1577.

446. Joujoux, J. M., Marty-Double, C., Godlewski, G., and Pignodel, C., 1986, Morphological aspects of parathyroid hyperplasia in patients with chronic renal insufficiency on dialysis, *Ann. Pathol.* **6**:164–169.

447. van Diemen-Steenvoorde, R., Donckerwolcke, R. A., Bosch, R., Visser, W. J., Raymakers, J. A., and Duursma, S. A., 1985, Treatment of renal osteodystrophy in children with dihydrotachysterol and 24,25-dihydroxyvitamin D3, *Clin. Nephrol.* **24**:292–299.

448. Shany, S., Rapoport, J., Zuili, I., Yankowitz, N., and Chaimovits, A., 1986, Enhancement of 24,25-dihydroxyvitamin D3 levels in patients treated with continuous ambulatory peritoneal dialysis, *Nephron* **42**:141–145.

449. Bettinelli, A., Bianchi, M. L., Aimini, E., Ortolani, S., Soldati, L., and Edefonti, A., 1986, Effects of 1,25-dihydroxyvitamin-D3 treatment on mineral balance in children with end-stage renal disease undergoing chronic hemofiltration, *Pediatr. Res.* **20**:5–8.

450. Coen, G., Mazzaferro, S., Bonucci, P., Massimetti, C., Donato, G., Landi, A., Smacchi, A., Della Rocca, C., and Cinotti, G. A., 1986, Treatment of secondary hyperparathyroidism of predialysis chronic renal failure with low doses of 1,25(OH)$_2$D3: Humoral and histomorphometric results, *Miner. Electrolyte Metab.* **12**:375–382.

451. Gordeladze, J. O., Mortensen, B., Nordal, K., Halse, J., Dahl, E., Aksnes, L., and Gautvik, K. M., 1987, The effect of parathyroid hormone (PTH) and 24,25-dihydroxy-vitamin D3 on adenyl cyclase of iliac crest biopsies: Diagnostic and prognostic tool for evaluation and treatment of uremic patients, *Scand. J. Clin. Lab. Invest.* **186**(Suppl.):13–20.

452. Lucas, P. A., Brown, R. C., Woodhead, J. S., and Coles, G. A., 1986, 1,25-Dihydroxycholecalciferol and parathyroid hormone in advanced chronic renal failure: Effects of simultaneous protein and phosphorus restriction, *Clin. Nephrol.* **25**:7–10.

453. Main, J., Velasco, N., Heyes, S. D., Whiting, P., Fraser, R. A., and Catto, G. R., 1986, The effect of dihydroxylated metabolites of vitamin D and dietary phosphate restriction on bone disease in uraemic rats, *Clin. Sci.* **71**:539–543.

454. Tessitore, N., Venturi, A., Adami, S., Roncari, C., Rugiu, C., Corgnati, A., Bonucci, E., and Maschio, G., 1987, Relationship between serum vitamin D metabolites and dietary intake of phosphate in patients with early renal failure, *Miner. Electrolyte Metab.* **13**:38–44.

455. Trachtman, H., and Gauthier, B., 1987, Parenteral calcitriol for treatment of severe renal osteodystrophy in children with chronic renal insufficiency, *J. Pediatr.* **110**:966–970.

456. Burnatowska-Hledin, M. A., Doyle, T. M., Eafie, M. J., and Mayor, G. H., 1986, 1,25-dihydroxyvitamin D3 increases serum and tissue accumulation of aluminum in rats, *J. Lab. Clin. Med.* **108**:96–102.

457. Slatopolsky, E., Weerts, C., Stokes, T., Windus, D., and Delmez, J., 1986, Alternative phosphate binders in dialysis patients: Calcium carbonate, *Semin. Nephrol.* **6**(Suppl. 1):35–41.

458. Gundberg, C. M., and Weinstein, R. S., 1986, Multiple immunoreactive forms of osteocalcin in uremic serum, *J. Clin. Invest.* **77**:1762–1767.

459. Cundy, T., Kanis, J. A., Earnshaw, M., and Woods, C. G., 1986, Comparative effects of alfacalcidol and parathyroidectomy with vitamin D in hyperparathyroid renal bone disease, *Q. J. Med.* **60**:659–670.

460. Fujimoto, Y., Obara, T., Ito, Y., Kodama, T., and Nishi, T., 1985, Surgical treatment of secondary hyperparathyroidism in patients with chronic renal failure: Reevaluation of indications for parathyroidectomy, *Endocrinol. Jpn.* **32**:863–874.

461. Levitt, M. D., Vivian, A. B., and Saker, B. M., 1986, Parathyroidectomy in chronic renal failure, *Aust. NZ J. Surg.* **56**:233–239.

462. Jansson, S., and Tisell, L. E., 1987, Autotransplantation of diseased parathyroid glands into subcutaneous abdominal adipose tissue, *Surgery* **101**:549–556.

463. Johnson, W. J., McCarthy, J. T., van Heerden, J. A., Sterioff, S., Grant, C. S., and Pao, P. C., 1988, Results of subtotal parathyroidectomy in hemodialysis patients, *Am. J. Med.* **84**:23–32.

464. Fiore, C. E., Lunetta, M., and Kanis, J. A., 1985, Long-term effects of histamine H$_2$-receptor antagonists on serum parathyroid hormone in chronic renal failure, *Clin. Endocrinol. (Oxf.)* **23**:277–282.

465. Hirschel-Scholz, S., Caverzasio, J., and Bonjour, J., 1985, Inhibition of parathyroid hormone secretion and parathyroid hormone-independent diminution of tubular calcium reabsorption by WR-2721, a uniquely hypocalcemic agent, *J. Clin. Invest.* **76**:1851–1856.

466. Parrish, C. M., and O'Day, D. M., 1986, Brown tumor of the orbit. Case report and review of the literature, *Arch. Ophthalmol.* **104:**1199–1202.
467. Bohlman, M. E., Kim, Y. C., Eagan, J., and Spees, E. K., 1986, Brown tumor in secondary hyperparathyroidism causing acute paraplegia, *Am. J. Med.* **81:**545–547.
468. Bogin, E., Chagnac, A., Juppner, H., and Levi, J., 1987, Effect of verapamil on plasma parathyroid hormone, *J. Clin. Chem. Clin. Biochem.* **25:**83–85.

12

Nutrition in Renal Disease

Bradley J. Maroni and William E. Mitch

1. Introduction

During the past 2 years, there has been an explosion of information attempting to identify the mechanism(s) whereby dietary protein restriction and pharmacologic agents influence progression in experimental models of renal disease. Experimental support for the beneficial effect of exercise on progression, exercise capacity, and intermediary metabolism emphasizes the importance of including exercise in the medical prescription for patients with renal disease. Long-term follow-up of kidney donors indicates that renal function is preserved in kidney donors, tempering concerns that renal dysfunction will progress following uninephrectomy. The utility of dietary protein restriction to reduce proteinuria and raise albumin stores in nephrotic patients has been reported, although its influence on nitrogen or protein balance remains to be determined. Preliminary experience with infusions of naturally occurring isotopes of amino acids to study the adaptive responses of normal subjects to dietary manipulation is available, but there is very little information on the response of uremic patients despite the widespread prescription of low-protein diets. The importance of measuring several indices of nutrition when assessing nutritional status during low-protein diet therapy has recently been emphasized.

Unfortunately, little insight has been gained into the mechanisms or importance of hyperlipidemia or vitamin and mineral requirements of patients with chronic renal failure (CRF). Similarly, there is little new information regarding therapeutic strategies for patients with acute renal failure (ARF). In this chapter, we review

BRADLEY J. MARONI and WILLIAM E. MITCH • Renal Division, Emory University School of Medicine, Atlanta, Georgia 30322 new information on progression and the developments in nutrition and renal disease just outlined.

2. Progression of Renal Disease

2.1. Experimental Renal Disease

2.1.1. Influence of Dietary Protein

For more than 50 years, it has been recognized that institution of a low-protein diet immediately following subtotal nephrectomy, but prior to the development of established renal disease, limits the development of proteinuria, glomerular sclerosis, and eventual mortality in rats. Recent studies have related progressive renal dysfunction to the adaptive increases in glomerular pressures and flows; the beneficial effect of a low-protein diet has been attributed to normalization of these parameters.[1] Criticisms of these studies are (1) the protein-restricted diet (6% protein) has been compared to a pharmacologic level of dietary protein (40%), rather than to a standard protein intake; (2) short-term studies do not address whether protein restriction, if instituted following established damage, would protect against progressive renal injury.

To address these questions, Nath et al.[2] maintained rats on an *ad libitum*, standard (24% protein) rat chow for 3 months after subtotal nephrectomy. Rats with >25 mg/day proteinuria were then paired by serum creatinine and fed isocaloric diets containing either 6% or 20% protein, but with identical electrolyte content; sucrose replaced protein in the 6% protein diet. The groups were not pair-fed. Renal hemodynamics 2 weeks following institution of the diets revealed no difference in single nephron glomerular filtration rates (SNGFR), but a significantly lower transcapillary hydraulic pressure (P_{GC}) and higher ultrafiltration coefficient (K_f) in rats fed the 6% protein diet. It was concluded that the reduction in P_{GC} resulted from relaxation of efferent arteriolar tone. In the 6% protein group, the increase in K_f counterbalanced the lower P_{GC}; consequently, SNGFR was the same in both groups. After 3 months (6 months following subtotal nephrectomy) and despite equivalent degrees of systolic hypertension, rats fed the 6% protein diet had higher GFRs and less proteinuria. Histologic change was not significantly different between groups. However, the fractional excretions of albumin and IgG were lower in the 6%-protein group, suggesting an improvement in the size- and charge-selective properties of the glomerulus. It was concluded that protein restriction instituted after established renal injury can preserve renal function in rats with subtotal nephrectomy.

To study glomerular injury following a less extensive reduction in renal mass, Hostetter et al. compared control, uninephrectomized, and 1⅓ nephrectomized rats.[3] Isocaloric diets containing high (40%) or low (6%) casein were fed for 4 to 8 months, but again, there was no pair feeding. At both intervals and at each level of renal mass, rats fed the high-protein diet had higher GFRs, but increased proteinuria; by 8 months, rats in all groups consuming the high-protein diet had more glomerular sclerosis. The extent of sclerosis and proteinuria was directly related to the initial loss of renal mass.

The age when renal mass is lost also affects subsequent deterioration in renal function. Okuda *et al.*[4] subjected rats at birth and at 2, 4, and 8 weeks to uninephrectomy. They were then fed a 22%-protein diet and followed for 48 weeks. Despite *ad libitum* feeding, weight gain and creatinine clearance were similar in all nephrectomized groups. The degree of proteinuria, hypoalbuminemia, and focal glomerular sclerosis was significantly greater in rats nephrectomized at 0, 2, or 4 weeks compared to those nephrectomized at 8 weeks. Compensatory renal hypertrophy was also greater in rats nephrectomized at 0 and 4 weeks compared to the 8-week group. These data may mean that the stimulus for hypertrophy affects the development of sclerosis. Recent abstracts are consistent with this conclusion.

Although protein restriction can limit progressive renal damage in experimental models of renal insufficiency, the level of protein used often retards growth. Friedman and Pityer[5] pair-fed isocaloric diets containing 6, 14, or 22% protein to three groups of rats (normal, sham-operated, and subtotal nephrectomy) and compared growth and renal function over 23 weeks. The 6% protein diet impaired growth in all groups; the 14 or 22% protein diet did not blunt growth. Rats subjected to subtotal nephrectomy and fed 22% protein died by 14 weeks. Despite more proteinuria in the 14% compared to the 6% group, creatinine clearance and survival were not significantly different, and it was concluded that the 14% protein maintains normal growth and improves survival in CRF rats. Although the experimental and control rats were pair-fed at each level of protein, the absolute intake of food was directly related to the level of dietary protein, so that the amount of protein eaten in the 6 and 14% groups was less. Unfortunately, the degree of histologic damage among the groups was not examined, and creatinine clearance may not be sufficiently sensitive to assess the extent of renal damage.

Okuda *et al.* have also examined the effects of three levels of dietary protein on renal function, histology, and nutritional status in another model of CRF, adriamycin-induced nephrotic syndrome.[6] The diets contained high (30%), low (10%), or very low (5%) protein; in order to provide equivalent quantities of energy, minerals, and electrolytes, each diet was allocated in proportion to body weight, based on the intake of the 5% protein group. By 24 weeks, rats fed 30% protein had developed massive proteinuria, progressive renal insufficiency, and extensive glomerular sclerosis. Animals fed 5% protein had substantially less proteinuria and stable serum creatinine and creatinine clearance, but their nutritional status worsened, as reflected by weight loss and hypoproteinemia. The 10% protein diet preserved renal function and was associated with less proteinuria and histologic damage, but weight did not increase normally and there was hypoproteinemia. This report highlights the need for more extensive investigation of the level of dietary protein that prevents progression while maintaining nutrition in the nephrotic syndrome.

El Nahas *et al.* present a different view of this seemingly unanimous agreement about a deleterious effect of high-protein diets.[7] In rats with nephrotoxic nephritis fed diets with identical mineral and caloric composition, only the 18% protein chow caused renal damage, while a low-casein (8%) and a high-casein (78%) diet protected the rats from renal failure. In contrast to either the 8% or 18% protein diets, the 78% casein diet was not associated with tubular calcification. With all three diets, there were strong correlations between glomerular sclerosis and tubular atrophy, although the slope of this relationship was less in rats receiving the high-casein diet. All three diets resulted in normal growth in control and impaired growth, but stable weight, in experimental rats, thereby excluding the possible influence of malnutrition on immune and/or inflammatory responses. The authors' interpretation was that there are separate glomerular and tubular contributions to the development of progressive renal dysfunction in rats.

To investigate whether protein derived from animal or vegetable sources influences the progression of experimental renal disease differently, Williams et al. compared a 24% soya protein diet to a 24% casein diet over 3 months in normal and 1⅓ nephrectomized rats.[8] Animals fed the soya had less proteinuria, hypertrophy, and histologic damage and improved survival compared to rats fed casein. Although the authors concluded that the source of dietary protein may be an important determinant of progressive renal damage, the lower protein quality and digestability of soya, as reflected by the lower urea nitrogen excretion, suggests that less soya protein may have been absorbed.

Regarding potential mediators of renal injury, Stahl et al. reported that in partially nephrectomized rats, a high-protein diet increased GFR and glomerular prostaglandin production (predominantly vasodilatory PGE_2) and that indomethacin administration reduced GFR.[9] With the low-protein diet, GFR and glomerular PGE_2 production were significantly lower, and no change in GFR was seen with indomethacin. Treatment with a thromboxane inhibitor had no effect on GFR. The authors suggest that the increased glomerular prostaglandins seen in response to the high-protein intake may modulate the increase in GFR. Fernandez-Repollet et al. reported that even short-term feeding of a low-protein diet to weanling rats resulted in marked decreases in GFR and RPF compared to rats fed 23% protein.[10] The hemodynamic change was attributed to a rise in renal vascular resistance and a dramatic reduction in vasodilatory prostaglandin PGE_2 excretion. Despite a reduced plasma renin activity and aldosterone, renal renin content was increased significantly, suggesting intrarenal activation of the renin system. Captopril prevented the intrarenal effect of low-protein feeding and raised GFR to the level of rats fed 23% protein. It was concluded that intrarenal angiotensin II and PGE_2 mediate the changes in renal hemodynamics induced by dietary protein restriction.

Another suggested mechanism is related to changes in the sensitivity of tubuloglomerular feedback (TGF) in response to changes in dietary protein. With high-protein feeding, a greater distal tubular flow rate is required to initiate TGF-mediated inhibition of SNGFR.[11] The mechanism appears to be related to enhanced loop of Henle absorption of sodium and chloride, so that tubular fluid at the macula densa has a lower sodium and chloride concentration compared to values seen with a low-protein intake. It is not known why sodium and chloride reabsorption are increased. Although these responses were seen in normal animals at extremes of dietary protein (40% vs. 6% casein), the influence of intermediate protein intakes and the importance of altered TGF in animals with experimental renal disease are unknown.

Most of the experimental evidence implicating dietary protein-induced glomerular "hyperfiltration" as the cause for progression in renal disease has been obtained from strains of rats that have a high incidence of spontaneous glomerular sclerosis with aging. Robertson *et al.* suggest that there may be an important species difference with respect to the influence of dietary protein on renal function and morphology.[12] They subjected 21 female beagle dogs to 75% nephrectomy (serum creatinine doubled) and maintained the animals for 4 years on diets containing 56, 27, or 19% protein. Although dogs fed 27 or 56% protein had significantly greater GFR and RPF than those consuming 19% protein, there was no deterioration of GFR or increase in proteinuria in any group. Furthermore, no animal developed hypertension, and although the incidence of glomerular pathology increased in proportion to dietary protein, in most dogs, pathology was minimal and there was no correlation between glomerular pathology and renal function. Two of nine dogs died with renal failure (one was fed 19% and the other 56% protein), but there was no relationship between renal failure or death and the level of dietary protein intake, suggesting that the response of dogs to loss of renal mass differs from that of rats. Whether dogs require more prolonged exposure to dietary protein and/or a greater reduction in renal mass to induce progressive renal dysfunction is unclear. In summary, changes in the renin–angiotensin axis, renal prostaglandins, and tubuloglomerular feedback are suggested contributors to the hemodynamic changes seen in response to a high-protein diet. However, species differences in the susceptibility to progressive glomerular sclerosis have been noted, and therefore, extrapolation of responses in rats to humans with renal disease may not be warranted.

2.1.2. Nonprotein Dietary Factors

Besides protein, other dietary constituents, including phosphate, carbohydrates, and lipids, reportedly influence progression of experimental renal disease. Although it has been suggested that a low-phosphate diet may delay progression in CRF patients as well as in rats with CRF, others have argued that this most likely reflects a concomitant reduction in food and/or protein intake.[1,13] Lumlertgul *et al.*[14] attempted to circumvent previous technical problems by feeding a normal diet supplemented with a phosphate binder. After 5/6 nephrectomy, rats were matched by serum creatinine and weight and subsequently pair-fed; weight gain and urinary urea nitrogen were comparable over the 3-month study. Rats receiving the phosphate binder developed hypophosphatemia, and at 6 weeks, they exhibited much less proteinuria and hyperlipidemia. By 12 weeks, renal function, histologic damage including nephrocalcinosis, and mortality were significantly less in rats supplemented with the phosphate binder. It was concluded that phosphate, independently of protein intake, limits progression and hyperlipidemia in the remnant kidney model. In the isolated perfused kidney of rats fed a phosphorus-restricted diet, Harris et al.[15] found a lower metabolic activity per nephron than that of rats fed the control diet. It was postulated that the beneficial effects of phosphate depletion on progression of CRF[14] are due in part to reduced metabolic demand. Although this conclusion raises the possibility that a stimulus for renal growth causes progression,[4] a cause-and-effect relationship has not been demonstrated between hypermetabolism and progression.

The role of dietary carbohydrate and lipid on progression of experimental renal disease remains controversial, in part due to mechanisms in study design. Klein-knecht et al. investigated carbohydrate restriction in rats following 5/6 subtotal nephrectomy.[16] Although the diets were designed to provide identical intake of all dietary constituents (except carbohydrates) per gram of food, food consumption remained lower in carbohydrate-restricted rats. Regardless, carbohydrate-restricted rats had reduced growth and higher urinary urea nitrogen excretion (implying increased endogenous protein catabolism); they also had lower serum creatinines, less histologic damage, and lower mortality rates. In another protocol, the type of carbohydrate was evaluated in adult rats subjected to less severe carbohydrate restriction (30 vs. 40%). Restriction of "simple" (glucose), but not complex (starch), carbohydrate was found to reduce mortality and after 9 weeks was associated with a lower plasma creatinine and less histologic damage. Thus, restriction of simple, but not complex, carbohydrates favorably influenced renal function and survival. Limitations of the study include (1) a high (50–80%) mortality, (2) hetero-genous degrees of renal insufficiency among groups, and (3) probable differences in intake of other dietary constituents including protein. In previous studies, restricting food intake of obese Zucker rats has also been shown to reduce the severity of spontaneous glomerular sclerosis. Unfortunately, this could not be attributed to carbohydrates since both calories and protein were restricted. In a study with a more complex design, Kasiske et al. alternated carbohydrate-restricted or replete diets every 3 weeks for 27–30 weeks to young and old, obese and lean Zucker rats.[17] Carbohydrate restriction reduced body and kidney weight, proteinuria, and glomerular area in young obese Zucker rats, but glomerular damage was not altered. In older obese Zucker rats with established renal damage, carbohydrate restriction did not reduce albuminuria or prevent the progression of glomerular injury. Since the carbohydrate was predominantly cornstarch, a beneficial effect of limiting sim-ple carbohydrates cannot be excluded. Interestingly, there was a significant correla-tion between elevated serum cholesterol and triglycerides and mesangial matrix expansion in young and old obese Zucker rats. This finding supports the possibility that lipids should be added to the list of factors causing progression in rats with subtotal nephrectomy (see following and Ref. 13).

Support for hyperlipidemia as an etiologic factor in progression of renal insuf-ficiency was provided by Diamond and Karnovsky.[18] In puromycin-induced nephrosis, rats fed a cholesterol- and cholic acid–supplemented diet had more proteinuria, lower inulin clearances, and, histologically, a greater percentage of mesangial foam cells, cellular proliferation, and glomerular sclerosis/hyalinosis.

Although this dietary regimen preferentially elevates serum cholesterol, the mechanism responsible for these findings and whether correction of hyperlipidemia will confer protection from progression is not known. In summary, reports in 1986–1987 hint that nonprotein dietary factors influence renal damage, at least in rats. Potential mechanisms for their effects are obscure. A more extensively investigated area is that of polyunsaturated fatty acids.

Diets rich in omega-3, polyunsaturated fatty acids (PUFA) can reduce serum lipids and prolong the bleeding time and are associated with reduced risk of cardiovascular disease. Since fish oils alter serum lipids and tromboxane synthesis and can prevent proteinuria and increase survival in NZB/NZW mice,[1] Scharschmidt *et al.* tested the utility of a fish oil–supplemented diet on progression in rats following subtotal nephrectomy.[19] The experimental diet was associated with functional and histologic deterioration in spite of a reduction in hyperlipidemia and glomerular thromboxane production. Why dietary supplementation with omega-3 PUFA seems to benefit immune-mediated (and, hence, inflammatory) renal disease, but not the remnant kidney model, is unknown. The difference could be that the lipooxygenase products are more important as inflammatory mediators in experimental lupus nephritis. Based on the foregoing, the results of Heifets *et al.*, showing that dietary supplementation with linoleic acid ameliorated hypertension, loss of renal function, and glomerular damage in rats with subtotal nephrectomy, was unexpected.[20] The linoleic acid supplement did increase the linoleic content of membranes in the renal cortex and medulla, but there was no significant change in urinary excretion of PGE_2, thromboxane, or their metabolites. How differing PUFAs can produce conflicting effects on renal function is unknown; possibly, the reason is linked to complex changes in prostaglandin production, as well as the pathogenesis of the experimental renal disease. For humans, the usefulness of PUFAs to slow progression must be regarded as unproven; the conflicting results in rats emphasize the importance of considering effects of dietary intervention on all body systems.

2.1.3. Nondietary Approaches to Arresting Progression

Angiotensin converting enzyme (ACE) inhibitors have been reported to slow progression in rats after subtotal nephrectomy, with or without supplemental chronic glucocorticoid therapy, and in diabetes. To test the hypothesis that systemic hypertension must be transmitted to the glomerular capillary for structural damage to occur, Anderson *et al.*[21] compared the efficacy of triple antihypertensive therapy (reserpine, hydralazine, plus hydrochlorothiazide) to enalapril. After subtotal nephrectomy, rats were fed standard chow *ad lib*, and 4 weeks later, a subset underwent micropuncture. Enalapril normalized systemic blood pressure and lowered glomerular capillary pressure (P_{GC}) to near normal. Despite the lower P_{GC}, SNGFR remained high because of an increase in blood flow which was due to efferent arteriolar vasodilatation and an increase in the ultrafiltration coefficient (K_f). Triple drug therapy also normalized systemic hypertension, but did not lower P_{GC}. Twelve weeks following renal ablation, enalapril-treated rats had less proteinuria and strikingly fewer glomerular lesions. Despite an equivalent reduction in systemic blood pressure, triple drug therapy failed to reduce glomerular capillary hypertension and was associated with histologic damage comparable to that in untreated rats with reduced renal mass. To determine whether enalapril or a low-protein diet can limit glomerular injury *after* established glomerular damage, Meyer et al.[22] maintained ⅚ nephrectomized rats on 24% protein chow for 8 weeks and then allocated them to control, enalapril, or low-protein (12% casein) therapy for an additional 12 weeks. Enalapril normalized systemic and intraglomerular pressures, prevented a further increment in proteinuria, and limited the prevalence of glomerular sclerosis. The low-protein diet normalized glomerular, but not systemic, hypertension, stabilized proteinuria, and reduced sclerosis to a level intermediate between the enalapril-treated and untreated control rats. Thus, both therapies limit the progression of glomerular injury in rats with established glomerular damage. The success of ACE inhibitors appears to be influenced by the duration and degree of preexisting injury. Beukers et al. tested captopril in uninephrectomized rats over 8 months.[23] Captopril was associated with minimal proteinuria and a low incidence of glomerular sclerosis, confirming prior studies. In contrast, if captopril was initiated 7 months postnephrectomy, when substantial proteinuria was present, it did not arrest the progression of proteinuria or glomerular sclerosis. Other evidence for a beneficial effect of ACE inhibitors was presented by Garcia et al.,[24] who showed that chronic, pharmacologic glucocorticoid therapy (equivalent to approximately 1 mg/kg per day) increased the already high SNGFR in rats subjected to partial renal ablation and accelerated the development of proteinuria and glomerular sclerosis. Concomitant treatment with an ACE inhibitor normalized glomerular pressure, minimized proteinuria, and markedly reduced the incidence of glomerular lesions. ACE therapy was shown to reduce efferent greater than afferent arteriolar resistance, thereby reducing glomerular pressure toward normal and protecting against disease progression.

Verapamil has been reported to benefit renal function in acute renal failure [25]; this has been attributed to improved mitochondrial respiratory function and inhibition of calcium accumulation. Moreover, verapamil has been shown to decrease nephrocalcinosis and tubular ultrastructure abnormalities after subtotal nephrectomy.[26] However, the latter study was stopped after 3 weeks when renal function was identical in control and verapamil-treated rats. To examine the long-term effect of verapamil on renal function and survival, Harris et al. paired ⅚ nephrectomized rats by blood pressure, weight, and renal function and administered daily verapamil or vehicle subcutaneously.[27] Despite progressive proteinuria and independent of any effect on systemic blood pressure, chronic verapamil therapy limited renal functional and histologic damage, as well as nephrocalcinosis, and improved survival. These same authors have subsequently shown that oxygen consumption in the isolated perfused remnant kidney is elevated threefold, but is not linked to changes in net sodium reabsorption, GFR, or glucose production.[15] Perfusing with verapamil lowered oxygen consumption and, hence, metabolic activity of the remnant kidney. It was proposed that the tubular adaptation to nephron loss may be a factor in progression of chronic renal disease.

Finally, exercise training can ameliorate progressive renal disease in rats with moderate CRF despite the persistence of systolic hypertension.[28] GFR was higher and proteinuria and glomerular sclerosis less in exercised rats compared to sedentary uremic controls. Furthermore, exercise reduced plasma triglycerides and low-density-lipoprotein cholesterol to values indistinguishable from those in nonuremic sedentary controls. Although the mechanisms for these changes are not known, this report complements previous studies showing that exercise can improve glucose and lipid metabolism, hypertension, and anemia, as well as work capacity and the sense of well-being in patients with renal failure (Ref. 13, and Section 4).

2.1.4. Experimental Diabetic Nephropathy

A protective effect of ACE inhibitors on progressive diabetic glomerulopathy has been reported by Zatz et al.[29] After streptozotocin, diabetic and age-and-weight-matched control rats were allocated to receive either tap water alone or enalapril. All rats were fed 24% protein chow, and diabetic rats received daily insulin in order to maintain moderate hyperglycemia (approximately 350 mg/dl). Micropuncture performed at 4–6 weeks poststreptozotocin revealed high glomerular pressures in the untreated rats, which were the only group to develop progressive proteinuria. Renal histology performed after 14 months revealed a comparable degree of glomerular damage in enalapril-treated diabetic rats and nondiabetic controls. In contrast, untreated diabetic rats had more glomerular damage. The protective effect of normalizing glomerular pressure despite persistent hyperglycemia lends support to the importance of hemodynamic factors in the pathogenesis of diabetic glomerulopathy. It does not, however, exclude the possibility that strict metabolic control could benefit renal function in diabetes. In fact, Jensen et al.[30] reported that strict metabolic control (defined as normal weight gain and blood glucose and the absence of glycosuria) normalized the high glomerular pressures and whole kidney GFR of diabetic rats. The lower P_{GC} was due to an increase in the ratio of afferent to efferent arteriolar resistances. These results were obtained only 2 weeks after induction of diabetes when renal function was normal, and histologic confirmation of a beneficial influence of strict metabolic control was not provided.

Bank et al. have suggested that elevations in glomerular pressure per se do not accelerate glomerular pathology or proteinuria in experimental diabetes.[31] Normotensive (WKY) and spontaneously hypertensive (SHR) rats were given streptozotocin; a subset of the SHR rats was treated with chlorothiazide, reserpine, and hydralazine. Micropuncture was performed at 1 week or 4 months and histology examined after 6 months. Experimental diabetes resulted in elevated glomerular pressure in both WKY and SHR rats, albeit to a greater degree in the latter. Systolic blood pressure remained high in SHR diabetic animals, but was normal in WKY diabetic rats and low in SHR diabetic animals receiving antihypertensive therapy. After 6 months of follow-up and despite a plasma glucose of ~450 mg/dl, no difference in proteinuria or histologic damage could be found in the kidneys of untreated SHR or normotensive WKY diabetic animals. The controversy over the importance of elevated glomerular pressures in experimental diabetic nephropathy is unresolved, but it is interesting that histologic damage in the Bank et al. study was limited by the same antihypertensive regimen that was associated with histologic damage in the Anderson et al. study.[21]

Bank and associates[32] have also reported that a disturbance in vascular smooth muscle calcium transport may be responsible for the renal vasodilatation and hyperfiltration found in experimental diabetes. To test this hypothesis, renal hemodynamics were measured 7–10 days following induction of streptozotocin diabetes during the intrarenal infusion of insulin with or without calcium. The amount of insulin and calcium infused did not alter arterial glucose or calcium levels or the function of the contralateral kidney. Infusions of insulin or calcium alone had no effect on hyperfiltration of the diabetic kidney. In contrast, when insulin and calcium were infused together, SNGFR, P_{GC}, and renal plasma flow decreased to normal levels; simultaneous infusion of verapamil returned these values to the previous hyperfiltering levels. It appears that the hyperfiltration of early experimental diabetic nephropathy may be related to decreased vascular tone caused by defective calcium transport into smooth muscle.

2.2. Progression in Humans

The importance of frequent clinical follow-up in retarding progression of CRF has recently been highlighted by Bergstrom et al.[33] When rates of progression before and after study entry were compared in patients eating an unrestricted diet, the rate of progression decreased by approximately 50% with more frequent clinic visits. This was correlated with a slight (~2 mm Hg), but significant, reduction in diastolic blood pressure. Although these findings do not exclude a beneficial effect of protein restriction on progression, they emphasize the importance of considering a "clinic" effect in the design of studies of dietary intervention.

Dietary regimens for treating progressive CRF include (1) a conventional lowprotein diet containing 0.6 g/kg per day, and (2) a very-low-protein diet (VLPD) containing 0.3 g/kg per day of predominantly vegetable proteins supplemented with either essential amino acids (EAA) or a mixture of EAA and ketoanalogs of EAA (KA). The advantages of each regimen in terms of abating progression have been debated, although Barsotti et al.'s experience suggested a ketoacid-supplemented diet can slow progression in patients who progress while consuming a conventional low-protein diet.[34] Support for a therapeutic advantage to a ketoacid-based diet was provided by Walser et al.[35] In five compliant patients with defined rates of loss of GFR while consuming a VLPD plus EAA diet and whose serum creatinine was less than 7.4 mg/dl, a significant slowing of progression was seen after switching to a

VLPD–KA diet. In contrast, progression was unabated in six patients whose serum creatinine exceeded 7.5 mg/dl at crossover. Nutrition was well maintained in all patients, as assessed by body weight, serum proteins, and urinary creatinine excretion.

The importance of assessing nutritional status was highlighted by Lucas et al. [36] They treated 12 patients with only 0.2 g protein/kg per day and about 50% of the amount of KA used by others[1,35] for 6–12 months. Although 11 of 12 subjects had a serum creatinine greater than 7.5 (mean 10.2 mg/dl), four maintained stable renal function for over 12 months. Therapy was associated with an improved sense of well-being and with significant decreases in serum urea, phosphate, parathyroid hormone (PTH) and calcium–phosphate product. However, despite stable serum albumin and transferrin levels, body weight, creatinine excretion, and an-thropometrics decreased significantly, suggesting loss of lean body mass with this overly restrictive regimen. This study also points out that changes in plasma pro-teins should not be used as the sole index of nutritional status.

Meisinger and Strauch have compared a KA regimen based on "Rose" re-quirements for EAA with a preparation containing an increased amount of KAs of branched-chain amino acids (BCAA); both groups received a 30-g-protein diet.[37] Body weight and serum proteins were maintained in both groups, but patients receiving the supplement containing more KAs of BCAA had normalization of plasma BCAA concentrations, stabilization of renal function, and lower serum urea, calcium, and phosphate levels. Even though no information regarding dietary compliance was provided, this regimen warrants further study since the results suggest that amino acid requirements of uremic patients are different from those of normal subjects. KA may exert other unexpected effects. Calcium salts of KA plus VLPD can blunt hyperparathyroidism in nondialysis patients, but this may be linked to dietary phosphorus restriction.[13] However, when hemodialysis patients consum-ing a high-phosphorus, unrestricted-protein diet were given calcium salts of KAs, secondary hyperparathyroidism was shown to improve, as reflected by a decrement in serum phosphorus and PTH.[38] It appears that the effect on PTH could not be attributed to a reduction in calcium and phosphorus intake, suggesting that it was specific for ketoacids.

Maschio et al.[39] have updated their experience with conventional low-protein diets in 349 CRF patients treated between 1972 and 1985. All were maintained on a diet containing 0.6 g/kg per day of protein, 40 kcal/kg per day, 700 mg phos-phorus, and 1–1.5 g calcium plus antihypertensive medications as required. Over a mean follow-up of 35 months (range 6–156 months), two-thirds of the patients had no further deterioration of renal function. The likelihood of success varied with the underlying disease; the best renal survival occurred with hypertensive nephrosclero-sis, whereas chronic glomerulonephritis (GN) and polycystic kidney disease (PCKD) patients had the worse prognosis. Hypertension adversely influenced the rate of progression, and proteinuria was a poor prognostic factor. No evidence of progressive protein depletion or malnutrition was observed. This study, like most others, used changes in serum creatinine to measure progression. Because several factors influence creatinine in renal disease,[33,40] the results cannot be considered conclusive.

A combined program using VLPD–KA and once-weekly hemodialysis was found to be an acceptable alternative to thrice-weekly hemodialysis in selected patients with advanced CRF.[41] Body weight, serum protein, and a sense of well-being were all maintained for an average of 18 months, confirming a previous report.[42]

2.2.1. Protein and Renal Function in Humans

Following acute ingestion of protein or with infusion of amino acids, GFR can increase in some normal subjects. In subjects with a baseline GFR below 50 ml/min per 1.73 M^2,[43] GFR did not increase after acute protein ingestion, and it was suggested that this demonstrated an absence of renal reserve, i.e., a state of "hyper-filtration" whereby available nephrons were functioning maximally. Hostetter[44] reported that a blunted response of GFR is not restricted to CRF patients. After a very large protein load (3.5 g/kg), only 6 of 10 patients had an increase in GFR; the average increase was 15% and not statistically different from zero. Schaap et al. determined GFR and RPF after 4 weeks of a low-protein (30–40 g protein/day) and, subsequently, a high-protein (80–90 g protein/day) diet in 24 subjects with CRF.[45] Consumption of the higher-protein diet was associated with a 20% increase in GFR, and the increment was independent of the baseline GFR, as reported by others.[1,46] In patients with a solitary kidney with or without superimposed renal insufficiency (GFR 23–70 ml/min), there was a significantly greater percentage increase in GFR following acute protein ingestion than in normal controls.[47] Thus, patients with renal insufficiency do experience changes in GFR with chronic changes in dietary protein. In contrast, acute protein loading of diabetic patients has been associated with a paradoxical decrease in GFR.[48] The decrease occurred despite stable blood pressure, renal plasma flow (RPF), and renal vascular resistance. Whether this means that protein ingestion changed the ultrafiltration coefficient or the efferent arteriolar tone is not known. In contrast to acute loading, it appears that diabetic patients with an elevated creatinine clearance experience a change in GFR similar to that of normal subjects in response to chronic changes in protein intake.[49] Following a reduction in dietary protein from 3.5 to 1.5 g/kg per day, GFR decreased to normal levels, suggesting that the high GFR in diabetic patients may be in part related to their increased protein intake with commonly prescribed diabetic diets. Changes in GFR associated with acute protein ingestion appears to be dependent upon the type of protein ingested. Casilan, a milk-based protein, did not acutely increase creatinine clearance but did raise it after 3–4 days.[50]

The mechanism(s) responsible for an increase in GFR and renal blood flow (RBF) with protein ingestion or amino acid infusion is not clear, although altera-tions in renal metabolism, tubuloglomerular feedback, and modulation by a hor-mone(s) have been suggested. Increased extraneuronal dopamine production has been shown to correlate with changes in renal function caused by protein ingestion in humans.[51] In this study, a 60-g protein load raised plasma dopa (in the presence of the dopamine decarboxylase inhibitor, carbidopa) and was associated with natriuresis and increased osmolar clearance. In the absence of carbidopa, there was no rise in plasma dopamine, but a prompt increase in dopamine excretion. Based on those findings and the ability of both protein and dopamine to increase RBF and GFR, as well as solute clearance, it was suggested that intrarenal dopamine is the mediator of several of the dietary protein–induced renal responses.

Dietary protein or amino acid infusion is known to stimulate glucagon, insulin, and growth hormone release, while infusions of pharmacologic doses of glucagon and growth hormone can increase GFR and RBF.[1] When somatostatin plus amino acids was infused into normal subjects, the amino acid–induced increase in GFR and RBF was blocked.[52] Concomitant infusion of insulin, glucagon, and growth hormone at rates that mimic the elevated blood levels seen with amino acid infusion, like the amino acid infusion alone, caused a rise in GFR and RBF. These results suggest that one or more of these hormones are responsible for the increase in GFR following amino acid infusion. However, it must be recognized that somatostatin inhibits the secretion of many hormones. Since physiologic and pharmacologic levels of hyperinsulinemia do not change GFR or RBF, a role for insulin *per se* seems unlikely. A role for growth hormone also seems unlikely since infusion of arginine HCl increased GFR and RPF to a comparable degree in normal subjects and growth hormone–deficient subjects[53]; plasma growth hormone levels rose only in normal subjects, while plasma glucagon increased in both groups. Although these results suggest a role for glucagon, this is not settled because pharmacologic concentrations of glucagon are required to increase RBF and GFR in dogs and a greater response occurs when glucagon is infused directly into the portal vein.[54] The latter observation supports the hypothesis that hyperfiltration following protein ingestion is mediated by some unidentified, vasoactive substance secreted by the liver. In fact, Dratwa *et al.* have reported that acute protein ingestion did not increase GFR in 10 patients with cirrhosis or in one patient with acute hepatitis.[55] After the patient with hepatitis recovered, he displayed a normal increment in GFR following protein ingestion. Interestingly, the increment in GFR and RBF in response to amino acid infusion into normal subjects is abolished by a low-sodium diet (20 meq/day); captopril restored the reduced hemodynamic response.[56] Inhibition of prostaglandin synthesis with indomethacin in subjects receiving a normal sodium intake can also blunt the amino acid effect on renal hemodynamics.[56] These results suggest a role for prostaglandins and/or the renin system in the hemodynamic response to amino acid infusion.

To extend these studies to CRF patients, Rosenberg *et al.* examined the influence of low (0.55 g/kg per day) and high (2 g/kg per day) protein diets on glomerular function and hormone production in 12 adults with a variety of glomerular diseases.[57] The low-protein diet rapidly improved glomerular permselectivity as reflected by decreased fractional excretion of albumin and IgG and large neutral dextrans. The high-protein diet was associated with higher plasma renin and aldosterone levels, as well as urinary excretion of prostaglandin E and 6-keto-PGF_1, suggesting that alterations in these hormones may be involved in mediating the beneficial effects of a low-protein diet. In summary, the mechanism(s) responsible for the inconsistent increase in GFR in response to acute protein load is undefined, but when present, it appears to be modulated by the level of dietary protein intake, protein source, volume status, and underlying disease process. How this change in GFR is related to progression of CRF is unknown.

2.2.2. Diabetic Renal Disease

A substantial proportion of patients with insulin-dependent diabetes develop renal failure; why some, but not all, patients are at risk is not known. Micro-albuminuria seems to be a marker for individuals at high risk for development of clinical diabetic nephropathy,[58] and young, diabetic patients with an increased GFR appear to lose glomerular function more rapidly than those with ''normal'' values for GFR.[59] Besides a high GFR, hypertension accelerates the diabetic nephropathy whereas effective antihypertensive therapy can slow the decline in renal function.[1,60] Short-term dietary protein restriction has been shown to reduce GFR and fractional excretion of albumin, independently of blood pressure or glycemic control in diabetic patients with microalbuminuria.[61,62] These clinical studies are consistent with experimental work suggesting that altered glomerular hemodynamics are important in the pathogenesis of diabetic nephropathy (see Section 2.1.4) and that lowering glomerular pressure can retard the progression of diabetic glomerulopathy despite persistent hyperglycemia. Recent data suggest that an elevated GFR in diabetic patients is seen only in a subgroup whose renal response to hyperglycemia is quantitatively different from that of diabetic patients with ''normal'' GFR. Only subjects with a persistently high baseline GFR increased their GFR in response to hyperglycemia induced by a glucose infusion; there also was an increase in RBF and filtration fraction, suggesting that hyperglycemia increased glomerular pressure.[63]

Whether intensive insulin therapy designed to achieve euglycemia can prevent or ameliorate diabetic complications, including nephropathy, has been intensely debated; furthermore, only the DCCT trial has attempted to address the question of primary prevention.[64] With respect to progression of kidney disease, results have been inconclusive, in part owing to patient heterogeneity, small sample size, and short-term follow-up. The Oslo study, designed to examine the effect of intensive therapy prospectively in patients with diabetes associated with less pronounced complications, reported no significant change in albuminuria during 2 years of follow-up in either the conventional or intensive insulin treatment group.[65] There was a small, but significant, decline in GFR in subjects treated with the insulin pump. It should be recognized that the intraindividual coefficient of variation in albumin excretion was large (e.g., mean of 45–62% by group), and that blood pressure and serum creatinine were normal and did not change during the study. The Kroc Study Group used a posthoc subgroup analysis to demonstrate that insulin pump therapy caused a significant decline in albuminuria in patients who entered the study with albumin excretion rates greater than 12 μg/min (the upper limit of normal).[66] Although results at 1 year in the Steno trial were inconclusive, after 2 years of follow-up, patients with incipient diabetic nephropathy (dipstick negative, but urine albumin 30–300 mg/24 hr) revealed a benefit from insulin pump over conventional therapy.[67] Albumin excretion exceeding 300 mg/24 hr developed in 5 of 18 conventionally treated patients, but in none of the 18 treated with the insulin pump ($p < 0.05$). Changes in fractional albumin clearance corroborated these findings; diastolic blood pressure increased only in conventionally treated subjects and was positively correlated with albumin excretion. In the insulin infusion group, GFR fell modestly (from 109 to 99 ml/min per 1.73 M^2), yet serum creatinine decreased significantly, suggesting that stricter metabolic control may have changed glomerular hemodynamics. Again, the confidence intervals for individual urinary albumin excretion rates were large, and albuminuria at entry in the five conventionally treated subjects who subsequently developed clinical proteinuria was higher than in those who did not develop clinical albuminuria. Following a 1-year baseline period, Bending et al. treated 12 matched subjects with intermittent albuminuria by albustix (mean duration of diabetes ~20 years) for a year with either conventional or insulin pump therapy.[68] Despite excellent blood pressure and glycemic control, GFR fell significantly in both groups; urinary albumin excretion varied widely at entrance and throughout the study and was not influenced by glycemic control. In both the Kroc and Steno trials, insulin pump therapy was associated with an increased incidence of diabetic ketoacidosis, and preliminary results from the DCCT have shown a statistically significant increase in severe hypoglycemic episodes.

In summary, no report has appeared demonstrating the utility of strict glycemic control in the primary prevention of diabetic complications. Short-term secondary intervention trials in patients with established diabetic complications have provided conflicting results and have not settled whether intensive insulin therapy retards complications. The effects of strict control on proteinuria have not been uniform, and it is unknown whether such therapy will prevent or retard the development of progressive renal failure. In view of the substantial investment in time and effort required for the insulin pump, as well as the increased risk of ketoacidosis and severe hypoglycemia, efficacy must be well demonstrated before intensive therapy can be advocated as standard diabetic care.

2.2.3. Progression in Kidney Donors

Donation of a kidney causes renal hypertrophy and an augmentation of GFR to approximately 75% of the preoperative value. Because of experimental evidence of hemodynamically mediated renal injury following subtotal nephrectomy and because of the association of focal glomerular sclerosis and proteinuria with unilateral renal agenesis,[69] concern has been raised that kidney donation may be detrimental. To date, several reports with follow-up exceeding 10 years have been published.[70–]

[75] The incidence of hypertension ranges from 15 to 48% (mean 22%); however, the proportion attributable to nephrectomy *per se* may be much less. For example, Anderson *et al.*[70] reported that, except for males aged 50–69, the incidence of hypertension was similar to that of the general population. Talseth *et al.*[71] noted that only 3 of 10 donors found to be hypertensive could be considered completely normotensive preoperatively, and Williams *et al.*[72] found no increase in hypertension when compared to siblings. In contrast, Hakim *et al.*[73] noted increased diastolic blood pressure in donors compared to age-matched controls. Proteinuria (>150 mg/24 hr) has been reported to occur in 13–25% (mean 20%) of kidney donors, but only 4% of 240 patients excreted >500 mg/day; patients who excreted >1 g/day appeared to have other medical disorders or acquired renal disease. Thus, even though proteinuria occurs in approximately 20% of kidney donors, it is typically mild and appears to be nonprogressive. Serum creatinine is reportedly stable over 10 years of follow-up.[76]

In summary, some (but not all) studies report an increased incidence of hypertension and there is modest, but nonprogressive, proteinuria in kidney donors. To date, there is no evidence of progressive renal dysfunction in donors followed for an average of 11–16 years postnephrectomy and, therefore, no compelling reason to stop recruiting living, related donors.

3. Metabolism in Chronic Renal Failure

3.1. Carbohydrate Metabolism

Previous investigations of insulin receptor function in uremia have yielded conflicting results: normal receptor number and binding to circulating monocytes and adipocytes vs. decreased receptor number on erythrocytes.[1] To investigate cellular mechanisms of insulin resistance and the impact of dialysis, insulin binding and action were examined in adipocytes from patients before and after initiation of continuous ambulatory peritoneal dialysis (CAPD).[77] All subjects had impaired glucose tolerance, fasting hyperglycemia, and hyperinsulinemia. From Scatchard analysis, insulin receptor number was decreased, but because receptor affinity was increased, maximum insulin binding was normal. Following 3 months of CAPD, maximum insulin binding fell owing to a decrease in both receptor affinity and number. Despite these abnormalities, baseline insulin-stimulated lipogenesis did not differ from that in control subjects, and CAPD did not influence insulin-stimulated glucose uptake or lipogenesis. These results contrast with the normal insulin binding and impaired glucose uptake reported to occur in adipocytes from chronically uremic rats.[78] In view of the well-documented decrease in muscle sensitivity to insulin in uremia,[1] Taylor *et al.*'s report suggests a difference between adipose tissue and muscle; an alternate explanation for the difference in muscle and adipocytes is that circulating inhibitors of insulin action are not detected by *in vitro* assays.

Suppression of hepatic glucose uptake and production is normal in uremic patients, but hepatocytes from CRF rats exhibit insulin resistance with respect to lipid synthesis and amino acid transport.[1,79] Because circulating inhibitors of insulin action may affect *in vitro* adipocyte function,[1] primary cultures of normal rat hepatocytes were incubated with serum from nondialyzed uremic patients.[79] No abnormality in insulin binding or processing, receptor structure, autophosphorylation, or receptor kinase activity was found. However, incubating normal hepatocytes for 20 hr with uremic sera inhibited insulin stimulation of pyruvate dehydrogenase activity and decreased maximum responsiveness of lipid synthesis and sensitivity of amino acid uptake to insulin. These studies lend further support for an inhibitor of insulin action. In summary, whether altered insulin binding contributes to insulin resistance in uremia is unsettled and may be tissue-specific. The predominant abnormality seems to occur at some point beyond interaction of insulin with its receptor.

A propensity for spontaneous or propranolol-induced hypoglycemia has been described in some uremic patients, which may be related to an abnormality in the response to the counterregulatory hormone glucagon. Baylor et al.[80] examined the influence of graded infusions of glucagon on glucose homeostasis in the presence or absence of propranolol. In uremic subjects, propranolol reduced the hepatic glycemic response to glucagon and the insulin secretory response to hyperglycemia. These results suggest a modulating effect of beta-adrenergic tone on glucose homeostasis in uremic patients, and that beta-blockade may impair counterregulatory responses. In 10 subjects with advanced uremia, therapy with a VLPD–KA regimen improved glucose tolerance and reduced peripheral insulin resistance, as reflected by increased sensitivity to insulin and a higher rate of maximum glucose disposal.[81] These results, as well as reports of improved glucose utilization after beginning hemodialysis, add support to the argument for a protein-derived toxin contributing to insulin resistance in uremia.

Exercise training can increase insulin sensitivity and responsiveness of muscle to glucose uptake and glycolytic utilization in rats with moderate renal insufficiency.[82] The influence of exercise on glucose metabolism can now be added to the growing list of favorable benefits of exercise on progression and other aspects of intermediary metabolism.

Few studies have examined the caloric requirements or whether the ability to adapt to a reduced caloric intake is intact in CRF patients. Kopple et al. varied the energy intake of six CRF patients between 15 and 45 kcal/kg per day (mean 24 days) while they received a constant intake of 0.55–0.60 g protein/kg per day.[83] Energy intake was positively correlated with nitrogen balance and changes in body weight and inversely correlated with urea nitrogen appearance, consistent with a protein-sparing effect of increasing caloric intake. When corrected for unmeasured nitrogen losses (0.5 g/day), nitrogen balance was negative in one of four patients fed 45, one of five fed 35, three of five fed 25, and two of two ingesting 15 kcal/kg per day. Based on these findings, the linear regression analysis of nitrogen balance vs. energy intake, and results from resting energy expenditure, it was concluded that 35 kcal/kg per day would be prudent for most stable CRF patients. Interestingly, changes in body weight and anthropometrics were more sensitive indicators of the adequacy of caloric intake than serum proteins, highlighting again the importance of following several nutritional parameters when evaluating dietary adequacy.

When CRF and hemodialysis patients were compared to normal subjects, energy expenditure (EE) during rest and exercise were not different, suggesting that the low energy intake of uremic patients is not an adjustment to a lower energy requirement, but rather is maladaptive.[84] Furthermore, when caloric intake was decreased, EE did not fall. Although it is possible that a reduction in EE might occur with a more drastic restriction of energy or with longer follow-up, it is also possible that CRF patients do not conserve energy normally.[83]

These experiments were the first systematic investigation of energy requirements and expenditure by uremic subjects and emphasize the need for additional studies of energy metabolism in uremia. It would be important in future studies to consider the influence of cigarette smoking in view of the recent report that energy expenditure increases 10% with smoking; this effect was not related to activity level or resting metabolic rate.[85]

3.2. Amino Acid and Protein Metabolism

Besides decreased urea clearance, an increase in urea appearance has been shown to account for 30–60% of the increase in blood urea nitrogen (BUN) following diuretic-induced sodium depletion.[86] The diuretic effect was associated with approximately a twofold increase in amino acid nitrogen release from peripheral tissues, suggesting that changes in protein turnover in skeletal muscle are responsible. Urea appearance was also increased by diuretics in sodium-depleted, adrenalectomized rats, excluding a role for glucocorticoids or epinephrine.

Persistent azotemia despite normal GFR and moderate dietary protein intake has been described in occasional patients, suggesting altered urea transport. Conte et al. described 14 such subjects who had increased urinary osmolarity and free water reabsorption, localizing the defect to the papillary collecting duct.[87] They suggested that reduced renal prostaglandin E_2 production may participate by altering medullary urea recycling.

The nitrogen-sparing effect of glucose is well documented in fasting subjects and animals and has been attributed to inhibition of the release of amino acids from peripheral tissues (e.g., muscle). Although substrate supply to the liver is clearly a regulator of urea production, a recent study in normal subjects demonstrated that glucose infusion also spares nitrogen by diminishing the ureagenic response of the liver, in part by inhibiting hepatic gluconeogenesis and probably by suppressing urea cycle activity.[88] On the other hand, glucose infusion into septic patients has failed to reduce urea production or hepatic gluconeogenesis,[89] so the utility of glucose infusions in sparing nitrogen in various catabolic conditions, including uremia, remains unsettled.

In isolated hepatocytes from CRF rats, urea production from gluconeogenic amino acids, alanine, glutamine, and serine has been shown to be increased, yet gluconeogenesis was decreased.[90] The former was associated with increased activity of glutaminase and serine hydratase; the carbons accumulated as lactate, pyruvate, and glutamate. Interestingly, metabolic acidosis also increased ureagenesis from glutamine in this same system, and when phlorhizin was given to normal rats in order to increase the plasma glucagon/insulin ratio, isolated hepatocytes exhibited metabolism similar to that of hepatocytes from uremic rats. However, these changes were seen only with pharmacologic concentrations of amino acids (10 mM); since the K_m values for these enzymes are in the millimolar range, it appears that the proposed changes in enzyme activity caused by uremia would have only minor effects on amino acid utilization.

Using the perfused hemicorpus preparation, Li and Wassner found that when CRF rats with mild azotemia were studied in the fed state, either in the presence or in the absence of insulin, muscle protein synthesis and degradation rates were normal.[91] In contrast, N-methylhistidine release, reflecting degradation of structural proteins, was clearly increased. When fasted, CRF rats lost more weight and had lower rates of protein synthesis, higher rates of protein degradation, and a greater degree of negative nitrogen balance. Body lipid content was decreased in CRF rats fed *ad libitum* and was correlated inversely with body weight and protein degradation, suggesting that decreased adipose stores may contribute to the exaggerated catabolic response occurring during periods of stress (e.g., fasting). This study extends our appreciation of how intercurent stress, such as starvation, may result in impaired growth and enhanced protein catabolism in uremia.

In contrast to Li and Wassner's report, Davis *et al.* reported that CRF increases muscle protein degradation *in vitro* but does not alter protein synthesis.[92] Exercise training reduced the elevated muscle protein catabolism caused by acute exercise and/or uremia, and it augmented the action of insulin on muscle protein turnover. These data add further support for a beneficial effect of exercise on intermediary metabolism. They also provide support for a postreceptor defect in insulin action.

Work from our laboratory has highlighted the importance of metabolic acidosis on muscle protein turnover and amino acid metabolism. When metabolic acidosis was induced in normal rats by gavage-feeding diets with or without ammonium chloride (NH_4Cl), acidosis stunted growth and increased urinary nitrogen and corticosterone excretion. Acidosis also increased protein degradation in incubated muscle by a glucocorticoid-dependent mechanism; it had no effect on muscle protein synthesis.[93] Since muscle glutamine production was not stimulated, it was suggested that proteolysis may play a role in the defense against metabolic acidosis by providing amino acid nitrogen from muscle which is converted to glutamine by the liver. To examine the role of metabolic acidosis in the abnormal protein metabolism of CRF, May *et al.* compared CRF rats (BUN 110 mg/dl) with spontaneous metabolic acidosis ($HCO_3 < 21$ mM) to pair-fed, sham-operated rats.[94] CRF was associated with increased urea appearance and corticosterone excretion, enhanced muscle protein degradation, and diminished insulin-stimulated protein synthesis. Sodium bicarbonate corrected the increased rate of muscle protein degradation, even though corticosterone excretion remained elevated and axotemia was unchanged. In contrast, sodium bicarbonate did not improve the defect in insulin-stimulated muscle protein synthesis.

Branched-chain amino acid (BCAA) metabolism is abnormal in uremia and ketoacidosis, two catabolic conditions associated with metabolic acidosis. To determine whether acidosis *per se* influenced BCAA, as well as protein metabolism in muscle, gavage-fed normal rats were given either NH_4Cl or NH_4 acetate.[95] Metabolic acidosis (mean HCO_3 = 19 mM) was associated with a significant reduction in plasma and muscle intracellular BCAA levels and with increased oxidation of valine and leucine. These differences were associated with an increase in the activated form and total enzyme concentration of branched-chain ketoacid dehydrogenase (BCKAD), the rate-limiting enzyme for BCAA metabolism in muscle. It was concluded that acidosis increases BCAA flux through the transminase and directly stimulates oxidative catabolism. Similarly, the spontaneous metabolic acidosis accompanying CRF was associated with decreased plasma BCAA and lower intracellular valine concentrations, as well as increased muscle BCAA oxidation.[96] Correction of the metabolic acidosis of CRF by $NaHCO_3$ normalized the elevated rate of BCAA decarboxylation; there also was an increase in plasma and intracellular BCAA concentrations. Thus, in CRF, even mild metabolic acidosis appears to cause important alterations in protein and amino acid metabolism, providing experimental evidence for the observation that sodium bicarbonate improves nitrogen balance in uremic patients.[97]

Ketoacids have been shown to serve as dietary substitutes for the corresponding EAA and are utilized therapeutically as supplements to protein-restricted diets in patients with CRF. Once ingested, KA are transaminated to yield their respective EAA, or irreversibly oxidized; the fate varies depending on the tissue, nutritional status, and coexistence of other diseases. Because these variables influence the nutritional efficiency of KA, it would be important to assess the efficiency of substitution. Recently, a clever, yet simple, method for assessing the nutritional efficiency of KAs has been devised and shown to yield the same results as growth experiments. By comparing the ratio of orally administered, radiolabeled KA and EAA to their ratio in body protein, the nutritional efficiency (R value) of the administered KA can be determined. Using this technique, Tungsanga *et al.*[98] reported that alpha-ketoisocaproate (KIC), the ketoanalog of leucine, was utilized more efficiently by CRF rats than by pair-fed controls. The R value varied from tissue to tissue (range 0.59–0.81) in CRF animals; an average whole-body value indicated that approximately 64% more KIC than leucine would be required in CRF, as opposed to 104% more in control animals. The reason for the better utilization of KIC as a precursor for leucine in CRF is not clear. It was also reported that the nutritional efficiency of KIC relative to leucine in normal rats varied inversely with dietary protein intake,[99] and that the whole-body nutritional efficiency of KIC could be predicted confidently from the R values determined in protein from kidney and muscle (R^2 = 0.99). Since BCKAD activity (the enzyme responsible for irreversible BCAA decarboxylation) is proportional to dietary protein intake, it is likely that the decreased efficiency with higher protein intakes reflects, in part, changes in BCKAD activity.

KA are typically provided either as the calcium or basic amino acid salts; whether nutritional efficiency differs between these two salts has not been examined. Funk *et al.* compared growth of rats and concluded that the basic amino acids used with BCAA ketoacids do not significantly affect utilization of the KA, with the possible exception of the lysine salt of KIC.[100] However, the relative inefficiency of this latter compound may simply have reflected the lower food intake of rats fed this supplement when compared to those receiving the ornithine or histidine KIC salts. Overall, nutritional efficiency of KA, when compared to their respective EAA, was 40–50%.

Over the last few years, the validity of the traditional concept of nutritionally indispensable amino acids has been questioned. It has become clear that some "nonessential" amino acids may become indispensable under certain clinical conditions and that nitrogen balance, as well as growth, are improved when both essential and nonessential amino acid nitrogen are provided. Laidlow and Kopple[101] have summarized the evidence supporting this viewpoint and have offered a modification of Jackson's[102] classification of indispensable amino acids based on insights gained from recent improvements in our understanding of the biochemistry and metabolism of the amino acids.

3.3. Lipid Metabolism

Previous editions[1,13] have discussed in depth the plasma lipid patterns in uremic hyperlipidemia, their pathogenesis, and therapeutic strategies. Little insight has been gained in this area over the past 2 years, but we will highlight several reports of particular interest.

Cholesterol transport from cell membranes to plasma, its esterification by lecithin cholesterol acetyltransferase (LCAT) [associated with high-density lipoprotein (HDL)], and its subsequent transfer to low-density lipoprotein (LDL) and very-low-density lipoprotein (VLDL) is important in the maintenance of cholesterol homeostasis. These processes are dependent on (1) the concentration gradient for nonesterified cholesterol between cell membranes and plasma, which is maintained by LCAT reaction, and (2) the gradient for cholesterol at the surface of VLDL and LDL. An elegant study by Dieplinger *et al.* examined the metabolism of cholesterol in normolipemic patients with ESRD receiving maintenance hemodialysis or CAPD.[103] Using an *in vitro*, fibroblast-based system, a reversed net transport of cholesterol from plasma to cells was demonstrated in hemodialysis patients. This was due to two distinct effects: (1) a low rate of cholesterol ester formation due to a reduction in circulating, activated LCAT, and (2) ineffective transfer of cholesterol esters to VLDL and LDL due to saturation of these lipoproteins with cholesterol. In contrast, CAPD patients had normal lipoprotein composition and cholesterol metabolic rates. The reason for the differences seen with the differing modes of dialytic therapy is unknown, but highlights a potentially important defect in cholesterol metabolism that is present even in normolipemic hemodialysis patients. The study did not address whether abnormalities in cholesterol metabolism are present in hyperlipemic CAPD subjects, a frequent occurrence in that population.

Recent studies have suggested that plasma levels of apolipoproteins may be better predictors of coronary artery disease than plasma lipids. Accordingly, Attman *et al.* have documented the presence of a characteristic lipoprotein profile in hyperlipidemic, predialysis CRF patients; the pattern differs from that of normal or nonuremic type IV hyperlipidemic subjects.[104] If confirmed, this pattern might be used to predict the risk of atherosclerotic complications in hyperlipidemic uremic subjects.

Hyperlipidemia is characteristic of the nephrotic syndrome[1,13] and is due to a combination of increased hepatic synthesis and reduced clearance of lipids. Since serum lipids are negatively correlated with serum protein concentrations, it seems logical that hyperlipidemia reflects a coordinate increase in both albumin and lipoprotein synthesis. Surprisingly, a recent study indicates that serum cholesterol and, to a large degree, triglyceride levels are independent of the rate of albumin synthesis; the major determinant of albumin synthesis was the degree of proteinuria.[105]

3.4. Treatment of Hyperlipidemia

Although the contribution of hyperlipidemia to arteriosclerosis in nephrotic patients is controversial, the association of coronary disease and hyperlipidemia in otherwise normal subjects has prompted investigators to explore potential therapeutic strategies in nephrotic subjects. Probucol and colestipol, utilized in short-term studies, reportedly reduce total and LDL cholesterol levels and exert variable changes in serum triglycerides.[106,107] Unfortunately, serum HDL cholesterol levels were also reduced by probucol, thereby tempering enthusiasm.

In view of evidence suggesting that potentially atherogenic remnant lipoproteins (IDL) accumulate in uremia,[13] a drug such as clofibrate, which enhances the catabolism of VLDL and IDL to LDL, should benefit hyperlipidemic, CRF patients. Clofibrate has been used to treat hyperlipidemia in CRF patients, but muscle toxicity and a potential for accelerating renal failure have been reported.[1,13] Gemfibrozil, a recently marketed analog of clofibrate, was given for 7 months to 18 CRF patients with hypercholesterolemia and hypertriglyceridemia in a single-blind crossover study design.[108] Therapy was associated with a 50% reduction in VLDL cholesterol and triglycerides and a 30% increase in HDL-C; lipoprotein changes occurred concomitantly with normalization of postheparin lipoprotein and hepatic lipases, just as with clofibrate. Unfortunately, 30% of the patients developed modest, but reversible elevations in serum CPK, and a muscle biopsy from one patient revealed focal necrosis of muscle fibers.

A VLPD diet supplemented with a KA mixture has been shown to significantly reduce serum triglycerides in patients when compared to values measured during therapy with a conventional low-protein diet or maintenance hemodialysis.[109] Since information on dietary composition and compliance was not provided, the influence of nonprotein dietary factors cannot be excluded. The salutary effect on serum triglycerides may also reflect improvement in insulin resistance and hyperparathyroidism, both of which have been reported with ketoacid-based regimens.[1,13,81]

Because of epidemiologic evidence reporting a low incidence of arteriosclerosis in populations consuming diets rich in omega-3 polyunsaturated fatty acids (fish oil) as well as their salutary effect on plasma lipids and platelet function, much interest has been generated into their therapeutic utility for reducing cardiovascular risk in selected populations.[110] When hemodialysis patients eating a normal diet received 20 ml/day (3.6 g) of fish oil (Max EPA) for 8 weeks, they experienced a 35% increase in HDL_2-C and a 35% decrease in serum triglycerides; there also was a significant reduction in blood pressure and platelet reactivity.[111] Therapy had to be discontinued because of flatulence and diarrhea in 20% of the patients, but the doses used were probably too high. Although these preliminary results are encouraging, long-term efficacy, dosage requirements, and effects on renal function are needed before supplemental fish oil can be recommended.

Interestingly, a diet rich in monounsaturated fats appears to be at least as effective in lowering total LDL cholesterol in hypercholesteremic subjects as a low-fat diet containing equal quantities of saturated, monosaturated, or polyunsaturated fatty acids.[112] In fact, whereas the high-monounsaturated diet did not change serum triglycerides or HDL-C, a low-fat diet raised triglycerides and reduced HDL-C. The increased carbohydrate content of the isocaloric low-fat diet probably is responsible for the latter, since isocaloric substitution of carbohydrate for fat increases plasma triglycerides.[1,13] The results emphasize our limited understanding of how various types of dietary fat change plasma lipids.

In summary, until it is settled whether hyperlipidemia in patients with CRF truly contributes to their excess cardiovascular morbidity and mortality, we can only advocate exercise and reducing the content of saturated fat to a P/S ratio greater than or equal to 1.[13]

4. Nutritional Management of CRF Patients

The therapeutic goal of conservative management of CRF patients includes correction of hypertension, metabolic acidosis, and calcium–phosphorus metabolism plus restriction of dietary protein to a level compatible with maintenance of body protein stores. Although previous studies emphasize the common occurrence of protein–calorie malnutrition in patients entering maintenance hemodialysis, if patients are closely monitored while consuming protein-restricted regimens that produce neutral nitrogen balance, indices of nutrition are maintained during long-term therapy.[1,13] Assessment of nutritional status in CRF is complicated by a lack of appropriate reference values, and factors other than nutritional status can influence the parameters being monitored.[1,13] Furthermore, recent reports[36,113] suggest there can be a dichotomy between changes in anthropometrics and plasma proteins, making nutritional evaluation even more difficult. No single parameter provides a reliable index of nutritional state, but multiple indices provide a more accurate assessment of nutrition. We recommend serial weights, anthropometric measurements, serum albumin, and transferrin to monitor patients treated with low-protein diets.[114] Clearly, additional research using complementary, reproducible measures of nutritional status are needed to assess accurately the long-term nutritional response to dietary manipulation.

The application of stable isotope technology to assess amino acid and protein requirements and mechanisms of adaptation to changes in dietary protein intake represents a new technique.[115] The method is based on a continuous infusion of isotopically labeled (nonradioactive) essential amino acids (most commonly, leucine) and provides an estimate of the rates of whole-body protein synthesis, degradation, and oxidation. In view of the limitations of the nitrogen balance method, measurement of amino acid turnover allows independent assessment of homeostatic processes and can provide insight into mechanisms of adaptation to dietary manipulation.[115] For example, the major adaptations in normal subjects to a surplus of dietary protein are to increase amino acid oxidation markedly and protein synthesis modestly (especially in response to feeding). When dietary protein is clearly inadequate, the major metabolic response appears to be a marked reduction in whole-body protein synthesis and degradation, with a smaller decrease in amino acid oxidation; these responses result in more efficient utilization of dietary amino acids.[116] The mechanisms of adaptation to dietary protein restriction in CRF and whether abnormalities may contribute to protein wasting in uremic subjects have only recently begun to be examined.

Hou *et al.* reported that predialysis CRF subjects have a reduced flux of [^{15}N]glycine or of [^{15}N]NH$_4$Cl while consuming 1.2 g/kg per day of protein, and, paradoxically, when intake was reduced to 0.6 g/kg per day, whole-body glycine flux and estimates of protein synthesis and catabolism increased markedly to values approaching those of normal subjects.[117] In the same report, protein turnover in normal subjects did not change when protein intake was reduced, even though the subjects were in negative nitrogen balance. The explanation for these findings is obscure.

When well-nourished adult hemodialysis patients consuming the recommended dietary allowance of protein (1.0 g/kg per day and 30–40 kcal/kg per day) were compared with matched postabsorptive normal subjects, protein synthesis was lower, protein breakdown was normal, and leucine oxidation was increased. It was concluded that increased amino acid oxidation and decreased protein synthesis contribute to muscle wasting in hemodialysis patients.[118]

In the fed state, leucine oxidation was found to be lower both preceding and at 3 months after institution of CAPD when compared to values obtained in normal subjects. Whole-body leucine flux and protein breakdown decreased slightly, but protein synthesis was not different from rates measured in normal subjects. Before and at 3 months after beginning CAPD, anthropometrics and total body potassium were normal, but serum protein levels declined and plasma amino acid abnormalities worsened. As previous studies have suggested that CAPD patients need at least 1.1 and preferably 1.2–1.3 g/kg per day of protein,[119] the protein intake of CAPD patients in this study (0.96 g/kg per day) could explain why amino acid oxidation decreased and why there was a trend toward reduced leucine flux and protein breakdown. If this were true, it would suggest that adaptive mechanisms are intact in CAPD patients.

Although protein–calorie malnutrition may be common in dialysis patients, longitudinal evaluation suggests that when subjects adhere to the prescribed dietary intake, nutritional status is maintained.[1,13,120] During long-term follow-up nutritional indices may decline, particularly in CAPD patients consuming less than 1.2 g/kg per day of protein and inadequate calories.[121] Cell-mediated immunity assessed by skin testing improved with the institution of CAPD, and the frequency of peritonitis was greater in CAPD patients with hypoalbuminemia, suggesting an impairment in humoral immunity due to malnutrition.[121]

Therapeutic benefits of exercise training for hemodialysis subjects are well recognized.[1,13] When patients have persisted in an exercise program, exercise capacity, anemia, blood pressure, hyperlipidemia, glucose intolerance, and depression have improved.[122–124] A concern that exercise might aggravate metabolic acidosis and electrolyte abnormalities (specifically, hyperkalemia) has not been substantiated, even in subjects taking concomitant beta-blockers.[125,126] Interestingly, following transplantation, exercise capacity increases significantly, a finding that is not explained by conditioning or by changes in hematocrit, suggesting an inhibitory effect of uremia *per se.*[127,128]

5. Nephrotic Syndrome

High-protein diets (HPD) have been recommended for nephrotic patients in an attempt to increase albumin synthesis. The appropriateness of this recommendation is questionable in view of recent reports.[129] When albumin turnover and excretion were determined in nine nephrotic subjects being fed sequentially 1.6 (HPD) or 0.8 [low-protein diet (LPD)] g/kg per day of protein and 35 kcal/kg per day for 10–14 days, the LPD diet was associated with a significant reduction in albumin excretion (mean −2.74 g, range 0.1–7.4 g/day) and a modest increase in serum albumin (+0.2 g/dl). Albumin synthesis was decreased by LPD diet and was more than offset by a concomitant decrease in albumin catabolism and fractional albumin excretion. The reduction in fractional albumin excretion with dietary protein restriction suggests an improvement in glomerular hemodynamics or permselectivity properties, supporting the work of Rosenberg *et al.*[57] Albumin synthesis increased significantly with the HPD diet; unfortunately, half the albumin synthesized appeared in the urine. It might be expected that since albumin mass was preserved with the LPD and since albumin is often used to assess nutritional status, body protein stores were also preserved. However, it is entirely possible that body protein stores are degraded in catabolic conditions and that the amino acids are used to synthesize new visceral proteins; i.e., there can be a dichotomy between albumin turnover and that of other body proteins. Consequently, simultaneous measurements of nitrogen balance and other indices of nutritional status are needed before dietary protein restriction can be recommended for nephrotic patients. If safety were confirmed, the study would be especially important since nephrotic range proteinuria is suggested to be a poor prognostic sign in some glomerular diseases. Consequently, it is possible that the use of LPD to reduce proteinuria in nephrosis may favorably influence prognosis. Only control trials can answer this important question.

Angiotensin II (AII) has been implicated as an important modulator of glomerular hemodynamics and permselectivity, in both normal and disease states (see Sections 2.1.3 and 2.2.1). In rats with partial renal vein constriction, saralasin infusion almost eliminated proteinuria.[130] Regarding patients, Rosenberg et al.[57] noted improved glomerular permselectivity in adults with glomerular disease following institution of LPD. The improvement was associated with a reduced activity of the renin system and increased prostaglandin excretion. Further support for AII-mediated changes in glomerular function affecting proteinuria comes from experimental studies with ACE inhibitors. The report that proteinuria in nephrotic diabetic subjects decreases with captopril therapy has been confirmed in patients with other types of renal diseases.[131,132] Although mean arterial pressure and GFR fell with lisinopril, the fractional excretion of albumin decreased, suggesting improved glomerular hemodynamics or permselectivity. The finding that the fall in urinary protein is positively correlated with both the reduction in filtration fraction and renal vascular resistance was interpreted as being consistent with decreased intraglomerular pressures. Of note, in 8 of 13 patients, serum potassium increased >5.8 mM/liter.

In experimental nephrosis as well, albuminuria is reduced by dietary protein restriction and enalapril therapy.[133] When enalapril was given to nephrotic rats eating 40% protein, albumin excretion decreased to a level seen in rats fed 8% protein; enalapril did not reduce albuminuria in nephrotic rats fed 8% protein. In another protocol, proteinuria was reduced by enalapril therapy, even when instituted after proteinuria was already established. The rapidity with which proteinuria was reduced by ACE inhibitors after established nephrosis and the similarity between the response to ACE inhibitors and LPD therapy suggest that both therapies modify urinary albumin excretion by a similar mechanism. Whether this is related to AII, prostaglandin synthesis, or bradykinin degradation is unknown.

Prostaglandin synthesis inhibitors also decrease proteinuria, although the reduction is modest in some instances unless the individuals are sodium-depleted.[134] Attempts to determine the mechanism have yielded conflicting results; changes in GFR do not appear to be responsible.[135] Nephrotic patients treated with alternate-day steroids have significantly more proteinuria on treatment days.[136] This observation may be explained by a change in glomerular hemodynamics.[24]

6. Vitamins and Trace Elements

6.1. Vitamins

Water-soluble vitamins have been recommended for uremic patients based on studies demonstrating an intake below the recommended daily allowance, decreased intestinal absorption, impaired cellular function, circulating inhibitors, or increased losses during dialytic treatment.[1,13] A recent study has questioned the need for a water-soluble vitamin supplement in hemodialysis patients. When patients were followed for 1 year without a vitamin supplement, average values for blood and red blood cell levels of folate, niacin, vitamins B_1, B_6, and B_{12}, and vitamin C were normal.[137] Although the blood levels of several vitamins decreased significantly following discontinuance of the vitamin supplement, the values stabilized within 6 months, and most of the patients were able, by diet alone, to maintain normal levels. A few individuals were found to have blood levels of folate, B_6, thiamine, and niacin below the normal range. Clearly, further research in this area is needed to quantitate actual intake and dialytic losses.

Hemodialysis patients have elevated blood oxalate levels without vitamin C supplementation, but with vitamin C, the levels rise even further.[138] Moreover, in one hemodialysis patient who decided to take 2.6 g of vitamin C daily for 7 years, excessive oxalate deposition was noted in a bone biopsy.[139]

In summary, the need for water-soluble vitamins for many hemodialysis patients has been questioned recently, and clarification of this issue is needed. At present, we recommend that a water-soluble vitamin supplement formulated to meet the estimated requirements of renal patients (e.g., Nephrocaps) be given. In view of the reports of peripheral nephropathy and hyperoxaloemia with high-dose pyridoxine therapy and vitamin C supplementation, respectively, "megavitamin" therapy should be avoided.[1,13]

In contrast to water-soluble vitamins, plasma vitamin A (retinol) levels are invariably increased in CRF patients.[1,13] Since its specific carrier protein, retinol-binding protein, is also increased in uremia, free retinol levels are normal; tissue levels of vitamin A are reported to be normal, increased, or decreased. Whether vitamin A actually contributes to anemia, dry skin, pruritus, and possibly hepatic dysfunction in uremia is still controversial.[1,13] Vitamin A toxicity has been reported in three CRF patients receiving parenteral nutrition, including a standard multivitamin supplementation (containing 1500 μg vitamin A); toxicity resolved with discontinuance of the vitamin supplementation.[140] It is generally agreed that vitamin A supplements should not be given to CRF patients, and vitamin supplements for parenteral nutrition solutions should be screened for vitamin A before use in CRF patients.

When the water supply of a dialysis unit was found to contain excess chlorine and patients exhibited evidence of oxidant-induced hemolytic anemia, vitamin E levels were found to be reduced.[141] Vitamin E levels normalized upon removal of chloramine, suggesting that vitamin E was important as an antioxidant in this setting. Increased erythrocyte membrane lipid peroxidation associated with decreased erythrocyte vitamin E levels has also been reported, and it was suggested that oxidant stress to membranes may be, in part, responsible for an increased red cell turnover in uremia.[142] Since plasma vitamin E levels have generally been reported as normal and since it has not been documented that vitamin E supplements increase erythrocyte survival, we cannot recommend vitamin E supplementation.

6.2. Trace Elements

The literature on trace elements in uremia is controversial and may reflect differences in analysis technique and/or standardization.[1] Although zinc deficiency has been suggested to be responsible for certain uremic symptoms and supplemental zinc may improve taste and immune function, the data are not uniform.[1,13] Following an oral zinc challenge, diminished zinc absorption was seen in hemodialysis patients compared to normal subjects. Coadministration of ferrous sulfate or aluminum hydroxide inhibited zinc absorption 28 and 75%, respectively, suggesting that these commonly prescribed agents may further impair zinc absorption in uremia.[143]

Tissue distribution of trace elements is abnormal in postmortem studies of uremic patients, although in most instances, it is not clear whether these abnormalities are clinically important.[13] In one group of hemodialysis patients, plasma nickel levels were markedly elevated, which was attributed to a contaminated dialysate water supply.[1] Elevated plasma cobalt levels are correlated with left ventricular dysfunction in uremic subjects.[1,13] In CAPD patients, plasma and erythrocyte bromide levels were found to be low, possibly because of dialysate losses, while very high (20- to 50-fold) serum chromium levels could be linked to high concentrations in the dialysate.[144] In summary, abnormalities in the concentration and distribution of trace elements can occur in uremia, but their clinical importance has not yet been demonstrated. It would seem prudent that dialysis water and peritoneal dialysate be closely monitored for excessive concentrations of trace elements.

7. Nutrition and Renal Transplantation

Whether a patient's nutritional status improves following successful transplantation has not been carefully examined. When dialysis patients were followed for 23 ± 24 months after successful transplantation (mean serum creatinine 1.6), they exhibited a significant increase in body weight, and in diabetic patients, serum albumin also improved significantly.[145] Prior to transplantation, diabetic patients appeared more malnourished than nondiabetic subjects (81 ± 8 vs. $91 \pm 15\%$ of ideal weight, respectively) and despite improvements in both groups following transplantation, weight was still significantly less in diabetic patients ($95 \pm 9\%$ vs. $108 \pm 16\%$). A surprisingly high percentage of the patients with or without diabetes (25 and 50%, respectively) had mean upper arm muscle circumference values below the fifth percentile, suggesting that a substantial prevalence of protein depletion remained posttransplantation. The mean prednisone dose averaged 17 mg/day at the time of evaluation and may have contributed to these findings. It will be important in future studies to follow patient longitudinally from transplantation utilizing several independent measures (Section 4) to assess the long-term nutritional response to successful renal transplantation.

Interestingly, body adipose distribution and skeletal muscle ultrastructure are altered by glucocorticoid therapy.[146] When body adiposity was assessed by computed tomography, the pattern in dialysis patients mimicked that seen in transplant patients and subjects with other diseases taking glucocorticoids. Sex-related differences in body adiposity were absent in patients receiving prednisone or being treated by dialysis. Although it is commonly assumed that glucocorticoids result in truncal obesity at the expense of peripheral stores, midthigh fat area was normal or increased, while estimates of muscle area were reduced in dialysis and renal transplant recipients.[146] Thus, corticosteroids, uremia, and the nutritional state can all adversely influence nutriture in transplant patients.

Renal transplant patients receiving maintenance doses of prednisone have a 30% reduction in the cross-sectional area of muscle fibers due predominantly to a decrease in myofibril volume; intracellular glycogen and lipid concentrations were increased 20 and 70%, respectively.[147] It was suggested that the decrease in muscle myofibrils might contribute to muscle weakness seen in some renal transplant recipients.

8. Acute Renal Failure

Little information is available on changes in plasma amino acid concentrations or the pharmacokinetics of their elimination in acute renal failure (ARF). When Druml *et al.* administered a standard parenteral amino acid solution to 12 clinically stable patients with ARF, characteristic alterations in the plasma aminogram and elimination profiles were seen.[148] Specific defects in metabolism accounting for these abnormalities were not identified, but the results suggest that standard amino acid preparations based on ''Rose'' requirements can adversely influence the plasma amino acid profile.

Defective amino acid transport might be one factor contributing to the abnormal amino acid concentrations and distributions seen in acute uremia. Since protein synthesis is dependent on an adequate supply of intracellular amino acids, defective amino acid transport could prove rate-limiting. To examine whether impaired amino acid transport into muscle is part of the ARF syndrome, the function of specific transporters was measured. Since insulin stimulates neutral amino acid transport in most tissues exclusively through System A, Maroni *et al.* confirmed the specificity of methylaminoisobutyrate for System A in muscle and investigated the influence of acute uremia on this transport system.[149] In the absence or presence of insulin, System A transport was significantly reduced in muscle from acutely uremic rats, yet the percent stimulation by insulin was similar to that in control muscle. Likewise, the insulin dose–response relationship confirmed that physiologic concentrations of insulin increased transport to a similar degree; at pharmacologic concentrations of insulin, there was a plateau in System A transport in ARF, but not in controls. ARF caused no detectable abnormality in the other two neutral amino acid transport systems, ASC and L.[150] Therefore, the major abnormality in transport appeared to be a depressed basal rate of System A transport, whereas stimulation of System A by physiologic concentrations of insulin was preserved. The degree of the defect makes it unlikely that changes in amino acid transport contribute to defective protein synthesis in muscle.

The level of dietary protein intake consumed before induction of renal ischemia reportedly has a dramatic influence on the degree of subsequent renal damage.[151] Whereas 70–90% of animals maintained on 20 or 60% protein died within days following renal ischemia, 90% of animals consuming 5% protein chow before ischemia survived. The maximum degree of protection required about 1 week of a low-protein diet before ischemia. Unfortunately, changing the diet immediately following ischemia had no influence on renal function or survival.

References

1. Druml, W. and Mitch, W. E., 1987, Nutrition in renal disease, in: *Contemporary Nephrology*, Volume 4 (S. Klahr and S. G. Massry, eds.), Plenum Press, New York.
2. Nath, K. A., Kren, S. M., and Hostetter, T. H., 1986, Dietary protein restriction in established renal injury in the rat. Selective role of glomerular capillary pressure in progressive glomerular dysfunction, *J. Clin. Invest.* **78**:1199.
3. Hostetter, T. H., Meyer, T. W., Rennke, H. G., and Brenner, B. M. 1986, Chronic effects of dietary protein in the rat with intact and reduced renal mass, *Kidney Int.* **30**:509.
4. Okuda, S., Motomura, K., Sanai, T., Tsuruda, H., Oh, Y., Onoyama, K., and Fujishima, M., 1987, Influence of age on deterioration of the remnant kidney in uninephrectomized rats, *Clin. Sci.* **72**:571.
5. Friedman, A. L. and Pityer, R., 1986, Beneficial effect of moderate protein restriction on growth, renal function and survival in young rats with chronic renal failure, *J. Nutr.* **116**:2466.
6. Okuda, S., Motomura, K., Sanai, T., Hirakata, H., Nanishi, F., Onoyama, K., and Fujishima, M., 1987, Effect of different levels of protein intake on renal deterioration and nutritional state in experimental renal disease, *Clin. Sci.* **73**:33.
7. El Nahas, A. M., Zoob, S. N., Evans, D. J., and Rees, A. J., 1987, Chronic renal failure after nephrotoxic nephritis in rats: Contributions to progression, *Kidney Int.* **32**:173.
8. Williams, A. J., Baker, F., and Walls, J., 1987, Effect of varying quantity and quality of dietary protein intake in experimental renal disease in rats, *Nephron* **46**:83.
9. Stahl, R. A. K., Kudelka, S., and Helmchen, U., 1987, High protein intake stimulates glomerular prostaglandin formation in remnant kidneys, *Am. J. Physiol.* **252**:F1083.
10. Fernandez-Repollet, E., Tapia, E., and Martinez-Maldonado, M., 1987, Effects of angiotensin-converting enzyme inhibition on altered renal hemodynamics induced by low protein diet in the rat, *J. Clin. Invest.* **80**:1045.
11. Seney, F. D., Jr., Persson, A. E. G., and Wright, F. S., 1987, Modification of tubuloglomerular feedback signal by dietary protein, *Am. J. Physiol.* **252**:F83.
12. Robertson, J. L., Goldschmidt, M., Kronfeld, D. S., Tomaszewski, J. E., Hill, G. S., and Bovee,

K. C., 1986, Long-term renal responses to high dietary protein in dogs with 75% nephrectomy, *Kidney Int.* **29:**511.

13. Maroni, B. J. and Mitch, W. E., 1985, Nutrition in renal disease in: *Contemporary Nephrology,* Volume 3 (S. Klahr and S. G. Massry, eds.), Plenum Press, New York.

14. Lumlertgul, D., Burke, T. J., Gillum, D. M., Alfrey, A. C., Harris, D. C., Hammond, W. S., and Schrier, R. W., 1986, Phosphate depletion arrests progression of chronic renal failure independent of protein intake, *Kidney Int.* **29:**658.

15. Harris, D. C. H., Chan, L., and Schrier, R. W., 1988, Remnant kidney hypermetabolism and progression of chronic renal failure, *Am. J. Physiol.* **254:**F267.

16. Kleinknecht, C., Laouari, D., Hinglais, N., Habib, R., Dodu, C., Lacour, B., and Broyer, M., 1986, Role of amount and nature of carbohydrates in the course of experimental renal failure, *Kidney Int.* **30:**687.

17. Kasiske, B. L., Cleary, M. P., O'Donnell, M. P., and Keane, W. F., 1986, Effects of carbohydrate restriction on renal injury on the obese Zucker rat, *Am. J. Clin. Nutr.* **44:**56.

18. Diamond, J. R. and Karnovsky, M. J., 1987, Exacerbation of chronic aminonucleoside nephrosis by dietary cholesterol supplementation, *Kidney Int.* **32:**671.

19. Scharschmidt, L. A., Gibbons, N. B., McGarry, L., Berger, P., Axelrod, M., Janis, R., and Ko, Y. H., 1987, Effects of dietary fish oil on renal insufficiency in rats with subtotal nephrectomy, *Kidney Int.* **32:**700.

20. Heifets, M., Morrissey, J. J., Purkerson, M. L., Morrison, A. R., and Klahr, S., 1987, Effect of dietary lipids on renal function in rats with subtotal nephrectomy, *Kidney Int.* **32:**335.

21. Anderson, S., Rennke, H. G., and Brenner, B. M., 1986, Therapeutic advantage of converting enzyme inhibitors in arresting progressive renal disease associated with systemic hypertension in the rat, *J. Clin. Invest.* **77:**1993.

22. Meyer, T. W., Anderson, S., Rennke, H. G., and Brenner, B. M., 1987, Reversing glomerular hypertension stabilizes established glomerular injury, *Kidney Int.* **31:**752.

23. Beukers, J. J. B., van der Wal, A., Hoedemaeker, P. J., and Weening, J. J., 1987, Converting enzyme inhibition and progressive glomerulosclerosis in the rat, *Kidney Int.* **32:**794.

24. Garcia, D. L., Rennke, H. G., Brenner, B. M., and Anderson, S., 1987, Chronic glucocorticoid therapy amplifies glomerular injury in rats with renal ablation, *J. Clin. Invest.* **80:**867.

25. Burke, T. J., Arnold, P. E., Gordon, J. A., Bulger, R. E., Dobyan, D. C., and Schrier, R. W., 1984, Protective effect of intrarenal calcium membrane blockers before or after renal ischemia, *J. Clin. Invest.* **74:**1830.

26. Goligorsky, M. S., Chaimovitz, C., Rapaport, J., Goldstein, J., and Kol, R., 1985, Calcium metabolism in uremic nephrocalcinosis: Preventive effect of verapamil, *Kidney Int.* **27:**774.

27. Harris, D. C. H., Hammond, W. S., Burke, T. J., and Schrier, R. W., 1987, Verapamil protects against progression of experimental chronic renal failure, *Kidney Int.* **31:**41.

28. Heifets, M., Davis, T. A., Tegtmeyer, E., and Klahr, S., 1987, Exercise training ameliorates progressive renal disease in rats with subtotal nephrectomy, *Kidney Int.* **32:**815.

29. Zatz, R., Dunn, B. R., Meyer, T. W., Anderson, S., Rennke, H. G., and Brenner, B. M., 1986, Prevention of diabetic glomerulopathy by pharmacological amelioration of glomerular capillary hypertension, *J. Clin. Invest.* **77:**1925.

30. Jensen, P. K., Christiansen, J. S., Steven, K., and Parving, H. H., 1987, Strict metabolic control and renal function in the streptozotocin diabetic rat, *Kidney Int.* **31:**47.

31. Bank, N., Klose, R., Aynedjian, H. S., Nguyen, D., and Sablay, L. B., 1987, Evidence against increased glomerular pressure initiating diabetic nephropathy, *Kidney Int.* **31:**898.

32. Bank, N., Lahorra, M. A., and Aynedjian, H. S., 1987, Acute effect of calcium and insulin on hyperfiltration of early diabetes, *Am. J. Physiol.* **252:**E13.

33. Bergstrom, J., Alvestrand, A., Bucht, H., and Gutierrez, A., 1986, Progression of chronic renal failure in man is retarded with more frequent clinical follow-ups and better blood pressure control, *Clin. Nephrol.* **25:**1.

34. Barsotti, G., Guiducci, A., Ciardella, F., and Giovannetti, S., 1981, Effects on renal function of a

low-nitrogen diet supplemented with essential amino acids and ketoanalogues and of hemodialysis and free protein supply in patients with chronic renal failure, *Nephron* **27**:113.

35. Walser, M., LaFrance, N. D., Ward, L., and VanDuyn, M. A., 1987, Progression of chronic renal failure in patients given ketoacids following amino acids, *Kidney Int.* **32**:123.

36. Lucas, P. A., Meadows, J. H., Roberts, D. E., and Coles, G. A., 1986, The risks and benefits of a low protein-essential amino acid–keto acid diet, *Kidney Int.* **29**:995.

37. Meisinger, E. and Strauch, M., 1987, Controlled trial of two keto acid supplements on renal function, nutritional status, and bone metabolism in uremic patients, *Kidney Int.* **22**:S-170.

38. Lindenau, K., Kokot, F., and Frohling, P. T., 1986, Suppression of parathyroid hormone by therapy with a mixture of keto analogues/amino acids in hemodialysis patients, *Nephron* **43**:84.

39. Maschio, G., Oldrizzi, L., Rugiu, C., Valvo, E., Lupo, A., Loschiavo, C., Tessitore, N., Fabris, A., Gammaro, L., and Panzetta, G., 1987, Factors affecting progression of renal failure in patients on long-term dietary protein restriction, *Kidney Int.* **32**:S-49.

40. Mitch, W. E., 1986, Measuring the rate of progression of renal insufficiency, in: *The Progressive Nature of Renal Disease* (W. E. Mitch, ed.), Churchill-Livingstone, New York.

41. Morelli, E., Baldi, R., Barsotti, G., Ciardella, F., Cupisti, A., Dani, L., Mantovanelli, A., and Giovannetti, S., 1987, Combined therapy for selected chronic uremic patients: Infrequent hemodialysis and nutritional management, *Nephron* **47**:161.

42. Mitch, W. E. and Sapir, D. G., 1981, An evaluation of reduced dialysis frequency using nutritional therapy, *Kidney Int.* **20**:122.

43. Bosch, J. P., Lauer, A., and Glabman, S., 1984, Short-term protein loading in assessment of patients with renal disease, *Am. J. Med.* **77**:873.

44. Hostetter, T. H., 1986, Human renal response to a meat meal, *Am. J. Physiol.* **250**:F613.

45. Schaap, G. H., Bilo, H. J. G., Alferink, T. H. R., Oe, P. L., and Donker, A. J. M., 1987, The effect of a high protein intake on renal function of patients with chronic renal insufficiency, *Nephron* **47**:1.

46. Viberti, G., Bognetti, E., Wiseman, M. J., Dodds, R., Gross, J. L., and Keen, H., 1987, Effect of a protein-restricted diet on renal response to a meat meal in humans, *Am. J. Physiol.* **253**:F388.

47. Rugiu, C., Oldrizzi, L., and Maschio, G., 1987, Effects of an oral protein load on glomerular filtration rate in patients with solitary kidneys, *Kidney Int.* **32**:S-29.

48. Bosch, J. P., Lew, S., Glabman, S., and Lauer, A., 1986, Renal hemodynamic changes in humans. Response to a protein loading in normal and diseased kidneys, *Am. J. Med.* **81**:809.

49. Kupin, W. L., Cortes, P., Dumler, F., Feldkamp, C. S., Kilates, M. C., and Levin, N. W., 1987, Effect on renal function of change from high to moderate protein intake in type I diabetic patients, *Diabetes* **36**:73.

50. Jones, M. G., Lee, K., and Swaminathan, R., 1987, The effect of dietary protein on glomerular filtration rate in normal subjects, *Clin. Nephrol.* **27**:71.

51. Williams, M., Young, J. B., Rosa, R. M., Gunn, S., Epstein, F. H., and Landsberg, L., 1986, Effect of protein ingestion on urinary dopamine excretion. Evidence for the functional importance of renal decarboxylation of circulating 3,4-dihydroxyphenylalanine in man, *J. Clin. Invest.* **78**:1687.

52. Castellino, P., Coda, B., and DeFronzo, R. A., 1986, Effect of amino acid infusion on renal hemodynamics in humans, *Am. J. Physiol.* **251**:F132.

53. Hirschberg, R. and Kopple, J. D., 1987, Role of growth hormone in the amino acid-induced acute rise in renal function in man, *Kidney Int.* **32**:382.

54. Premem, A. J., 1985, Importance of the liver during glucagon-mediated increases in canine renal hemodynamics, *Am. J. Physiol.* **249**:F319.

55. Dratwa, M., Burette, A., van Gossum, M., Collart, F., Wens, R., Charlier, L., Tielemans, C., and Deltenre, M., 1987, No rise in glomerular filtration rate after protein loading in cirrhotics, *Kidney Int.* **32**:S-32.

56. Ruilope, L. M., Rodicio, J., Robles, R. G., Sancho, J., Miranda, B., Granger, J. P., and Romero,

J. C., 1987, Influence of a low sodium diet on the renal response to amino acid infusions in humans, *Kidney Int.* **31**:992.

57. Rosenberg, M. E., Swanson, J. E., Thomas, B. L., and Hostetter, T. H., 1987, Glomerular and hormonal responses to dietary protein intake in human renal disease, *Am. J. Physiol.* **253**:F1083.

58. Mogensen, C. E., 1987, Microalbuminuria as a predictor of clinical diabetic nephropathy, *Kidney Int.* **31**:673.

59. Mogensen, C. E. and Christensen, C. K., 1984, Predicting diabetic nephropathy in insulin-dependent patients, *N. Engl. J. Med.* **311**:89.

60. Parving, H., Andersen, A. R., Smidt, U. M., Hommel, E., Mathiesen, S. R., and Svendsen, P. A., 1987, Effect of antihypertensive treatment on kidney function in diabetic nephropathy, *Br. Med. J.* **294**:1443.

61. Cohen, D., Dodds, R., and Viberti, G., 1987, Effect of protein restriction in insulin dependent diabetics at risk of nephropathy, *Br. Med. J.* **294**:795.

62. Evanoff, G. B., Thompson, C. S., Brown, J., and Weinman, E. J., 1987, The effect of dietary protein restriction on the progression of diabetic nephropathy, *Arch. Intern. Med.* **147**:492.

63. Wiseman, M. J., Mangili, R., Alberetto, M., Keen, H., and Viberti, G., 1987, Glomerular response mechanisms to glycemic changes in insulin-dependent diabetics, *Kidney Int.* **31**:1012.

64. The DCCT Research Group, 1988, Are continuing studies of metabolic control and microvascular complications in insulin-dependent diabetes mellitus justified? *N. Engl. J. Med.* **318**:246.

65. Dahl-Jorgensen, K., Brinchmann-Hansen, O., Hanssen, K. F., Ganes, T., Kierulf, P., Smeland, E., Sandvik, L., and Aagenaes, O., 1986, Effect of near normoglycemia for two years on progression of early diabetic retinopathy, nephropathy, and neuropathy: The Oslo study, *Br. Med. J.* **293**:1195.

66. Kroc Collaborative Study Group, 1984, Blood glucose control and the evolution of diabetic retinopathy and albuminuria, *N. Engl. J. Med.* **311**:365.

67. Feldt-Rasmussen, B., Mathiesen, E. R., and Deckert, T., 1986, Effect of two years of strict metabolic control on progression of incipient nephropathy in insulin-dependent diabetes, *Lancet* **2**:1300.

68. Bending, J. J., Viberti, G. C., Watkins, P. J., and Keen, H., 1986, Intermittent clinical proteinuria and renal function in diabetes: Evolution and the effect of glycemic control, *Br. Med. J.* **292**:83.

69. Kiprov, D. D., Colrin, R. B., and McCluskey, R. T., 1982, Focal and segmental glomerulosclerosis and proteinuria associated with unilateral renal agenesis, *Lab. Invest.* **46**:275.

70. Anderson, C. F., Velosa, J. A., and Frohnert, P. P., 1985, The risks of unilateral nephrectomy: Status of kidney donors 10 to 20 years postoperatively, *Mayo Clin. Proc.* **60**:367.

71. Talseth, T., Fauchald, P., Skrede, S., Djoseland, O., Berg, K. J., Stenstrom, J., Heilo, A., Brodwall, E. K., and Flatmark, A., 1986, Long-term blood pressure and renal function in kidney donors, *Kidney Int.* **29**:1072.

72. Williams, S., Oler, J., and Jorkasky, D. K., 1986, Long-term renal function in kidney donors: A comparison of donors and their siblings, *Ann. Intern. Med.* **105**:1.

73. Hakim, R. M., Goldszer, R. C., and Brenner, B. M., 1984, Hypertension and proteinuria: Long-term sequelae of uninephrectomy in humans, *Kidney Int.* **25**:930.

74. Vincenti, F., Amend, W. J. C., Jr., and Kaysen, G., 1983, Long-term renal function in kidney donors: Sustained compensatory hyperfiltration with no adverse effects, *Transplantation* **36**:626.

75. Smith, S., Laprad, P., and Grantham, J., 1985, Long-term effect of uninephrectomy on serum creatinine concentration and arterial blood pressure, *Am. J. Kidney Dis.* **6**:143.

76. Bay, W. H. and Hebert, L. A., 1987, The living donor in kidney transplantation, *Ann. Intern. Med.* **106**:719.

77. Taylor, R., Heaton, A., Hetherington, C. S., and Alberti, K. G. M. M., 1986, Adipocyte insulin binding and insulin action in chronic renal failure before and during continuous ambulatory peritoneal dialysis, *Metabolism* **35**:430.

78. Maloff, B. L., McCaleb, M. L., and Lockwood, D. H., 1983, Cellular basis of insulin resistance in chronic uremia, *Am. J. Physiol.* **245**:E178.

79. Folli, F., Sinha, M. K., Brancaccio, D., and Caro, J. F., 1986, Insulin resistance in uremia: *In vitro* model in the rat liver using human serum to study mechanisms, *Metabolism* **35**:989.

80. Baylor, P., Shilo, S., Zonszein, J., and Shamoon, H., 1986, Beta-adrenergic contribution to glucagon-induced glucose production and insulin secretion in uremia, *Am. J. Physiol.* **251**:E322.

81. Aparicio, H. G. M., Potaux, L., de Precigout, V., Bouchet, J. L., and Aubertin, J., 1987, Low protein and low phosphorus diet in patients with chronic renal failure: Influence on glucose tolerance and tissue insulin sensitivity, *Metabolism* **36**:1080.

82. Davis, T. A., Klahr, S., and Karl, I. E., 1987, Glucose metabolism in muscle of sedentary and exercised rats with azotemia, *Am. J. Physiol.* **252**:F138.

83. Kopple, J. D., Monteon, F. J., and Shaib, J. K., 1986, Effect of energy intake on nitrogen metabolism in nondialyzed patients with chronic renal failure, *Kidney Int.* **29**:734.

84. Monteon, F. J., Laidlaw, S. A., Shaib, J. K., and Kopple, J. D., 1986, Energy expenditure in patients with chronic renal failure, *Kidney Int.* **30**:741.

85. Hofstetter, A., Schutz, Y., Jequier, E., and Wahren, J., 1986, Increased 24-hour energy expenditure in cigarette smokers, *N. Engl. J. Med.* **314**:79.

86. Kamm, D. E., Wu, L., and Kuchmy, B. L., 1987, Contribution of the urea appearance rate to diuretic-induced azotemia in the rat, *Kidney Int.* **32**:47.

87. Conte, G., Dal Canton, A., Terribile, M., Cianciaruso, B., Di Minno, G., Pannain, M., Russo, D., and Andreucci, V. E., 1987, Renal handling of urea in subjects with persistent azotemia and normal renal function, *Kidney Int.* **32**:721.

88. Jahoor, F. and Wolfe, R. R., 1987, Regulation of urea production by glucose infusion *in vivo*, *Am. J. Physiol.* **253**:E543.

89. Shaw, J. H. F., Klein, S., and Wolfe, R. R., 1985, Assessment of alanine, urea and glucose interrelationships in normal subjects and in patients with sepsis with stable isotopic tracers, *Surgery* **97**:557.

90. Klim, R. A., Albajar, M., Hems, R., and Williamson, D. H., 1986, Effects of chronic uremia on the formation of glucose and urea plus ammonia from L-alanine, L-glutamine and L-serine in isolated rat hepatocytes, *Clin. Sci.* **70**:627.

91. Li, J. B. and Wassner, S. J., 1986, Protein synthesis and degradation in skeletal muscle of chronically uremic rats, *Kidney Int.* **29**:1136.

92. Davis, T. A., Klahr, S., and Karl, I. E., 1987, Insulin-stimulated protein metabolism in chronic azotemia and exercise, *Am. J. Physiol.* **253**:164.

93. May, R. C., Kelly, R. A., and Mitch, W. E., 1986, Metabolic acidosis stimulates protein degradation in rat muscle by a glucocorticoid-dependent mechanism, *J. Clin. Invest.* **77**:614.

94. May, R. C., Kelly, R. A., and Mitch, W. E., 1987, Mechanisms for defects in muscle protein metabolism in rats with chronic uremia. Influence of metabolic acidosis, *J. Clin. Invest.* **79**:1099.

95. May, R. C., Hara, Y., Kelly, R. A., Block, K. P., Buse, M. G., and Mitch, W. E., 1987, Branched-chain amino acid metabolism in rat muscle: Abnormal regulation in acidosis, *Am. J. Physiol.* **252**:E712.

96. Hara, Y., May, R. C., Kelly, R. A., and Mitch, W. E., 1987, Acidosis, not azotemia, stimulates branched-chain, amino acid catabolism in uremic rats, *Kidney Int.* **32**:808.

97. Papadoyannakis, N. J., Stefanidis, C. S., and McGeown, M., 1984, The effect of the correction of metabolic acidosis on nitrogen and potassium balance of patients with chronic renal failure, *Am. J. Clin. Nutr.* **40**:623.

98. Tungsanga, K., Kang, C. W., and Walser, M., 1986, Utilization of alpha-ketoisocaproate for protein synthesis in uremic rats, *Kidney Int.* **30**:891.

99. Kang, C. W., Tungsanga, K., and Walser, M., 1986, Effect of the level of dietary protein on the utilization of alpha-ketoisocaproate for protein synthesis, *Am. J. Clin. Nutr.* **43**:504.

100. Funk, M. A., Lowry, K. R., and Baker, D. H., 1987, Utilization of the L- and DL-isomers of alpha-keto-beta-methylvaleric acid by rats and comparative efficacy of the keto analogs of branched-chain amino acids provided as ornithine, lysine and histidine salts, *J. Nutr.* **117**:1550.

101. Laidlaw, S. A. and Kopple, J. D., 1987, Newer concepts of the indispensable amino acids, *Am. J. Clin. Nutr.* **46**:593.

102. Jackson, A. A., 1983, Amino acids: Essential and non-essential? *Lancet* **1**:1034.

103. Dieplinger, H., Schoenfeld, P. Y., and Fielding, C. J., 1986, Plasma cholesterol metabolism in end-stage renal disease. Difference between treatment by hemodialysis or peritoneal dialysis, *J. Clin. Invest.* **77**:1071.

104. Attman, P. O., Alaupovic, P., and Gustafson, A., 1987, Serum apolipoprotein profile of patients with chronic renal failure, *Kidney Int.* **32**:368.

105. Kaysen, G. A., Gambertoglio, J., Felts, J., and Hutchison, F. N., 1987, Albumin synthesis, albuminuria and hyperlipidemia in nephrotic patients, *Kidney Int.* **31**:1368.

106. Valeri, A., Gelfand, J., Blum, C., and Appel, G. B., 1986, Treatment of the hyperlipidemia of the nephrotic syndrome: A controlled trial, *Am. J. Kidney Dis.* **13**:388.

107. Iida, H., Izumino, K., Asaka, M., Fujita, M., Nishino, A., and Sasayama, S., 1987, Effect of probucol on hyperlipidemia in patients with nephrotic syndrome, *Nephron* **47**:280.

108. Pasternack, A., Vanttinen, T., Solakivi, T., Kuusi, T., and Korte, T., 1987, Normalization of lipoprotein lipase and hepatic lipase by gemfibrozil results in correction of lipoprotein abnormalities in chronic renal failure, *Clin. Nephrol.* **27**:163.

109. Ciardella, F., Morelli, E., Niosi, F., Caprioli, R., Baldi, R., Cupisti, A., Petronio, G., Carbone, C., and Barsotti, G., 1986, Effects of a low phosphorus, low nitrogen diet supplemented with essential amino acids and ketoanalogues on serum triglycerides of chronic uremic patients, *Nephron* **42**:196.

110. Knapp, H. R., Reilly, I. A. G., Alessandrini, P., and Fitzgerald, G. A., 1986, In vivo indexes of platelet and vascular function during fish-oil administration in patients with atherosclerosis, *N. Engl. J. Med.* **314**:937.

111. Rylance, P. B., Gordge, M. P., Saynor, R., Parsons, V., and Weston, M. J., 1986, Fish oil modifies lipids and reduces platelet aggregability in hemodialysis patients, *Nephron* **43**:196.

112. Grundy, S. M., 1986, Comparison of monounsaturated fatty acids and carbohydrates for lowering plasma cholesterol, *N. Engl. J. Med.* **314**:745.

113. Goodship, T. H. J., Lloyd, S., Clague, M. B., Bartlett, K., Ward, M. K., and Wilkinson, R., 1987, Whole body leucine turnover and nutritional status in continuous ambulatory peritoneal dialysis, *Clin. Sci.* **73**:463.

114. Blumenkrantz, M. J., Kopple, J. D., Gutman, R. A., Chan, Y. K., Barbour, G. L., Roberts, C., Shen, F. H., Gandhi, V. C., Tucker, C. T., Curtis, F. K., and Coburn, J. W., 1980, Methods for assessing nutritional status of patients with renal failure, *Am. J. Clin. Nutr.* **33**:1567.

115. Young, V. R., 1987, McCollum Award Lecture, Kinetics of human amino acid metabolism: nutritional implications and some lessons, *Am. J. Clin. Nutr.* **46**:709.

116. Motil, K. J., Matthews, D. E., Bier, D. M., Burke, J. F., Munro, H. N., and Young, V. R., 1981, Whole-body leucine and lysine metabolism: response to dietary protein intake in young men, *Am. J. Physiol.* **240**:E712.

117. Hou, J. C., Zhou, J., Zhu, H., Wu, J. Z., Wu, J. C., and Zhang, M., 1986, Dynamic aspects of whole-body nitrogen metabolism in uremic patients on dietary therapy, *Nephron* **44**:288.

118. Berkelhammer, C. H., Baker, J. P., Leiter, L. A., Uldall, R., Whittall, R., Slater, A., and Wolman, S. L., 1987, Whole-body protein turnover in adult hemodialysis patients as measured by ^{13}C-leucine, *Am. J. Clin. Nutr.* **46**:778.

119. Blumenkrantz, M. J., Kopple, J. D., Moran, J. K., and Coburn, J. W., 1982, Metabolism balance studies and dietary protein requirements in patients undergoing continuous ambulatory peritoneal dialysis, *Kidney Int.* **21**:849.

120. Carvounis, C. P., Carvounis, G., and Hung, M. H., 1986, Nutritional status of maintenance hemodialysis patients, *Am. J. Clin. Nutr.* **43**:946.

121. Young, G. A., Young, J. B., Young, S. M., Hobson, S. M., Hildreth, B., Brownjohn, A. M., and Parsons, F. M., 1986, Nutrition and delayed hypersensitivity during continuous ambulatory peritoneal dialysis in relation to peritonitis, *Nephron* **43**:177.

122. Carney, R. M., Templeton, B., Hong, B. A., Harter, H. R., Hagberg, J. M., Schechtman, K. B., and Goldberg, A. P., 1987, Exercise training reduces depression and increases the performance of pleasant activities in hemodialysis patients, *Nephron* **47**:194.

123. Goldberg, A. P., Geltman, E. M., Gavin, J. R., III, Carney, R. M., Hagberg, J. M., Delmez, J. A., Naumovich, A., Oldfield, M. H., and Harter, H. R., 1986, Exercise training reduces coronary risk and effectively rehabilitates hemodialysis patients, *Nephron* **42**:311.

124. Painter, P. L., Nelson-Worel, J. N., Hill, M. M., Thornbery, D. R., Shelp, W. R., Harrington, A. R., and Weinstein, A. B., 1986, Effects of exercise training during hemodialysis, *Nephron* **43**: 87.

125. Latos, D. L., Strimel, D., Drews, M. H., and Allison, T. G., 1987, Acid-base and electrolyte changes following maximal and submaximal exercise in hemodialysis patients, *Am. J. Kidney Dis.* **10**:439.

126. Lundin, A. P., Stein, R. A., Brown, C. D., LaBelle, P., Kalman, F. S., Delano, B. G., Heneghan, W. F., Lazarus, N. A., Krasnow, N., and Friedman, E. A., 1987, Fatigue, acid-base and electrolyte changes with exhaustive treadmill exercise in hemodialysis patients, *Nephron* **46**: 57.

127. Painter, P., Hanson, P., Messer-Rehak, D., Zimmerman, S. W., and Glass, N. R., 1987, Exercise tolerance changes following renal transplantation, *Am. J. Kidney Dis.* **10**:452.

128. Painter, P., Messer-Rehak, D., Hanson, P., Zimmerman, S. W., and Glass, N. R., 1986, Exercise capacity in hemodialysis, CAPD, and renal transplant patients, *Nephron* **42**:47.

129. Kaysen, G. A., Gambertoglio, J., Jimenez, I., Jones, H., and Hutchison, F. N., 1986, Effect of dietary protein intake on albumin homeostasis in nephrotic patients, *Kidney Int.* **29**:572.

130. Yoshioka, T., Mitarai, T., Kon, V., Deen, W. M., Rennke, H. G., and Ichikawa, I., 1986, Role for angiotensin II in an overt functional proteinuria, *Kidney Int.* **30**:538.

131. Taguma, Y., Kitamoto, Y., Futaki, G., Ueda, H., Monma, H., Ishizaki, M., Takahashi, H., Sekino, H., and Sasaki, Y., 1985, Effect of captopril on heavy proteinuria in azotemic diabetics, *N. Engl. J. Med.* **313**:1617.

132. Heeg, J. E., DeJong, P. E., van der Hem, G. K., and De Zeeuw, D., 1987, Reduction of proteinuria by angiotensin converting enzyme inhibition, *Kidney Int.* **32**:78.

133. Hutchison, F. N., Schambelan, M., and Kaysen, G. A., 1987, Modulation of albuminuria by dietary protein and converting enzyme inhibition, *Am. J. Physiol.* **253**:F719.

134. Alavi, N., Lianos, E. A., Venuto, R. C., Mookerjee, B. K., and Bentzel, C. J., 1986, Reduction of proteinuria by indomethacin in patients with nephrotic syndrome, *Am. J. Kidney Dis.* **8**:397.

135. Zoja, C., Benigni, A., Verroust, P., Ronco, P., Bertani, T., and Remuzzi, G., 1987, Indomethacin reduces proteinuria in passive Heymann nephritis in rats, *Kidney Int.* **31**:1335.

136. Wetzels, J. F. M., Gerlag, P. G. G., Sluiter, H. E., Hoitsma, A. J., and Koene, R. A. P., 1986, Prednisone-induced fluctuations of proteinuria in patients with a nephrotic syndrome, *Nephron* **44**: 344.

137. Ramirez, G., Chen, M., Boyce, H. W., Jr., Fuller, S. M., Ganguly, R., Brueggemeyer, C. D., and Butcher, D. E., 1986, Longitudinal follow-up of chronic hemodialysis patients without vitamin supplementation, *Kidney Int.* **30**:99.

138. Ono, K., 1986, Secondary hyperoxalemia caused by vitamin C supplementation in regular hemodialysis patients, *Clin. Nephrol.* **26**:239.

139. Ott, S., Andress, D. L., and Sherrard, D. J., 1986, Bone oxalate in a long-term hemodialysis patient who ingested high doses of vitamin C, *Am. J. Kidney Dis.* **13**:450.

140. Gleghorn, E. E., Eisenberg, L. D., Hack, S., Parton, P., and Merritt, R. J., 1986, Observations of vitamin A toxicity in three patients with renal failure receiving parenteral alimentation, *Am. J. Clin. Nutr.* **44**:107.

141. Cohen, J. D., Viljoen, M., Clifford, D., de Oliveira, A. A., Veriava, Y., and Milne, F. J., 1986, Plasma vitamin E levels in a chronically hemolyzing group of dialysis patients, *Clin. Nephrol.* **25**: 42.

142. Taccone-Gallucci, M., Giardini, O., Ausiello, C., Piazza, A., Spagnoli, G. C., Bandino, D., Lubrano, R., Taggi, F., Evangelista, B., Monaco, P., Tabilio, M. R., Valeri, M., Citti, G., and Casciani, C. U., 1986, Vitamin E supplementation in hemodialysis patients: effects on peripheral blood mononuclear cells lipid peroxidation and immune response, *Clin. Nephrol.* **25**:81.

143. Abu-Hamdan, D. K., Mahajan, S. K., Migdal, S. D., Prasad, A. S., and McDonald, F. D., 1986, Zinc tolerance test in uremia. Effect of ferrous sulfate and aluminum hydroxide, *Ann. Intern. Med.* **104:**50.

144. Wallaeys, B., Cornelis, R., Mees, L., and Lameire, N., 1986, Trace elements in serum, packed cells, and dialysate of CAPD patients, *Kidney Int.* **30:**599.

145. Miller, D. G., Levine, S. E., D'Elia, J. A., and Bistrian, B. R., 1986, Nutritional status of diabetic and nondiabetic patients after renal transplantation, *Am. J. Clin. Nutr.* **44:**66.

146. Horber, F. F., Zurcher, R. M., Herren, H., Crivelli, M. A., Robotti, G., and Frey, F. J., 1986, Altered body fat distribution in patients with glucocorticoid treatment and in patients on long-term dialysis, *Am. J. Clin. Nutr.* **43:**758.

147. Horber, F. F., Hoppeler, H., Herren, D., Claassen, H., Howald, H., Gerber, C., and Frey, F. J., 1986, Altered skeletal muscle ultrastructure in renal transplant patients on prednisone, *Kidney Int.* **30:**411.

148. Druml, W., Burger, U., Kleinberger, G., Lenz, K., and Laggner, A., 1986, Elimination of amino acids in acute renal failure, *Nephron* **42:**62.

149. Maroni, B. J., Karapanos, G., and Mitch, W. E., 1986, System A amino acid transport in incubated muscle: effects of insulin and acute uremia, *Am. J. Physiol.* **251:**F74.

150. Maroni, B. J., Karapanos, G., and Mitch, W. E., 1986, System ASC and sodium-independent neutral amino acid transport in muscle of uremic rats, *Am. J. Physiol.* **251:**F81.

151. Andrews, P. M. and Bates, S. B., 1986, Dietary protein prior to renal ischemia dramatically affects postischemic kidney function, *Kidney Int.* **30:**299.

13

Dialysis

Lee W. Henderson

1. Erythropoietin

Probably the single most noteworthy scientific event that has occurred in the interval since my last writing for *Contemporary Nephrology* 2 years ago is the availability of erythropoietin for clinical trials[1,2] in our end-stage renal disease (ESRD) patient population. This much heralded event is the logical "outgrowth" of recombinant DNA technology[3-5] coupled with a long-standing perceived need of the clinician/researcher[6]; it is evident from the studies in Britain of Winearls *et al.*[1] and in the United States by Eschbach *et al.*[2] and in Switzerland by Stutz *et al.*[7] that recombinant human erythropoietin (rHuEpo) (25–100 units/kg body weight, i.v., thrice weekly) restores hematocrit to the 35–40% range with striking enhancement of patient well-being, energy level, and appetite. Erythropoietin levels in the serum returned to the normal range related to the hematocrit on these doses, i.e., 33 ± 8 μ/ml.

At the present there have been remarkably few side effects: a mild increase of blood pressure, "functional" iron deficiency, slightly higher predialysis potassium and creatinine levels, and one episode of grand mal seizure which was considered to be more temporally than etiologically linked to rHuEpo treatment. To date there are no reported cases of the development of antibodies to the rHuEpo. Concern has been raised by earlier studies, such as those performed by Babb *et al.*[8] that creatinine and potassium, which dwell within the cell water, will permeate the red cell wall slowly enough to slow the clearance of these solutes by the dialyzer. In addition, the red cell component of whole blood has only a 70% water content as

LEE W. HENDERSON • Extramural Grant Research, Baxter Healthcare Corporation, Renal Therapy Division, Round Lake, Illinois 60073.

contrasted with plasma at 90%, which means that for every ml/min of blood flow across the hemodialysis membrane, at hematocrit 40–45% (as opposed to 25–30%), less solute-containing water is available to be cleared of uremic toxins. Even if the solute moves incredibly swiftly across the cell wall of the erythrocyte, as is the case, for example, for urea,[9,10] there will still be a small (4–5%) reduction in clearance due to the higher volume per milliliter of whole blood occupied by proteins, such as hemoglobin. For solutes that traverse red cell membranes more slowly, such as creatinine, the reduction in clearance may be more striking (10–15%). The studies to date do not provide transport studies to help quantify this effect. The small rises in predialysis creatinine and potassium reported by Eschbach *et al.* do not seem to warrant our concern because of the increase in dietary intake associated with the rise in hematocrit, which could in part or totally explain the higher plasma concentrations. The data reported so far support only a minor reduction in clearance and are consonant with the calculated reduction (10–15%) based on the higher volume of blood water occupied by protein. Whether charge-bearing solutes, such as phosphate, will show greater reduction in clearance remains to be tested.

It is interesting to identify that patients who, in their pre rHuEpo treatment, were normotensive appear to stay that way after their hematocrit returns toward normal[11] as contrasted with those entering the study with hypertension. Winerals *et al.*[1] report an episode of hypertensive encephalopathy in 1 of their 10 study subjects. Eschbach *et al.*,[2] in their 17-subject study, report a single grand mal seizure in a subject with hypertension who presumably had had a prior and unrelated (to rHuEpo) episode of seizure. Stutz *et al.*[7] do not report such an event in their eight subjects. Herein lies a problem with the clinical trials so far reported. There has not been a control group studied in parallel. It may well have been that those conducting the trial felt comfortable with historical controls of hemoglobin/hematocrit in the ESRD population. The disservice to their science is, of course, in the incidence of stroke, hypertension, or other untoward events that arise in their rHuEpo-treated group and in learning whether these events are to be expected in the observed frequency with maintenance dialysis or are rHuEpo related. My personal experience suggests that this incidence of seizures is outside of that expected for a comparable maintenance dialysis control group.

Winerals *et al.*[1] report that two of their subjects had problems of increased clotting in their fistulae (one clotted off completely). Casati *et al.*[11] also report fistula thrombosis in 2 of 14 subjects and a cerebral ischemic lesion in one. Further work by the Milan group[12] is of interest as it examines the uremic hemostatic defect as measured by prolonged bleeding times and reduced adhesion of platelets to vascular endothelium. Seven uremic patients with low hematocrit (<23%) and prolonged (>19 min) bleeding times were reexamined after treatment with rHuEpo and restoration of their hematocrits toward normal. There was a pronounced shortening of the bleeding time and their platelets showed a greatly increased adherence to the *in vitro* test material (human umbilical arterial wall).

A long-standing question that rHuEpo should provide an answer for is whether circulating uremic toxins are inhibitory to bone marrow function. There are recent studies from Saito et al.[13] in support of their presence in spent dialysis fluid. This work is at odds with the implications of Eschbach et al.[2] and others, who show a normal response with respect to the level of the hematocrit for administered rHuEpo which would imply no inhibitors. Furthermore, work by Eschbach et al.[14] with a uremic sheep model failed to identify such inhibitors. (It should be duly noted that ruminants that are herbivorous are different in respect to their diet and metabolic waste products than are carnivores or omnivores like humans. For example, the anephric sheep that continues eating becomes alkalemic rather than acidemic owing to the alkaline nature of the herbivorous diet which provides bicarbonate in excess of the generation of metabolic hydrogen ion.) Morra et al.[15] studied normal red cell precursors *in vitro* and the effect of uremic plasma introduced into the culture media. Predialysis uremic serum inhibits their replication, but when postdialysis uremic serum was introduced, the precursor cells showed normal growth. Precursor cells taken from uremic serum showed a uniform depression in replicative activity. Similar work by Delwiche et al.[16] supports the presence of inhibitors of all three marrow progenitor cell lines when serum creatinine concentrations were greater than 7 mg/dl in the serum tested. At present, the *in vitro* data suggest the presence of inhibitors in uremic patients' serum. Whether there are specific inhibitors of erythropoiesis that contribute to the anemia in uremic humans remains moot. Studies with rHuEpo should resolve this question in the next few years.

Two recent studies support improved erythropoiesis on treatment with continuous ambulatory peritoneal dialysis (CAPD).[17,18] Chandra et al.[17] report a rise in plasma erythropoietin levels in a single patient showing an improvement in hematocrit when switched from hemodialysis to peritoneal dialysis. More impressive is the work of Coles and Cavill,[18] who studied 15 patients with chronic renal failure using sensitive ferrokinetic techniques. In the face of unchanging levels of plasma erythropoietin they were able to show that on switching to CAPD there was significant prolongation of red cell half-life in three of their subjects and an increase in marrow turnover of iron in another subset of three. One must again question whether circulating inhibitors of normal erythropoiesis and their improved removal across the peritoneal membrane underlie these observations.

A question that arises with rHuEpo and peritoneal dialysis subjects relates to their independence and self-determination for details of treatment that so strongly underlie the psychologic advantage of CAPD. This trades off against the need, certainly to begin with, for monitoring of hemoglobin/hematocrit and blood pressure levels that would compromise this independence when rHuEpo is prescribed. Whether an intraperitoneal route of administration is feasible (it seems likely) remains to be determined.

Finally, insight into the dynamics of the erythropoiesis/hematocrit relationship in uremia may be taken from the work of Walle et al.[19] and Besarab et al.[20] The first study shows that in a stable uremic patient with anemia the normal feedback relationship that results in release or suppression of erythropoietin by reduction or increase in hematocrit remains intact in uremia, but operates at a much lower level of both erythropoietin and hematocrit. The second article traces the response of this feedback system into the posttransplant setting and identifies that uremic anemia "corrects in an orderly manner" in response to receipt of a functioning graft which restarts the normal feedback relationship between erythropoietin and hematocrit. Supernormal levels of hormone give way to normal values as hematocrit rises to normal. This process is blocked by delayed function and/or acute rejection of the graft and returns only with restored renal excretory function.

2. New Middle Molecules

Most readers will appreciate that I carry a long-standing belief in both the presence and pathophysiologic important of "middle molecules" in the syndrome of uremia. It is, therefore, of considerable interest to me that several new candidates for this designation have been identified in the 2 years since my last writing. I shall try to be even-handed in my description of this new work, recognizing that many of my well-informed peers may well consider middle molecules to be the flying saucers of nephrology.

There has been strong recent interest in atrial natriuretic factor (ANF), β-2-microglobulin (β-2-M), and interleukin 1 (IL-1) and their role in uremia.

2.1. Atrial Natriuretic Factor

Work on natriuretic hormones has indeed been extensive since de Wardener's pioneering original observations in dogs.[21] During the 1950s to the late 1960s an inordinate (in my view) amount of time and taxpayer dollars were invested in the search for a hormonal regulator other than aldosterone that, coupled with variations in glomerular filtration rate, modulated the body regulation of sodium balance, especially in the physiologic circumstance of sodium retention in edema-forming states. During this period, serious investigators of high stature could be cited at national meetings or in the literature as pro or con on the problem, depending on their state of personal intellectual evolution, creating a scientific climate not too dissimilar from that now surrounding the middle molecule. The work of such staunch believers as Buckalew[22] was given impetus by the recent outcome of studies tracking the early observation of de Bold[23,24] that changes in fluid and electrolyte balance altered the number of granules present in the cardiac atria in an orderly manner. The link between sodium/volume status and the heart conjured hypotheses of a volume regulatory reflex, which on test have resulted in the discovery of the family of atrial peptides that not only alter renal sodium handling, but act at physiologic concentration as potent vasorelaxants and antagonists for norepinephrine as well as suppressants of the renin–angiotensin system.[25–28] While the structures of these atrial natriuretic factors have been completely worked out, their function and, in particular, their detailed physiologic and pathophysiologic actions are still under investigation. See Buckalew[29] for a recent concise review.

For our purposes, it is of particular interest to note that increased right atrial stretch results in the release of a 28-amino-acid (3000-dalton) polypeptide that can result in peripheral vasodilatation as well as antagonize native vasopressors, such as norepinephrine, and suppress the release of angiotensin. As our patients enter for dialysis in a fluid-expanded state, they should show high levels of ANF. Work by Rascher et al.[30] in children with chronic renal failure as well as Saxenhofer et al.[31] in adults on maintenance dialysis show marked elevation of ANF in blood taken just predialysis, i.e., 447 ± 50 pg/ml predialysis vs. 167 ± 31 pg/ml in normal subjects (mean $\pm$ SEM).[32-34] Other workers confirm this observation and make the case that patients with chronic renal failure and normal volume status show somewhat elevated values over normal, whereas those with demonstrable fluid overload have values even higher than the predialysis values in the maintenance dialysis patients.[34] There is some variability in the absolute numbers reported by various investigators for their normal populations, suggesting that differences in assay technique are common. See, for example, the normal values reported by Zoccali et al.,[35] whose normal subjects had levels of 14 ± 2 pg/ml, ($n = 7$), whereas those of Hasegawa et al.[36] were 37.6 ± 1.9 pg/ml ($n = 59$) and of Larochelle et al.[33] 65.3 ± 2.9 pg/ml ($n = 40$). These are to be contrasted with the value of 167 ± 31 pg/ml reported by Saxenhofer et al.[31] This makes for difficulties in close comparison of absolute values for maintenance dialysis subjects but not in the above-reported relative values. A question addressed by several of these workers relates to the possibility of having abnormal ANF fragments circulating in uremic subjects. With one exception,[37] studies to address this question have shown a single peak on size separation methodology (gel permeation chromatography) applied to plasma.[31,36]

Could ANF account for symptomatic hypotension during the course of dialysis? The work by Saxenhofer and others just cited finds against this attractive hypothesis, as ANF levels fall with dialysis treatment. For example, the levels in one study ($n = 42$) fell on average to 164 ± 24 pg/ml at the close of hemodialysis from 447 ± 50 and therefore should not contribute to symptomatic hypotension in the third and fourth hours of treatment.[31] Of interest are the accompanying cardiodynamic data reported for their hemodialysis subjects. The hemofiltration subjects were not reported. Total peripheral resistance fell significantly ($p < 0.05$) over the 3.8 ± 0.5 hour treatment from 1158 ± 97 to 1013 ± 82 dyn.sec.cm^5, whereas cardiac index rose numerically, but not significantly (4.25 ± 0.31 to $4.4 \pm .27$ liters/min per m^2) as a result of an increase in heart rate (80 ± 3 to 88 ± 5 BPM, $p < 0.01$). Right atrial pressure fell from $8 \pm .05$ mm Hg to 0.8 ± 0.5 mm Hg ($p < 0.01$). While heart rate and right atrial pressure correlate with ANF release, the influence of atrial pressure would be expected to predominate in this circumstance. An additional crucial point in all of this is the short half-life (high endogenous clearance rate) for ANF in humans, i.e., 3.2 min (a clearance of 2.4 liters/min) reported by Yandle et al.[38] The latter figure absolutely dwarfs the artificial kidney clearance whether by hemodialysis or hemofiltration. These data mean we must look elsewhere for the difference in acute cardiovascular morbidity noted between hemodialysis and hemofiltration.[39,40]

Even with the major reduction in plasma ANF levels observed with hemodialysis, this reduction in plasma concentration of a potent vasodilator did not permit total peripheral resistance to rise after removal of excess total body water at the end of treatment, as would be considered normal.

Although there is conflict as to the amount of ANF cleared by cuprophane hemodialysis,[31,33] with reported values ranging from 0 (probably too low) to 25 ml/min, I reiterate that even 14 ml/min (if the value was correct) would make a negligible impact on total removal given an endogenous clearance of 2.4 liters/min.

Finally, this study does not address a potentially interesting hypothesis: namely, that cuprophane membrane activates complement-mediated pulmonary hypertension to occur in the first 20 min of hemodialysis in sheep,[41] swine,[42] and humans.[43] Acute early pulmonary hypertension would presumably increase the ANF levels, and this might account for shock occurring in the first 30 min of dialysis, an event that, while not common, does occur and is difficult to explain on a purely sodium/volume basis.

More work clearly needs to be done on this interesting molecule.

2.2. β-2-Microglobulin

Gejyo et al.[44] and Gorevic et al.[45] have identified β-2-M as the major constituent of the "amyloid" seen in the carpal tunnel syndrome of patients who have been maintained on dialysis for a prolonged time. Others have noted an upswing in incidence of this distressing dialysis syndrome at 10 years of maintenance or thereafter.[46] These new observations have led to resurgence of interest in this molecule, which was first identified by Berggard and Bearn[47] in 1968. A substantial body of knowledge already in hand on β-2-M has accumulated over the years. It is clearly a middle molecule (11,800 daltons) consisting of 100 amino acids and containing a single disulfide bridge.[48] β-2-M is the light chain of the Class I major histocompatibility antigens HLA-A, -B, and -C. As such, it is present on all cell surfaces. The plasma concentration of β-2-M is the result of the balance between cell surface "shedding" and the almost exclusive loss from the plasma of β-2-M (in normals) through glomerular filtration. Normally, after filtration, almost all (95%) of the β-2-M is reabsorbed in the proximal tubule, metabolized, and returned to the plasma as amino acids.[49] This explains our awareness of increased β-2-M levels in the urine as indicative of proximal tubular dysfunction, e.g., aminoglycosides especially gentamycin,[50–53] heavy metal toxicity,[54–56] Fanconi syndrome,[56] upper urinary tract infection,[57] and so forth. Diseases with high cell number and/or turnover rates, e.g., multiple myeloma, show high plasma levels as well.[58]

Plasma levels in ESRD patients maintained on cuprophane dialysis are more than a log order higher than normal, i.e., 40–50 mg/liter vs. 2–3 mg/liter for the normal.[44] This high plasma level undoubtedly reflects the loss of nephron mass in the ESRD patient. Whether cell shedding rate is different from normal in the uremic population remains to be determined. In addition, there may be new excretory paths or minor normal pathways that are now hypertrophied that contribute to the elimination of β-2-M in the ESRD patient.

Clearance across the cuprophane membrane at a molecular weight of 11,800 daltons would be expected to be negligible (<3 ml/min) when compared with normal glomerular clearance at 100–110 ml/min.

Given this background and precious little (i.e., none) published information on β-2-M kinetics in the maintenance dialysis population, we are asked to make judgments about reported plasma levels on cuprophane membrane dialysis (50.7 ± 3.9 mg/liter) that are higher than on polyachrylonitrile (PAN–Hospal) membrane dialysis.[59] The amount of β-2-M generated in a day (150–200 mg) certainly exceeds what can be removed by cuprophane hemodialysis, where 1–2 ml/min clearance would likely be a maximum removal rate.[60] PAN–Hospal dialysis, on the other hand, might be expected to remove considerably more, due in no small measure to the convective element of clearance inherent in dialysis with highly water permeable membranes like PAN[61]; i.e., 10–20 ml/min would yield 120–240 mg/hr of treatment, which may equate to 1 day's generation of β-2-M but not enough to balance the books for the full week. The intriguing question of whether the release of inflammatory mediators such as C3a and, in particular, C5a might increase cell shedding of β-2-M remains to be proven. Conceptually, the direct stimulation of both polymorphs and monocytes might increase shedding of these cell types, but the release of monokines of the interleukin family as well as tumor necrosis factor might also play a role.[62,63] Further investigation will undoubtedly be forthcoming.

It remains of interest that we have what by classical definition is a uremic toxin, i.e., a substance normally present in low concentration in the plasma that is dependent on renal excretory capacity to be eliminated from the body and that produces a toxic syndrome when nephron mass is lost. It is of particular interest to this writer that its molecular structure is well characterized and its molecular size falls between conventional small uremic toxins and albumin. It remains to be determined whether the presence of an elevated level of β-2-M is the sole etiology of the carpal tunnel syndrome or whether this is simply an epiphenomenon to another, more basic uremic disturbance of the target tissues.

2.3. Interleukin-1

Since the original hypothesis that IL-1 may be relevant to some of the syndromes associated with the treatment of uremia by dialysis,[62] there has been the demonstration of IL-1 release from monocytes that have been exposed to hemodialysis.[64–66] This has given rise to additional speculation and experimentation to try and determine what, if any, of the specific features of the uremic syndromes may be explained by this 17,000 to 18,000-dalton solute. IL-1 must be considered a family of polypeptides with at least two well-characterized species in the human. These two forms represent two distinct gene products. One is acidic and the other neutral. The latter accounts for 98% or more of that present in human plasma. Both forms have very similar biologic activities in spite of sharing only a 26% amino acid homology.[67] There are many potential areas that IL-1's presence would help to explain with regard to uremia,[68] but as of this writing none have been proven. I cite

- Dialysis somnolence—IL-1 increases slow wave sleep in rabbits.[69]
- Muscle wasting—IL-1 exerts a catabolic influence on muscle tissue.[70]
- Dialysis hypotension—IL-1 releases tissue PGE_2, a known potent vasodilator.[71]
- Dialysis osteopenia—IL-1 induces an active resorption of bone matrix.[72]

This powerful inflammatory mediator, in order to be qualified as a uremic toxin, must be shown to underlie one or more of these events. It may well be classed as an iatrogenic toxin if its presence relates only to use of a complement-activating membrane or stems from dialysate impurities. It is clear, because of its molecular size, that removal by dialysis will be slow to absent using conventional dialyzers with cuprophane membrane. Filtration and/or adsorption would seem to be required to effect a quantitatively significant removal. For IL-1, as for ANF, the endogenous clearance likely exceeds what we will be able to effect with dialysis techniques. Possibly a more important effort will be to improve our understanding of why the elevations occur and how the underlying process(es) may be blocked.

3. Biocompatibility of Synthetic Membranes

Two new, more complement-kind membranes have been introduced since my last writing.[73,74] This suggests a genuine concern about the bad performance of cuprophane in the complement arena. Hemophan, introduced by Enka Corporation, is a modification of Cuprophan, which has tertiary amino groups added to the hydroxyl groups of the cellulose. Only about 5% of the hydroxyl groups have had the addition of the tertiary amino end group and yet comparative studies show that peak levels of C3a desarg, the *in vivo* index of complement activation, are only 60% of those seen with unsubstituted Cuprophan. The reduction in leukocyte count at 15 min shows a comparable 60% reduction. These values are quite similar to those seen, for example, with the cellulose acetate membranes.[63] The polycarbonate membrane offers a comparative value for C3a generation of 50% with only a 22% reduction in polymorphs as compared with Cuprophan. Schohn et al. report that invasive cardiodynamic studies during hemodialysis with polycarbonate membrane do not produce the rise in pulmonary artery pressure noted with Cuprophan.[43] Hemophan has not yet been tested this way. Cheung et al.[42] have shown that C5a given intravenously in normal swine produces a rise in pulmonary artery pressure comparable to that seen with Cuprophan. One may speculate that not enough C5a is generated by the polycarbonate membrane to both saturate white blood cell receptors[75] and have enough left over to produce vasoconstriction in the pulmonary circuit. A second paper, by Cheung et al.,[76] shows that certain membranes take up (adsorb) C3a and C5a from the blood. Polyachrylonitrile membrane (Hospal) was the most active, with 90% of radiolabeled C3a and 80% of C5a absorbed. Cellulose acetate (Daicel) was not too far behind, with 80% of C3a and 60% of C5a absorbed. Cuprophan and reused Cuprophan showed less than 30% uptake. This property would be important in the net biologic consequences of employing a membrane, and testing of Hemophan polycarbonate and other membranes for this property will be important.

Of further interest in the Cheung et al. study is a lack of diffusive transport for these middle molecules (~10,000 daltons) for even the Hospal membrane, the most "open" of those studied.

There is an interesting disagreement in the literature on the presumed effects of bioincompatibility on the gas transport characteristics of the lung. Bouffard et al.[77] examined 13 mechanically ventilated patients during 24 dialyses for acute renal failure. Cuprophan membrane with acetate bath was compared with poly-achrylonitrile (Hospal) membrane with acetate and with bicarbonate baths. They conclude that measurement of the oxygen gradient across the alveolar membrane cannot be used to determine the difference in treatment technique. Vanholder et al.,[78] on the other hand, studying 12 stable chronic dialysis patients with first use and reused cuprophan, were able to show a 10 mm Hg reduction in arterial oxygen tension at 20 min into the procedure and a reduction in carbon monoxide lung diffusion capacity and transfer factor that temporally coincided with the reduced oxygen tension. This is not a new controversy: Ralph et al.[79] and Jacob et al.[80] agree with Bouffard et al. and De Backer et al.[81] and Dolan et al.[82] agree with Vanholder et al. While there are many differences in the study subject population, i.e., acute vs. chronic uremia, differences in the animal models employed (dog and rabbit), it remains unclear to this writer just how best to reconcile these differences. One might glibly dismiss the newest set of conflicting studies by pointing out that 12 of the 13 study subjects examined by Bouffard et al.[77] were septicemic and, as such, presumably had ongoing classical pathway activation of complement trig-gered by antigen–antibody complexes. As such, their polymorph population, while larger than the number of nonsepticemic chronic uremic patients, would have poly-morph C5a receptor down-regulation, as reported to occur by Skubitz et al.[83] and Lewis et al.[75] As such, pulmonary leukosequestration would not occur; however, the fall in leukocytes that they measure with the Cuprophan membrane negates this easy explanation. Something of this sort, however, must be operative and needs to be unveiled. I remain persuaded that the maintenance dialysis patient does show a small C5a-mediated reduction in arterial oxygen tension and diffusion capacity, as suggested by Vanholder et al.[78] and De Backer et al.[81] I am uncertain about this in the acute renal failure population.

An interesting side issue in the Bouffard et al.[77] article is the strong evidence for an increase in oxygen consumption during the 4-hr dialysis. While acetate metabolism could account for some of this increased oxygen uptake, the lesser, but still significant, increase with bicarbonate-containing dialysate indicates something more is present. The Cuprophan acetate bath combination showed the largest increase in oxygen utilization, with polyachrylonitrile acetate bath showing distinctly less utilization. Could this be the catabolic stimulus reported by Borah et al.[84] and confirmed by others[85] that attends hemodialysis and is likely mediated by the monokines IL-1 and tumor necrosis factor?

Maggiore et al.[86] tells us something that we might suspect but would have a hard time quantitating, namely, that blood cooling by 10°C (35–25° in the dialyzer) abrogates almost completely the generation of C5a and the leukopenia of hemodialysis. It seems unlikely to me that this lack of complement activation underlies their prior observation of increased cardiovascular stability on cool dialysis. (See Section 5 on the hemodynamic response to dialysis for further discussion of this point.)

Turning to cell elements in the blood, we have seen the demonstration of IL-1 production from monocytes during the coarse of hemodialysis by Bingel et al.[64] and Luger et al.,[65] lending credence to the original speculation that it should be present.[62] The significance of these findings in terms of clinical response needs study. Kay and Raij[87] report an interesting, if preliminary, observation on the response of human natural killer lymphocytes to exposure to Cuprophan and polycarbonate membrane. Cuprophan exposure produced a significant reduction in their killer function whereas polycarbonate membrane exposure did not. The test system used by these authors is free of the effects of complement activation and hence presumably is reflective of direct interactions between the lymphocyte and the membrane. This observation may underlie the nonselective increased incidence of neoplasms[88–90] in the maintenance of the hemodialysis population as natural killer cells are felt to be part of the immune surveillance system.

4. Peritoneal Dialysis

With respect to understanding the mechanism of transport across the peritoneal membrane, I recommend the work from the Missouri group on the importance of lymphatic drainage from the peritoneal cavity.[91,92] Those of you who have utilized the peritoneum as a conduit for the placement of red cells into the vascular space in children with aplastic anemia and thrombosed peripheral veins know that something other than diffusion across a semipermeable membrane is going on. In their editorial review[92] they identify work done in the 1950s and 1960s that confirms a nonsize discriminatory movement of water, protein, and cell elements from the peritoneal space to the blood via the lymphatics[93–95] and note that von Recklinghausen,[96] well before that, had identified stomata opening from the peritoneal membrane directly into end lymphatics. The right side of the diaphragm is particularly richly endowed with these openings. In the presently reported experiments with the rat, the loss of peritoneal fluid volume by lymphatic absorption at the 2-hr time point, when 15% dextrose-containing dialysis solution was used, accounted for 25% of the actual cumulative total ultrafiltration volume; i.e., at 120 min 40 ml of ultrafiltrate had been formed but 10 ml had left the cavity via the lymphatics.[91] The surprising thing was the magnitude of the lymphatic flow rate and, with time, the significant detriment in ultrafiltrate measured as drained volume that this lymphatic uptake causes. An additional interesting element of this fluid movement is its apparent independence from the force that drives the arrival of capillary ultrafiltrate into the peritoneal space, namely, the osmolality of the dialysis solution; 15% dextrose–containing dialysis solution, a superclinical osmolar driving force applied in this rat model, did not show any difference from an isoosmolar lactated Ringer's solution in terms of cumulative lymphatic flow rate when factored per 100 g body weight of the animal. Earlier work by this group[97] showed that when 15% dextrose solution is employed, there is no alteration in either the morphology or the transport characteristics of the membrane. Earlier work by Zink and Greenway[98] found the same independence from osmotic gradient in disappearance rate of fluid from the peritoneal cavity of cats.

Two points of concern arise in my mind with regard to this work. The first involves the method for determining lymph flow rate. The lymphatic flow rate calculation hangs on the assumption that lymphatic drainage is the only mechanism for a macromolecular index solute to depart the peritoneal cavity aside from its diffusive loss. Both Zink and Greenway[98] and Flessner et al.[99] have shown that macromolecular constituents of instilled peritoneal solutions find their way into adjacent tissues, but do not find their way into the blood for prolonged periods, i.e., 3–4 hr. This is at odds with our expectation for lymphatic drainage. Flessner et al.[99] indicate the magnitude of loss of a radiolabeled macromolecule (fibrinogen) is substantial (50%) and hence the magnitude of true lymphatic flow would be reduced by the same magnitude. Second, as noted by Morris et al.,[100] the rate of loss from the peritoneal cavity of cells and protein is dependent on the rate of respiration (diaphragmatic movement). As body size and respiratory rate hold a rough inverse correlation, it will be important to examine the quantitative importance of this mechanism in a 70+ kg man as contrasted with the rat. With these reservations in mind, the importance of this alternative mechanism for solute and water movement out of the peritoneal space must be accounted for in any modeling of transport.

Several articles of interest address the peritonitis problem. Fenton et al.[101] have examined infection rates in 277 patients coming for treatment to the Toronto General Hospital for the time period March 1978 through December 1985. A mean duration of 25 patient-months per patient was noted. The message from this work may be found in its title. The fact that they see no improvement in the rate of infection (0.95 episodes/year) over time (from 1981 to 1985) is distressing, particularly in light of the deliberate use of a series of "improved" connection devices. Fenton et al.[101] note a balancing between constant reduction in incidence of infection in the low-risk group and the deliberate adding of larger numbers of high-risk patients to their program. As this is a large and long-standing program, their results are likely to be reflective of the experience of others. Their rate of infection is numerically better than the 1.4 episodes/year reported by the National Registry[102] and the large experience reported from the network coordinating council of Southern California and Southern Nevada (NCC #4)[103] of 1.3 episodes/year. The variability between centers in these multicenter studies make a statistical difference between these numbers unlikely. Fenton et al. have not addressed this point.[101]

Two variants of the "Y" set that have stemmed from work by Maiorca et al.[104] and Buoncristiani and Di Paolo[105] have been reported.[106,107] The report by Lempert et al.[106] on the "O" set shows a numerical (but not statistical) reduction from baseline historical controls (3 months leading into O-set use) of 0.99 episode of peritonitis/year to 0.72 episode. They correctly point out that their baseline incidence is sufficiently low that it is clear that the 10 participating centers have selected low-risk patients (76 in number) for the study. This system employed sodium hypochlorite (0.5%) as a disinfectant within the Y connector. This material found its way into the peritoneal space on 22 occasions over the two 6-week evaluation periods employed. In addition to the positive reception by the patient of this "bagless" system, the authors note that their results point to infectious sources that lie outside the lumen of the catheter and "connectology"-related contamination. Interestingly, they suggest that the performance of the system without disinfectant should be examined as a means to eliminate inadvertent (or "vertent" in small quantities) patient exposure to this toxin and to shorten exchange time. Suki et al.,[107] in reporting a Y-set variant in which an adhesive based "third hand" device was used to enhance the rigor of the sterile connections and in which no sterilant was used, suggested that it would be of interest to try this with use of a disinfectant. The infection rate during use of the Y set for the 30 patients (six trial centers) observed for a minimum of 6 weeks was 0.52 episode/year. In this study, peritonitis recurring within 21 days of onset of a prior episode, or within 10 days of completing a coarse of antibiotic or yielding the same organism (or no growth) as the prior episode, is considered a single episode. While these are rational criteria, they are probably a point of difference from the previously noted studies that would favor the numerically lower incidence reported. Unfortunately, the design of the present study does not permit a valid statistical comparison using the patient as his own control; one is left with using control figures from other studies.

The bottom line in my mind in the work so far reported on improved connection systems is that the improvement to be seen in the incidence of peritonitis when employed in low-risk patients is small and compares in magnitude with the differences reported between individual experience of centers using comparable hardware; that peritonitis remains a significant cause of the "dropout" rates reported, i.e., 40% for the Registry for all 7295 patients at the time of reporting,[102] and 41% for 254 patients at 24 months, reported by Nissenson from NCC #4[103]; that infection rates in the low-risk population are likely not to yield to new connection devices, but must await elucidation and improvement of the patient's immunologic defense[108,109]; and that new connection devices are likely to be most cost effective in the high-risk populations of diabetics, blacks, and the aged.[101,102]

5. Hemodynamic Response to Dialysis

Several articles have been published on this important subject but none shed any definitive light on the underlying cause(s).[109–111] London et al.[109] show an increase in left ventricular end-diastolic volume and increased ratio of left ven-

tricular radius to posterior wall thickness in 57 maintenance dialysis patients selected (from 116 patients) to be normotensive. In this careful prospective study, the
control group consisted of 40 matched nonuremic normotensive study subjects. The
identification of this anatomic abnormality did not correlate with functional derangements (i.e., reduced ejection fraction or velocity of circumferential fiber shortening) or with differences in blood volume from the control group. Extensive
correlation between this anatomic abnormality and indices of parathyroid hormone
(PTH) excess were present as well as a correlation with the degree of anemia.
although these correlations are of interest, one is left feeling that anemia, osteitis
fibrosa, and the anatomic derangements of the heart all are manifestations of the
uremic process and not likely to be etiologically linked to one another.

In a brilliant exposition of the cardiovascular response to hemofiltration, Henderson[110] systematically demonstrates in a group of 21 stable end-stage uremic
patients that episodes of shock during treatment fell by one-half (60% to 30%) when
switching from the control period of 3 months on cellulose membrane hemodialysis
to 3 months on polysulphone membrane predilution hemofiltration. Removal of
excess total body water was comparable with the two techniques. This is not a new
observation and, as such, would not merit publication.[112,113] New observations in
this work are the lack of correlation between reduction in episodes of symptomatic
hypotension and improvement in the baroreflex arc neuropathy of the afferent limb
noted in literally all of the 13 patients completing this portion of the protocol. This
neuropathy blocks or blunts the rise in heart rate that should defend against shock
from vascular volume depletion.[114] Furthermore, there was lack of correlation with
the presence of hypertension and whether it got worse or better on hemofiltration.
This is at odds with previously published work by others.[114] Furthermore, the fall in
incidence of shock did not correlate with changes in patient temperature, as has
been suggested in work from Maggiore et al.[115] Unfortunately, this paper does
nothing but destroy promising hypotheses about the underlying cause of shock
during treatment. We now must conclude that something other than curing the
neuropathy or changing the core temperature of the body underlies the reduction in
the incidence of shock seen with hemofiltration.

Finally, Teo et al.,[111] employing a protocol in which hemodialysis with
cuprophane or cellulose acetate membrane for 240 ± 0 min with acetate dialysis
fluid (35 mmol/liter acetate, 135 meq/liter sodium) in 10 patients was compared
with hemodiafiltration for 204 ± 10 min in the same patients in which the 6 liters of
ultrafiltrate were generated using a polyacrylonitrile membrane (Hospal). This was
replaced with a hypertonic solution of sodium bicarbonate/chloride. This short-
time, low-filtrate-volume hemodiafiltration was associated with a significantly
higher cardiac ejection fraction and fractional circumferential fiber bundle shortening. There was a corresponding difference in the increase of the velocity of circumferential fiber shortening and in the end-systolic diameter. This impedance and
echocardiographic study is also somewhat disappointing in that there are easily four
and likely more explanations for the differences noted, i.e., improved calcium
and/or bicarbonate concentrations, loss of an unidentified vasodepressor substance
with hemodiafiltration, the switch away from the cardiodepressor acetate, and the

use of a more biocompatible (as assessed by complement activation) membrane during hemodiafiltration. We need to know whether there is something special about the filtration techniques that preserves a more normal cardiovascular response to vascular volume depletion.

6. Shortening Treatment Time

For this chapter 2 years ago, I spent considerable time on the details of reported experience using short-treatment-time protocols with various dialysis equipment packages. I had expected to find more on this subject in the literature in the intervening 2 years since that writing. My informal awareness that many dialysis units have embarked on protocols involving more permeable (than cuprophane) membranes and higher (400 ± 50 ml/min) blood flow rates supported my expectation in this regard. Surprisingly, although many seem to be employing this short (3 hr) treatment time prescription, not much has been published on the subject. Rubin et al.[116] report their experience in 12 maintenance dialysis patients used as their own control for 6 months of hemodialysis with (presumably but not stated) Cuprophan and conventional flow rate values vs. 6 months on polyacrylonitrile membrane (Hospal) using a 400 ml/min blood flow rate and a 500 ml/min dialysate flow rate. A 4-hr control treatment was contrasted with a 3-hr experimental period. This experimental treatment prescription reportedly provides, on average, a 1.08 normalized clearance value (kt/v). In this short follow-up experience there was no significant change in pretreatment blood urea nitrogen, creatinine, bicarbonate, calcium, alkaline phosphate, potassium, hematocrit, albumin, n-terminal PTH, mean midarm circumference, or triceps skinfold thickness. Phosphate rose from 5.4 ± 0.3 to 5.9 ± 0.4 mg/dl at the end of the experimental period.

Raja et al.[117] report the survival rate (%) at 10 years for 69 patients (seven were lost to transplantation) undergoing 8–12 hr of treatment per week to be 35%. The dialysis time for the 17 10-year survivors was, on average, 9.6 ± 0.6 hr/week. This retrospective report is short on technical details, indicating only that "large surface area" coils were used for the first 3 years and Travenol CF 1511 dialysers for the last 7 years. Blood flow rates were 250–275 ml/min. All one may learn from this report is that the survival figure for these patients is comparable to that of some other reports, e.g., Neff et al.,[118] but is by no means exemplary. Not remarkable is the identification that high levels of blood pressure and plasma triglyceride are negative risk factors.

It is hoped that at the next writing we will have the results of some prospectively designed studies to examine.

7. Filtration Modalities

Kaplan has studied predilution continuous arteriovenous hemofiltration (CAVH) using vacuum-assisted filtration.[119] One is initially put off by the introduction of greater technical complexity to what has been a delightfully simple method. When one identifies that in the five study subjects the clearance for urea (averaged over the duration of their therapy) was 18 ml/min, i.e., at least half again more than is his experience with conventional CAVH and comparable to that reported by Ronco *et al.*[120] employing both diffusive and convective modalities for this technique, one comes away impressed. This means the technique can be employed with success even in the high-catabolic-rate cases that normally required augmentation with conventional hemodialysis.

I believe that with identification, that uremia *per se* does not blunt the energy needs of the patient,[121] that acute renal failure imposes an incredible nutritional stress,[122] and that CAVH and related techniques that make "vascular space" available for aggressive nutritional treatment will be required in order to improve mortality in this distressingly fragile group of patients.

8. Access

Vanholder *et al.*[123] review their 10-year experience with single-needle dialysis using a double-headed blood pump of their design in 98 patients; 76 of these patients were studied using standard single-pool urea kinetic modeling. Comparison of their results with control data taken from the literature show urea kinetic parameters indistinguishable from those reported by the National Cooperative Dialysis Study. No distinction could be made between the single-needle population and an adequately dialyzed twin-needle population as regards hematocrit hospitalization rate and cumulative survival. Fistula survival was felt to be somewhat better than average, although the sensitivity of this parameter to the technique of needle placement makes the use of control data taken from the literature inappropriate. The intellectual appeal of single-needle dialysis remains in my mind, and I am surprised that in this day of the informed patient that patient preference has not driven this technique into wider application.

Interesting preliminary work on a self-sealing dialysis blood access prosthesis is offered by Schanzer *et al.*[124] They have used two coaxial polytetrafluoroethylene (PTFE) tubes with a layer of silicone sealant configured between these coaxial tubes. The needle then transverses PTFE, then silicone sealant, and finally the PTFE tube in contact with the blood. In dogs blood loss on needle withdrawal was half that of a control device consisting of two coaxial PTFE tubes without the sealant, which in turn was even more strikingly less than a control observation using conventional PTFE grafts. If clinical trials confirm these results, this triple-wall device would seem to be a worthwhile choice. We still need a nonthrombogenic prosthetic material.

A logical evolution is reported by Schwab *et al.*,[125] who describe the use of percutaneous transinminal angioplasty (PTA) for correction of venous stenosis in PTFE vascular access grafts. Fourteen of seventeen stenoses at the vein/PTFE junction or proximal portion of the vein anastomosed thereto were successfully treated by PTA. Of the remaining three, two yielded to surgery, indicating, as one might anticipate, that PTA is a powerful adjunctive technique in the preservation of PTFE vascular accesses.

References

1. Winearls, C. G., Oliver, D. O., Tippard, M. J., Reid, C., Downing, M. R., and Cotes, P. M., 1986, Effective human erythropoietin derived from recombinant DNA on the anemia of patients maintained by chronic hemodialysis, *Lancet* **2**:1175.
2. Eschbach, J. W., Egrie, J. C., Downing, M. R., Browne, J. K., and Adamson, J. W., 1987, Correction of anemia of end stage renal disease with recombinant human erythropoietin results of a phase I and II clinical trial, *N. Engl. J. Med.* **316**:73.
3. Jacobs, K., Shoemaker, C., Rudersdorf, R, Neill, S. D., Kaufman, R. J., Mufson, A., Seehra, J., Jones, S. S., Hewich, R., Fritsch, E. F., Kawakita, M., Shimizu, T., and Miyake, T., 1985, Isolation and characterization of genomic and cDNA clones of human erythropoietin, *Nature* **313**: 806.
4. Lin, F. K., Suggs, S., Lin, C. H., Browne, J., Smalling, R., Egrie, J. C., Chen, K. K., Fox, G. M., Martin, F., Stabinsky, Z., Babrawi, S. M., Lai, P., and Goldwasser, E., 1985, Cloning and expression of the human erythropoietin gene, *Proc. Natl. Acad. Sci. USA* **82**:7580.
5. Lai, P. H., Everett, R., Wang, F. F., Arakawa, T., and Goldwasser, E., 1986, The primary structure of human erythropoietin, *J. Biol. Chem.* **261**:3116.
6. Jacobson, L. O., Goldwasser, E., Fried, W., and Plzak, L., 1957, Role of the kidney and erythropoesis, *Nature* **179**:633.
7. Stutz, B., Rhyner, K., Vogtli, J., and Binswanger, U., 1987, Successful treatment of anemia in hemodialysis patients using recombinant human erythropoietin. Maintenance dosage and serum concentration, *Schweiz. Med. Wochenschr.* **117**:1397.
8. Babb, A. L., Popovich, R. P., Farrell, T. C., and Blagg, C. R., 1972, Effects of erythrocyte mass transfer rates on solute clearance measurement during hemodialysis, *Proc. Eur. Dial. Transplant Assoc.* **9**:303.
9. Cheung, A. K., Alford, M. F., Wilson, M. M., Leypoldt, J. K., and Henderson, L. W., 1983, Urea Movement across erythrocyte membrane during artificial kidney treatment, *Kidney Int.* **23**: 866.
10. Colton, C. K., Smith, K. A., Merrill, E. W., and Reece, J. M., 1970, Diffusion of organic solutes in stagnant plasma and erythrocyte suspensions, *Chem. Eng./Progress Symp.* Series 66:85.
11. Casati, S., Passerini, P., Campise, M. R., Graziani, G., Cesana, B., Perisic, M., and Ponticelli, C., 1987, Benefits and risks of protractive treatment with human recombinant erythropoietin in patients having hemodialysis, *Br. Med. J. Clin. Res.* **295**:1017.
12. Moia, M., Mannucci, P. M., Vizzotto, L., Casati, S., Cattaneo, M., and Ponticelli, C., 1987, Improvement in the hemostatic defect of the uremia after treatment with the recombinant human erythropoietin, *Lancet* **2**:1227.
13. Saito, A., Suzuki, I., Chung, T. G., Okamoto, T., and Hotta, T., 1986, Separation of an inhibitor of erythropoiesis in "middle molecules" from hemodialysate from patients with chronic renal failure, *J. Clin. Chem.* **32**:1938.
14. Eschbach, J. W., Mladenovic, J., Garcia, J. F., Wahl, P. W., and Adamson, J. W., 1984, Anemia of chronic renal failure in sheep; response to erythropoietin rich plasma *in vivo*, *J. Clin. Invest.* **74**: 434.
15. Morra, L., Ponassi, A., Gurreri, G., Moccia, F., Caristo, G., Mela, G. S., and Sacchetti, C., 1987, Alterations of erythropoiesis in chronic uremic patients treated with intermittent hemodialysis, *Biomedicalpharmacotherapy (France)* **41**(7):396.
16. Delwiche, F., Segal, G. M., Eschbach, J. W., and Adamson, J. W., 1986, Hematopoietic inhibitors in chronic renal failure; lack of *in vitro* specificity, *Kidney Int.* **29**:641.

17. Chandra, M., McVicar, M., Clemons, G., Mossey, R. T., and Wilkes, B. M., 1987, Role of erythropoietin in the reversal of anemia of renal failure with continuous ambulatory peritoneal dialysis, *Nephron* **46:**312.

18. Coles, G. A., and Cavill, I., 1986, Erythropoiesis in the anemia of chronic renal failure; response to CAPD, *Nephrol. Dial. Transplant.* **1:**170.

19. Walle, A. J., Wong, G. Y., Clemons, G. K., Garcia, J. F., and Niedermayer, W., 1987, Erythropoietin–hematocrit feedback circuit in the anemia of end stage renal disease, *Kidney Int.* **31:**205.

20. Besarab, A., Caro, J., Jarrell, B. E., Francos, G., and Erslev, A. J., 1987, Dynamics of erythropoiesis following renal transplantation, *Kidney Int.* **32:**526.

21. de Wardener, A. G. and Clarkson, E. M., 1985, Concept of natriuretic hormone, *Physiol. Rev.* **65:** 658.

22. Buckalew, V. M., Jr. and Gruber, K. A., 1984, Natriuretic hormone, *Annu. Rev. Physiol.* **46:**343.

23. de Bold, A. J., 1978, Heart atria granularity affects of changes in water–electrolyte balance, *Proc. Soc. Exp. Biol. Med.* **161:**508.

24. de Bold, A. J., Borenstein, H. B., Veress, A. T., and Sonnenberg, H., 1981, A rapid and potent naturiuretic response to intravenous injection of atrial myocardial extract in rats, *Life Sci.* **29:**89.

25. Needleman, P., Adam, S. P., Cole, D. R., Currie, M. G., Geller, D. M., Michener, M. L., Saper, C. B., Schwartz, D., and Standaert, D. G., 1985, Atriopeptins as cardiac hormones, *Hypertension* **7:**469.

26. Maack, T., Camargo, M. J. F., Kleinert, H. D., Laragh, J. H., and Atlas, S. A., 1985, Atrial natriuretic factor; structure and functional properties, *Kidney Int.* **27:**607.

27. Needleman, P. and Greenwald, J. E., 1986, Atriopeptin, a cardiac hormone intimately involved in fluid electrolyte and blood pressure homeostasis, *N. Engl. J. Med.* **314:**828.

28. Buckalew, V. M. Jr., Morris, M., and Hamilton, R. W., 1987, *Atrial natriuretic* factor, *Adv. Intern. Med.* **32:**1.

29. Buckalew, V. M. Jr., 1987, The natriuretic hormones, *AKF Neph. Lett.* **4:**1.

30. Rascher, W., Tulassay, T., and Lang, R. E., 1985, Atrial natriuretic peptide in plasma of volume overloaded children with chronic renal failure, *Lancet* **2:**303.

31. Saxenhofer, H., Gnadinger, M. P., Weidmann, P., Shaw, S., Schohn, D., Hess, C., Uehlinger, D. E., and Jahn, H., 1987, Plasma levels and dialysance of atrial natriuretic peptide in terminal renal failure, *Kidney Int.* **32:**554.

32. Hodsman, G. P., Jackson, B., DeBrevi, L. M., Ogawa, K., and Johnston, C. I., 1987, Atrial natriuretic factor in chronic renal failure; studies in man and the rat, *J. Clin. Exp. Pharmacol. Physiol.* **14:**247.

33. LaRochelle, P., Beroniade, V., Gutkowska, J., Cusson, J. R., Lecrivain, A., du-Souich, P., Cantin, M., and Genest, J., 1987, Influence of hemodialysis on the plasma levels of the atrial natriuretic factor in chronic renal failure, *J. Clin. Invest. Med.* **10:**350.

34. Shenker, Y., Port, F. K., Swartz, R. D., Gross, M. D., and Grekin, R. J., 1987, Atrial natriuretic hormone secretion in patients with renal failure, *Life Sci.* **41:**1635.

35. Zoccali, C., Ciccaielli, M., Mallamaci, F., Delfino, D., Salnitro, F., Parlongo, S., and Maggiore, Q., 1986, Affect of ultrafiltration on plasma and concentrations of atrial natriuretic peptide in hemodialysis patients, *J. Neph. Dial. Transplant.* **1:**188.

36. Hasegawa, K., Matsushita, Y., Inoue, T., Morii, H., Ishibashi, M., and Yamaji, T., 1986, Plasma levels of atrial natriuretic peptide in patients with chronic renal failure, *J. Clin. Endocrinol. Metab.* **63:**819.

37. Ogawa, K., Smith, A. I., Hodsman, G. P., Jackson, B., Woodcock, E. A., and Johnston, C. I., 1987, Plasma atrial natriuretic peptide; concentrations and circulating forms in normal man and patients with chronic renal failure, *J. Clin. Exp. Pharmacol. Physiol.* **14:**95.

38. Yandle, T. G., Richards, A. M., Nicholls, M. G., Cuneo, R., Espiner, E. A., and Livesey, J. H., 1986, Metabolic clearance rate and plasma half-life of alpha human atrial natriuretic peptide in man, *Life Sci.* **38:**1827.

39. Shaldon, S., Baldamus, C. A., Koch, K. M., and Lysaght, M. J., 1983, Of sodium symptomatology and syllogism, *Journal of Blood Purification* **1**:16.

40. Baldamus, C. A., Ernst, W., Fassbinder, W., and Koch, K. M., 1980, Differing hemodynamic stability due to differing sympathetic response; comparison of ultrafiltration hemodialysis and hemofiltration, *Proc. Eur. Dial. Transplant Assoc.* **17**:205.

41. Walker, J. F., Lindsay, R. M., Peters, S. D., Sibbald, W. J., and Linton, A. L., 1983, A sheep model to examine the cardiopulmonary manifestations of blood–dialyzer interactions, *ASAIO* **3**: 123.

42. Cheung, A. K., LeWinter, N., Chenoweth, D. E., Lew, W. Y. W., and Henderson, L. W., 1986, Cardiopulmonary effects of cuprophane-activated plasma in the swine, *Kidney Int.* **29**:799.

43. Schohn, D. C., Jahn, H. A., Eber, M., and Hauptmann, G., 1986, Biocompatibility and hemodynamic studies during polycarbonate vs. cuprophane membrane dialysis, *Journal of Blood Purification* **4**:102.

44. Gejyo, F., Yamada, T., Odani, S., Nakagawa, Y., Arakawa, M., Kunitomo, T., Kataoka, H., Suzuki, M., Hirasama, Y., Shirahama, T., Cohen, A. S., and Schmid, K., 1985, A new form of amyloid protein associated with chronic hemodialysis was identified as beta-2-microglobulin, *Biochem. Biophys. Res. Commun.* **29**:701.

45. Gorevic, P. D., Casey, T. T., Stone, W. J., DiRaimondo, C. R., Prelli, F. C., and Frangione, B., 1985, Beta-2-microglobulin is an amyloidogenic protein in Man, *J. Clin. Invest.* **76**:2425.

46. Charra, B., Calemard, E., Uzan, M., Terrat, J. C., Vanel, T., and Laurent, G., 1984, Carpal tunnel syndrome shoulder pain and amyloid deposits in long term hemodialysis patients, *Proc. Eur. Dial. Transplant Assoc.* **21**:291.

47. Berggard, I. and Bearn, A. G., 1968, Isolation and properties of a low molecular weight beta-2-globulin occurring in human biological fluids, *Biochemistry* **243**:4095.

48. Cunningham, B. A., Wang, J. L., Berggard, I., and Peterson, P. A., 1973, The complete amino acid sequence of beta-2-microglobulin, *Biochemistry* **12**:4811.

49. Statius van Eps, L. W. and Schardijn, G. H. C., 1983, Beta-2-microglobulin and the renal tubule, in: *Non-invasive Diagnosis of Kidney Disease* (G. Lubec, ed.), *Karger*, Basel, p. 103.

50. Cabrera, J., Arroyo, V., Ballesta, A. M., Rimola, A., Gual, J., Elena, M., and Rodes, J., 1982, Aminoglycoside nephrotoxicity in cirrhosis, *Gastroenterology* **82**:97.

51. Gatell, J. M., San Miguel, J. G., Zamora, L., Araujo, V., Castells, C., Moreno, A., Jimenez de Anta, M. T., Marin, J. L., Elena, M., and Ballesta, A., 1985, Tobramycin and amikacin nephrotoxicity: Value of serum creatinine versus urinary concentration of Beta-2-microglobulin *Nephron* **41**:337.

52. Fleming, J. J., Child, J. A., Cooper, E. H., Hay, A. M., Morgan, D. B., and Parapia, L., 1980, Renal tubular damage without glomerular damage after cytotoxic drugs and aminoglycosides, *Biol. Med.* **33**:251.

53. Tulkens, P. M., 1986, Experimental studies on nephrotoxicity of aminoglycosides at low doses, *Am. J. Med.* **80** (Suppl. 6B):105.

54. Taniguchi, N., Tanaka, N., Kishihara, C., Ohno, H., Kondo, T., Matsuda, I., Fujino, T., and Harada, M., 1979, Determination of carbonic anhydrase C and beta-2-microglobulin by radioimmunoassay in urine of heavy metal exposed, subjects and patients with renal tubular acidosis, *Environ. Res.* **20**:154.

55. Sorensen, P. G., Nissen, M. H., Groth, S., and Rorth, M., 1985, Beta-2-microglobulin excretion; an indicator of long term nephrotoxicity during cisplatinum treatment, *Cancer Chemother. Pharmacol.* **14**:247.

56. Statius van Eps, L. W. and Schardijn, G. H. C., 1984, Value of determination of beta-2-microglobulin in toxic nephropathy and interstitial nephritis, *Klin. Wochenschr.* **18**:673.

57. Schardijn, G. H. C., Statius van Eps, L. W., Stout-Zonneveld, A. A. M., Kager, J. C. G. M., and Persijn, J. P., 1980, Urinary beta-2-microglobulin in urinary tract infections, *Acta Clin. Belg.* **35** (Suppl. 10):21.

58. Wibell, L., 1976, Studies on beta-2-microglobulin in patients and normal subjects, *Acta Clin. Belg.* **31** (Suppl. 8):14.

59. Hauglustaine, D., Waer, M., Michielsen, P., Goebels, J., and Vandeputte, M., 1986, Hemodialysis membranes, serum beta-2-microglobulin, and dialysis amyloidosis, *Lancet* **1**:1211.

60. Karlsson, F. A., Groth, T., Sege, K., Wibell, L., and Peterson, P. A., 1980, Turnover in humans of beta-2-microglobulin; constant chain of HLA-antigens, *Eur. J. Clin. Invest.* **10**:293.

61. Schmidt, M., Baldamus, C. A., and Schoeppe, W., 1984, Backfiltration in hemodialyzers with highly permeable membranes. An *in vitro* and *in vivo* investigation, *Journal of Blood Purification* **2**:108.

62. Henderson, L. W., Koch, K. M., Dinarello, C. A., and Shaldon, S., 1983, Hemodialysis hypotension; the Interleukin hypothesis, *Journal of Blood Purification* **1**:3.

63. Henderson, L. W., and Chenoweth, D., 1987, Biocompatibility of artificial organs; an overview, *Journal of Blood Purification* **5**:100.

64. Bingel, M., Lonnemann, G., Shaldon, S., Koch, K. M., and Dinarello, C. A., 1986, Human interleukin I production during hemodialysis, *Nephron* **43**:161.

65. Luger, A., Kovarik, J., Hans-Krister, S., Urbanska, A., and Luger, T. A., 1987, Blood membrane interaction in hemodialysis leads to increased cytokine production, *Kidney Int.* **32**:84.

66. Port, F. K., Van De Kerkhove, K. M., Kunkel, S. L., and Kluger, M. J., 1987, The role of dialysate in the stimulation of interleukin-I production during clinical hemodialysis, *Am. J. Kidney Dis.* **10**:118.

67. Auron, P. E., Rosenwasser, L. J., Matsushima, K., Copeland, T., Dinarello, C. A., Oppenheim, J. J., and Webb, A. C., 1985, Human and murine interleukin I possess sequence and structural similarities, *Mol. Cell* **2**:169.

68. Dinarello, C. A., 1983, The biology of interleukin I and its relevants to hemodialysis, *Journal of Blood Purification* **1**:197.

69. Krueger, J. M., Dinarello, C. A., and Chedid, L., 1983, Promotion of slow wave sleep by a purified Interleukin I preparation, *Fed. Proc.* **42**:356.

70. Baracos, B., Rodemann, H. P., Dinarello, C. A., and Goldberg, A. L., 1983, Stimulation of muscle protein degridation by leucocyte pyrogen, *N. Engl. J. Med.* **308**:553.

71. Crossi, V., Breviario, F., Ghezzi, P., DeJana, E., and Mantovani, A., 1985, Interleukin I induces prostacyclin in vascular cells, *Science* **229**:1174.

72. Gowen, M., Wood, D. D., Ihrie, E. J., Meats, J. E., and Russess, R. G. G., 1984, Stimulation by human Interleukin I of cartiledge breakdown and production of collagenase proteoglycanase by human chondrocytes but not human osteoblasts in vitro, *Biochem. Biophys. Acta* **797**:186.

73. Schaefer, R. M., Horl, W. H., Kokot, K., and Heidland, A., 1987, Enhanced biocompatibility with a new cellulosic membrane; Cuprophan vs. Hemophan, *Journal of Blood Purification* **5**:262.

74. Konstantin, P. and Bailey, R. N., 1986, Polycarbonate–polyether flat sheet membrane; manufacture, structure and performance, *Journal of Blood Purification* **4**:6.

75. Lewis, S. L., Van Epps, D. E., and Chenoweth, D. E., 1987, Leukocyte C5A receptor modulation during hemodialysis, *Kidney Int.* **31**:112.

76. Cheung, A. K., Chenoweth, D. E., Otsuka, D., and Henderson, L. W., 1986, Compartmental distribution of complement activation products in artificial kidneys, *Kidney Int.* **30**:74.

77. Bouffard, Y., Viale, J. P., Annat, G., Guillaume, C., Percival, C., Bertrand, O., and Motin, J., 1986, Pulmonary gas exchange during hemodialysis, *Kidney Int.* **30**:920.

78. Vanholder, R. C., Pauwels, R. A., Vandenbogaerde, J. F., Lamont, H. H., Van Der Straten, M. E., and Ringoir, S. M., 1987, Cuprophan reuse and intra dialytic changes of lung diffusion capacity and blood gasses, *Kidney Int.* **32**:117.

79. Ralph D. D., Ott, S. M., Sherrard, D. J., and Hlastala, M. P., 1984, Inert gas analysis of ventilation-perfusion matching during hemodialysis, *J. Clin. Invest.* **73**:1385.

80. Jacob, A. J., Gavellas, G., Zarco, R., Perez, G., and Bourgoignie, J. J., 1980, Leucopenia hypoxia and complement function with different hemodialysis membranes, *Kidney Int.* **18**:505.

81. De Backer, W. A., Verpooten, G. A., Borgonjon, D. J., Vermeire, P. A., Lins, R. R., and De Broe, M. E., 1983, Hypoxemia during hemodialysis; effects of different membranes and dialysate composition, *Kidney Int.* **23**:738.

82. Dolan, M. J., Whipp, B. J., Davidson, W. D., Weitzman, R. E., and Wasserman, K., 1981,

Hypopnea associated with acetate hemodialysis; carbon dioxide–flow-dependent ventilation, *N. Engl. J. Med.* **305:**72.

83. Skubitz, K. M. and Craddock, P. R., 1981, Reversal of hemodialysis granulocytopenia in pulmonary leucostasis, *J. Clin. Invest.* **67:**1383.

84. Borah, M. F., Schoenfeld, P. Y., Gotch, F. A., Sargent, J. A., Wolfson, M., and Humphreys, M. H., 1979, Nitrogen balance during intermittent dialysis therapy of uremia, *Kidney Int.* **14:**491.

85. Ward, R. A., Shirlow, M. J., Hayes, J. M., Chapman, G. V., and Farrell, P. C., 1979, Protein catabolism during hemodialysis, *Am. J. Clin. Nutr.* **32:**2443.

86. Maggiore, Q., Enia, G., Catalano, C., Misefari, V., and Mundo, A., 1987, Effect of blood cooling on cuprophan-induced anaphylotoxin generation, *Kidney Int.* **32:**908.

87. Kay, N. E. and Raij, L. R., 1986, Immune abnormalities in renal failure in hemodialysis, *Journal of Blood Purification* **4:**120.

88. Sutherland, G. A., Glass, J., and Gabriel, R., 1977, Increased incidence of malignancy chronic renal failure, *Nephron* **18:**182.

89. Lindner, A., Farewell, V., and Sherrard, D., 1981, High incidence of neoplasia in uremic patients receiving long term dialysis, *Nephron* **27:**292.

90. Matas, A. J., Simmons, R. L., Kjellstrand, C. M., Buselmeier, T. J., and Najarian, J. S., 1975, Increased incidence of malignancy during chronic renal failure, *Lancet* **1:**883.

91. Nolph, K. D., MacTier, R., Khanna, R., Twardowski, Z. J., Moore, H., and McGary, T., 1987, The kinetics of ultrafiltration during peritoneal dialysis; the role of lymphatics, *Kidney Int.* **32:**219.

92. MacTier, R. A., Khanna, R., Twardowski, Z. J., and Nolph, K. D., 1987, Role of peritoneal cavity lymphatic absorbtion in peritoneal dialysis, *Kidney Int.* **32:**165.

93. Courtice, F. C. and Steinbeck, A. W., 1950, Lymphatic drainage of plasma in the peritoneal cavity of the cat, *Aust. J. Exp. Biol. Med. Sci.* **28:**161.

94. Simer, P. H., 1944, The drainage of particulant matter from the peritoneal cavity by lymphatics, *Anat. Rec.* **88:**175.

95. Raybuch, A. G., Allen, L., and Harms, W. S., 1960, Absorbtion of serum from the peritoneal cavity, *Am. J. Physiol.* **199:**201.

96. von Recklinghausen, F. T., Zur Fettre Sorption, 1863, *Archi. Pathol. Anat. Physiol.* **26:**172 (Abstract).

97. Levin, T. N., Ragden, L. B., Nielsen, L. H., Moore, H. L., Twardowski, Z. J., Khanna, R., and Nolph, K. D., 1987, Maximum ultrafiltration rates during peritoneal dialysis in rats, *Kidney Int.* **31:**731.

98. Zink, J. and Greenway, C. V., 1977, Control of ascites absorption in anesthetized cats; affects of intraperitoneal pressure, protein and furosimide diauresis, *Gastroenterology* **73:**1119.

99. Flessner, M. F. R., Parker, J., and Sieber, S. M., 1983, Peritoneal lymphatic uptake of fibrinogen and erythrocytes in the rat, *Am. J. Physiol.* **244** (*Heart Circ. Physiol.*) (13):H 89.

100. Morris, B., Murphy, M. J., and Bessie, M., 1970, The passage of red blood cells from the peritoneal cavity, in: *Lymphatics Lymph and Lymphoid Tissue* J. M. Yoffey and F. C. Courtice, (eds.), Academic Press, London, p. 303.

101. Fenton, S. S. A., Pei, Y., Delmore, T., Cattran, D. C., Bowman, C., Johnston, N., Campbell, L., Klarke, W. T., and Richardson, R. N. A., 1986, The CAPD peritonitis rate is not improving with time, *Trans. ASAIO* **32:**546.

102. Nolph, K. D., Cutler, S. J., Steinberg, S. M., and Novak, J. W., 1985, Continuous ambulatory peritoneal dialysis in the United States; a 3 year study, *Kidney Int.* **28:**198.

103. Nissenson, A. R., Gentile, D. E., Soderblom, R. E., Brax, C., and Medical Review Board NCC 4, Los Angeles, California, 1986, Long term outcome of continuous ambulatory peritoneal dialysis; Southern California/Southern Nevada experience, *Trans. ASAIO* **32:**560.

104. Maiorca, R., Cantaluppi, A., Cancarini, G. C., Scalamogna, A., Broccoli, R., Graziani, G., Brasa, S., and Ponticelli, C., 1983, Prospective and control trial of a Y connector and disinfection to prevent peritonities and continuous ambulatory peritoneal dialysis, *Lancet* **2:**642.

105. Buoncristiani, U., and Di Paolo, N., 1983, Auto sterilizing CAPD connection systems, *Nephron* **35:**244.

106. Lempert, K. D., Kolb, J. A., Swartz, R. D., Campese, V., Golper, T. A., Winchester, J. F., Nolph, K. D., Husserl, F. E., Zimmerman, S. W., Kurtz, S. B., and Mars, R., 1986, A multi center trial to evaluate the use of the CAPD "O" set, *Trans. ASAIO* **32:**557.

107. Suki, W. N., Walshe, J. J., Ashbrook, D. W., Gentile, D. E., Tucker, C. T., Ash, S. R., and Ahmad, S., 1986, Multi center evaluation of a bagless CAPD system, *Trans. ASAIO* **32:**572.

108. Kurz, P., Kohler, H., Meuer, S., Hutteroth, T., and Meyer zum Buschenfelde, K. H., 1986, Impaired cellular immune responses in chronic renal failure; evidence for a T cell defect, *Kidney Int.* **29:**1209.

109. London, G. M., Febiani, F., Marchais, S. J., Christine de Zernejoul, M., Guerin, A. P., Safar, M. E., Metivier, F., and Llach, F., 1987, Uremic cardiomyopathy; an inadequate left ventricular hypertrophy, *Kidney Int.* **31:**973.

110. Henderson, L. W., 1986, Heterogeneity of the cardiovascular response to hemofiltration, *Kidney Int.* **29:**901.

111. Teo, K. K., Basile, C., Ulan, R. A., Hetherington, M. D., and Kappogoda, T., 1987, Effects of hemodialysis and hypertonic hemodiafiltration on cardiac function compared, *Kidney Int.* **32:**399.

112. Quellhorst, E. A., Schuenemann, B., and Hildbrebrand, U., 1983, Morbidity and mortality in long term hemofiltration, *ASAIO J.* **6:**185.

113. Baldamus, C. A., 1983, Clinical value and technical feasability of long-term hemofiltration, *ASAIO J.* **6:**192.

114. Lilly, J., Golden, J., and Stone, R., 1976, Adrenergic regulation of blood pressure in chronic renal failure, *J. Clin. Invest.* **57:**1190.

115. Maggiore, Q., Pizzarelli, F., Sisca, S., Zoccali, C., Parlongo, S., Nicolo, F., and Creazzo, G., 1982, Blood temperature and vascular stability during hemodialysis and hemofiltration, *Trans. ASAIO* **28:**523.

116. Rubin, J. E., Friedmann, P., and Berlyne, G. M., 1986, Rapid blood flow short dialysis does not adversely effect the clinical, biochemical or nutrition status of patients, *Trans. ASAIO* **32:**377.

117. Raja, R., Kramer, M., Goldstein, S., Caruana, R., and Lerner, A., 1986, Short hemodialysis-10 year follow up, *Trans. ASAIO* **32:**374.

118. Neff, M. S., Eiser, A. R., Slifkin, R. F., Baum, M., Baez, A., Gupta, S., and Amarga, E., 1983, Patients surviving 10 years on hemodialysis, *Am. J. Med.* **74** (6):996.

119. Kaplan, A. A., 1986, Clinical trial with pre dilution and vacuum suction; enhancing the efficiency of the CAVH treatment, *Trans. ASAIO* **32:**49.

120. Ronco, C., Bragantini, L., Brendolan, A., Dell'Aquila, R., Fabris, A., Chiaramonte, S., Feriani, M., Laquaniti, L., and La Greca, G., 1985, Arterial venous hemodiafiltration combined with continuous arterial venous hemofiltration, *Trans. ASAIO* **31:**349.

121. Monteon, F. J., Laidlaw, S. A., Shaib, J. K., and Kopple, J. D., 1986, Energy expenditure in patients with chronic renal failure, *Kidney Int.* **30:**741.

122. Feinstein, E. J., Blumenkrantz, M. J., Healey, M., Koffler, A., Silberman, H., Massry, S. G., and Kopple, J. D., 1981, Clinical and metabolic response to perenteral nutrition in acute renal failure, *Medicine* **60:**124.

123. Vanholder, R., Hoenich, N., Bogaert, A. M., and Ringoir, S., 1986, Long term experience with the routine single needle dialysis; a review, *Trans. ASAIO* **32:**300.

124. Schanzer, H., Martinelli, G. P., Bock, G., and Peirce, E. C., 1986, PTFE-silicone self-sealing dialysis prosthesis, *Trans. ASAIO* **32:**297.

125. Schwab, S. J., Saeed, M., Sussman, S. K., McCann, R. L. L., and Stickel, D. L., 1987, Transluminal angioplasty of venous stenosis in polytetrafluoroethylene vascular access grafts, *Kidney Int.* **32:**395.

14

Renal Transplantation

Larry B. Melton and Terry B. Strom

1. Introduction

Transplantation is now well established as the preferred therapy for patients suffering from end-stage renal disease. The main obstacle still to be overcome is that of inducing allograft tolerance in recipients while avoiding over-immunosuppression with the attendant risks of opportunistic infection and malignancy. There is at present no consensus on the optimal protocol for immunosuppression, and many individual centers employing different regimens report excellent allograft and patient survival.

In designing an immunosuppressive program several principles must be considered. First is patient preparation and selection of the best available HLA match. There are now good data to support the notion that even well-matched kidneys that are shared between centers have a better outcome than do poorly matched kidneys transplanted locally.[1] Second is a multitiered approach to drug therapy which combines several agents, thus targeting different points in the sequence of T-cell activation. This minimizes the toxicity of individual drugs by keeping doses of each at a lower level than would otherwise be required. Third, it is clear that greater levels of immunosuppression are required to obtain engraftment than are necessary to maintain the transplant long term. This allows for tapering of the immunologic "poisons" that are the mainstay of drug therapy. Next is careful investigation of each episode of transplant dysfunction to distinguish between rejection, pharmacologic toxicity, and acute renal failure. One of the complicating features of clinical trans-

LARRY B. MELTON and TERRY B. STROM • Department of Medicine, Harvard Medical School, and Beth Israel Hospital, Boston, Massachusetts 02215.

plantation is that these three entities may be present singly or in combination with each other and therefore demand precise definition prior to initiation of treatment. Finally, appropriate reduction or withdrawal of an immunosuppressive agent is necessary when the risk : benefit ratio is no longer favorable to the patient.

2. Immunosuppression

2.1. Pretransplant Preparation

Candidates for cadaveric renal allografts have generally, for over a decade, received random donor blood transfusions before transplantation.[2,3,5-7] The improvement in allograft survival related to this routine is a matter of record,[2] although the precise mechanism by which it is accomplished is the subject of controversy. The potential mechanisms include transfusion-related selection of responder vs. nonresponder recipients, immunization against CMV, T-suppressor cell activation, iron overload, and production of immunosuppressive antibodies.[2,8]

Recently, with the widespread use of cyclosporine (CsA) in the pharmacologic armamentarium and the emergence of varied and intense immunosuppressive protocols, the use of pretransplant blood transfusions has come under increasing scrutiny. Many now deny a salubrious transfusion effect on allograft survival. Data from the International Collaborative Transplant Study (CTS) registry[9] and the Scandinavian Multicenter Study[10] indicate that, in the years since 1984, the use of third-party transfusions in CsA-treated patients does not facilitate allograft survival at 1 year. Other reports from individual centers[11] also show a diminished or absent transfusion effect in CsA-treated patients.

In contrast, data from UCLA during the same period shows a continued, albeit modest, improvement in allograft survival in transfused patients treated with CsA.[12] Reasons for this effect may relate to racial differences between the groups and to the number of HLA mismatches. When blacks and whites were considered separately in the UCLA data, the transfusion effect was apparent in blacks at 1 year but was lost at 3 years. In contrast, the effect in whites was only 5% at both 1 and 3 years (Table 1). Furthermore, the benefits obtained by pretransplant transfusions were most notable in patients receiving HLA mismatched grafts; i.e., if there were two or more mismatches at HLA-A,B, -B,DR, or any mismatches at HLA-DR. Melzer *et al.*[13] also maintain that in their patient population the transfusion effect is still present. Thus, there is some debate about the use of third-party transfusion in cadaver kidney recipients, but evidence suggests a diminishing effect in some selected patient populations.

The use of pretransplant donor-specific transfusions (DST) in living–related allografts may be a relic. Early studies demonstrated an improved survival and decreased number of rejection episodes in one-haplotype-matched kidneys[4] with DST. One unsolved problem, however, is the development of adverse sensitization against the donor.[14-16] Many groups have attempted to reduce the high rate of

Table I. Effect of Pretransplant Transfusions (TFS) on
Allograft Survival in Recipients Treated with Cyclosporine[a]

Recipient	n	TFS	Percent allograft survival		
			1 year	2 year	3 year
All	5308	+	79 ± 1	72 ± 1	66 ± 1
All	709	−	69 ± 2[b]	62 ± 2[b]	57 ± 3[b]
Black	649	+	72 ± 2	58 ± 3	51 ± 4
Black	170	−	55 ± 4[b]	49 ± 5	49 ± 5
White	3621	+	79 ± 1	73 ± 1	67 ± 1
White	415	−	74 ± 2[b]	67 ± 3	62 ± 4

[a]Reprinted with permission from Cecka et al.[12]
[b]Statistically significant differences.

sensitization by simultaneous administration of an immunosuppressive agent, usually azathioprine.[17−20] The preferable alternative is eliminating DST altogether, assuming no compromise in allograft survival results.

Concerning DST recipients treated with CsA, transplants undertaken from 1982 to 1984 and reported in the CTS suggested a beneficial effect of DST on allograft survival.[21] In contrast, Leivestad et al. reported that allograft survival in CsA-treated one-haplotype-matched grafts was not influenced by DST.[22] This finding was confirmed by the Scandinavian Multicenter Study[10] and now in a more recent report from the CTS.[9] Many centers, including Boston's Beth Israel Hospital, have now eliminated DST from their protocol.

2.2. Pharmacotherapy

The beneficial effect of corticosteroids in transplantation was initially described for skin grafts in rabbits.[23,24] The applicability of monodrug corticosteroid therapy in canine renal allografts was quickly evaluated and found to be effective.[25] However, combined corticosteroids plus azathioprine (Aza) produce a marked improvement in organ allograft survival.[26] Initially, relatively high doses of glucocorticoids were used. However, the adverse effects of high-dose therapy prompted investigations to evaluate the efficacy of lower doses of steroids. Low-dose steroids as an element in combination therapy produce equivalent rates of engraftment[27−29] while reducing the frequency and severity of steroid complications.

Recent investigations on the mechanisms of steroid immunosuppression have convincingly demonstrated that corticosteroids block production of interleukin-1 (IL-1) by accessory cells (macrophages)[30] at both the transcriptional[33,39] and posttranscriptional level,[39,40] thus abrogating at least one of the cytokine signals delivered from accessory cells necessary for primary T-cell activation and subsequent graft rejection. Since IL-1 provides an important signal leading to the activation of T cells, it is not surprising that steroids block production of IL-2 by inhibiting mRNA transcription[32,41] and may therefore block production of a second cytokine in the T-cell activation cascade. The effect of steroids on IL-2 production may be exerted on IL-1-producing macrophages—not on T-cells.

Aza, introduced in 1961, is a nitroimidazole derivative of 6-mercaptupurine, blocks nucleic acid synthesis, and hence interferes with T-cell activation/proliferation at a more distal stage than that influenced by steroids. The first demonstration of Aza's benefit in renal transplantation was obtained by Calne,[31,34] in which several transplanted dogs, although eventually dying of pneumonia, had essentially normal kidneys at the time of their death. Aza became a mainstay in pharmacologic immunosuppression.[35,36]

CsA was discovered in 1972, and its immunosuppressive effects were described by Borel *et al.* in 1976.[37] The ability of CsA as a single agent to prolong renal allografts in humans was confirmed.[38]

The first immunosuppressive property of CsA that was described was its ability to suppress T-cell-dependent B-cell activation.[37,42,43,44,47] Primary T-cell responses are inhibited by CsA, especially when the agent is present at the initiation of cultures.[45,46] Antigen-induced T-cell proliferation requires *de novo* synthesis of the IL-2 receptor and secretion of the T-cell growth factor IL-2. Miyawaki *et al.*[48] demonstrated that although CsA is able to block lectin-stimulated T-cell proliferation, there is no abrogation of surface expression of the IL-2 receptor but IL-2 production is dramatically inhibited.[46,49]

More recent studies in murine leukemic T cells,[50] human leukemic T cells,[50,51] and normal human T cells[41] demonstrate that CsA blocks transcription of . IL-2 and other lymphokine genes.[55-57] With strong stimulants, induction of the IL-2 receptor gene is not dramatically reduced.[41] However, other studies using weaker stimulants suggest that induction of IL-2R mRNA is completely blocked by CsA.[52-54] It is obvious that the action of CsA and the activation sequence of T lymphocytes are incompletely understood.

In any event, the advantage gained by using steroids, Aza, and CsA in concert is the result of targeting several steps in the activation process to obtain a much more powerful immunosuppression than is possible with a single agent. Furthermore, lower doses of these agents help to minimize the toxicity of each of them individually. The usual initial doses at our institution are prednisone 40 mg/day, Aza 1.5–2.0 mg/kg per day, and cyclosporine 8 mg/kg per day (or ⅓ of this dose intravenously). This protocol is used for both cadaveric and living donor kidneys. The dose of Aza usually remains stable but reductions are sometimes made in response to myelotoxicity. Prednisone and CsA, however, are gradually reduced so that at 1 year posttransplant the dose of prednisone is 10 mg/day and CsA is at the lowest dose required to maintain adequate allograft function with minimal nephrotoxicity—typically 100–200 mg/day. True immunologic tolerance has not yet been routinely achieved in clinical practice, but by the first anniversary of the transplant most patients enjoy immunosuppressive regimens that are significantly less aggressive than those required early to obtain engraftment.

2.3. Adverse Effects of Pharmacologic Therapy

While CsA has provided a powerful tool to the transplant physician, it comes at the price of frequent nephrotoxicity.[38,57] The nephrotoxicity of CsA is known to take two guises—acute and chronic toxicity. Acute toxicity appears as a decrease in renal blood flow causing decreased glomerular filtration (GFR).[58-61] Hyperkalemia is frequent.[61,62] Direct perfusion of the kidney with CsA causes a decrease in renal blood flow and an increase in renal vascular resistance.[63] These are abolished by phenoxybenzamine but not with captopril. This effect in a recent allograft must be mediated by circulating catecholamines since the transplanted kidney is not innervated. However, a direct effect of CsA on the renal vasculature is not excluded. Fortunately, this acute hemodynamic toxicity is readily reversible by decreasing the dose or discontinuing the administration of CsA.[58-61]

A second acute CsA-related injury takes the form of an arteriopathy, manifested by arteriolar and capillary thrombosis and resembling the hemolytic–uremic syndrome. It was first noted in allogeneic marrow transplantation.[65] Now, this lesion is well described in CsA-treated renal allograft recipients who developed acute renal failure (ARF).[66] On microscopic examination, intimal proliferation, luminal narrowing, intravascular thrombosis, and glomerular ischemia coupled with a microangiopathic hemolytic peripheral blood smear are noted. In one report, all but 1 of 16 patients with this lesion lost their transplanted kidneys.[66]

In patients with primary nonfunction, CsA is a particularly potent nephrotoxin. CsA does, in fact, cause a prolongation of the recovery time from primary nonfunction.[68,71] In one study[68] ARF in patients receiving CsA/prednisone lasted more than twice as long as in Aza/prednisone–treated patients (25.5 vs. 11.5 days). Interestingly, recent reports suggest that perfusion of the donated kidney with calcium channel blockers prior to transplantation decreases immediate posttransplant ARF.[72]

Chronic CsA toxicity is a distinct entity and has been best described in human cardiac transplant recipients. Using inulin clearance as a marker for GFR, Myers *et al.*[64] clearly demonstrated that cardiac transplant recipients treated with high doses of CsA/prednisone had a lower GFR by approximately 50% than did patients treated with Aza/prednisone. Five of these patients underwent renal biopsy to evaluate renal dysfunction. Glomerular changes noted consisted primarily of focal and segmental sclerosis. Severe tubulointerstitial damage present, disproportional to the glomerular injury, included tubular atrophy and loss, fibrosis of the interstitium, thickening of basement membranes, and other degenerative changes. These changes have been noted in several reports,[67,70] and the nephrotoxicity is dose related.[67] However, caution must be taken in attributing all interstitial fibrosis to CsA because this feature is also noted in some long-term renal transplants treated with Aza/prednisone[69] and can be the consequence of chronic rejection.

As follow-up in cardiac allograft recipients, after 12–24 months, 37 CsA-treated patients and 24 Aza-treated patients were selected for study.[69] Of the CsA group, 12 agreed to renal biopsy for evaluation of depressed renal function. Serum creatinine in CsA patients was 50% of that in patients on Aza and renal blood flow was depressed by 40% with a renal vascular resistance greater than twice noted that in Aza patients. In addition, there was prominent fibrosis and glomerular sclerosis in CsA-treated patients although no Aza controls were available for comparison.

Other adverse effects of CsA therapy include hirsutism, gingival hyperplasia, hypertension, glucose intolerance, hyperkalemia, tremors, paresthesias, hyperbilirubinemia, transaminase elevation, and lymphoma.[73]

3. Cellular Basis of Allograft Rejection

The primary function of the immune system is to protect the individual from invasion by microbes. All allogeneic transplants, recognized as nonself, are subjected to some degree of cellular infiltration by host lymphocytes. This interstitial nephritis must necessarily be viewed on a continuum of biologic responses in which subclinical "rejection" and irreversible rejection represent the two extremes. Rejection is the direct result of antigen recognition by host cells. The recognition process is not blocked by any of the current pharmacologic agents. However, the antigen-induced secretion of lymphokines and cellular proliferation can be inhibited in an adequately immunosuppressed recipient. Failure of immunosuppression allows activation of T lymphocytes, cellular proliferation, and the acute rejection process. The inflammatory infiltrate characteristic of rejection is a severe form of interstitial nephritis complete with hemorrhage, edema, and tubular infiltration, all of which are absent in subclinical rejection.

It is clear that the lymphocytes responsible for acute cellular rejection consist of several subsets that possess different functions.[74,75] The functions of the T-cell subsets have been defined, in part, by major histocompatibility (MHC) restriction characteristics. CD4+ cells are MHC class II restricted, i.e. recognize antigen plus self-class II, whereas CD8+ cells are MHC class I restricted, i.e., recognize antigen plus self-class I.[85]

Both CD4+ and CD8+ cells are present in the transplanted kidney.[78,81] Several groups have passively transferred selected lymphocyte subsets into T-cell-deficient hosts to identify those cells that are responsible for rejection. The initial studies were interpreted as identifying CD4+ cells to be solely responsible for the rejection process[74,76]; however, while CD4+ cells are of primary importance in the rejection process, CD8+ cells are required to experimentally reproduce the rapid temporal nature of clinical allograft rejection.[79,80] Nevertheless, elimination of either CD4+ or CD8+ subsets does not completely prevent rejection of class I and II mismatched allografts. Some CD4+ cells exert cytolytic function[82,85]; CD8+ cells can elaborate lymphokines necessary for cellular growth.[77] It is now accepted that, in general, CD4+ cells are required primarily to initiate rejection while CD8+ cells, activated by CD4+ dependent lymphokines, are primarily responsible for the cytolytic manifestations of the rejection process.[82]

Mild rejection episodes are characterized by a patchy interstitial infiltration of T cells, accompanied by modest infiltrations of the tubules.[81,84] While CD8+ cells are not abundant in the infiltrate associated with subclinical rejection, the more intense infiltrate in mild cellular rejection contains a balanced population of CD4+ and CD8+ T cells.[81] Prednisone, CsA, and Aza are all effective in routine immunosuppression for preventing the activation of lymphocytes, but in their usual doses they are not effective in abrogating the function of previously activated cells because these cells have progressed past the site of action of the drugs. Nevertheless, high-dose prednisone does exert significant suppressive action on lymphocytes involved in ongoing mild rejection. The exact role of steroids in reversing rejection is not well defined, but probably consists of several events, including inhibition of monokine (IL-1) and lymphokine release, reduced extravascular migration of lymphocytes, inhibition of cytotoxic T-cell function, and suppressed phagocytosis by monocytes.[83]

More severe rejection episodes are characterized by diffuse interstitial lymphocyte infiltration and an accompanying glomerular infiltration of T lymphocytes carrying the CD8+ marker.[81] In this form of rejection, the severity can be directly correlated with the extent of cellular infiltrate and with the proportion of CD8+ cells present.[81,84,86] These CD8+ cells are the predominant mononuclear cells in the interstitium, invading tubules, glomeruli, and the intima of vessels. In the most severe forms of cellular rejection CD8+ cells can be found lining the intima and invading the adventitia of medium-sized vessels.[81] In contrast, CD4+ cells seem to be concentrated in focal infiltrates in a perivascular or periglomerular location.[81,84] High proportions of CD8+ cells are associated with increasingly severe and more resistant rejections. For these rejections, more powerful therapies may be required.

Antithymocyte globulin has traditionally been used in patients with steroid-insensitive rejections. Recently, the monoclonal pan T-cell antibody OKT3 has become available and has proven highly effective as an antirejection therapy. The initial multicenter trial group utilized OKT3 for first rejection episodes in cadaveric renal transplants. With daily intravenous infusions of 5.0 mg, 94% of these first rejections were reversed.[87] OKT3 has now been shown to be effective in steroid-resistant rejections,[88,89] and in one study,[88] 82% of rejections resistant to both steroids and antithymocyte globulin responded to OKT3 therapy.

Other types of cellular rejection are even more resistant to therapy. These are characterized by extensive mononuclear cell infiltration which includes macrophages as well as T lymphocytes. Interestingly, B cells do not seem to be a prominent component of the infiltrate even in severe rejections.[81] By convention, therapy has been initiated with steroids for all rejection episodes. However, it seems reasonable to evaluate the extent and nature of mononuclear cell infiltration as a marker for severity before making a decision concerning a drug therapy. If the biopsy reveals a particularly angry, dense, mononuclear cell infiltrate, it is not unreasonable to initiate OKT3 treatment without use of prior steroid therapy.

4. Tomorrow's Shangri-la?

Currently available therapy for immunosuppressive treatment leaves much to be desired. The available agents are relatively nonspecific and, additionally, they target nonimmune cells for injury. Moreover, current more sophisticated therapeutic options are directed at all T cells. The ideal treatment would selectively target only those cells that are responding to the allograft and eliminate them from the immunologic arsenal. There are two hypothetical approaches to this ideal therapeutic option at the present time.

The first approach in more selective antirejection therapy has been to reduce the target population from all T cells, e.g., OKT3, to only those T cells that have been activated by exposure to the incompatable graft antigens. This approach has been explored by using a monoclonal antibody (mAb) to the IL-2 receptor (IL-2R). The mAb competes with IL-2 for binding sites and effectively targets activated T cells. In initial animal experiments, mice received orthotopic cardiac allografts. One group was treated with mAb M7/20, a mouse IgM mAb directed against the IL-2R. The mAb was administered by i.p. injection daily for 10 days beginning on the day of transplant. In five of six control mice the allografts were rejected by day 16 and the sixth was rejected on day 29. In contrast, two of six mice treated with M7/20 rejected their allografts on days 20 and 31, respectively, with the remaining four surviving for more than 90 days[90] (Fig. 1). A similar result was demonstrated in studies using the cardiac allograft model in rats, although graft survival in both experimental and control groups was not as long as in the mouse experiments.[91]

In monkeys receiving heterotopic renal allografts, an anti-IL-2R mAb, anti-Tac, given at 2 mg/kg every other day, was able to prolong allograft survival from a maximum of 7 days in control animals to 14 days in treated animals in one study[93] and from 14 days to 22 days in another study.[94]

This same approach has been utilized in clinical trials using a rat anti-human mAb, 33B3.1, against the IL-2R in cadaveric renal allograft recipients.[92] The mAb

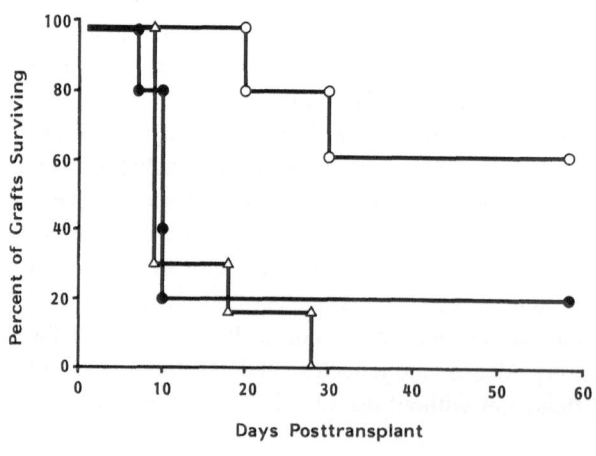

Fig. 1. Survival of C57BL/10 mice heart allografts in B10.AKM recipients. M7/20 treated grafts (○) had significantly longer survival than untreated controls (△) or those treated with a control IgM mAb that binds pre-B cells (RA3-2C2,●). (Reproduced from Kirkman et al.,[90] by copyright permission of the Rockefeller University Press.)

was administered to patients in addition to the usual doses of prednisone and Aza. One group received 5 mg i.v. daily for 14 days and the second group received 10 mg i.v. daily for the same period. CsA was initiated on day 14 of the mAb treatment. In groups receiving 33B3.1 there were fewer rejections than in an historical control group, although this reached statistical significance only in the patients receiving 10 mg daily. In our own unit, none of 14 cadaver donor recipients treated with a similar anti-IL-2R mAb, anti-Tac, experienced a rejection episode in the first 2 months posttransplantation.

A second approach to investigative immunotherapy has taken a more elegant twist. A chimeric gene consisting of a fusion between the cDNA encoding for IL-2 and a portion of the structural gene for diphtheria toxin in which the toxin receptor binding domain has been replaced by IL-2 sequences[95,96] has been constructed and transfected into *Escherichia coli,* resulting in the production of an IL-2 hybrid. The IL-2 portion of the molecule binds to the IL-2R expressed on activated T-cells. It is then internalized by receptor-mediated endocytosis into an acidic endosome where the molecule is cleaved and the toxic portion released. The toxin translocates to the cytoplasm and inhibits protein synthesis by ADP ribosylation of elongation factor 2. Furthermore, since the receptor recognition portion of the toxin is not encoded by the chimeric gene, there is no binding to cell surface receptors other than the IL-2R. Experiments using these chimeric toxins have clearly shown *in vitro* specificity for IL-2R+ cells, inhibition of protein synthesis, and, ultimately, cell death. In *in vivo* experiments in mice receiving heterotopic cardiac allografts and treated with IL-2-diphtheria toxin, 5 of 6 hosts receiving 1.0 μg/d as an i.p. injection kept their allografts for more than 50 days as compared to controls, all of whom rejected their grafts by day 10[98] (Fig. 2). A similar approach has been undertaken by another

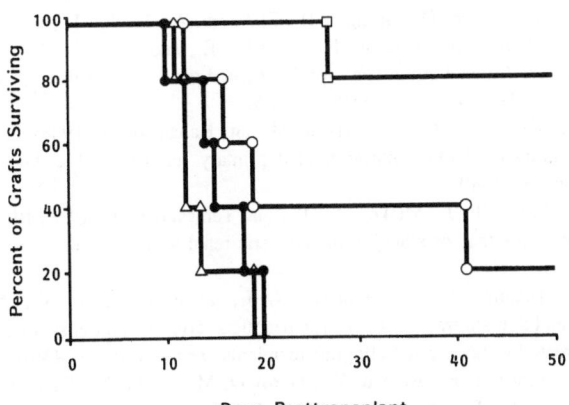

Fig. 2. Survival of B10.BR mice heart allografts in C57BL/10 recipients treated with an IL2-diphtheria toxin fusion protein. Untreated controls (●) and grafts treated with an inactive diphtheria toxin mutant (CRM-45, △) had significantly shorter survival than animals treated with 1 μg/day of IL-2 toxin (□). A dose of 0.5 μg/day (○) was less effective, although survival in 40% of the animals was prolonged over that of controls. (Reprinted from Kirkman *et al.,*[98] with permission.)

group but using *Pseudomonas* exotoxin instead of diphtheria toxin.[97] The IL-2 diphtheria toxin hybrid completely blocks delayed-type hypersensitivity reactions *in vivo* by eliminating IL-2R positive cells.[99] Data demonstrating the clinical efficacy of these toxins in human transplantation are not yet available and thus final pronouncement concerning their utilization in this circumstance is pending. However, studies to date are very promising in the development of more selective immunotherapies.

References

1. Opelz, G., 1988, The benefit of exchanging donor kidneys among transplant centers, *N. Engl. J. Med.* **318:**1289–1292.
2. Opelz, G., Sengar, D. P. S., Mickey, M. R., and Terasaki, P. I., 1973, Effect of blood transfusions on subsequent kidney transplants, *Transpl. Proc.* **5:**253–259.
3. Fehrman, I., Groth, C. G., Lundgren, G., and Moller, E., 1980, Improved renal allograft survival in transfused uremics, *Transplantation* **30:**324–327.
4. Salheim, B. G., Flatmark, A., Salvorsen, S., Juvell, J., Pape, J., and Thorsby, E., 1980, Effect of blood transfusion on renal transplantation, *Transplantation* **30:**281–284.
5. Fehrman, I., Gisth, C. G., Lundgren, G., Maynusson, G., and Moller, E., 1979, Pretransplant dialysis and blood transfusion—Correlation with cadaveric kidney graft survival, *Transpl. Proc.* **22:** 152–155.
6. Opelz, G. and Terasaki, P. I., 1978, Improvement of kidney graft survival with increased numbers of blood transfusion, *N. Engl. J. Med* **299:**799–803.
7. Vincenti, F., Duca, R., Cimend, W., Perkins, H. A., Cochrin, K. C., Feduska, J. J., and Salvatierra, O. 1978, Immunologic factors determining survival of cadaver kidney transplants. *N. Engl. J. Med.* **299:**793–798.
8. Sengar, D. P. S., Opelz, G., and Terasaki, P. I., 1973, Outcome of kidney transplants and suppression of mixed leukocyte culture by plasma, *Transpl. Proc.* **5:**641–647.
9. Opelz, G., 1987, Improved kidney graft survival in nontransfused recipients, *Transpl. Proc.* **19:** 149–152.
10. Lundgren, G., Albrechtsen, D., Brynger, H., Flatmark, A., Frodin, L., Gabel, H., Husberg, B., Klintmalm, G., Maurer, W., Persson, H., Thorsby, E., and Groth, C. G., 1986, Role of blood transfusions and HLA matching in cyclosporine-treated renal transplant recipients: A Scandinavian Multicenter Study, *Transpl. Proc.* **18:**1248–1255.
11. Kerman, R. H., Van Buren, C. T., Lovis, R. M., and Kahan, B. D., 1988, Successful transplantation of 100 untransfused cyclosporine-treated primary recipients of cadaveric renal allografts, *Transplantation* **45:**37–40.
12. Cecka, J. M., Cicciarelli, J., Mickey, M. R., and Terasaki, P. I., 1988, Blood transfusions and HLA matching—an either/or situation in cadaveric renal transplantation, *Transplantation* **45:**81–86.
13. Melzer, J. S., Husing, R. M., Feduska, N. J., Tomlanovich, F. V., Amend, W. J. C., Garovoy, M., and Salvatierra, O., 1987, The beneficial effect of pretransplant blood transfusions in cyclosporine-treated cadaver renal allograft recipients, *Transplantation* **43:**61–64.
14. Salvatierra, O., Vincenti, F., Amend, W., Garovoy, M., Iwaki, Y., Terasaki, P. I., Potter, D., Duca, R., Hopper, S., Slemmer, T., and Feduska, N., 1983, Four year experience with donor-specific blood transfusions, *Transpl. Proc.* **15:**924–931.
15. Takahaski, I., Otsubo, O., Nishimura, M., Maeda, T., Yanagisawa, T., Nozaki, H., Sugimoto, H., Kusaba, Y., Yamada, Y., Yamauchi, J., Sakai, A., and Inou, T., 1982, Prolonged graft survival by donor-specific blood transfusion (DSBT), *Transpl. Proc.* **14:**367–369.
16. Mendez, R., Iwaki, Y., Mendez, R. G., Bogaard, T., Self, B., Kanoeda, Y., and Terasaki, P. I.,

1982, Antibody response and allograft outcome with deliberate donor-specific blood transfusions, *Transpl. Proc.* **14**:378–382.

17. Newton, W. T. and Anderson, C. B., 1973, Planned immunosuppression of renal allograft recipients, *Surgery* **74**:430–436.

18. Anderson, C. B., Tyler, J. D., Sicard, G. A., Anderman, C. K., Rodey, G. E., and Etheredge, E. E., 1984, Pretreatment of renal allograft recipients with immunosuppression and donor-specific blood, *Transplantation* **38**:664–668.

19. Anderson, C. B., Sicard, G. A., and Etheredge, E. E., 1982, Pretreatment of renal allograft recipients with azathioprine and donor-specific blood products, *Surgery* **92**:315.

20. Glass, N. R., Miller, D. T., Sallinger, H. W. and Belzer, F. O., 1983, Comparative analysis of the DST and immuran-plus-DST protocols for live donor renal transplantation, *Transplantation* **36**: 636–641.

21. Opelz, G., 1985, Current relevance of the transfusion effect in renal transplantation, *Transpl. Proc.* **17**:1015–1022.

22. Leivestad, T., Flatmark, A., and Thorsby, E., 1985, Transplants of kidneys from one-haplotype-mismatched living related donors. Experience with donor-specific transfusions and cyclosporine, *Transpl. Proc.* **17**:2679–2680.

23. Billingham, R. E., Krohn, P. L., and Medawar, P. B., 1951, Effect of locally applied cortisone acetate on survival of skin homografts in rabbits, *Br. Med. J.* **2**:1049.

24. Billingham, R. E., Krohn, P. L., and Medawar, P. B., 1951, Effect of cortisone on survival of skin homografts in rabbits, *Br. Med. J.* **1**:1157.

25. Dempster, W. J., 1953, The effects of cortisone on the homotransplanted kidney, *Arch. Int. Pharmacol. Ther.* **95**:253.

26. Goodwin, W. E., Kauffman, J. J., Mims, M. M., Turner, R. D., Glassock, R., Goldman, R., and Maxwell, M. M., 1963, Human renal transplantation I. Clinical experiences with six cases of renal homotransplantation, *J. Urol.* **89**:13.

27. Chan, L., French, M. E., Oliver, D. O., and Morris, P. J., 1981, High and low dose prednisone, *Transpl. Proc.* **13**:336–338.

28. Buckels, J. A. C., Mackintosh, P., and Barnes, A. D., 1981, Controlled trial of low versus high dose oral steroid therapy in 100 cadaveric renal transplants, *Proc. Eur. Dial. Transpl. Assoc.* **18**: 394.

29. Salaman, J. R., Griffin, P. J. A., and Pierce, K., 1982, A controlled clinical trial of low-dose prednisone in renal transplantation, *Transpl. Proc.* **15**:103–104.

30. Snyder, D. S. and Unanue, F. R., 1982, Corticosteroids inhibit murine macrophage Ia expression and interleukin 1 production, *J. Immunol.* **129**:1803–1805.

31. Calne, R. Y., 1961, Inhibition of the rejection of renal homografts in dogs by purine analogs, *Transpl. Bull.* **28**:445–461.

32. Kaplan, M. P., Lysz, K., Rosenberg, S. A., and Rosenberg, J. C., 1983, Suppression of interleukin-2 production by methylprednisolone, *Transpl. Proc.* **15**:407–410.

33. Lew, W., Oppenheim, J. J., and Matsushima, K., 1988, Analysis of the suppression of IL-1 alpha and IL-1 beta production in human peripheral blood mononuclear adherent cells by a glucocorticoid hormone, *J. Immunol.* **140**:1895–1902.

34. Calne, R. Y., Alexander, G. P., and Murray, J. E., 1962. A study of the effects of drugs in prolonging survival of homologous renal transplant in dogs, *Ann. NY Acad. Sci.* **99**:743–761.

35. Murray, J. E., Merrill, J. P., Dammin, G. J., Dealy, J. B., Alexander, G. W., and Harrison, J. H., 1982, Kidney transplantation in modified recipients, *Curr. Surg.* **156**:337–355.

36. Murray, J. E., Merrill, J. P., Harrison, J. H., Wilson, R. E. I., and Dammin, G. J., 1963, Prolonged survival of human kidney homografts by immunosuppressive drug therapy, *N. Engl. J. Med.* **268**:1315–1323.

37. Borel, J. F., Feurer, C., Gubler, H. V., and Stahelin, H., 1976, Biological effects of cyclosporin A: A new antilymphocytic agent, *Agents Action* **6**:468–475.

38. Calne, R. Y., Thiru, S., McMaster, P., Craddock, G. N., White, D. J. G., Evans, D. B., Dunn, D.

C., and Pentlow, B. D., 1978, Cyclosporine A in patients receiving renal allografts from cadaver donors, *Lancet* **2:**1323–1327.

39. Knudsen, P. J., Dinarello, C. A., and Strom, T. B., 1987, Glucocorticoids inhibit transcriptional and post-transcriptional expression of interleukin 1 in U937 cells, *J. Immunol.* **139:**4129–4134.

40. Kern, J. A., Lamb, R. J., Reed, J. C., Daniele, R. P., and Nowell, P. C., 1988, Dexamethasone inhibition of interleukin 1 beta production by human monocytes, *J. Clin. Invest.* **81:**237–244.

41. Reed, J. C., Abidi, A. H., Alpers, J. D., Hoover, R. G., Robb, R. J., and Newell, P. C., 1986, Effect of cyclosporin A and dexamethasone on interleukin 2 receptor gene expression, *J. Immunol.* **137:**150–154.

42. Borel, J. F., Feurer, C., Magnee, C., and Stahelin, H., 1977, Effects of the new anti-lymphocytic peptide cyclosporin A in animals, *Immunology* **32:**1017–25.

43. Tosato, G., Pike, S. E., Koski, I. R., and Blaese, R. M., 1982, Selective inhibition of immunoregulatory cell functions by cyclosporine A, *J. Immunol.* **128:**1986–1991.

44. Paavonen, T. and Hayry, P., 1980, Effect of cyclosporin A on T-dependent and T-independent immunoglobulin synthesis *in vitro, Nature* **287:**542–544.

45. Borel, J. F., 1976, Comparative study of *in vitro* and *in vivo* drug effects on cell mediated cytotoxicity, *Immunology* **3:**631–641.

46. Hess, A. B., Tutschka, P. J., and Santos, G. W., 1982, Effect of cyclosporin A on human lymphocyte responses *in vitro*, III. CsA inhibits the production of T lymphocyte growth factors in secondary mixed lymphocyte responses but does not inhibit the response of primed lymphocytes to TCGF, *J. Immunol.* **128:**355–359.

47. Bird, A. G., McLachlan, S. M., and Britton, S., 1981, Cyclosporin A promotes spontaneous outgrowth in vitro of Epstein–Barr virus–induced B-cell lines, *Nature* **289:**300–301.

48. Miyawaki, T., Yachie, A., Ohzeki, S., Nagaoki, T., and Taniguchi, N., 1983, Cyclosporin A does not prevent expression of Tac antigen, a probable TCGF receptor molecule, on mitogen-stimulated human T cells, *J. Immunol.* **130:**2737–2742.

49. Hess, A. D., Tutschka, P. J., Pu, Z., and Santos, G. W., 1982, Effect of cyclosporin A on human lymphocyte responses in vitro. IV. Production of T cell stimulatory growth factors and development responsiveness to these growth factors in CsA-treated primary MLR cultures, *J. Immunol.* **128:**360–367.

50. Elliott, J. F., Lin, Y., Mizell, S. B., Bleackley, R. C., Harnish, D. G., and Paetkau, V., 1984, Induction of interleukin-2 messenger RNA inhibited by cyclosporin A, *Science* **226:**1439–1441.

51. Kronke, M., Leonard, W. J., Depper, J. M., Arya, S. K., Wong-Staal, F., Gallo, R. C., Waldmann, T. A., and Greene, W. C., 1984, Cyclosporin A inhibits T-cell growth factor gene expression at the level of mRNA transcription, *Proc. Natl. Acad. Sci. USA* **81:**5214–5218.

52. Gauchat, J. F., Khandjian, E. W., and Weil, R., 1986, Cyclosporin A prevents induction of the interleukin 2 receptor gene in cultured murine thymocytes, *Proc. Natl. Acad. Sci. USA* **83:**6430–6434.

53. Suthanthiran, M., 1987, Inhibitory activity of cyclosporine is dependent on the activating signal(s) provided to T cells, *J. Pediatr.* **111:**1008–1011.

54. Wiskocil, R., Weiss, A., Imbodin, J., Kamin-Lewis, R., and Stobo, J., 1985, Activation of a human T cell line: A two stimulus requirement in the pretranslational events involved in the coordinate expression of interleukin 2 and gamma interferon genes, *J. Immunol.* **134:**1599–1603.

55. Granelli-Piperno, A., Andrus, L., and Steinman, R. M., 1986, Lymphokine and nonlymphokine mRNA levels in stimulated human T cells, *J. Exp. Med.* **163:**922–937.

56. Herold, K. C., Lancki, D. W., Moldwin, R. L., and Fitch, F. W., 1986, Immunosuppressive effects of cyclosporine A on cloned T cells, *J. Immunol.* **136:**1315–1321.

57. Hamilton, D. V., Calne, R. Y., Evans, D. B., Henderson, R. B., Thiru, S., and White, D. J., 1981, The effect of long term cyclosporin A on renal function, *Lancet* **1:**1218–19.

58. Najarian, J. S., Ferguson, R. M., Sutherland, D. E., Rynasiewicz, J. T., and Simmons, R. L., 1983, A prospective trial of the efficacy of cyclosporine in renal transplantation at the University of Minnesota, *Transpl. Proc.* **15:**438–441.

59. Canadian Multicenter Transplant Group, 1983, A randomized clinical trial of cyclosporin in cadaveric renal transplantation, *N. Engl. J. Med.* **309:**809–815.

60. Merion, R. M., White, D. J. G., Thiru, S., Evans, D. B., and Calne, R. Y., 1984, Cyclosporine: Five years' experience in cadaveric renal transplantation, *N. Engl. J. Med.* **310:**148–154.

61. Adu, D., Turney, J., Michael, J., and McMaster, P., 1983, Hyperkalemia in cyclosporine treated renal allograft recipients, *Lancet* **2:**370–372.

62. Bantle, J. P., Nath, K. A., Sutherland, D. E., Najarian, J. S., and Ferris, T. F., 1985, Effects of cyclosporine in the renin–angiotensin–aldosterone system and potassium excretion in renal transplant recipients, *Arch. Intern. Med.* **145:**505–508.

63. Murray, B. M., Paller, M. S., and Ferris, T. F., 1985, Effect of cyclosporine administration on renal hemodynamics in conscious rats, *Kidney Int.* **28:**767–774.

64. Myers, B. D., Ross, J., Newton, L., Luetscher, J., and Perlroth, M., 1984, Cyclosporine-associated chronic nephropathy, *N. Engl. J. Med.* **311:**699–705.

65. Shulman, H., Striker, G., Deeg, H. J., Kennedy, M., Storb, R., and Thomas, E. D., 1981, Nephrotoxicity of cyclosporin A after allogeneic marrow transplantation, *N. Engl. J. Med.* **305:** 1392–1395.

66. Sommer, B. G., Innes, J. T., Whitehurst, R. M., Sharma, H. M., and Ferguson, R. M., 1985, Cyclosporine-associated renal arteriopathy resulting in loss of allograft function, *Am. J. Surg.* **149:** 756–764.

67. Klintmalm, G., Sundelin, B., Bohman, S. O., and Wilczek, H., 1984, Interstitial fibrosis in renal allografts after 12 to 46 months of cyclosporin treatment: beneficial effect of low doses in early posttransplantation period, *Lancet* **2:**950–954.

68. Hall, B. M., Tiller, D. J., Duggin, G. G., Horvath, J. S., Farnsworth, A., May, J., Johnson, J. R., and Sheil, A. G. R., 1985, Post-transplant acute renal failure in cadaver renal recipients treated with cyclosporine, *Kidney Int.* **28:**178–186.

69. Myers, B. D., Sibley, R., Newton, L., Tomlanovich, S. J., Boshkos, C., Stinson, E., Luetscher, J. A., Whitney, D. J., Krasny, D., Coplon, N. S., and Perlroth, M. G., 1988, The long-term course of cyclosporine-associated chronic nephropathy. *Kidney Int.* **33:**590–600.

70. Moran, M., Tomlanovich, S., and Myers, B. D., 1984, Cyclosporine-induced chronic nephropathy in human recipients of cardiac allografts. *Transpl. Proc.* **17** (Suppl. 1):185–190.

71. Neumayer, H.-H., Lopping, A., Velten, M., and Wagner, K., 1987, Effect of cyclosporine A on post-ischemic acute renal failure in conscious dogs: role of vasoactive renal hormones, *Transpl. Proc.* **19:**4035–4040.

72. Wagner, K. and Neumayer, H.-H., 1987, Influence of the calcium antagonist dilitiazem on delayed graft function in cadaveric kidney transplantation: results of a 6 month follow-up, *Transpl. Proc.* **19:** 1353–1357.

73. Cohen, D. J., Loertscher, R., Rubin, M. F., Tilney, N. L., Carpenter, C. B., and Strom, T. B., 1984, Cyclosporine: A new immunosuppressive agent for organ transplantation, *Ann. Intern. Med.* **101:**667–682.

74. Loveland, B. E. and McKenzie, I. F. C., 1982, Which T cells cause graft rejection? *Transplantation* **33:**217–221.

75. Loveland, B. E. and McKenzie, I. F. C., 1982, Cells mediating graft rejection in the mouse III. Ly-1+ precursor T cells generate skin graft rejection, *Transplantation* **33:**407–410.

76. Loveland, B. E. and McKenzie, I. F. C., 1982, Cells mediating graft rejection in the mouse IV. The Ly-5, 6 and 7 effector cell phenotype, *Transplantation* **33:**411–413.

77. MacDonald, H. R., Sekaly, R. P., Kanagawa, O., Thiernesse, N., Taswell, C., Cerottini, J. C., Weiss, A., Glasebrook, A. L., Engers, H. D., Kelso, A., Brunner, K. T., and Bron, C., 1982, Cytolytic T lymphocyte clones, *Immunobiology* **161:**84.

78. Renkonen, R., Soots, A., von Willebrand, E., and Hayry, P., 1983, Lymphoid cell subclasses in rejecting renal allograft in the rat, *Cell Immunol.* **77:**187–195.

79. Heidecke, C. D., Kupiec-Weglinski, J. W., Lear, P. A., Abbud-Filho, M., Araujo, J. L., Araneda, D., Strom, T. B., and Tilney, N. L., 1984, Interleukin-2 rich lymphokines produce

acute rejection of vascularized cardiac allografts in T cell deprived rats, *J. Immunol.* **133:**582–588.

80. Rosenberg, A. S., Mizuochi, T., Sharrow, S. O., and Singer, A., 1987, Phenotype, specificity, and function of T cell subsets and T cell interactions involved in skin allograft rejection, *J. Exp. Med.* **165:**1296–1315.

81. Bishop, G. A., Hall, B. M., Duggin, G. G., Horvath, J. S., Shiel, A. G. R., and Tiller, D. J., 1986, Immunopathology of renal allograft rejection analyzed with monoclonal antibodies to mononuclear cell markers, *Kidney Int.* **29:**708–717.

82. Cobbold, S. and Waldman, H., 1986, Skin allograft rejection by L3/T4+ and Lyt2+ T cell subsets, *Transplantation* **41:**634–649.

83. Fauci, A. S., Dale, D. C., and Balow, J. E., 1976, Corticosteroid therapy: Mechanisms of action and clinical consideration, *Ann. Intern. Med.* **84:**304–315.

84. Sanfilippo, F., Kobeck, P. C., Vaughn, W. K., and Bollinger, R. R., 1985, Renal allograft cell infiltrates associated with irreversible rejection, *Transplantation* **40:**679–695.

85. Sprent, J., Schaefer, M., Lo, D., and Korngold, R., 1985, Functions of purified L3T4+ and Lyt-2+ cells *in vitro* and *in vivo, Immunol. Rev.* **91:**195–218.

86. Tuazon, T. V., Schneeberger, E. E., Bhan, A. K., McCluskey, R. T., Cosimi, A. B., Schooley, R. T., Rubin, R. H., and Colvin, R. B., 1987, Mononuclear cells in acute allograft glomerulography, *Am. J. Pathol.* **129:**119–132.

87. Ortho Multicenter Transplant Study Group, 1985, A randomized clinical trial of OKT3 monoclonal antibody for acute rejection of cadaveric renal transplants, *N. Engl. J. Med.* **313:**337–342.

88. Norman, D. J., Barry, J. M., Bennett, W. M., Leone, M., Henell, K., Funnell, B., and Hubert, B., 1988, The use of OKT3 in cadaveric renal transplantation for rejection that is unresponsive to conventional anti-rejection therapy, *Am. J. Kidney Dis.* **11:**90–93.

89. Thistlewaite, J. R., Stuart, J. K., Mayes, J. T., Gaber, A. O., and Stuart, F. P., 1988, Use of a brief steroid trial before initiating OKT3 therapy for renal allograft rejection, *Am. J. Kidney Dis.* **11:**94–98.

90. Kirkman, R. L., Barrett, L. V., Gaulton, G. N., Kelley, V. E., Ythier, A., and Strom, T. B., 1985, Administration of an anti-interleukin-2 receptor monoclonal antibody prolongs cardiac allograft survival in mice, *J. Exp. Med.* **162:**358–362.

91. Kupiec-Weglinski, J. W., Diamantstein, T., Tilney, N. L., and Strom, T. B., 1985, Therapy with monoclonal antibody to interleukin 2 receptor spares suppressor T cells and prevents or reverses acute allograft rejection in rats, *Proc. Natl. Acad. Sci. USA* **83:**2624–2627.

92. Soulillou, J. P., LeMauff, B., Olive, D., Delaage, M., Peyronnet, P., Hourmant, M., Mawas, C., Hirn, M., and Jacques, Y., 1987, Prevention of rejection of kidney transplants by monoclonal antibody directed against interleukin 2, *Lancet* **1:**1339–1342.

93. Shapiro, M. E., Kirkman, R. L., Reed, M. H., Puskas, J. D., Majoujian, G., Letvin, N. L., Carpenter, C. B., Milford, E. L., Waldmann, T. A., Strom, T. B., and Schlossman, S. F., 1987, Monoclonal anti-IL-2 receptor antibody in primate renal transplantation, *Transpl. Proc.* **19:**594–598.

94. Reed, M. H., Shapiro, M. E., Strom, T. B., Milford, E. L., Carpenter, C. B., Letvin, N. L., Waldmann, T. A., and Kirkman, R. L., 1981, Prolongation of primate renal allografts with anti-Tac monoclonal antibody, *Current Surg.* **45:**28–30.

95. Williams, D. P., Parker, K., Bacha, P., Bishai, W., Borowski, M., Genbauffe, F., Strom, T. B., and Murphy, J. R., 1987, Diphtheria toxin receptor binding domain substitution with interleukin-2: Genetic construction and properties of a diphtheria toxin–related interleukin-2 fusion protein, *Protein Eng.* **1:**493–498.

96. Bacha, P., Williams, D. P., Waters, C., Williams, J. M., Murphy, J. R., and Strom, T. B., 1988, Interleukin 2 receptor–targeted cytotoxicity. Interleukin 2 receptor–mediated action of a diphtheria toxin–related interleukin 2 fusion protein, *J. Exp. Med.* **167:**612–622.

97. Lorberboum-Galski, H., FitzGerald, D., Chaudhary, V., Adhya, S., and Pastan, I., 1988, Cytotox-

ic activity of an interleukin-2 pseudomonas exotoxin chimeric protein produced in *Escherichia coli*, *Proc. Natl. Acad. Sci. USA* **85:**1922–1926.

98. Kirkman, R. L., Bacha, P., Barrett, L. V., Forte, S., Murphy, J. R., and Strom, T. B., 1988, Prolongation of cardiac allograft survival in murine recipients treated with a diphtheria toxin-related interleukin-2 fusion protein, *Transplantation* **47:**327–330.

99. Kelley, V. E., Bacha, P., Pankewycz, O. G., Nichols, J. C., Murphy, J. R., and Strom, T. B., 1988, Interleukin-2 diphtheria toxin fusion protein can abolish cell-mediated immunity *in vivo*, *Proc. Natl. Acad. Sci. USA* **4:**3980–3984.

15

Drugs and the Kidney

William M. Bennett

1. Introduction

Drug effects on the kidney and, in turn, the influence of renal disease on drug metabolism continue to play an important part of day-to-day clinical medicine for the nephrologist. This review updates current information in various areas of renal pharmacology emphasizing those recent advances with current or future clinical implications.

2. Pharmacologic Principles and the Effects of Renal Disease

A series of concise articles covering fundamental aspects of pharmacokinetics for clinicians has been published. Concepts of clearance, metabolic first-pass biliary excretion, and drug metabolism are reviewed in lucid fashion.[1-4] Welling discusses the use of graphic methods for analysis of pharmacokinetic data.[5] With increasing sophistication of analytic methods for drugs and their metabolites in body fluids, therapeutic monitoring of many drugs is now possible. Proper use of these data depends on a good understanding of sample timing and individual drug pharmacokinetics.[6] An automated immunoassay method was used to measure serum carbamazepine, digoxin, gentamicin, lidocaine, phenobarbital, phenytoin, quinidine, valproic acid, and vancomycin. These drugs could be accurately determined in the

---

WILLIAM M. BENNETT • Department of Medicine, Oregon Health Sciences University, Portland, Oregon 97201.

uremic milieu despite the presence of potentially interfering accumulated uremic metabolites.[7]

2.1. Effect of Renal Dysfunction and Age on Drug Pharmacokinetics

Drug absorption is reduced in renal failure as measured by D-xylose absorption. Although D-xylose volume of distribution and elimination half-life are increased in renal failure, the serum concentration obtained 1 hr after an oral dose is a valid measurement of intestinal function in uremic patients.[8] Aluminum-containing antacids are widely used for gastrointestinal phosphate binding. Phosphate binding is maximum at pH 2–3 and greater with liquid than with tablets or capsules.[9] Drug absorption may be affected by these preparations.

Gibson published a scholarly review of drug metabolic pathways in the presence of renal failure.[10] Since hepatic microsomal mixed-function oxidases may be altered in end-stage renal failure, even drugs or metabolites whose biotransformation is dependent on the liver, such as morphine or paracetamol, may produce adverse reactions in renal patients.[10] In addition, individual differences in highly polymorphic metabolic gene products may provide an explanation for idiosyncratic reactions and variable pharmacokinetics with medications used in renal patients such as sulfonamides[11] or antiarrhythmic drugs.[12]

Endogenous substances retained in renal failure have digitalis-like properties, such as inhibition of Na,K-ATPase. This inhibition of the sodium pump has a postulated role in adaptation to loss of renal function.[13] Hemodialysis may acutely increase plasma levels of these substances; however, long-term dialysis decreases these transport inhibitors.[13] Interpretation of serum digoxin levels may be difficult since these endogenous solutes may cross-react with the antidigoxin antibodies in various diagnostic kits, especially when these solutes accumulate in individuals with renal failure.[14] Also, cardioinactive metabolites of digoxin can increase immunoreactive digoxin.[15] Digitoxin measurement is not affected by the endogenous or exogenous compounds.[16] In dialysis patients not on cardiac glycosides, a sensitive radioimmunoassay gave values for digitalis-like factors of up to 0.25 ng/ml.[17] Assays for digitalis-like factors using [^{3}H]ouabain displacement or Na,K-ATPase are more sensitive than digoxin radioimmunoassay.[18] There is wide variability among commercial digoxin radioimmunoassay kits, and individual sera varied by as much as 0.6 ng/ml. Some assays detected low amounts of digitalis-like factors in 23% of patients not on cardiac glycosides, with the highest level being 0.5 ng/ml.[19]

As the population of patients treated for end-stage renal failure ages, those changes in pharmacokinetics secondary to healthy aging independent of renal dysfunction should also be considered. Pharmacogeriatric principles have been reviewed recently.[20,21] Drug-induced illness and drug interactions are common in the elderly, many related to physiologic changes occurring in the kidney.[22] An easy-to-remember formula relating creatinine clearance to age is $C_{cr} = 130 - age$.[23] A comprehensive list of drugs causing psychiatric symptoms is useful to consider in patients whose clinical deterioration is out of proportion to renal failure or chronologic age *per se*.[24] Decreased clearances of the components of the widely prescribed antihypertensives Dyazide and Maxide with age are closely correlated with reductions in renal function.[25] Fatal hyperkalemia can result, particularly if beta blockers or angiotensin converting enzyme inhibitors are prescribed concurrently.[26] Gentamicin disposition follows a similar pattern of decreased renal clearance with age.[27] Conversely, infants and children have increased clearance of cyclosporine compared to adult transplant recipients.[28]

2.2. Drug Binding in Renal Disease

Alpha-1 acid glycoprotein concentrations increase in chronic renal failure.[29] While the mechanism underlying the increase is unclear,[30] basic drugs may be increasingly bound, lowering "free" drug levels. Disopyramide is bound primarily to this plasma protein, instead of albumin, as is suggested by normal binding in nephrotic patients with massive albumin losses.[31]

Drug–protein binding is reduced for many acidic drugs in chronic renal failure.[32] Gulyassy and colleagues have further characterized the binding inhibitors in uremic serum that compete with acidic drugs for binding sites on serum proteins. Binding inhibitory activity is due to a family of aromatic amino acids including hippurate, β-*m*-hydroxyphenyl-hydracrylate and *P*-hydroxyphenylacetate.[33] Mabuchi and Nakahashi isolated additional serum inhibitors, 3-carboxy-4-methyl-5 propyl-furapropanoic acid, which is a constituent of normal urine,[34] as well as indoxylsulfate, 2-hydroxybenzoylglycine, and 3-indolacetic acid.[35] Based on these considerations, the use of free drug concentrations for therapeutic drug monitoring clinical practice was reviewed.[36] There are currently insufficient data to justify adoption of this more complicated methodology for routine nephrologic patients.

2.3. Renal Drug Transport Processes

Cimetidine is excreted into the urine after substantial active transport from peritubular blood by proximal tubular epithelial cells. In brush border membrane vesicles, this transport is mediated by organic cation–proton exchange. pH-stimulated uptake of [^{3}H]cimetidine was inhibited by quinidine, procainamide, and excess unlabeled cimetidine, but not by probenecid.[37] Cimetidine inhibited hepatic cytochome P-450 enzymes in the liver and competed with ranitidine and triamterene for tubular secretion in healthy subjects, but did not compete with organic anions or zwitterions.[38,39] This suggests selectivity for a common cationic secretory transport system. The clinical correlates of these interactive processes have been summarized.[40,41] In addition to renal excretory mechanisms, alterations in hepatic blood flow and metabolizing activity contribute to numerous interactions which need to be considered by the prescribing physician.

Active penicillin uptake and secretion was inhibited by organic acids, including therapeutically relevant sulfonamides, salicylate, thiazides, and indomethacin.[42] Quinidine and quinine are stereoisomers; however, quinidine is preferred in a ratio of 4–5 to 1 over quinine by this stereoselective renal drug transport process for organic bases.[43] Tubular secretion is a major pathway of renal digoxin elimination. Tubular transport of digoxin is independent of defined anionic and cationic transport systems and does not depend on the Na^+,K^+-ATPase receptor. Secretion can be modulated by calcium antagonists and spironolactone.[44]

3. Drug Effects on Renal Function

Calcium antagonists dramatically improve renal hemodynamics in experimental renal ischemia. This property may ultimately prove useful in clinical situations such as acute renal failure, cadaver organ preservation, and modification of toxic nephropathy. Calcium antagonists produce vasodilatation in these situations with preservation of glomerular filtration rate (GFR), presumably because of their selective action on afferent arteriolar resistance vessels.[45] In patients with essential hypertension, diltiazem produces increases in GFR and effective renal plasma without a change in filtration fraction. The authors suggested attenuated intrarenal effects of angiotensin and norepinephrine.[46] Micropuncture studies in rats with renal nerve stimulation support this hypothesis.[47] Diltiazem produced less stimulation of plasma renin activity and catecholamines than nifedipine in anesthetized dogs.[48] Felodopine, a new calcium antagonist, increases sodium and calcium excretion while lowering filtration fraction and preserving GFR.[49]

Low-dose dopamine improves renal function as measured by GFR and effective renal plasma flow (ERPF) in normals and patients with renal disease, although no effect was noted if the baseline GFR was less than 50 ml/min per 1.73m². This is presumably due to a maximally utilized renal reserve filtration capacity.[50] High doses of the dopamine antagonist metoclopramide decrease renal plasma flow and could potentiate cisplatin nephrotoxicity when used to alleviate symptoms in cancer chemotherapy regimes.[51]

Postsynaptic binding sites for α and α_2 adrenoreceptor agonists are found in the renal cortex, with α_2 sites predominating.[52] α_2 Agonists such as the antihypertensive agents guanabenz and clonidine can induce a diuresis and natriuresis or at least counterbalance α_1-stimulated sodium reabsorption.[53]

4. Prescribing for Patients with Renal Dysfunction

Updated recommendations for the use of relevant drugs in patients with varying degrees of renal dysfunction are available.[54–57] Bjornsson has published a nomogram for the rapid determination of a dosage adjustment factor if the fraction of a drug dose normally excreted unchanged by the kidney is known.[58] Principles of drug dosing in organ transplant recipients were summarized by Burckart.[59] Use of antibiotics in renal failure has been summarized by Van Scoy and Wilson.[60]

Central to most dosing recommendations is some determination of renal function usually based on serum creatinine. It should be recognized that second- and third-generation cephalosporins, such as cefoxitin, ceforanide, ceftizoxime, ceftriaxone, and moxalactam, can falsely elevate serum creatinine and reduce creatinine clearance.[61,62] Trimethoprim given to patients with chronic renal failure elevated serum creatinine by 35% by inhibition of tubular creatinine secretion.[63]

Hearing loss may be associated with renal failure. In addition, many drugs that cause ototoxicity have renal dysfunction as a major risk factor. Ototoxic drugs used by nephrologists include aminoglycosides, loop diuretics, nonsteroidal antiinflammatory drugs, and chemotherapeutic agents.[64]

5. Removal of Drugs by Extracorporeal Means and Peritoneal Dialysis

Nephrologic practice frequently involves consultation regarding the use of extracorporeal techniques for removing drugs and poisons in overdose situations. Cutler *et al.* and Choi and Johnson have published concise reviews of drugs removed by hemodialysis and hemoperfusion.[65,66] The continued important role of activated charcoal in the management of some overdoses was emphasized by Derlet and Albertons.[67] For example, charcoal hemoperfusion is effective for methotrexate toxicity.[68]

Extracorporal therapy with continuous arteriovenous hemofiltration (CAVH) is now widely applied to critically ill patients and patients with acute renal failure. Drug losses during the procedure, while usually small, may be of clinical importance in a critical-care patient.[69,70] Removal is dependent on ultrafiltrate flow rate and the sieving coefficient.[71] Vancomycin, ordinarily not removed during conventional hemodialysis because of high protein binding and a molecular weight of 1200 daltons, is lost during hemofiltration.[72,73] Serum level monitoring and dosage supplementation are necessary. Both CAVH and hemoperfusion were more effective than hemodialysis in removing procainamide metabolites,[74,75] but Torasemide is not significantly eliminated from the blood by these techniques.[76] Hemofiltration has been used successfully in a digoxin overdose.[77] Many drugs, such as aminoglycosides, are predictably removed by hemofiltration according to their known plasma protein binding.[78,79] Some charged molecules can be bound to the membrane of the hemofilter, reducing their effective blood levels.[80]

The pharmacokinetics of drugs during continuous ambulatory peritoneal dialysis (CAPD) is a fertile area for clinical investigation inasmuch as intraperitoneal antibiotics are routinely used to treat peritonitis. The diagnosis and management of CAPD is the subject of an official position statement by the British Society of Antimicrobial Chemotherapy.[81]

Janicke *et al.* have developed a simplified modeling method which accounts for bidirectional transfer of drugs given to CAPD patients.[82] After a single intravenous dose of vancomycin, dialysate concentration averaged 8 ng/ml for 3 days and 4 ng/ml for 6 days despite extremely low peritoneal clearance.[83] A 30 mg/kg intraperitoneal dose of vancomycin produced therapeutic serum and end-dwell dialysate concentrations over a 1-week period.[84] Teicoplanin has similar penetration into peritoneal fluid after intravenous doses.[85] Peritonitis enhances drug entry into the peritoneum by both intravenous and intraperitoneal administration routes.[86,87] Ten to twelve percent of the total clearance of intravenous acyclovir is through peritoneal dialysis in CAPD patients.[88] There is 91% bioavailability of intraperitoneal acyclovir.[89] Tobramycin absorption from the peritoneal space is increased with peritonitis[90] and averages about 60% of a dose. Gentamicin is removed in amounts requiring dosage supplementation in intermittent peritoneal dialysis.[91] Insignificant amounts of cefamandole, tocainide, ranitidine, and procainamide are removed through CAPD, and dosage supplements are not required.[92-95]

However, pharmacokinetic studies with clindamycin, moxalactam, ceftriaxone, and cefotaxime reveal similar data to previous CAPD publications, namely, that adequate intraperitoneal concentrations are achieved after intravenous dosing but that bioavailability is 30–70% with intraperitoneal dose absorption.[96-99] Using a crossover pharmacokinetic analysis, Walshe and Janicke showed that a 1–3 mg/kg intraperitoneal load of tobramycin, followed by 0.6–1.2 mg/kg every 24 hr (based on lean body weight), gave adequate fluctuating peak serum and dialysate levels. The more constant plasma level obtained with 8 µg/ml in each 2-liter exchange, as is conventionally done, is theoretically more ototoxic and may be more expensive.[100] Oral ciprofloxacin absorption is delayed in CAPD patients by phosphate-binding antacids. Long dwell times are necessary to achieve adequate peritoneal drug concentrations.[101] Amphotericin but not dipyridamole increased peritoneal fluid and solute clearances during peritoneal dialysis.[102,103]

Although hemodialysis may remove thiocyanate generated by prolonged infusions of nitroprusside, hydroxocobalamin intramuscularly may help reverse cyanide toxicity produced by overdoses of this drug. Metabolic acidosis and drug tachyphylaxis are poor prognostic signs during short-term, high-dose nitroprusside use (total dose 1.5 mg/kg).[104] Small amounts of ibuprofen metabolites, but little parent drug, are found in the dialysate of patients receiving regular dialysis, suggesting ibuprofen removal is primarily by metabolic pathways.[105] Isosorbide was effectively removed by hemodialysis but not peritoneal dialysis.[106]

6. Aspects of Specific Drugs in Patients with Renal Disease

6.1. Aminoglycosides

Aminoglycoside nephrotoxicity incurred a cost of $2500 over and above other hospital costs in a case-control study designed to assess the impact of this common toxic nephropathy.[107] Dosing of aminoglycosides to achieve targeted peak and trough serum levels continues to be a therapeutic challenge for clinicians. The cost effectiveness of computerized dosing programs using multiple serum levels for individualized pharmacokinetics is unclear. A high incidence of toxicity has been reported when aminoglycosides are dosed by nonpharmacokinetic methods.[108] Alanine aminopeptidase increase in the urine occurs as early as the first day of therapy, especially when aminoglycosides are combined with vancomycin.[109] Although high baseline serum creatinine and elevated trough levels are associated with nephrotoxicity, this does not imply a cause-and-effect relationship. In fact, it is likely that drug accumulation is due to renal dysfunction.[110] In a prospective study, basing dosing on published population-based kinetics, an acceptable toxicity profile was achieved with targeted peak and trough levels in 81% of subjects.[111] Comparisons of a simpler individualized approach using Bayesian principles with the more expensive Sawchuk–Zaske method requiring multiple serum levels were equivalent in predicting steady-state trough tobramycin concentrations.[112] To further complicate aminoglycoside dosing, Nahata *et al.* point out the interlot variability of gentamicin and tobramycin in commercial preparations of aminoglycosides.[113] In dogs with subclinical renal dysfunction, three-times-daily dosing is less efficacious and more toxic than the same daily dose given less frequently.[114]

Steady-state accumulation of netilmicin in renal tissue is higher than accumulation of tobramycin using a crossover design in normal volunteers. If intracellular aminoglycoside concentrations translate into more nephrotoxicity, these differences in pharmacokinetics could be important.[115] However, compelling evidence for this in patients is lacking, and at present the differences in experimental nephrotoxicity among relevant aminoglycosides do not justify use of any single agent over a less expensive alternative. Habekacin, a new semisynthetic aminoglycoside similar to amikacin, demonstrates pharmacokinetic behavior similar to other available aminoglycosides.[116] No new aminoglycoside has been proven to be superior to conventional drugs. When gentamicin resistance is a problem, amikacin is the agent of choice.[117]

6.2. Carbapenems

Carbapenems are a new class of β-lactam antibiotics, of which imipenem is the first clinically available congener. They differ from penicillins in that the 1-sulfur atom is replaced by a carbon and there is an extra double bond in the molecule.[118] When cilastatin, a dehydropeptidase I inhibitor, is coadministered with imipenem, urinary excretion of the active antibiotic increases markedly.[119] Decreased renal function causes reduced elimination of both imipenem and cilastatin necessitating decreased dosage for end-stage renal disease patients. Seizures may occur when high serum levels occur.[120] These drugs have a broad antimicrobial spectrum and may replace the nephrotoxic aminoglycosides for some indications. Patients allergic to penicillins should also be considered to be allergic to carbapenems.[121]

6.3. Cephalosporins and Monobactams

Cephalosporins continue to be heavily prescribed because of their relative safety and efficacy even in complicated patients. As pointed out in an excellent short summary, the cost of these drugs has to be justified by favorable comparisons to older drugs in this class.[122] The pharmacokinetic properties of this class of antibiotics were succinctly reviewed by Bergan.[123] Cefotetan is a broad-spectrum agent with high activity against gram-negative organisms, even strains producing β-lactamase. The drug is renally excreted without active metabolites but can be converted to a tautomer with antibacterial properties similar to those of the parent cefotetan. In severe renal failure the dose interval should be spread to 48 hr after a 1 to 2 g load.[124] Supplemental doses are needed after hemodialysis but not for peritoneal dialysis.[125] Similar kinetic considerations apply to cefmenoxime[126,127] and ceftazidime.[128]

Cefonicid is a once-a-day, second-generation drug which is comparable to cefazolin ceforanide and cefamandole for urinary infections. It is not dialyzable.[129,130] Ceforanide is a new second-generation parenteral cephalosporin which can be given twice daily. Except for a prolonged half-life, it has no particular therapeutic advantage. It is dialyzable, as opposed to cefonicid.[131] Cefoxitin given to patients with renal failure penetrates pleural fluid extremely well.[132] Cefixime is an oral, extended-half-life, broad-spectrum cephalosporin whose dose interval must be increased when creatinine clearance falls below 20 ml/min per 1.73 m².[133] Cephadroxil is effective in a once- or twice-daily oral regimen, as opposed to the similar drugs cephalexin and cephradine, which require more frequent dosing.[134] Cefsulodin is a narrow-spectrum, third-generation cephalosporin which has anti-pseudomonal properties. It has a prolonged half-life in renal failure and significant amounts of drug are removed during hemodialysis.[135] Cefpiramide total body clearance stays constant as renal function declines despite a fall in renal clearance. Non renal routes of elimination become more important as renal disease progresses.[136]

Platelet dysfunction and hypoprothrombinemia may be troublesome for renal patients who already had an enhanced propensity to bleed. The pharmacokinetics of a 1-methyl 1-H-tetrazole-5-thiol side chain of cefamandole, which inhibits prothrombin precursors, was reviewed by Aronoff *et al.* They found that the side chain had reduced protein binding in renal failure predisposing to this side effect.[137] Babiak and Ryback reviewed the hemotological effects of β-lactam antibiotics.[138] Encephalopathy occurred due to cefazolin in a uremic patient in whom dosage was excessive for the degree of renal insufficiency.[139]

Azthreonam is the first monobactam approved in the United States. It has excellent activity against gram-negative bacteria because the drug binds to a high-affinity binding protein in the cell wall of these organisms. Most β-lactamases will not inactivate azthreonam. The usual half-life of 1.7 hr is extended to 6 hr in anephric patients. Hemodialysis and peritoneal dialysis both remove significant amounts of azthreonam. There is little cross-allergenicity with penicillins or cephalosporins. Azthreonam has little gram-positive or anaerobic coverage. Dosage should be cut to 25–50% of normal in patients with severe renal failure.[140,141]

6.4. Penicillins

The combination of a penicillin with an inhibitor of β-lactamase has been used with efficacy in intraabdominal and gynecologic infections. The combination as ampicillin with sulbactam is the latest to become available. Sulbactam does not affect the pharmacokinetics of ampicillin. The combination given parenterally has 1 g of sulbactam to 2 g of ampicillin. The half-life of sulbactam is 1 hr, which is extended in renal failure.[142–144] The combination of amoxicillin and clavulanic acid can be given orally as well as parenterally. In renal failure amoxicillin clearance is reduced to a greater extent than clavulanic acid. Dosage intervals should not exceed 12 hr to maintain effective concentrations of the β-lactamase inhibitor.[145] Similar kinetic considerations apply to the combination of clavulanic acid with ticarcillin.[146–148] A concise review of the penicillins has been published by Wright and Wilkowske.[149]

Fluorinated quinoline antibiotics are exciting new agents for treatment of gram-positive and gram-negative infections. Importantly, they have significant activity against anaerobes and *Pseudomonas* species. As opposed to the chemically related nalidixic acid, development of resistance is unusual. The primary mechanism of action is inhibition of DNA gyrase, which interferes with a conformational change in bacterial DNA necessary for protein synthesis.[150–152] Efficacy has been shown in complicated urinary tract infections, even those caused by *Pseudomonas* and other multiply resistant organisms.[153] These drugs can be given orally with excellent results. Ciprofloxacin is 2–4 times more active than norfloxacin or ofloxacin against the usual urinary tract pathogens. Adverse reactions are minor and are largely confined to transitory nausea, vomiting, or diarrhea. A single case of reversible nephrotoxicity has been reported.[154] The new fluoroquinolones may interfere with hepatic P-450-mediated theophylline metabolism. Solubility of these drugs decreases with alkaline pH, and patients should be monitored for urinary crystal deposition. Aluminum-containing antacids reduce ciprofloxacin absorption.[155] An intravenous preparation is available which is eliminated from the body primarily by renal clearance.[156] Lode *et al.* summarized the comparative pharmacokinetics of this exciting new class of antibiotics.[157] Pharmacokinetic parameters relating to the five most clinically imminent quinolones are depicted in Table I.[158]

Dose adjustment of ciprofloxacin and other congeners is necessary in patients with reduced GFR as well as ambulatory elderly subjects because of extended drug half-life. Dose intervals of 12–24 hr should be used.[159,160] No adjustment is necessary for hemodialysis[161] or peritoneal dialysis, although oral ciprofloxacin may produce drug levels in peritoneal fluid sufficient to treat CAPD-associated peritonitis.[161a] Use of fluorinated quinolones in pregnancy is contraindicated.[162] A single case of reversible acute renal failure associated with norfloxacin has been

Table I. Pharmacokinetic Parameters Related to Fluorinated Quinoline Antibiotics[a]

	% of dose excreted unchanged	Usual $t^{1/2}$ (hr)	ESRD $t^{1/2}$ (hr)	Protein binding (%)	Dose internal in ESRD[b] (hr)	Removal by dialysis
Ciprofloxacin	40–60	3.5–5	10–15	30	12–24	No
Enoxacin	60	4–6	24–36	18	24	No
Norfloxacin	30	3–7	10–18	15	12–24	No
Ofloxacin	>90	3.5–9	24–36	30	24–48	No
Pefloxacin	10–15	8–12	24–48	<30	24–48	No

[a]See Refs. 155, 164–167.
[b]ESRD = end-stage renal disease.

reported. Renal biopsy showed interstitial edema and lymphocyte infiltrate without eosinophils.[163]

6.5. Vancomycin–Teicoplanin

Vancomycin-like antibiotics are widely used in nephrology because of their favorable gram-positive coverage and their prolonged half-life in renal failure. Recent extensive reviews have been published.[167,168] The renal handling of vancomycin, not previously studied, showed major excretion by glomerular filtration and concentration dependent nonrenal clearance in normal volunteers.[169] In normal subjects there was a high incidence of "red man syndrome," consisting of generalized erythema, pruritus, and angioedema with hypotension when a 1-g dose is delivered over less than 1 hr.[170,171] A small amount of hydrocortisone in the intravenous infusion may minimize this syndrome.[172] In renal disease, even slow administration of vancomycin can lead to this complication.[173] True allergic reactions, although extremely rare, are prolonged in renal failure patients.[174] Oral vancomycin is useful in renal patients for the treatment of antibiotic-associated colitis. Unless daily doses are greater than 2 g or duration of therapy is prolonged for 10 days, serum levels are not usually in the toxic range.[175]

Teicoplanin is a new glycopeptide antibiotic with an antimicrobial spectrum similar to that of vancomycin against gram-positive aerobic and anaerobic bacteria. Elimination half-life is markedly prolonged in renal failure.[176] In end-stage renal disease a single 6 mg/kg dose can be given every 3 days.[177] Wide individual differences in teicoplanin clearance were noted in critically ill patients in addition to reduced clearance due to renal insufficiency.[178] Little drug is lost by hemodialysis or peritoneal dialysis and thus dosage adjustment after dialysis is unnecessary.

6.6. Other Antimicrobial Agents Used by Nephrologists

Wilson and Cockerill have reviewed the use of tetracyclines, chloramphenicol, erythromycin, and clindamycin.[179] The elimination half-life and total clearance of erythromycin do not depend on renal function.[180] Consistent with the ototoxicity observed in patients with renal failure, Kanfer *et al.* have demonstrated higher maximum serum concentrations and increased area under the time–concentration curves for erythromycin in renal failure. They suggested enhanced bioavailability of erythromycin in chronic renal failure predisposing to ototoxicity.[181]

Pentamidine has undergone a resurgence of use due to its activity against *Pneumocystis carinii* infections in acquired immune deficiency syndrome. Hypotension and nephrotoxicity occur frequently despite recommended doses. The interval between doses should be extended to 36–48 hr in renal insufficiency.[182] The drug has a large volume of distribution, which decreases in patients given intravenous, as opposed to intramuscular, dosing.[183] Renal toxicity, affecting 25% of patients, is usually manifested by reversible rises in blood urea nitrogen and creatinine. The need for dialysis is unusual.

A new combination of sulfadiazine with trimehtoprim, co-trimazine, was compared to conventional sulfamethoxazole–trimethoprim. More sulfonamide and acetylated metabolite are present in the urine with the new combination. Any reductions in sulfonamide in the new combination are of doubtful clinical importance.[184] Pharmacokinetic analysis of intravenous trimethoprim–sulfamethoxazole during hemodialysis suggests that 50% of a usual maintenance dose should be supplemented after each dialysis.[185]

The use of antiviral drugs is increasing. Concise reviews are available.[186,187] Acyclovir used intravenously in high doses can cause neurotoxicity and reversible acute renal failure.[188] This can occur after only one or two doses.[189] Clearance of acyclovir is exclusively renal, with a half-life of 20 hr in anuric patients.[190] Ganciclovir, a congener of acyclovir, has activity against cytomegalovirus in immunocompromised hosts. Daily doses of 3–15 mg/kg are effective in clearing viremia in approximately 80% of cases. The normal half-life of 4.2 hr is extended in renal failure.[191] Another antiviral drug, 9-[2 hydroxy-(1-hydroxy-methyl) ethoxymethyl] guanine also has a beneficial action in cytomegalovirus infections. Dosage reduction is necessary in renal insufficiency.[192]

Renal failure impairs total body and renal clearance of ethambutol. An anephric patient should receive a normal initial dose of 15 mg/kg and 7 g/kg daily thereafter.[193] Antituberculous drugs have been reviewed.[194] Treatment for systemic fungal infections was concisely summarized.[195,196] Antihelminthics used widely around the world have also been recently reviewed.[197] For severe helminthic infections, praziquantel has become the drug of choice. Few data on use in renal patients are available. Albendazole is useful for treatment of hydatid cysts.[198] Dapsone is used widely for leprosy, malaria prophylaxis, and dermatologic disorders. The drug is extensively metabolized and should not accumulate in renal failure.[199]

6.7. Antiarrhythmic and Cardiac Drugs

A variety of effective new antiarrhythmic compounds have become available in the last few years. Because they themselves may produce serious rhythm disturbances, attention to proper use is extremely important in renal patients who may demonstrate altered pharmacokinetics. Useful brief reviews are available.[200,201] Mexilitine, originally developed as an anticonvulsant, has a structural similarity to lidocaine. Renal failure has little effect on elimination half-life.[202] However, excretion is markedly reduced in alkaline urine.[203] Tocainide, also structurally like lidocaine, needs dosage adjustment in renal failure as well as supplemental doses posthemodialysis.[204] Flecainide has a prolonged half-life in renal failure, and lower initial and maintenance doses are advisable.[205,206] Treatment with flecainide may be associated with prolonged PR and QRS intervals,[205,207] and blood level monitoring to ensure flecainide concentrations less than 750 ng/ml is recommended.[207] Encainide undergoes extensive metabolism to pharmacologically active metabolites, particularly in individuals who demonstrate an extensive metabolizer phenotype for debrisoquin 4-hydroxylation. Parent drug and active metabolite clearance are reduced in renal failure.[208] Treatment should begin with one-third the usual dose when there is impaired renal function.[209,210]

An older drug, disopyramide, which has an antiarrhythmic profile similar to that of quinidine and procainamide, has been reappraised.[211,212] Protein binding is increased in uremia owing to increases in α_1 acid glycoprotein. Although dosage must be reduced in patients with creatinine clearances less than 50 ml/min, little drug is lost during hemodialysis.[212] Amiodarone is extremely lipid soluble and accumulates in tissues.[213] The drug is excreted in the bile with an extremely long half-life. Little is excreted by the kidney or is removed by dialysis.[214] When high concentrations of α_1 acid glycoprotein are present, as in renal failure or after myocardial infarction, binding of basic drugs such as quinidine or dispyramide may be increased. Under these circumstances high total serum levels may actually be "therapeutic" since the free fraction is unchanged.[215] Propafenone is a new class I antiarrhythmic drug which can be given orally or intravenously. Renal failure should not affect drug pharmacokinetics, although limited data are available.[216]

Because of the multiple alternatives available, procainamide use in patients with renal failure should be limited. N-acetyl procainamide, a pharmacologically active metabolite, can have rebound increases in plasma levels even after prolonged dialysis for overdose.[217] The development of IgG antiguanosine antibodies correlates with the manifestations of procainamide-induced systemic lupus erythematosus.[218]

New positive inotropic agents are helpful in many critically ill patients. Amrinone and milrinone improve short-term cardiac performance and are structurally unrelated to cardiac glycosides or sympathomimetics. Both drugs have substantial renal excretion and have decreased systemic clearance in severe heart failure due to compromised renal hemodynamics.[219,220] Dobutamine and ibopamine are catecholamine-like drugs which increase low cardiac output. Both agents are being evaluated for long-term use.

In a critical review of the use of dipyridamole as an antithrombotic agent in cardiac patients, Oates et al. concluded that caution was warranted in extrapolating animal studies to humans. In humans, an antithrombotic effect additional to that of aspirin has not been convincingly demonstrated.[221]

With a renewed interest in organic nitrates for treatment of angina and congestive failure, recent literature has detailed their pharmacokinetic behavior. Glyceryltrinitrate is metabolized in the liver, and predominantly inactive metabolites are excreted in the urine.[222] There is also extensive extrahepatic metabolism. With transdermal preparations, blood levels are maintained for 24 hr and thus any attenuation of action occurs for more fundamental pharmacodynamic reasons.[223] Isosorbide 5-nitrate is unaffected by renal failure and clinical dialysis.[224,225]

6.8. Antihypertensives

Antihypertensive drugs affect sexual function frequently in both male and female patients. A recent list of offending agents has been published.[226] Angiotensin converting enzyme inhibitors, calcium channel blockers, and vasodilators are rarely implicated, as compared to other drug groups. A brief, balanced summary of available therapeutic drugs for chronic hypertension with dosages and adverse effects is useful for clinical practice.[227]

New drugs with α_1-receptor antagonist properties similar to those of prazosin have become available. Indoramin reduces blood pressure by peripheral vasodilatation without drop in cardiac output. In normotensive subjects the drug does not adversely affect renal function or electrolyte excretion.[228] Terazosin, another postsynaptic α_1-adrenoreceptor blocker, has a longer half-life than prazosin, allowing once-daily dosing. Also, gastrointestinal absorption is more complete than with prazosin.[229,230] Terazosin dosing does not need to be altered in renal insufficiency.[231] Doxazosin, another longer-lasting congener, has similar pharmacokinetics in normals and renal failure patients.[232] The antihypertensive effect of prazosin may be more pronounced in renal failure patients, although this effect is not explained by altered pharmacokinetics.[233]

Labetolol with selective α_1-blocking properties combined with modest beta blockade is widely used in nephrology practice. Little drug is lost during regular dialysis.[234] Transdermal clonidine allows good blood pressure control in renal insufficiency despite apparent insensitivity to blood levels higher than those achieved in patients with normal renal function.[235] Nephrotic syndrome and new-onset diabetes are rare complications of clonidine therapy.[236] Guanfacine and guanabenz are centrally acting agents which can be substituted for the more familiar clonidine or methyldopa.[237,238] Guanfacine can be given once daily in the elderly and without dose adjustment in patients with renal failure.[239]

6.9. Beta Blockers

Beta blockers continue to be widely used in nephrologic practice for management of hypertension. Esmolol, an ultra-short-acting, cardioselective β-adrenoreceptor antagonist, will be most useful in critical care situations.[240–242] This titratable intravenous analog has a half-life of only 9 min. After a 500 μg/kg loading dose infused over 1–4 min, a maintenance infusion of 50–200 μg/kg per min is usually effective.[240,243] The renal hemodynamic effects of single doses of conventional beta blockers were studied in hypertensive patients.[244] A 10–20% drop in GFR and effective renal plasma flow was observed except with pindolol and teratolol.[245] Other studies have shown no change in renal function with Betaxolol, a new β_1-selective agent, and nadolol.[246] The clinical significance of these hemodynamic changes is unclear, but most likely are of little consequence.

The subject of lipophilicity of beta blockers and relationship to central nervous side effects was reviewed by Drayer.[247] Poorly lipid-soluble congeners such as atenolol, sotalol, and nadolol are excreted unchanged in the urine with accumulation in renal failure.[248] More lipid-soluble compounds generally have their pharmacokinetics unaltered by renal failure.[248] For example, penbutalol, a nonselective beta blocker with a long elimination half-life, needs no adjustment in renal failure. This drug lowers blood pressure without bradycardia due to intrinsic agonist activity.[249] The cardioselective beta blocker bevantolol and the nonselective penbutolol do not have altered pharmacokinetics in renal failure and do not reduce renal function.[250,251] Bevantolol does not appear to cause peripheral vasoconstriction due to a partial action on alpha adrenoreceptors.[252] Sotalol does not have intrinsic sympathomimetic activity, membrane stabilizing properties, or cardioselectivity. Its lack of propensity to depress ventricular function could be useful in hypertensive renal patients.[253] Celiprolol is a new cardioselective beta blocker with partial agonist action and some vasodilating properties. It does not cause bronchoconstriction and seems to preserve tissue blood flow. If the favorable properties of celiprolol are confirmed in further studies, this drug may be a very useful addition to currently available beta blockers.[254]

6.10. Angiotensin Converting Enzyme Inhibitors

Angiotensin converting enzyme inhibitors have rapidly achieved an important place in the management of hypertension and congestive heart failure because of impressive efficacy and improvement of renal hemodynamics combined with a favorable side effect profile.[255,256] Captopril acts as a direct inhibitor of the enzyme, while enalapril must be converted to the active drug enalaprilic acid in the liver. Enalapril is much longer acting, allowing once-daily doses, and its bioavailability is unaffected by food.[257] When large doses of converting enzyme inhibitors are used to treat patients with advanced congestive heart failure, the prolonged hypotensive effects of enalapril may be a disadvantage with respect to renal and cerebral perfusion.[258] Renal excretion of captopril and the active enalapril moiety are reduced in renal failure and the elderly. Dosage reduction is recommended in most of these patients.[259–262] However, as with most drugs used to treat hypertension with renal insufficiency, drug dosing is governed by blood pressure response, not pharmacokinetic considerations. If large doses are used, however, the patient should be carefully monitored for hyperkalemia, particularly with diabetes or in patients on beta blockers. Enalapril pharmacology and clinical use have been extensively reviewed by Cleary and Taylor[263] and Borek *et al.*[264]

Various nephrologic syndromes caused by angiotensin converting enzyme inhibitors were reviewed by Donker. Rare cases of allergic interstitial nephritis have been reported with captopril and enalapril. If one congener causes a reaction, the patient may tolerate a different angiotensin converting enzyme inhibitor. Proteinuria and membranous nephropathy may develop in some patients treated with captopril in high doses.[265] This is extremely rare, being reported in less than 0.1% of patients treated. More common is reversible acute renal failure in patients with renal artery stenosis given angiotensin converting enzyme inhibitors. Renal dysfunction is presumably due to loss of angiotensin effect on efferent arteriolar resistance vessels.[266] It appears prudent to check the renal function of patients at risk, i.e., older patients with diffuse vascular disease, patients with solitary functioning kidneys, and patients on concomitant diuretics,[267] 2–3 weeks after commencing therapy. In renal transplant artery stenosis, renal failure may be irreversible.[268,269] Caution is warranted in the use of converting enzyme inhibition for renal transplant recipients.[270]

Both captopril and enalapril are associated with a dry cough in 1–2% of patients. In healthy subjects, captopril shifts the dose–response curve to a standard cough challenge, with capsaicin to the left.[271] This disappears when the drug is stopped.[272–274] Captopril raises serum digoxin levels by reducing renal clearance of cardiac glycosides.[275]

Ramipril, like enalapril, has to be activated to the liver to an active metabolite.[276,277] A lysine analog of enalaprilic acid, lisinopril, and pentopril are effective antihypertensive drugs in patients with renal failure.[278,279] Alacepril, another new angiotensin converting enzyme inhibitor, is converted to captopril in the liver.[280]

6.11. Calcium Antagonists

There has been an explosion of knowledge concerning the utility of calcium antagonists in the management of hypertension and other cardiovascular conditions treated by renal physicians. Verapamil, nifedipine, and diltiazem pharmacokinetics have been reviewed.[281,282] These currently available drugs, although different in chemical structure, have similar pharmacokinetic properties. They have high systemic clearances dependent on liver blood flow. Renal disease has little effect on the pharmacokinetics of verapamil and diltiazem; however, the elimination half-life of nifedipine is increased in advanced renal failure owing to an altered volume of distribution. Verapamil inhibits the renal and extrarenal clearance of digoxin, raising serum levels of the cardiac glycoside. Diltiazem does not affect digoxin levels, although this drug impairs hepatic oxidation reactions.[283,284] Verapamil also impairs the metabolism of quinidine raising serum levels.[285] In healthy elderly subjects, verapamil elimination is impaired. This factor should be considered when prescribing for older hypertensive patients, particularly those with renal impairment.[286] Verapamil did not change endogenous noradrenergic activity, sodium-volume state, or the renin–angiotensin system in patients with essential hypertension.[287] Dialysis does not influence the pharmacokinetics of calcium antagonists.[288] Nifedipine has rarely been associated with hypokalemia,[289] and a single case of agranulocystis has been described in a dialysis patient.[290] Although sublingual nifedipine has been used in hypertensive crises, biting the capsule followed by swallowing of its contents gives faster absorption and higher plasma levels.[291]

Several new calcium antagonists will soon become available for clinical use. Nicardipine is an effective drug for hypertension when used as monotherapy and may be associated with less fluid retention than other vasodilators.[292,293] Effective dosage is 20–40 mg in three divided doses. The drug seems to blunt aldosterone secretion in response to increased plasma renin activity.[294] Nitrendipine is effective as an antihypertensive with once-daily doses of 5–20 mg. This drug has predominantly peripheral rather than coronary vasodilatory actions and thus induces impressive lowering of diastolic pressure.[295] These actions contrast with the potent coronary vasodilator bepridil, whose long half-life allows prolonged antianginal action with once-daily dosing.[296] The calcium antagonist nisoldipine protects the kidney against experimental ischemic and glycerol-induced acute renal failure.[297,298] The "second generation" dihydropyridine calcium antagonists were reviewed by Freedman and Waters.[299]

6.12. Diuretics

Diuretic drugs continue to be an integral part of the therapeutic armamentarium of nephrologists. The pharmacology of new agents and the loop diuretics was reviewed by Imbs *et al.* and Beermann and Grind.[300,301] These valuable drugs inhibit a transport system for sodium, potassium, and chloride in cell membranes of the thick ascending limb of Henle's loop, causing natriuresis.[302] Loop diuretics are known to maintain efficacy in patients with renal insufficiency. Brater *et al.* have shown that remnant nephrons of diseased kidneys have an exaggerated response to furosemide. The maximal response to an intravenous dose is with 120–160 mg.[303] Piretanide is a new loop diuretic with potency, on a weight basis, six times that of furosemide, which is useful in severe congestive heart failure.[304] In renal failure, drug delivery into the tubule is reduced in proportion to the decrease in creatinine clearance.[305] Torasemide has similar properties, with a potency factor five times that of furosemide. The influence of torasemide on urinary volume and sodium excretion is reduced by probenecid, suggesting that, like other loop diuretics, secretion into the tubular fluid is a major requirement for drug response.[306] For bumetanide, drug efficacy does not differ between the oral and intravenous routes of administration.[307] Cumulative sodium excretion in renal insufficiency was greater with intravenous furosemide than bumetanide. The potency ratio of furosemide to bumetanide is reduced to 20 in renal failure compared to 40 in normal subjects.[308]

Amiloride pharmacology has been summarized. Its mechanism of action relates to its inhibition of sodium ion movement by an effect on transport proteins, including a sodium–hydrogen antiporter. Amiloride increases calcium reabsorption and by its effect on sodium reabsorption is potassium sparing.[309] Triamterene may induce crystaluria and casts in acid urine even in healthy subjects. Alkalinization of the urine may prevent these changes.[310] Acute renal failure due to crystal deposition can occur with thiazide–triamterene combination drugs.[311] A case of agranulocytosis due to spironolactone has been reported.[312]

6.13. Analgesics, Antiinflammatory Drugs, and Drugs Used in Gout

It has been widely recognized by clinicians that patients with renal failure are often "sensitive" to morphine. Even small doses may produce profound respiratory depression and decreased level of consciousness. By modern analytic methods, morphine itself does not accumulate; however, there is retention of pharmacologically active metabolites, such as morphine-6-glucuronide, which may be of etiologic importance.[313–315] Morphine-6-glucuronide is four times as active as morphine in mice with a prolonged duration of action.[316] The half-lives of absorption and elimination of morphine itself are actually shortened in renal failure.[317] In renal transplant recipients with initial allograft dysfunction, plasma morphine concentrations are higher than in living donor recipients and nonanesthetized controls. The authors of these reports reject technical artifacts of their assay as an explanation for morphine retention.[318] They propose that the kidney is a major organ of morphine metabolism, based on studies in the isolated perfused rat kidney.[319]

Meperidine has a prolonged elimination half-life in renal failure owing to a lower plasma clearance and an increased volume of distribution. An active metabolite normeperidine also has decreased excretion.[320] Prolonged effects of codeine are also reported. The accumulation of metabolites is the probable explanation for the adverse effects of all opioid analgesics in renal insufficiency.[321]

Nonnarcotic analgesics and antiinflammatory drugs are widely prescribed in renal patients. Acetaminophen and aspirin have been comprehensively reviewed.[322,323] Acetaminophen is well tolerated and produces fewer side effects than aspirin but has little antiinflammatory effect owing to lack of action on peripheral cyclooxygenase.[322] Salsalate, a nonacetylated salicylate, is removed by regular hemodialysis.[324] A direct comparison of ibuprofen, now available without a prescription, with aspirin revealed a low incidence of renal dysfunction with both drugs.[325] Patients on diuretics are at increased risk of renal dysfunction with drugs that inhibit cyclooxygenase. Brogden reviewed nonsteroidal antiinflammatory drugs.[326] All of these drugs have the potential to cause fluid and sodium retention, thus antagonizing diuretic drugs. Sulindac, piroxicam, and naproxen did not differ in their ability to inhibit serum thromboxane and 6-keto prostaglandin $F_{1\alpha}$. Due to less renal cyclooxygenase inhibition, blood pressure was lower with sulindac than with the other drugs.[327] Sulindac did inhibit bumetanide-induced sodium and water excretion.[328] Ibuprofen interfered with blood pressure control in patients with mild–moderate hypertension as compared to acetaminophen controls.[329]

Prescription of nonsteroidal drugs to patients with renal insufficiency often causes transient, reversible decreases in renal plasma flow and GFR.[330,331]

Sulindac has been considered as relatively renal sparing since the kidney inactivates the pharmacologically active sulfide metabolite.[332] Renal failure impairs the reduction of sulindac to the active sulfide, but does not affect oxidation to inactive sulfone.[333,334] This provides another explanation for the purported renal-sparing properties of sulindac.

Etodolac is a new nonsteroidal analgesic with a reportedly low incidence of gastric irritant side effects.[335] Less than 2% of patients with arthritis receiving etodolac developed renal dysfunction.[336] Members of the chemically novel oxicam family are effective agents with long half-lives, allowing once-daily dosing.[337,338] Piroxicam elimination is impaired in elderly patients with abnormal renal function,[337] but tenoxicam pharmacokinetics are not affected.[339] Piroprofen, ketoprofen, and carprofen are new proprionic acid derivatives with no particular pharmacokinetic or pharmacodynamic advantages over standard agents.[340–342] Proquazone and nabumetone, unlike other nonsteroidal drugs, do not have free acidic groups in their structure.[334,344] No adjustments are necessary for renal insufficiency.[345] They demonstrate no definite increase in therapeutic index but may have less gastric irritation. There is not enough dialysis loss of indomethacin to require supplemental postdialysis doses.[346]

Nephrotic syndrome is rarely reported as a complication of nonsteroidal antiinflammatory drugs, such as naproxen and indomethacin.[347] Although remission of minimal-change pathology is usual when the offending drug is withdrawn, a relapse without further naproxen exposure has been described.[348] Reversible drug-induced membranous nephropathy was associated with ketoprofen.[349] Suprofen has been withdrawn from the market in the United States and European countries because of numerous reports of severe flank pain and acute renal failure. These reactions have largely occurred in previously healthy males after a single or a few doses.[350–352] Acute uricosuria has been the postulated mechanism, and of interest in this regard is the structural similarity between suprofen and the uricosuric thiazide diuretic ticrynafen, which also caused this syndrome.[353] Other cases of suprofen-induced acute renal failure were due to interstitial nephritis.[354]

Allopurinol pharmacokinetics were summarized by Murrell and Rapeport.[355] The major metabolite of allopurinol, oxypurinol undergoes renal excretion with retention in renal failure. Thus, renal failure patients are predisposed to severe hypersensitivity reactions, including fatal exfoliative dermatitis, unless dosage is decreased. In addition, allopurinol inhibits azathioprine metabolism, which may result in severe posttransplant bone marrow depression.[355] Elevation of plasma colchicine levels in renal failure may cause proximal muscle weakness and axonal polyneuropathy, which can be mistaken for uremic neuropathy. Discontinuation of colchicine, if done early, can result in marked improvement.[356]

6.14. Miscellaneous Drugs

Cancer chemotherapy and immunosuppression are increasingly offered to patients with coexistent illness and renal dysfunction. Levin reviewed pharmacokinetic considerations as applied to anticancer pharmacology,[357] and drug indications and toxicities have been concisely summarized.[358] Etoposide and teniposide are semisynthetic derivatives of podophyllotoxin which are increasingly used by clinical oncologists. These drugs damage the DNA in tumors.[359] The role of the kidney in drug excretion is controversial, since only some studies have shown reduced drug clearance in renal failure.[360] Interleukin-2 in combination with autologous lymphokine-activated killer cells has produced encouraging remissions in patients with advanced metastatic cancer. This therapy was complicated by reversible fluid retention, azotemia, and oliguria with low fractional sodium excretion. The precise mechanism of this drug-induced prerenal azotemia is unclear.[361] Hemodynamic measurements strongly suggest a "capillary leak" syndrome.[362] High-dose methotrexate is often associated with tubular dysfunction and occasionally acute renal failure.[363] Salicylate and probenecid decrease plasma protein binding and renal tubular secretion of methotrexate.[364]

Azathioprine is rapidly converted to 6-mercaptopurine (6-MP) *in vivo*. There are marked interindividual differences in azathioprine metabolism. This suggests that monitoring of 6-MP might be clinically useful in dose adjustment.[365] A thorough summary of azathioprine use in renal transplantation has been published. Renal dysfunction does not alter azathioprine disposition.[366]

New intravenous anesthetics and neuromuscular blocking drugs are useful in complex renal failure patients. Metabolism of vecuronium and atracurium is organ independent, which allows safe use in renal and hepatic failure.[367–370] Intravenous azathioprine may slightly antagonize the neuromuscular blockade of vecuronium and atracurium.[371] Mujais reviewed the renal effects of general anesthetics.[372] Rarely, acute renal failure follows halothane-induced hepatitis.[373] Dantrolene is useful in the treatment of the malignant hyperthermia syndrome and its associated myoglobinuria. It has also been given to patients with heat stroke and neuroleptic malignant syndrome. Dantrolene acts within skeletal muscle fibers by inhibiting calcium release.[373a]

Cyclosporine has become a mainstay in most transplant immunosuppressive regimens. Constant intravenous infusions of cyclosporine reach a plateau concentration at 24 hr. Doses of 10 mg/kg per day are cleared more slowly than lower doses, suggesting a finite hepatic capacity for cyclosporine metabolism.[374] Interestingly, cyclosporine impairs prednisolone metabolism, potentially increasing steroid side effects.[375]

Many drugs that alter hepatic P-450 metabolism modify cyclosporine pharmacokinetics. Recently, a somatostatin analog used to reduce pancreatic exocrine secretions markedly reduced cyclosporine blood levels, necessitating a 50% increase in dosage.[375a]

6.15. Drugs Used for Neurologic, Psychiatric, and Anxiety Disorders

Balant-Gorgia and Balant reviewed the relevant pharmacokinetics of antipsychotic drugs.[376] Little specific information exists for any agent in patients with renal disease. The first of a new class of agents, the benzamides, as represented by sulpiride, has a prolonged half-life in renal failure. It is also removed during hemodialysis, and postdialysis dosage supplementation may be needed.[376] Fluoxetine is a new antidepressant which enhances serotinergic neurotransmission.[377] Renal dysfunction has no effect on its clearance rate or half-life.[378] When tricyclic antidepressant levels are measured in patients with chronic renal failure, they are not different from those of control subjects. However, conjugated metabolites do accumulate and may be responsible for side effects inasmuch as glucuronide metabolites of tricyclic antidepressants have pharmacologic activity.[379] The pharmacokinetics of buspirone, an anxiolytic with a unique chemical structure, are little changed in the presence of renal disease.[380] Liver disease, however, affects total body clearance of most anxiolytic drugs, including benzodiazepines.[381] Hypercalcemia and increases in immunoreactive parathyroid hormone (PTH) concentrations are regularly noted in patients treated for affective disorders with lithium carbonate. *In vitro* lithium makes parathyroid tissue less sensitive to calcium and may stimulate parathyroid growth. Serum calcium should be monitored periodically during lithium treatment.[382]

Cholinesterase inhibitor pharmacokinetics have been extensively reviewed.[383] Pyridostigmine and neostigmine elimination half-life and plasma clearance are reduced in anephric patients. This may lead to a longer duration of neuromuscular blockade. Neostigmine is probably the agent of choice as it is extensively metabolized independent of renal function.[383] Cedarbaum has provided an extensive review of the clinical pharmacokinetics of antiparkinsonian drugs. Renal disease has a major effect on amantidine pharmacokinetics and doses should be lowered in proportion to a reduction in creatinine clearance.[384]

6.16. Gastrointestinal Drugs

Histamine-2 (H_2) receptor antagonists are widely prescribed. New analogs have similar pharmacokinetics as standard agents such as ranitidine and cimetidine.[385] They are secreted by the renal tubule and have extended half-lives in renal failure.[386] Famotidine, the most recently released, is 20 times more potent than cimetidine and 7.5 times more potent than ranitidine on a weight basis in decreasing basal and gastrin-stimulated acid secretion. It does not have antiandrogenic effects, nor does it alter hepatic drug metabolism. The drug was not significantly removed by hemodialysis[387]; however, dose adjustment is necessary in renal insufficiency.[388] Omeprazole inhibits gastric acid secretion by interacting with H^+,K^+-ATPase in the pareital cells and appears more effective than H_2-receptor antagonists for duodenal ulcer. This drug is extensively metabolized by the liver and its pharmacokinetics are unaffected by renal failure.[389]

6.17. Lipid-Lowering Agents

Hyperlipidemia and subsequent accelerated atherosclerosis are major risk factors for premature death in patients with end-stage renal disease, nephrotic syndrome, renal transplants, and essential hypertension. Diet and conventional drugs such as nicotinic acid, clofibrate, probucol, colestipol, cholestryamine, and gemfibrosil are marginally effective and present major compliance problems because of unpleasant side effects. Lovostatin, the first of a new class of hypolipidemic agents, acts as a competitive inhibitor of the rate-limiting enzyme in chosterol biosynthysis, 3-hydroxy-3 methylglutaryl-coenzyme A reductase.[390,391] This drug preferentially lowers low-density-lipoprotein cholesterol and is remarkably effective in nephrotic hyperlipidemia. The usual effective dose in this situation is 20 mg bid.[392] In early clinical trials occasional asymptomatic rises in muscle enzymes and, rarely, rhabdomyolysis have been noted.

When using cholestyramine to treat hyperlipidemia, the clinician should be aware that absorption of other medications such as hydrochlorothiazide may be decreased.[393] The best time to give the binding resin is 4 hr after the thiazide diuretic. Benzafibrate and fenofibrate are new lipid-lowering drugs chemically related to clofibrate which must have their dosage reduced markedly in patients with renal insufficiency.[394,395] As with clofibrate, muscle necrosis and rhabdomyolysis are reported.[396] Omega-3 polyunsaturated fatty acids in the form of fish oil have a marked hypolipidemic effect, which may be useful in patients on continuous ambulatory peritoneal dialysis.[397]

6.18. Other Drugs Used in Nephrologic Practice

Patients with renal disease, particularly after renal transplantation, frequently develop insulin resistance and glucose intolerance. Ferner and Chaplin reviewed oral hypoglycemic drugs.[398] Drugs with long half-lives, such as chlorpropamide, or with renally excreted active metabolites, such as acetohexamide, can cause prolonged fatal hypoglycemia, particularly in patients with renal disease. Biguanides, such as phenformin or metformin, produce lactic acidosis. Metformin may cause this problem less often since it does not undergo extensive metabolism. However, metformin is renally excreted and therefore needs dosage adjustment in renal failure.[398] Glyburide kinetics and clearance are minimally affected by renal failure.[399] Sorbinil and potentially other aldose reductase inhibitors may be effective in prevention of diabetic complications such as neuropathy and retinopathy. Beneficial effects on experimental diabetic nephropathy await further data and clinical confirmation.[400] Human insulin has no disadvantages compared to porcine products and has become the preferred choice for all new diabetics.[401]

Warfarin anticoagulants continue to be used in nephrologic practice. The long half-life (35 hr) is unaffected by renal failure.[402] However, nephrotic patients have a shorter half-life of approximately 18 hr.[403] Increased hepatic protein synthesis may also cause an increase in vitamin-dependent clotting factors in nephrosis. Both these factors combine to make dosage requirements of warfarin different in patients with nephrotic syndrome.[404]

Pentoxifylline is an oral drug used to reduce blood viscosity and decrease the potential for platelet aggregation and thrombus formation. Clearance from the plasma is reduced in severe renal failure.[405] Accumulation of the drug and its metabolites may cause severe nausea and vomiting.[406] Ticlopidine inhibits platelet action and aggregation. It is extensively metabolized and thus unlikely to produce problems in renal patients.[407] However, troublesome gastrointestinal, hepatic, and dermatologic side effects may limit the utility of this drug. Buflomedil is a vasoactive drug which inhibits alpha adrenoreceptors and platelet activation. It also reduces blood viscosity. Based on limited data, dosage adjustment in renal failure is unnecessary.[408] Using platelet function assays, dipyridamole inhibited platelet aggregation only at high doses and 1 hr after administration, when plasma concentrations were highest. Implications of these data for clinical therapy are unclear.[409]

A new, nonsedating antihistamine, astemizole, has been released. Like terfenadine, it appears safe in renal patients without dose adjustment. It can be administered once daily.[403] Enprostil, a synthetic analog of prostaglandin E_2, is effective in management of peptic ulcer disease. Diarrhea may be troublesome.[410] Nedocromil, related to sodium cromgolycate, is useful in reversible obstructive airways disease. No data on use in renal patients are reported.[411]

Mannitol pharmacokinetics were studied by Cloyd et al. Elimination half-life was 71 min and disposition was biphasic. Neither mannitol concentration nor change in serum osmolarity correlated with dose. Doses greater than 1.5 g/kg produced sustained elevations of serum osmolarity and could produce hypertonic dehydration unless appropriate fluids were administered.[412] Recent evidence suggesting that chronic lead exposure may lead to heretofore unexplained chronic renal failure has focused attention on EDTA chelation therapy in individuals with compromised renal function. Chronic renal failure per se does not cause lead accumulation.[413] A 1-g dose of $Ca_2 Na_2$ EDTA has a clearance highly correlated with creatinine clearance. Urinary lead excretion correlated with initial blood lead. Subjects with abnormal renal function had greater blood lead decreases in 4 days when compared to normals. No deterioration of renal function due to EDTA was noted.[414]

7. Drug Nephrotoxicity

Hospital-acquired acute renal failure is a serious illness, with a case fatality rate still approaching 40–60%. A recent case-control study showed that exposure to aminoglycoside antibiotics and radiologic contrast media were risk factors, along with age, sepsis, and congestive heart failure. Patients in that report were matched with controls for baseline renal function.[415] A large retrospective study implicated nephrotoxins in approximately 7% of acute renal failure. However, interstitial nephritis due to drugs was considered separately.[416]

Recent literature regarding common nephrotoxins encountered by clinicians is covered in this section. Interstitial nephritis thought to be on an allergic or immunologic basis is still encountered, with nonsteroidal antiinflammatory drugs, cimetidine antibiotics, and allopurinol as frequent offenders. Improvement in renal function after drug withdrawal, a characteristic renal biopsy, and peripheral blood increases of IgE and eosinophils are consistent with a hypersensitivity mechanism.[417] Drug-induced hyperkalemia is a significant problem in elderly patients, particularly those with renal dysfunction. This subject was reviewed by Cannon-Babb and Schwartz.[418]

7.1. Radiographic Contrast Media

Contrast nephropathy, as a consequence of angiography or pyelography, continues to be emphasized in patients at increased risk, including those with renal failure and diabetes. However, a prospective study of 125 patients undergoing translumbar aortography did not reveal reduction in renal function in any group of patients, including diabetics. Mannitol and fuoresemide did not add extra protection to that achieved with volume repletion alone.[419] In cardiac angiography, there was a 23% incidence of a rise in serum creatinine of 1 mg/dl or greater in 139 patients with baseline serum creatinine of at least 2 mg %. Contract nephropathy was independently associated with class IV heart failure, multiple exposures to contrast within 72 hr, total dose of contrast medium, and diabetes.[420] Fairley and Ihle reported thrombotic microangiopathy in a renal transplant patient receiving aortofemoral angiography.[421]

The pharmacology of intravascular radio contrast media was reviewed by Morris and Fischer.[422] Metabolic clearance of the new, low-ionic ioxaglate is higher than of conventional agents in the renal failure patient.[423] Although some studies have shown the new agents to be less nephrotoxic as measured by enzymuria,[424,425] frank acute renal failure has been reported.[426] Whether any alleged differences in nephrotoxicity offset the 20-fold greater cost must be settled by further studies.[427–429]

Studies on the pathogenesis of contrast nephropathy have lagged behind the clinical recognition of this entity. In dogs, the major physiologic effect observed was an osmotically mediated vasodilatation. Tubular morphologic effects were absent.[430] *In vitro,* sodium and meglumine diatrizoate induces renal artery contraction independent of endothelium or andrenergic nerves.[431] Suppression of oxygen free radicals with allopurinol prevented declines in GFR.[432] Diatrizoate aggravated the degree of cell injury induced by hypoxia in isolated proximal tubular cell fragments.[433]

7.2. Angiotensin Converting Enzyme Inhibitors

With increasing use of angiotensin converting enzyme (ACE) inhibitors, reversible acute renal dysfunction in patients with bilateral renal artery stenosis and transplant artery stenosis is familiar to most nephrologists. When concomitant diuretics are used, this complication can be observed in patients with unilateral renal artery stenosis[434] and severe congestive heart failure.[435] Prostaglandin-mediated sodium excretion enhanced by the diuretic may underlie the hemodynamic changes.[436] In patients with congestive heart failure, filtration fraction falls with converting enzyme inhibition and azotemia can result despite a drop in renal vascular resistance.[437] This is not a toxic effect but instead results from hemodynamic changes that can be reversed by judicious sodium repletion.[438] ACE inhibitors may be associated with occlusion of the renal artery in unilateral renal artery stenosis despite stability of serum creatinine measurements.[439] In the experimental two-kidney, one-clip model of renovascular hypertension, converting enzyme inhibition produced tublointerstitial changes in the clipped kidney. These changes were greatly magnified when the unclipped kidney was removed.[440]

7.3. Aminoglycoside Nephrotoxicity

Aminoglycosides continue to be investigated as the major group of clinically relevant nephrotoxins.[441] Despite numerous new alternative agents, this class of compounds remains widely used because of their proven efficacy. Based on experimental data, novel approaches to dosing using single large daily doses may maximize efficacy by taking advantage of concentration-dependent bacterial killing and the postantibiotic effect while minimizing toxicity.[442,443] The latter, well established in animals,[443,444] has been suggested by DeBroe et al. in humans since, for any daily dose, renal cortical aminoglycoside concentrations are greater with constant infusions compared to conventional intermittent dosing.[445] Renal accumulation of gentamicin, however, was shown to enhance sterilization of kidneys in Escherichia coli pyelonephritis.[446] In addition to age, duration of therapy, and underlying renal function,[447] liver disease has emerged as a significant risk factor for aminoglycoside nephrotoxicity.[448] Sawyers et al. have developed a bedside scoring system which identifies high- and low-risk patients for nephrotoxicity if aminoglycosides are prescribed.[449] Further trials comparing various aminoglycosides with regard to nephrotoxic potential have appeared. Tobramycin and netilmicin, both combined with piperacillin, produced 11 and 17% nephrotoxicity, respectively, in oncology patients (not statistically significant); however, there was less ototoxicity with netilmicin.[450] Gentamicin appeared less nephrotoxic and ototoxic than amikacin[451]; however, differences were slight and probably do not offset the wide cost differential. Using electron microscopy of the urine, Mandal et al. showed that the finding of myeloid bodies in addition to necrotic tubular cells suggests the specific etiology for a patient's acute renal failure.[452] A syndrome of renal potassium and magnesium wasting with activation of the renin–angiotensin system was reported with prolonged gentamicin therapy.[453]

Ototoxicity due to aminoglycosides has been thought to be similar to nephrotoxicity in that there was preferential concentration in the inner ear as compared to plasma. Recent data suggest instead that both inner ear tissues and renal cortex demonstrate rapid and saturable uptake without excessive concentration. Gentamicin can be transported against a concentration gradient in the mouse.[454] Penetration of drug into intracellular compartments from which disappearance is slow is probably more important than accumulation per se in either nephrotoxicity or ototoxicity.[455,456]

Conventional wisdom has related aminoglycoside nephrotoxicity to their ability to interact with phospholipids after specific adsorptive pinocytosis into the lysomes of proximal tubular cells.[457,458] Lysosomes accumulating gentamicin may demonstrate impaired fusion with pinocytotic vesicles.[459] Aminoglycosides are also accumulated within lysosomes of cultured skin fibroblasts with the formation of osmiophilic myeloid bodies. However, no evidence of lysosomal dysfunction could be detected. Membrane lipid metabolism was disturbed, however.[460] Similar absence of lysosomal dysfunction was observed in rat cortex.[458]

The extent and kinetics of cortical uptake are said to be related to the relative nephrotoxicity of various congeners. However, polyamino acids, such as polyaspartic acid (PAA), which inhibit renal brush border and basolateral membrane binding *in vitro,* completely protect the kidney *in vivo* from aminoglycoside nephrotoxicity despite massive accumulation of the aminoglycoside inside the tubular cell.[461,462] Lipid peroxidation is reduced in PAA-treated animals.[463] Ramsammy *et al.* have convincingly shown, however, that lipid peroxidation is a consequence, not a primary cause, of gentamicin-induced tubular cell injury.[464]

Aminoglycosides produce abnormalities of phosphoinositide metabolism which may be responsible for abnormalities in cell calcium handling and response to PTH.[465–467] In cultured human proximal tubular cells, gentamicin induces myeloid bodies, competitively inhibits acid sphingomyelinase (pH optimum 5.6) in the lysosomal fraction, and inhibits noncompetitively neutral sphingomyelinase (pH optimum 7.4) in the microsomal/plasma membrane. Magnesium stimulates the activity of the neutral sphingomyelinase.[468] In proximal tubule brush border vesicles of rabbits, gentamicine inhibits Na-dependent glucose transport.[469] Chronic gentamicin treatment inhibited energy-linked functions of renal cortical mitochondria, probably by impairment of rate-limiting synthesis of respiratory enzymes. This suggest that aminoglycoside-induced cell injury could be analogous to the antibacterial effect of these drugs to interfere with ribosomal protein synthesis.[470]

Although the majority of cell injury due to aminoglycosides occurs in the proximal tubule, Toubeau *et al.* reported ultrastructural evidence of lysosomal phospholipidosis in distal and collecting tubules.[471] *E. coli* endotoxin can enhance the accumulation of [^{3}H]tobramycin in all nephron segments.[472] In view of the adverse consequences of *E. coli* toxins on isolated tubular cells,[473] it is possible that studies in infected animals may be necessary to gain better insights about human nephrotoxicity from animal models. Bernard *et al.* showed that gentamicin competes with exogenous and endogenous cationic proteins for binding sites on tubular membranes. The lysosomal enzymuria used as a marker for nephrotoxicity may represent a rather nonspecific increased exocytosis.[474]

In addition to the effects of polyamino acid mentioned earlier, other experimental maneuvers modify aminoglycoside nephrotoxicity. Thyroxine, presumably by stimulation of Na,K-ATPase or acceleration of membrane repair, confers partial protection against aminoglycosides and other nephrotoxins.[475] Experimental diabetes mellitus quantitatively reduces renal cortical accumulation of aminoglycosides, although transport is qualitatively similar to that observed in normal animals.[476] Calcium entry blockers such as verapamil and nitrendipine give conflicting results, with some studies showing no protection and others some improvement in function.[477,478] Cephem and β-lactam antibiotics modify experimental aminoglycoside nephrotoxicity possibly by the Na content of the adjunctive drug.[479,480] Pyridoxal phosphate, which complexes with amino groups of potentially toxic substances, reduces the LD_{50} of gentamicin.[481] Conversely, pyridoxal phosphate depletion by other drugs or illness may potentiate nephrotoxicity of appropriate doses of gentamicin.[482] Long-term treatment with gentamicin may cause chronic tubulointerstitial changes even though glomerular filtration rate remains near normal.[483]

7.4. Cisplatin

Nephrotoxicity continues to be the limiting factor of cancer chemotherapy with cisplatin. Hydration, volume expansion, and mannitol modify acute decreases in renal function, but chronic progressive declines in renal function may be observed from 2 to 6 months following treatment.[484] As measured by excretion of urinary enzymes such as N-acetylglucosaminidase and γ-glutamyl transferase, cumulative nephrotoxicity occurs with multiple courses of cisplatin.[485,486] Urinary $β_2$-microglobulin was not as useful.[487] Renal magnesium wasting developed in 19 of 28 patients treated with a total of 82 doses of cisplatin. Hypomagnesemia was universally present.[488] The protective maneuvers used to prevent acute nephrotoxicity were reviewed by DeBroe and Wedeen. Thiosulfate may detoxify circulating cisplatin by forming thiosulfate–cisplatin complexes as well as producing osmotic diuresis.[489] Hyperuricemia and hypoalbuminemia correlate inversely with rises in serum creatinine.[490] Individualization of therapy based on free levels of ultrafilterable platinum was suggested as a means to limit cisplatin nephrotoxicity.[491]

Insights into the pathogenesis of cisplatin nephrotoxicity have been derived from experimental models. Changes in mitochondrial respiration and calcium accumulation occur secondary to cisplatin therapy.[492] In experimental models, urinary enzymes increase prior to the development of frank azotemia.[493] Hypomagnesemia and renal magnesium wasting persist after therapy is stopped. These functional abnormalities correlate with morphologic abnormalities in the S3 segment of the proximal tubular.[494] In animals, platinum levels remain measurable in kidney tissue for periods up to 1 month after the drug is stopped. This tissue platinum retention can be correlated with chronic tubulointerstitial changes, including cyst formation.[495] Increased renal prostaglandin synthesis following cisplatin therapy may account for the cisplatin-induced concentrating defect.[496] In animals, atrial natriuretic peptide and sulfur nucleophiles, such as diethyldithiocarbamate, protect against renal dysfunction.[497–499]

7.5. Cyclosporine

The most frequent and potentially limiting consequence of cyclosporine immunosuppression is nephrotoxicity.[500] Attempts to experimentally reproduce the clinical syndromes described in patients have not been completely successful. The only cyclosporine effects for which acceptable animal models exist are acute renal dysfunction and hypertension. Doses required to mimic clinically observed phenomena are larger than those used in clinical transplantation, raising questions about their relevance. Nonetheless, some insights into the pathogenesis of cyclosporine nephrotoxicity have been obtained in animal models.

Primary nonfunction of renal transplants necessitating dialysis is more frequent with cyclosporine immunosuppression than with azathioprine, largely because of high initial cyclosporine doses (>15 mg/kg). Ischemic injury to the kidney due to adverse procurement conditions potentiates this problem.[501] In some patients, cyclosporine must be discontinued because of persistent acute renal failure. Even after function ultimately improves, cyclosporine-treated patients have approximately twice as long a period of oligoanuria as with azathioprine.[502] There is evidence that cadaver kidneys experiencing prolonged oligoanuria have inferior 1- and 2-year survival despite the fact that serum creatinine often returns to normal following the oliguric period. There is an analogous period of acute renal failure following heart transplantation presumably due to high initial cyclosporine doses interacting with ischemic renal injury produced by heart bypass.[503]

Monitoring of cyclosporine blood levels during the period of oligoanuria is crucial for minimization of this problem. In patients with nonfunction for more than 3 weeks, empiric dose reduction is indicated even if blood concentrations are in the "therapeutic" range. Biopsy of renal allografts in this situation can be helpful to exclude clinically silent rejection so that antirejection treatment can be instituted.

Many transplant patients treated with cyclosporine develop one or more episodes of acute renal insufficiency. Since these episodes rapidly improve within a few days after cyclosporine dosage is reduced and since they occur in recipients of nonrenal allografts, they have been presumed to be due to cyclosporine. In the renal transplant recipient these episodes are difficult to distinguish from rejection, particularly in the absence of fever, allograft tenderness, and oliguria. Both conditions may be associated with decreased fractional sodium excretion and isosthenuria. Often the correct diagnosis of these episodes can be made only after observation of the patient's response to a therapeutic maneuver such as antirejection therapy or cyclosporine dose reduction. Although trough cyclosporine levels are often high in patients subsequently proven to have acute cyclosporine nephrotoxicity, a normal or low level does not exclude the diagnosis. In some circumstances, cyclosporine can act synergistically with rejection to produce renal dysfunction. Biopsy of the easily accessible renal allograft during episodes of acute renal dysfunction often is helpful in documenting the absence of treatable rejection. If the transplant biopsy fails to show acute rejection, particularly if arteriolar hyalinosis is present, dose reduction regimens are indicated in an attempt to avoid chronic tubulointerstitial fibrosis, which has been noted in many patients with frequent episodes of reversible cyclosporine-induced creatinine rises.

The precise mechanism of cyclosporine's nephrotoxic effect is unclear. Experimentally, morphologic evidence of vacuoles in proximal tubular cells has suggested direct tubular cell toxicity. However, proximal tubular function remains intact, and tubular cell necrosis is conspicuously absent when renal function is markedly depressed by cyclosporine.[504] Even enzymuria, thought to be a sensitive marker of tubular cell injury, has been absent in most studies. Short-term experiments with parenteral cyclosporine have demonstrated renal vasoconstriction with marked elevations of renal vascular resistance. Suggested hormonal mediators for cyclosporine-induced renal vasoconstriction are angiotensin II, catecholamines, and alteration in renal prostaglandin metabolism. It is possible that in the clinical situation vasoconstriction produced by cyclosporine is additive to renal ischemia and rejection-mediated renal hemodynamic changes.

Progressive renal insufficiency is well documented in transplant recipients receiving cyclosporine for over 12 months. While this process can be attributed to chronic allograft rejection in renal transplant recipients, in nonrenal recipients and in patients with autoimmune disease, it is most certainly due to a nephrotoxic effect of cyclosporine. Long-term cyclosporine-treated recipients as a group have lower GFRs than comparable patients immunosuppressed with azathioprine.[505] In a series of heart transplant recipients the decline in renal function could not be attributed to cardiac dysfunction since cardiac performance was normal and similar to that of azathioprine-treated heart recipients. Similar chronic renal dysfunction has been described in long-term liver transplant recipients[506] and patients receiving long-term cyclosporine therapy for autoimmune uveitis.[507] While excessive initial doses of cyclosporine may play a role in chronic nephrotoxicity, the condition may be progressive despite dose reduction. In some patients, however, stopping cyclosporine altogether after a year of treatment results in rapid improvement in renal hemodynamics and function.[508] Whether permanent structural damage remains is unknown. Several patients have required dialysis for end-stage renal disease due to chronic cyclosporine nephrotoxicity. Clinically, hypertension and proteinuria are noted even in nonrenal recipients, excluding rejection as an explanation for the findings.

No good animal model exists that reproduces the chronic effects of cyclosporine treatment as described in human patients. Some recent information suggests that cyclosporine stimulates interstitial fibroblastic proliferation.[509] Rogers et al. have suggested that infiltrating macrophages could be a possible source of vasoconstrictive prostaglandins.[510] Activated macrophages could also stimulate various growth factors for fibroblasts and lymphokines, providing a theoretical link between the acute vasoconstriction due to cyclosporine and the more chronic interstitial changes observed in patients.

In some patients cyclosporine is associated with fulminant acute renal failure and thrombocytopenia. This syndrome, reported primarily in bone marrow transplant recipients, also occurs de novo in renal transplantation.[511] In renal transplantation, this vasculopathy confers a poor prognosis on the allograft despite absence of pathologic changes of acute rejection. Histologic examination of the kidneys reveals arteriolar lesions similar to the hemolytic–uremic syndrome with thrombotic microangiopathy and occasionally afferent arteriolar thrombosis. Plasmapheresis has been used to induce hematologic remission and renal recovery.[511] This clinical and pathologic picture can be reproduced in experimental animals pretreated with bacterial endotoxin and then given cyclosporine.[512] Cyclosporine also enhances platelet aggregation.[513]

Increases of blood pressure either *de novo* or from previously hypertensive levels are frequently seen in cyclosporine-treated patients.[514,515] In cardiac transplantation where renal rejection is not present, the majority of cyclosporine-treated patients are hypertensive compared to historical azathioprine-treated patients.[516] Although renal function is usually also decreased, this is not uniformly true. In both cardiac and renal allograft recipients plasma renin activity is low and relatively unresponsive to stimulatory maneuvers such as captopril challenge.[517] Conventional approaches to antihypertensive therapy are often ineffective, necessitating multiple-drug regimens. Neurologic symptoms unrelated to hypertension, including focal convulsions and hemiplegia, can be noted with cyclosporine immunosuppression.[518]

Calcium channel blockers reversibly increase cyclosporine levels and careful monitoring of blood levels should be available when these drugs are used in antihypertensive regimens.[519]

7.6. Lithium

The development of renal tubular dysfunction with moderate declines in glomerular filtration rate has been associated with long-term lithium therapy for affective disorders.[520] Minor reductions in overall renal function may be of limited clinical importance over a 5- to 10-year period on the drug despite evidence of tubular dysfunction.[521-523] In animals, chronic renal tubulointerstial disease definitely results from long-term lithium therapy.[524] Close observation and serum level monitoring of lithium-treated patients is warranted, although based on present evidence, the drug should not be withheld where clinically indicated. Neonatal diabetes insipidus has been reported due to maternal use of lithium during pregnancy.[525] Metronidazole may raise plasma lithium levels and thereby potentiate renal dysfunction.[526] An in-depth review of lithium-induced renal effects emphasizes the efficacy of amiloride in the management of polyuria. Amiloride may prevent lithium-induced polyuria by reducing intracellular lithium accumulation.[527]

7.7 Nonsteroidal Antiinflammatory Drugs and Analgesic Nephropathy

Analgesic-associated nephropathy remains a preventable, but still underappreciated, cause of chronic renal failure. The major pathologic lesion is renal papillary necrosis, which is often difficult to detect clinically until a very advanced stage. Bach and Bridges have exhaustively reviewed a large experimental literature on chemically induced renal papillary necrosis.[528] Evidence is strong that combinations of antipyretic analgesics taken over many years can cause chronic renal failure.[529] Acetaminophen alone or aspirin may cause this syndrome if taken habitually[530,531] Compounds such as salicylates can be metabolized to reactive intermediates which bind to cellular organelles, producing toxic damage.[532] Renal pelvic and renal cell cancer are increased in prevalence in analgesic abusers with papillary necrosis.[532a,532b] Chronic dialysis patients with analgesic nephropathy have higher plasma aluminum levels presumably due to gastric hyperacidity which enhances aluminum absorption from phosphate binders.[533]

Renal effects of nonsteroidal antiinflammatory drugs (NSAID) continue to be the subject of published symposia,[534,535] review articles,[536,537] and editorials.[538] Renal failure was due to analgesics and NSAIDs in 37% of 398 drug-associated renal failures in a 1-year study from 58 nephrology units in France.[539] Intravenous aspirin given to patients in an intensive care unit caused a 41% decline in inulin clearance.[540] Asymptomatic declines in renal function are probably extremely common in rheumatology clinics.[541] Reversible nonoliguric renal failure is reported with the phenylbutazone-related drug azapropazone. In addition to effects on renal hemodynamics, uricosuria and interstitial nephritis are seen in these cases.[542] Uricosuria is a primary mechanism proposed for suprofen and other nephropathy from NSAIDs.[543,544] The alleged renal-sparing properties of sulindac have generated many clinical studies.[545] Further experience is consistent with little adverse effect on renal function in chronic renal insufficiency.[546–548] Ibuprofen, but not piroxicam or sulindac, produced renal deterioration in one study.[549] In patients with cirrhosis, sulindac reduced renal vasodilatory prostaglandins and renal function.[550,551] Etodolac, even in high doses, produced only transient reversible renal dysfunction.[552] Prolonged treatment produced a syndrome of hypoprostaglandinism with hyperkalemia, low plasma aldosterone, and hypertension.[553] Mefenamic acid may produce acute renal failure by a variety of mechanisms, including interstitial nephritis and papillary necrosis.[544,554] In patients taking over-the-counter ibuprofen, acute cortical necrosis,[555] interstitial nephritis, and nephrotic syndrome have been reported.[556–558]

Minimal-change nephrotic syndrome can be caused by NSAIDs with or without renal failure and interstitial nephritis. The minimal-change lesion can progress to focal glomerular sclerosis even when the offending drug is stopped.[559] The use of NSAIDs to reduce proteinuria in nephrotic syndrome has been studied further. In short-term studies, indomethacin and diclofenac reduce proteinuria without major adverse effects. Long-term follow-up is not available to ascertain the overall effect of this strategy on renal functional outcome.[560,561]

7.8. Miscellaneous Nephrotoxins

Penicillamine has been used to treat serious disorders such as Wilson's disease, cystinuria, severe rheumatoid arthritis, and scleroderma. Netter et al. reviewed its pharmacokinetic properties.[562] Rapidly progressive glomerulonephritis successfully treated with pulse methylprednisolone has been reported as one of the many types of penicillamine nephropathy.[563] In addition, interstitial nephritis and nephrotic syndrome proved by rechallenge were noted in a rheumatoid patient given penicillamine.[564] IgM deposition in glomeruli was reported in a similar nephrotic patient.[565] When necessary for hemodialysis patients, penicillamine can be given in 250-mg doses after each dialysis.[566] Oral gold has less tendency to produce proteinuria and nephrotic syndrome than injectable forms of gold and should be used preferentially in renal patients.[567] Gold-induced proteinuria resolves completely over 6–40 months without specific therapy. Although creatinine clearance declined by 20%, no patient developed progressive renal failure.[568] When ε-aminocaproic acid is used to treat hematuria in patients with clotting disorders, acute flank pain, fever, and acute renal failure can occur due to clot obstruction. A delayed dense nephrogram on intravenous pyelography is characteristic.[569] When renacidin, a stone-dissolving agent composed of gluconic and citric acid plus their magnesium salts, is used, the clinician should be alert for hypermagnesemia and worsening renal function.[570]

Rifampin is an uncommon, but important, cause of acute renal failure. Oliguric renal failure preceded by a prodromal illness characterized by fever, chills, and musculoskeletal pain is most frequent. Intermittent or interrupted rifampin therapy and a predominantly interstitial nephritis suggest an immunologic pathogenesis.[571] Rapidly progressive glomerulonephritis with nephrotic syndrome has been reported.[572] Acute interstitial nephritis and cholestatic jaundice were caused by trimipramize, a tricyclic antidepressant.[573] Hydralazine-induced renal dysfunction is produced by focal and segmental necrotizing glomerulonephritis in 1–2% of patients treated for long periods of time (average 6.5 years). Renal damage may be permanent unless the drug is promptly withdrawn when nephritis is diagnosed.[574] Nomifensine overdosage can cause acute renal failure without myoglobinuria and intravascular hemolysis, although most cases demonstrate these features.[575]

Addo and Poon-King reported a 72% survival rate among 72 patients treated for paraquat poisoning with a dexamethasone and cyclophosphamide regimen designed to depress reactive oxygen species from white blood cells and macrophages.[576] Renal dysfunction and hypokalemia are common, the latter probably due to forced diuresis.[576] The management of ethylene glycol overdose consists of correction of metabolic acidosis with sodium bicarbonate, ethyl alcohol to inhibit glycol metabolism, and hemodialysis to remove the poison. Although oliguric acute renal failure may occur, dialysis is indicated even if renal failure is not present.[577] A bicarbonate dialysis bath should be used to maximally remove glycolic acid and improve acidemia.[578] Mannitol used to treat acute glaucoma can produce acute worsening of preexisting renal insufficiency.[579]

In a variety of drug-induced interstitial nephritides, the inflammatory infiltrate had a predominance of suppressor/cytotoxic lymphocytes.[580] Others have found predominance of macrophage/monocyte cells.[581] Isolated cases of drug-induced interstitial nephritis continue to be reported as uncommon manifestations of frequently prescribed drugs such as cefoxitin and amoxicillin.[582,583] The sensitivity eosinophiluria as a diagnostic feature of drug-induced interstitial nephritis is substantially increased by the use of Hansel's stain as compared to the standard Wright's stain.[584]

Amphotericin remains the treatment of choice for systemic fungal infections. Usually, declines in renal function are preceded by hypokalemia and renal tubular abnormalities. A more abrupt, but reversible renal failure syndrome has been reported recently.[585] This is at least partially due to renal vasoconstriction produced by amphotericin, independent of the sympathetic nervous system and the renin–angiotensin system.[586]

Mitomycin C used in cancer chemotherapy can cause thrombotic micro-angiopathy involving the kidneys and pulmonary vessels. Evidence of disseminated intravascular coagulation is usually absent.[587] Chemotherapy should be discontinued if the syndrome develops. Plasmapheresis and fresh frozen plasma therapy has been unsuccessful in reversing renal failure.[588] Other chemotherapeutic agents can occasionally cause this syndrome.[589] Adriamycin is an anthracycline anti-neoplastic drug which causes glomerular and tubular lesions in animals and occasionally in humans. Tubulointerstitial inflammatory changes, rather than consequences of drug-induced proteinuria, seem to be the major determinant of progressive renal damage.[590] The molecular mechanisms of Adriamycin damage may be related to enhanced membrane lipid peroxidation.[591]

Reid and Muther described a rapidly reversible deterioration in renal function in a patient with severe congestive heart failure treated with nitroprusside for afterload reduction. They postulated a "steal" of blood from the kidney due to preferential dilatation of other vascular beds.[592] Chronic laxative abuse, like analgesic abuse, may cause irreversible tubulointerstitial nephropathy and renal failure.[593]

References

1. Gibaldi, M., 1986, The basic concept: Clearance, *J. Clin. Pharmacol.* **26:**330–331.
2. Pang, K. S., 1986, Metabolic first-pass effects, *J. Clin. Pharmacol.* **26:**580–582.
3. Jordan, R. A. and Woolf, T. F., 1987, Basic concepts in drug metabolism: Part II, *J. Clin. Pharmacol.* **27:**87–90.
4. Gregus, Z. and Klaassen, C. D., 1987, Biliary excretion, *J. Clin. Pharmacol.* **27:**537–541.
5. Welling, P. G., 1986, Graphic methods in pharmacokinetics: The basics, *J. Clin. Pharmacol.* **26:** 510–514.
6. Bayer, W. H., 1986, Therapeutic drug monitoring, *West. J. Med.* **145:**524–527.
7. Sedman, A. J., Molitoris, B. A., Nakata, L. M., and Gal, J., 1986, Therapeutic drug monitoring in patients with chronic renal failure: Evaluation of the Abbott TDx™ drug assay system, *Am. J. Nephrol.* **6:**132–134.
8. Worwag, E. M., Craig, R. M., Jansyn, E. M., Kirby, D., Hubler, G. L., and Atkinson, A. J, Jr., 1987, D-Xylose absorption and disposition in patients with moderately impaired renal function. *Clin. Pharmacol. Ther.* **41:**351–357.
9. Balasa, R. W., Murray, R. L., Kondelis, N. P., and Bischel, M. D., 1987, Phosphate-binding properties and electrolyte content of aluminum hydroxide antacids, *Nephron* **45:**16–21.
10. Gibson, T. P., 1986, Renal disease and drug metabolism: An overview, *Am. J. Kidney Dis.* **8:**7–17.
11. Shear, N. H., Spielberg, S. P., Grant, D. M., Tang, B. K., and Kalow, W., 1986, Differences in metabolism of sulfonamides predisposing to idiosyncratic toxicity, *Ann. Intern. Med.* **105:**179–184.

12. Siddoway, L. A., Thompson, K. A., McAllister, C. B., Wang, T., Wilkinson, G. R., Roden, D. M., and Woosley, R. L., 1987, Polymorphism of propafenone metabolism and disposition in man: Clinical and pharmacokinetic consequences, *Circulation* **75**:785–791.

13. Kelly, R. A., O'Hara, D. S., Mitch, W. E., Steinman, T. I., Goldszer, R. C., Solomon, H. S., and Smith, T. W., 1986, Endogenous digitalis-like factors in hypertension and chronic renal insufficiency, *Kidney Int.* **30**:723–729.

14. Fitzsimmons, W. E., 1986, Influence of assay methodologies and interferences on the interpretation of digoxin concentrations, *Drug Intell. Clin. Pharm.* **20**:538–542.

15. Vlasses, P. H., Besarab, A., Lottes, S. R., Conner, D. P., Green, P. J., and Gault, M. H., 1987, False-positive digoxin measurements due to conjugated metabolite accumulation in combined renal and hepatic dysfunction, *Am. J. Nephrol.* **7**:355–359.

16. Walker, J. A., Bialy, G. B., Cronin Walker, V., Sherman, R. A., and Eisinger, R. P., 1987, Digoxin-like immunoreactive substance in chronic hemodialysis patients: Effect on digitoxin radioimmunoassay, *Am. J. Nephrol.* **7**:300–302.

17. Gault, H., Vasdev, S., Vlasses, P., Longerich, L., and Dawe, M., 1986, Interpretation of serum digoxin values in renal failure, *Clin. Pharmacol. Ther.* **39**:530–536.

18. Vasdev, S., Johnson, E., Longerich, L., Prabhakaran, V. M., and Gault, M. H., 1987, Plasma endogenous digitalis-like factor is in healthy individuals and in dialysis dependent and kidney transplant patients, *Clin. Nephrol.* **27**:169–174.

19. Greenway, D. C. and Nanji, A. A., 1986, Digoxin-like immunoreactive substance in renal failure: A reappraisal, *Nephron* **44**:108–110.

20. Greenblatt, D. J., Abernethy, D. R., and Shader, R. I., 1986, Pharmacokinetic aspects of drug therapy in the elderly, *Ther. Drug. Monit.* **8**:249–255.

21. Cohen, J. L., 1986, Pharmacokinetic changes in aging, *Am. J. Med.* **80**(Suppl. 5A):31–38.

22. Brown, W. W., David, B. B., Spry, L. A., Wongsurawat, N., Malone, D., and Domoto, D. T., 1986, Aging and the kidney, *Arch. Intern. Med.* **146**:1790–1796.

23. Keller, F., 1987, Kidney function and age. *Nephrol. Dial. Transp.* **2**:382.

24. Drugs that cause psychiatric symptoms. 1986. *The Medical Letter* **28**:81–86.

25. Williams, R. L., Thornhill, M. D., Upton, R. A., Blume, C., Clark, T. S., Lin, E., and Benet, L. Z., 1986, Absorption and disposition of two combination formulations of hydrochlorothiazide and triamterene: Influence of age and renal function, *Clin. Pharmacol. Ther.* **40**:226–232.

26. Stemmer, C. L., Perez, G. O., and Oster, J. R., 1987, Impairment of β-$_2$-Adrenoceptor-stimulated potassium uptake in end-stage renal disease, *J. Clin. Pharmacol.* **27**:628–631.

27. Matzke, G. R., Jameson, J. J., and Halstenson, C. E., 1987, Gentamicin disposition in young and elderly patients with various degrees of renal function, *J. Clin. Pharmacol.* **27**:216–220.

28. Yee, G. C., Lennon, T. P., Gmur, D. J., Kennedy, M. S., and Deeg, H. J., 1986, Age-dependent cyclosporine: Pharmacokinetics in narrow transplant recipients, *Clin. Pharmacol. Ther.* **40**:438–443.

29. Docci, D., 1986, Serum alpha-1-acid glycoprotein (AAG) in chronic renal failure, *Nephron* **42**:347.

30. Rolan, P. E., Muirhead, M., and Clarkson, A. R., 1986, Increased plasma levels of alpha-1-acid glycoprotein in chronic renal failure are unlikely to be due to decreased renal elimination, *Nephron* **42**:345–346.

31. Echizen, H., Saima, S., Umeda, N., and Ishizaki, T., 1986, Protein binding of disopyramide in liver cirrhosis and in nephrotic syndrome, *Clin. Pharmacol. Ther.* **40**:274–280.

32. Vanholder, R., Van Landschoot, N., De Smet, R., Ringoir, S., and Hakim, R., 1986, Inhibition of drug protein binding (PB) during chronic renal failure, *Proc. Am. Soc. Nephrol.* **19**:64a (Abstract).

33. Gulyassy, P. F., Bottini, A. T., Stanfel, L. A., Jarrard, E. A., and Depner, T. A., 1986, Isolation and chemical identification of inhibitors of plasma ligand binding, *Kidney Int.* **30**:391–398.

34. Mabuchi, H. and Nakahashi, H., 1986, Isolation and characterization of an endogenous drug-binding inhibitor present in uremic serum, *Nephron* **44**:277–281.

35. Mabuchi, H. and Nakahashi, H., 1986, Profiling of endogenous ligand solutes that bind to serum proteins in sera of patients with uremia, *Nephron* **43**:110–116.

36. Svensson, C. K., Woodruff, M. N., Baxter, J. G., and Lalka, D., 1986, Free drug concentration monitoring in clinical practice. Rationale and current status, *Clin. Pharmacol.* **11**:450–469.

37. McKinney, T. D. and Kunnemann, M. E., 1987, Cimetidine transport in rabbit renal cortical brush-border membrane vesicles, *Am. J. Physiol.* **242**:F525–F535.

38. Muirhead, M. R., Somogyi, A. A., Rolan, P. E., and Bochner, F., 1986, Effect of cimetidine on renal and hepatic drug elimination: Studies with triamterene, *Clin. Pharmacol. Ther.* **40**:400–407.

39. Van Crugten, J., Bochner, F., Keal, J., and Somogyi, A., 1985, Selectivity of the cimetidine-induced alterations in the renal handling of organic substrates in humans. Studies with anionic, cationic and zwitterionic drugs, *J. Pharmacol. Exp. Ther.* **236**:481–487.

40. Somogyi, A. and Muirhead, M., 1987, Pharmacokinetic interactions of cimetidine 1987, *Clin. Pharmacol.* **12**:321–366.

41. Nazario, M., 1986, The hepatic and renal mechanisms of drug interactions with cimetidine, *Drug. Intell. Clin. Pharm.* **20**:342–348.

42. Nierenberg, D. W., 1986, Drug inhibition of penicillin tubular secretion: Concordance between *in vitro* and clinical findings, *J. Pharmacol. Exp. Ther.* **240**:712–716.

43. Notterman, D. A., Drayer, D. E., Metakis, L., and Reidenberg, M. M., 1986, Stereoselective renal tubular secretion of quinidine and quinine, *Clin. Pharmacol. Ther.* **40**:511–517.

44. Koren, G., 1987, Clinical pharmacokinetic significance of the renal tubular secretion of digoxin. *Clin. Pharmacokinet.* **13**:334–343.

45. Loutzenhiser, R. and Epstein, M., 1987, Calcium antagonists and the kidney, *Hosp. Pract.* **22**: 63–76.

46. Sunderrajan, S., Reams, G., and Bauer, J. H., 1986, Renal effects of diltiazem in primary hypertension, *Hypertension* **8**:238–242.

47. Pelayo, J. C., 1986, Modulation of renal adrenergic effector mechanisms by calcium entry blockers, *Am. J. Physiol.* **252**:F613–F620.

48. Blackshear, J. L., Orlandi, C., Williams, G. H., and Hollenberg, N. K., 1986, The renal response to diltiazem and nifedipine: Comparison with nitroprusside, *J. Cardiol. Pharmacol.* **8**: 37–43.

49. Schmitz, A., 1987, Acute renal effects of oral felodipine in normal man, *Eur. J. Clin. Pharmacol.* **32**:17–22.

50. ter Wee, P. M., Smit, A. J., Rosman, J. B., Sluiter, W. J., and Donker, A. J. M., 1986, Effect of intravenous infusion of low-dose dopamine on renal function in normal individuals and in patients with renal disease, *Am. J. Nephrol.* **6**:42–46.

51. Israel, R., O'Mara, V., Austin, B., Bellucci, A., and Meyer, B. R., 1986, Metoclopramide decreases renal plasma flow, *Clin. Pharmacol. Ther.* **39**:261–264.

52. Strandhoy, J. W., 1985, Role of alpha-2 receptors in the regulation of renal function, *J. Cardiovasc. Pharmacol.* **7**:S28–S33.

53. Goldberg, M. and Gehr, M., 1985, Effects of alpha-2 agonists on renal function in hypertensive humans, *J. Cardiovasc. Pharmacol.* **7**:S34–S37.

54. Bennett, W. M., Aronoff, G., Golper, T. A., Morrison, G., Singer, I., and Brater, D. C., 1987, *Drug Dosing in Renal Failure: Guidelines for Adults*. American College of Physicians, Philadelphia.

55. Reed, W. E., Jr. and Sabatini, S., 1986, The use of drugs in renal failure, *Semin. Nephrol.* **6**: 259–295.

56. Bennett, W. M. and Golper, T. A., 1987, Drug therapy in renal disease, in: *Scientific American Medicine*. Scientific American Publishers, New York, Appendix A1–A29.

57. Brater, D. C., 1987, *Drug Use in Clinical Medicine*. B. C. Decker, Toronto.

58. Bjornsson, T. D., 1986, Nomogram for drug dosage adjustment in patients with renal failure, *Clin. Pharmacol.* **11**:164–170.

59. Burckart, G. J., 1987, Drug kinetics and dosing in organ transplant patients, *Trans. Immun. Lett.* **4**:1–12.

60. Van Scoy, R. E. and Wilson, W. R., 1987, Antimicrobial agents in adult patients with renal insufficiency: Initial dosage and general recommendations, *Mayo Clin. Proc.* **62:**1142–1145.

61. Piveral, K., Miller, S. C., Baird, D. R., and Pleasants, R. A., 1986, Apparently raised serum creatinine levels due to cephalosporins, *JAMA* **255:**323–324.

62. Guay, D. R. P., Meatherall, R. C., and Macaulay, P. A., 1983, Interference of selected second- and third-generation cephalosporins with creatinine determination, *Am. J. Hosp. Pharm.* **40:**435–438.

63. Myre, S. A., McCann, J., First, M. R., and Cluxton, R. B., Jr., 1987, Effect of trimethoprim on serum creatinine in healthy and chronic renal failure volunteers, *Ther. Drug Monit.* **9:**161–165.

64. Rybak, L. P., 1986, Drug ototoxicity, *Am. Rev. Pharmacol. Toxicol.* **26:**79–99.

65. Cutler, R. E., Forland, S. C., St. John Hammond, P. G., and Evans, J. R., 1987, Extracorporeal removal of drugs and poisons by hemodialysis and hemoperfusion, *Annu. Rev. Pharmacol. Toxicol.* **27:**169–191.

66. Choi, L. and Johnson, C. A., 1987, Dialyzability of drugs, *Dialysis Transpl.* **16:**537–540.

67. Derlet, R. W. and Albertson, T. E., 1986, Activated charcoal-past, present and future, *West. J. Med.* **146:**493–496.

68. Bouffet, E., Frappaz, D., Laville, M., Finaz, J., Pinkerton, C. R., Philip, T., and Brunat-Mentigny, M., 1986, Charcoal haemoperfusion and methotrexate toxicity, *Lancet* **1:**1497.

69. Bosch, J. P., 1986, Continuous arteriovenous hemofiltration (CAVH): Operational characteristics and clinical use, *AKF Nephrol. Lett.* **3:**15–26.

70. Golper, T. A., Wedel, S. K., Kaplan, A. A., Saad, A. M., Donta, S., and Paganini, E. P., 1985, Drug removal during continuous arteriovenous hemofiltration: Theory and clinical observation, *Int. J. Artif. Organs* **8:**307–313.

71. Lau, A. H., Kronfol, N. O., and Barakat, M., 1987, Effect of blood and ultrafiltrate flow rates on drug sieving during continuous hemofiltration, *Trans. Am. Soc. Artif. Intern. Organs* **33:**297–299.

72. Matzke, G. R., O'Connell, M. B., Collins, A. J., and Keshaviah, P. R., 1986, Disposition of vancomycin during hemofiltration, *Clin. Pharmacol. Ther.* **40:**425–430.

73. Lau, A. H., Kronfol, N. O., and John, E., 1987, Increased vancomycin elimination with continuous hemofiltration, *Trans. Am. Soc. Artif. Intern. Organs* **33:**772–774.

74. Domoto, D. T., Brown, W. W., and Bruggensmith, P., 1987, Removal of toxic levels of N-acetylprocainamide with continuous arteriovenous hemofiltration or continuous arteriovenous hemodiafiltration, *Ann. Intern. Med.* **106:**550–552.

75. Braden, G. L., Fitzgibbons, J. P., Germain, M. J., and Ledewitz, H. M., 1986, Hemoperfusion for treatment of N-acetylprocainamide intoxication, *Ann. Intern. Med.* **105:**64–65.

76. Loute, G., Adam, A., Heremans, C., and Willems, B., 1986, The influence of haemodialysis and haemofiltration on the clearance of torasemide in renal failure, *Eur. J. Clin. Pharmacol.* **3** (Suppl.):53–55.

77. Lai, K. N., Swaminathan, R., Pun, C. O., and Vallance-Owen, J., 1986, Hemofiltration in digoxin overdose, *Arch. Intern. Med.* **146:**1219–1221.

78. Zarowitz, B. J., Anandan, J. V., Dumler, F., Jayashankar, J., and Levin, N., 1986, Continuous arteriovenous hemofiltration of aminoglycoside antibiotics in critically ill patients, *J. Clin. Pharmacol.* **26:**686–689.

79. Golper, T. A., Saad, A.-M. A., and Morris, C. D., 1986, Gentamicin and phenytoin sieving through hollow-fiber polysulfone hemofilters, *Kidney Int.* **30:**937–943.

80. Kronfol, N., Lau, A., and Barakat, M., 1987, Aminoglycoside binding to polyacrylonitrile hemofilter membranes during continuous hemofiltration, *Trans. Am. Soc. Artif. Intern. Organs* **33:**297–299.

81. British Society of Antimicrobial Chemotherapy, 1987, Working Party Report: Diagnosis and management of peritonitis in continuous ambulatory peritoneal dialysis, *Lancet* **1:**845–850.

82. Janicke, D. M., Morse, G. D., Apicella, M. A., Jusko, W. J., and Walshe, J. J., 1986, Pharmacokinetic modeling of bidirectional transfer during peritoneal dialysis, *Clin. Pharmacol. Ther.* **40:**209–218.

83. Whitby, M., Edwards, R., Aston, E., and Finch, R. G., 1987, Pharmacokinetics of single dose intravenous vancomycin in CAPD peritonitis, *J. Antimicrob. Chemother.* **19**:351–357.

84. Morse, G. D., Farolino, D. F., Apicella, M. A., and Walshe, J. J., 1987, Comparative study of intraperitoneal and intravenous vancomycin pharmacokinetics during continuous ambulatory peritoneal dialysis, *Antimicrob. Agents Chemother.* **31**:173–177.

85. Traina, G. L., Gentile, M. G., Fellin, G., Rosina, R., Cavenaghi, L., Buniva, G., and Bonati, M., 1986, Pharmacokinetics of teicoplanin in patients on continuous ambulatory peritoneal dialysis, *Eur. J. Clin. Pharmacol.* **31**:501–504.

86. Harford, A. M., Sica, D. A., Tartaglione, T., Polk, R. E., Dalton, H. P., and Poyner, W., 1986, Vancomycin pharmacokinetics in continuous ambulatory peritoneal dialysis patients with peritonitis, *Nephron* **43**:217–222.

87. Walshe, J. J. and Morse, G. D., 1986, The influence of peritonitis on the pharmacokinetics of intraperitoneal vancomycin, *Proc. Am. Soc. Nephrol.* **19**:99a (Abstract).

88. Shah, G. M., Winer, R. L., and Krasny, H. C., 1986, Acyclovir pharmacokinetics in a patient on continuous ambulatory peritoneal dialysis, *Am. J. Kidney Dis.* **7**:507–510.

89. Boelaert, J., Schurgers, M., Daneels, R., Van Landuyt, H. W., and Weatherley, B. C., 1987, Multiple dose pharmacokinetics of intravenous acyclovir in patients on continuous ambulatory peritoneal dialysis, *J. Antimicrob. Chemother.* **20**:69–76.

90. Rubin, J., Deraps, G. D., Walsh, D., Adair, C., and Bower, J., 1986, Protein losses and tobramycin absorption in peritonitis treated by hourly peritoneal dialysis, *Am. J. Kidney Dis.* **8**:124–127.

91. Indraprasit, S., Ukaravichien, V., Pummangura, C., and Kaojarern, S., 1986, Gentamicin removal during intermittent peritoneal dialysis, *Nephron* **44**:18–21.

92. Bliss, M., Mayersohn, M., Arnold, T., Logan, J., Michael, U. F., and Jones, W., 1986, Disposition kinetics of cefamandole during continuous ambulatory peritoneal dialysis, *Antimicrob. Agents Chemother.* **29**:649–653.

93. Raehl, C. L., Moorthy, A. V., and Beirne, G. J., 1986, Procainamide pharmacokinetics in patients on continuous ambulatory peritoneal dialysis, *Nephron* **44**:191–194.

94. Sica, D. A., Comstock, T., Harford, A., and Eshelman, F., 1987, Ranitidine pharmacokinetics in continuous ambulatory peritoneal dialysis, *Eur. J. Clin. Pharmacol.* **32**:587–591.

95. Raehl, C. L., Beirne, G. J., Moorthy, A. V., and Patel, A. K., 1987, Tocainide pharmacokinetics during continuous ambulatory peritoneal dialysis, *Am. J. Cardiol.* **60**:747–750.

96. Heim, K. L., Halstenson, C. E., Comty, C. M., Affrime, M. B., and Matzke, G. R., 1986, Disposition of cefotaxime and desacetyl cefotaxime during continuous ambulatory peritoneal dialysis, *Antimicrob. Agents Chemother.* **30**:15–19.

97. Albin, H., Ragnaud, J. M., Demotes-Mainard, F., Vincon, G., Couzineau, M., and Wone, C., 1986, Pharmacokinetics of intravenous and intraperitoneal ciftriaxone in chronic ambulatory peritoneal dialysis, *Eur. J. Clin. Pharmacol.* **31**:479–483.

98. Albin, H., Ragnaud, J. M., Demotes-Mainard, F., Vincon, G., and Wone, C., 1986, Pharmacokinetics of intravenous and intraperitoneal ciftriaxone in chronic ambulatory peritoneal dialysis, *Eur. J. Clin. Pharmacol.* **30**:299–302.

99. Schwartz, M. T., Kowalsky, S. F., McCormick, E. M., Parker, M. A., and Echols, R. M., 1986, Clindamycin phosphate kinetics in subjects undergoing CAPD, *Clin. Nephrol.* **26**:303–306.

100. Walshe, J. J. and Janicke, D. M., 1986, Crossover pharmacokinetic analysis comparing intravenous and intraperitoneal administration of tobramycin, *J. Infect. Dis.* **153**:796–799.

101. Golper, T. A., Hartstein, A. I., Morthland, V. H., and Christensen, J. M., 1987, Effects of antacids and dialysate dwell times on multiple-dose pharmacokinetics of oral ciprofloxacin in patients on continuous ambulatory peritoneal dialysis, *Antimicrob. Agents Chemother.* **31**:1787–1790.

102. Reams, G. P., Young, M., Sorkin, M., Twardowski, Z., Gloor, H., Moore, H., and Nolph, K. D., 1985–86, Effects of dipyridamole on peritoneal clearances, *Uremia Invest.* **9**:27–33.

103. Maher, J. F., Kirszel, P., Chakrabarti, E., and Bennett, R. R., 1986, Contrasting effects of amphotericin B and the solvent sodium desoxycholate on peritoneal transport, *Nephron* **43**:38–42.

104. Kayser, S. R. and Kurisu, S., 1986, Hydroxocobalamin in nitroprusside-induced cyanide toxicity, *Drug Intell. Clin. Pharm.* **20**:365–366.

105. Antal, E. J., Wright, C. E., III, Brown, B. L., Albert, K. S., Aman, L. C., and Levin, N. W., 1986, The influence of hemodialysis on the pharmacokinetics of ibuprofen and its major metabolites, *J. Clin. Pharmacol.* **26**:184–190.

106. Evers, J., Bonn, R., Boertz, A., Cawello, W., Luckow, V., Fey, M., Aboudan, F., and Dickmans, H-A., 1987, Pharmacokinetics of isosorbide-*t*-nitrate during haemodialysis and peritoneal dialysis, *Eur. J. Clin. Pharmacol.* **32**:503–505.

107. Eisenberg, J. M., Koffer, H., Glick, H. A., Connell, M. L., Loss, L. E., Talbot, G. H., Shusterman, N. H., and Strom, B. L., 1987, What is the cost of nephrotoxicity associated with aminoglycosides? *Ann. Intern. Med.* **107**:900–909.

108. Mathews, A. and Bailie, G. R., 1989, High incidence of nephrotoxicity with aminoglycosides dosed by non-pharmacokinetic methods, *Nephron* (in press).

109. Rybak, M. J., Frankowski, J. J., Edwards, D. J., and Albrecht, L. M., 1987, Alanine aminopeptidase and β_2-microglobulin excretion in patients receiving vancomycin and gentamicin, *Antimicrob. Agents Chemother.* **31**:1461–1464.

110. Cimino, M. A., Rotstein, C., Slaughter, R. L., and Emrich, L. J., 1987, Relationship of serum antibiotic concentrations to nephrotoxicity in cancer patients receiving concurrent aminoglycoside and vancomycin therapy, *Am. J. Med.* **83**:1091–1097.

111. Keller, F., Wagner, K., Borner, K., Kemmerich, B., Lode, H., Offermann, G., and Distler, A., 1986, Aminoglycoside dosage in hemodialysis patients, *J. Clin. Pharmacol.* **26**:690–695.

112. Rodvold, K. A. and Blum, R. A., 1987, Predictive performance of Sawchuk–Zaske and Bayesian dosing methods for tobramycin, *J. Clin. Pharmacol.* **27**:419–427.

113. Nahata, M. C., Hipple, T. F., and Clotz, M., 1986, Interlot variability in gentamicin and tobramycin concentration and its possible significance, *Ther. Drug. Monit.* **8**:256–258.

114. Frazier, D. L. and Riviere, J. E., 1987, Gentamicin dosing strategies for dogs with subclinical renal dysfunction, *Antimicrob. Agents Chemother.* **31**:1929–1934.

115. Winslade, N. E., Adelman, M. H., Evans, E. J., and Schentag, J. J., 1987, Single-dose accumulation pharmacokinetics of tobramycin and netilmicin in normal volunteers, *Antimicrob. Agents Chemother.* **31**:605–609.

116. Fillastre, J. P., Leroy, A., Humbert, G., Moulin, B., Bernadet, P., and Josse, S., 1987, Pharmacokinetics of habekacin in patients with renal insufficiency, *Antimicrob. Agents Chemother.* **31**:575–577.

117. Edson, R. S. and Terrell, C. L., 1987, The aminoglycosides: Streptomycin, kanamycin, gentamicin, tobramycin, amikacin, netilmicin, and sisomicin, *Mayo Clin. Proc.* **62**:916–920.

118. Wise, R., 1986, *In vitro* and pharmacokinetic properties of the carbapenems, *Antimicrob. Agents Chemother.* **30**:343–349.

119. Rogers, J. D., Meisinger, A. P., Ferber, F., Calandra, G. B., Demetriades, J. L., and Bland, J. A., 1985, Pharmacokinetics of impipenem and cilastatin in volunteers, *Ann. Infect. Dis.* **7**:S435–S634.

120. Anon., 1986, Imipenem-cilastatin sodium (primaxin), *Med. Lett.* **28**:29–32.

121. Clissold, S. P., Todd, A., and Campoli-Richards, D. M., 1987, Imipenem/cilastatin. A review of its antibacterial activity, pharmacokinetic properties and therapeutic efficacy, *Drugs* **33**:183–241.

122. Thompson, R. L., 1987, Cephalosporin, carbapenem, and monobactam antibiotics, *Mayo Clin. Proc.* **62**:821–834.

123. Bergan, T., 1987, Pharmacokinetic properties of the cephalosporins, *Drugs* **34**:89–104.

124. Smith, B. R., LeFrock, J. L., Thyrum, P. T., Doret, B. A., Yeh, C., Onesti, G., Schwartz, A., and Zimmerman, J. J., 1986, Cefotetan pharmacokinetics in volunteers with various degrees of renal function, *Antimicrob. Agents Chemother.* **29**:887–893.

125. Browning, M. J., Holt, H. A., White, L. O., Chapman, S. T., Banks, R. A., Reeves, D. S., and

Yates, R. A., 1986, Pharmacokinetics of cefotetan in patients with end-stage renal failure on maintenance dialysis, *J. Antimicrob. Chemother.* **18:**103–106.

126. Konishi, K., 1986, Pharmacokinetics of cefmenoxime in patients with impaired renal function and in those undergoing hemodialysis, *Antimicrob. Agents Chemother.* **30:**901–905.

127. Campoli-Richards, D. M. and Todd, P. A., 1987, Cefmenoxime. A review of its antibacterial activity, pharmacokinetic properties and therapeutic use, *Drugs* **34:**188–221.

128. van Dalen, R., Baars, A. M., and Termond, E., 1986, Dosage adjustment for ceftazidime in patients with impaired renal function, *Eur. J. Clin. Pharmacol.* **30:**597–605.

129. Phelps, R. G. and Conte, J. E., Jr., Multiple-dose pharmacokinetics of cefonicid in patients with impaired renal function, *Antimicrob. Agents Chemother.* **29:**913–917.

130. Saltiel, E. and Brogden, R. N., 1986, Cefonicid. A review of its antibacterial activity, pharmacological properties and therapeutic use, *Drugs* **32:**222–259.

131. Campoli-Richards, D. M., Lackner, T. E., and Monk, J. P., 1987, Ceforanide. A review of its antibacterial activity, pharmacokinetic properties and clinical efficacy, *Drugs* **34:**411–437.

132. Barrueco, M., Otero, M. J., Garcia, M. J., Lanao, J. M., and Dominguez-Gil, A., 1986, Pleural fluid levels of cefoxitin in patients with renal impairment, *Int. J. Clin. Pharm. Ther. Toxicol.* **24:**485–489.

133. Guay, D. R. P., Meatherall, R. C., Harding, G. K., and Brown, G. R., 1986, Pharmacokinetics of cefixime (CL 284,635; FK 027) in healthy subjects and patients with renal insufficiency, *Antimicrob. Agents Chemother.* **30:**485–490.

134. Tanrisever, B. and Santella, P. J., 1986, Cefadroxil. A review of its antibacterial, pharmacokinetic and therapeutic properties in comparison with cephalexin and cephradine, *Drugs* **32:**1–16.

135. Wright, D. B., 1986, Cefsulodin, *Drug Intell. Clin. Pharm.* **20:**845–849.

136. Conte, J. E., Jr., 1987, Pharmacokinetics of cefpiramide in volunteers with normal or impaired renal function, *Antimicrob. Agents Chemother.* **31:**1585–1588.

137. Aronoff, G. R., Wolen, R. L., Obermeyer, B. D., and Black, H. R., 1986, Pharmacokinetics and protein binding of cefamandole and its 1-methyl-1 H-tetrazole-5-thiol side chain in subjects with normal and impaired renal function, *J. Infect. Dis.* **153:**1069–1074.

138. Babiak, L. M. and Rybak, M. J., 1986, Hematological effects associated with beta-lactam use, *Drug Intell. Clin. Pharm.* **20:**833–836.

139. Josse, S., Godin, M., and Fillastre, J. P., 1987, Cefazolin-induced encephalopathy in a uraemic patients, *Nephron* **45:**72.

140. Childs, S. J. and Bodey, G. P., 1986, Aztreonam, *Pharmacotherapy* **6:**138–152.

141. Anon., 1987, Aztreonam (Azactam), *Med. Lett.* **29:**45–48.

142. Anon., 1987, Ampicillin/sulbactam (Unasyn), *Med. Lett.* **29:**79–82.

143. Campoli-Richards and Brogden, R. N., 1987, Sulbactam/Ampicillin. A review of its antibacterial activity, pharmacokinetic properties, and therapeutic use, *Drugs* **33:**577–609.

144. Foulds, G., 1986, Pharmacokinetics of sulbactam/Ampicillin in humans: A review, *Rev. Infect. Dis.* **8:**S503–S511.

145. Horber, F. F., Frey, F. J., Descoeudres, C., Murray, A. T., and Reubi, F. C., 1986, Differential effect of impaired renal function on the kinetics of clavulanic acid and amoxicillin, *Antimicrob. Agents Chemother.* **29:**614–619.

146. Dalet, F., Amado, E., Donate, T., and del Rio, G., 1986, Pharmacokinetics of the combination if ticarcillin with clavulanic acid in renal insufficiency, *J. Antimicrob. Chemother.* **17:**57–64.

147. Jungbluth, G. L., Cooper, D. L., Doyle, G. D., Chudzik, G. M., and Jusko, W. J., 1986, Pharmacokinetics of ticarcillin and clavulanic acid (Timentin) in relation to renal function, *Antimicrob. Agents Chemother.* **30:**896–900.

148. Watson, I. D., Boulton-Jones, M., Stewart, M. J., Henderson, I., and Payton, C. D., 1987, Pharmacokinetics of clavulanic acid-potentiated ticarcillin in renal failure, *Ther. Drug. Monit.* **9:**139–147.

149. Wright, A. J. and Wilkowske, C. J., 1987, The penicillins, *Mayo Clin. Proc.* **62:**806–820.

150. Terp, D. K. and Rybank, M. J., 1987, Ciprofloxacin, *Drug Intell. Clin. Pharm.* **21:**568–74.

151. Marble, D. A. and Bosso, J. A., 1986, Norfloxacin: A quinoline antibiotic, *Drug Intell. Clin. Pharm.* **20**:261–6.
152. Rowen, R. C., Michel, D. J., and Thompson, J. C., 1987, Norfloxacin: Clinical pharmacology and clinical use, *Pharmacotherapy* **7**:92–110.
153. Gasser, T. C., Ebert, S. C., Graversen, P. H., and Madsen, P. O., 1987, Ciprofloxacin pharmacokinetics in patients with normal and impaired renal function, *Antimicrob. Agents Chemother.* **31**:709–712.
154. Gerritisen, W. R., Peters, A., Henry, F. C., and Brouwers, J., 1987, Cirprofoxacin-induced nephrotoxicity, *Nephrol. Dialysis Transpl.* **2**:382–383.
155. Dudley, M. N., 1987, Pharmacokinetic and pharmacodynamic properties of new quinoline antiinfectives, *Hosp. Formul.* **22**:9–15.
156. Drusano, G. L., Weir, M., Forrest, A., Plaisance, K., Emm, T., and Standiford, H. C., 1987, Pharmacokinetics of intravenously administered ciprofloxacin in patients with various degrees of renal function, *Antimicrob. Agents Chemother.* **31**:860–864.
157. Lode, H., Höffken, G., Prinzing, C., Glatzel, R., Olschewski, W. P., Sivers, B., Reimnitz, D., Borner, K., and Koeppe, P., 1987, Comparative pharmacokinetics of new quinolones, *Drugs* **34**:21–25.
158. Wise, R., Lister, D., McNulty, C. A. M., Griggs, D., and Andrews, J. M., 1986, The comparative pharmacokinetics of five quinolones, *J. Antimicrob. Chemother.* **18**:71–81.
159. LeBel, M., Barbeau, G., Bergeron, M. G., Roy, D., and Vallée, F., 1986, Pharmacokinetics of ciprofloxacin in elderly subjects, *Pharmacotherapy* **6**:87–91.
160. Webb, D. B., Roberts, D. E., Williams, J. D., and Asscher, A. W., 1986, Pharmacokinetics of ciprofloxacin in healthy volunteers and patients with impaired kidney funtion, *J. Antimicrob. Chemother.* **18**:83–87.
161. Singlas, E., Taburet, A. M., Landru, I., Albin, H., and Ryckelinck, J. Ph., 1987, Pharmacokinetics of ciprofloxacin tablets in renal failure; Influence of haemodialysis. *Eur. J. Clin. Pharmacol.* **31**:589–593.
161a. Shalit, I., Greenwood, R. B., Marks, M. I., Pederson, J. A., and Frederick, D. L., 1986, Pharmacokinetics of single-dose oral ciprofloxacin in patients undergoing chronic ambulatory peritoneal dialysis, *Antimicrob. Agents Chemother.* **30**(1):152–156.
162. Anon., 1987, Safety of antimicrobial drugs in pregnancy, *Med. Lett.* **29**:61–63.
163. Boelaert, J., de Jaegere, P. P., Daneels, R., Schurgers, M., Gordts, B., and van Landuyt, H. W., 1987, Case report of renal failure during norfloxacin therapy, *Clin. Nephrol.* **27**:272.
164. Monk, J. P. and Campoli-Richards, D. M., 1987, Ofloxacin. A review of its antibacterial activity, pharmacokinetic properties and therapeutic use, *Drugs* **33**:346–391.
165. Fillastre, J. P., Leroy, A., and Humbert, G., 1987, Ofloxacin pharmacokinetics in renal failure, *Antimicrob. Agents Chemother.* **31**:156–160.
166. Bury, R. W., Becker, G. J., Kincaid-Smith, P. S., Moulds, R. W., and Whitworth, J. A., 1987, Elimination of enoxacin in renal disease, *Clin. Pharmacol. Ther.* **41**:434–8.
167. Rybak, M. J. and Boike, S. C., 1986, Monitoring vancomycin therapy, *Drug Intell. Clin. Pharm.* **20**:757–761.
168. Cheung, R. P. F. and DiPiro, J. T., 1986, Vancomycin: An update, *Pharmacotherapy* **6**:153–169.
169. Golper, T., Noonan, H., Anderson, J., Elzinga, L., Brummeh, R., Andersen, J. L., Gilbert, D., and Bennett, W., 1988, Vancomycin pharmacokinetics: renal handling and nonrenal clearances in normal subjects, *Clin. Pharmacol. Ther.* **43**:565–570.
170. Healy, D. P., Polk, R. E., Garson, M. L., Rock, D. T., and Comstock, T. J., 1987, Comparison of steady-state pharmacokinetics of two dosage regimens of vancomycin in normal volunteers, *Antimicrob. Agents Chemother.* **31**:393–397.
171. Southorn, P. A., Plevak, D. J., Wright, A. J., and Wilson, W. R., 1986, Adverse effects of vancomycin administered in the perioperative period, *Mayo Clin. Proc.* **61**:721–724.
172. Hermans, P. E. and Wilhelm, M. P., 1987, Vancomycin, *Mayo Clin. Proc.* **62**:901–905.

173. Arroyo, J. C., Rosansky, S. J., and Rosenzweig, P. N., 1986, Correspondence, *Am. J. Kidney Dis.* **7:**511.

174. Packer, J., Olshan, A. R., and Schwartz, A. B., 1987, Prolonged allergic reaction to vancomycin in end-stage renal disease, *Dialysis Transpl.* **16:**86–88.

175. Matzke, G. R., Halstenson, C. E., Olson, P. L., Collins, A. J., and Abraham, P. A., 1987, Systemic absorption of oral vancomycin in patients with renal insufficiency and antibiotic-associated colitis, *Am. J. Kidney Dis.* **9:**422–425.

176. Bonati, M., Traina, Villa, G., Salvadeo, A., Gentile, M. G., Fellin, G., Rosina, R., Cavenaghi, L., and Buniva, G., 1987, Teicoplanin pharmacokinetics in patients with chronic renal failure, *Clin. Pharmacol.* **12:**292–301.

177. Falcoz, C., Ferry, N., Pozet, N., Cuisinaud, G., Zech, P. Y., and Sassard, J., 1987, Pharmacokinetics of teicoplanin in renal failure, *Antimicrob. Agents Chemother.* **31:**1255–1262.

178. Domart, Y., Pierre, C., Clair, B., Garaud, J. J., Regnier, B., and Gibert, C., 1987, Pharmacokinetics of teicoplanin in critically ill patients with various degrees of renal impairment, *Antimicrob. Agents Chemother.* **31:**1600–1604.

179. Wilson, W. R. and Cockerill, F. R., III., 1987, Tetracyclines, chloramphenicol, erythromycin, and clindamycin, *Mayo Clin. Proc.* **62:**906–915.

180. Disse, B., Gundert-Remy, U., Weber, E., Andrassy, K., Sietzen, W., and Lang, A., 1986, Pharmacokinetics of erythromycin in patients with different degrees of renal impairment, *Int. J. Clin. Pharm. Ther. Toxicol.* **24:**460–464.

181. Kanfer, A., Stamatakis, G., Torlotin, J. C., Fredj, G., Kenouch, S., and Méry, J. Ph., 1987, Changes in erythromycin pharmacokinetics induced by renal failure, *Clin. Nephrol.* **27:**147–150.

182. Goa, K. L. and Campoli-Richards, D. M., 1987, Pentamidine isethionate. A review of its antiprotozoal activity, pharmacokinetic properties and therapeutic use in pneumocystic carinii pneumonia, *Drugs* **33:**242–258.

183. Conte, J. E., Upton, R. A., Phelps, R. T., Wofsy, C. B., Zurlinden, E., and Lin, E. T., 1986, Use of a specific and sensitive assay to determine pentamidine pharmacokinetics in patients with AIDS, *J. Infect. Dis.* **154:**923–929.

184. Bergan, T., Örtengren, B., and Westerlund, D., 1986, Clinical pharmacokinetics of co-trimazine, *Clin. Pharm.* **11:**372–386.

185. Nissenson, A. R., Wilson, C., and Holazo, A., 1987, Pharmacokinetics of intravenous trimethoprim-sulfamethoxazole during hemodialysis, *Am. J. Nephrol.* **7:**270–274.

186. Wood, M. J. and Geddes, A. M., 1987, Antiviral therapy, *Lancet* **2:**1189–1192.

187. Hermans, P. E. and Cockerill, F. R., 1987, Antiviral agents, *Mayo Clin. Proc.* **62:**1108–1115.

188. Jones, P. G. and Beier-Hanratty, S. A., 1986, Acyclovir: Neurologic and renal toxicity, *Ann. Intern. Med.* **104:**892.

189. Spiegal, D. M. and Lau, K., 1986, Acute renal failure and coma secondary to acyclovir therapy, *JAMA* **255:**1882–1883.

190. Dorsky, D. I. and Crumpacker, C. S., 1987, Drugs five years later: Acyclovir, *Ann. Intern. Med.* **107:**859–874.

191. Laskin, O. L., Cederberg, D. M., Mills, J., Eron, L. J., Mildvan, D., and Spector, S. A., 1987, Ganciclovir for the treatment and suppression of serious infections caused by cytomegalovirus, *Am. J. Med.* **83:**201–207.

192. Fletcher, C., Sawchuk, R., Chinnock, B., de Miranda, P., and Balfour, H. H., Jr., 1986, Human pharmacokinetics of the antiviral drug DHPG, *Clin. Pharmacol. Ther.* **40:**281–286.

193. Varughese, A., Brater, D. C., Benet, L. Z., and Lee, C-S. C., 1986, Ethambutol kinetics in patients with impaired renal function, *Am. Rev. Respir. Dis.* **134:**34–38.

194. Van Scoy, R. E. and Wilkowske, C. J., 1987, antituberculous agents, *Mayo Clin. Proc.* **62:**1129–1136.

195. Anon., 1986, Drugs for treatment of systemic fungal infections, *Med. Lett.* **28:**41–44.

196. Terrell, C. L. and Hermans, P. E., 1987, Antifungal agents used for deep-seated mycotic infections, *Mayo Clin. Proc.* **62:**1116–1128.

197. Katz, M., 1986, Anthelmintics. Current concepts in the treatment of helminthic infections, *Drugs* **32:**358–371.
198. Marriner, S. E., Morris, D. L., Dickson, B., and Bogan, J. A., 1986, Pharmacokinetics of albendazole in man, *Eur. J. Clin. Pharmacol.* **30:**705–708.
199. Zuidema, J., Hilbers-Modderman, E. S. M., and Merkus, F. W. H. M., 1986, Clinical pharmacokinetics of dapsone, *Clin. Pharm.* **11:**299–315.
200. Anon., 1986, Drugs for cardiac arrhythmias, *Med. Lett.* **28:**111–116.
201. Kreeger, R. W. and Hammill, S. C., 1987, New antiarrhythmic drugs: Tocainide, mexiletine, flecainide, encainide, and amiodarone, *Mayo Clin. Proc.* **62:**1033–1050.
202. Oates, J. A., Wood, A. J. J., and Campbell, R. W. F., 1987, Drug therapy. Mexiletine, *N. Engl. J. Med.* **316:**29–34.
203. Anon., 1986, Mexiletine for arrhythmias, *Med. Lett.* **28:**65–68.
204. Roden, D. M. and Woosley, R. L., 1986, Drug therapy. Tocainide, *N. Engl. J. Med.* **315:**41–45.
205. Roden, D. M. and Woosley, R. L., 1986, Drug therapy. Flecainide, *N. Engl. J. Med.* **315:**36–40.
206. Braun, J., Kollert, J. R., and Becker, J. U., 1987, Pharmacokinetics of flecainide in patients with mild and moderate renal failure compared with patients with normal renal function, *Eur. J. Clin. Pharmacol.* **31:**711–714.
207. Salerno, D. M., Granrud, G., Sharkey, P., Krejci, J., Larson, T., Erlien, D., Berry, D., and Hodges, M., 1986, Pharmacodynamics and side effects of flecainide acetate, *Clin. Pharmacol. Ther.* **40:**101–107.
208. Bergstrand, R. H., Wang, T., Roden, D. M., Stone, W. J., Wolfenden, H. T., Woosley, R. L., Wilkinson, G. R., and Wood, A. J. J., 1986, Encainide disposition in patients with renal failure, *Clin. Pharmacol. Ther.* **40:**64–70.
209. Tordjman, T. and Estes, N. A. M., 1987, Encainide: Its electrophysiologic and antiarrhythmic effects, pharmacokinetics, and safety, *Pharmacotherapy* **7:**149–163.
210. Brogden, R. N. and Todd, P. A., 1987, Encainide. A review of its pharmacological properties and therapeutic efficacy, *Drugs* **34:**519–538.
211. Brogden, R. N. and Todd, P. A., 1987, Disopyramide. A reappraisal of its pharmacodynamics and pharmacokinetic properties, and therapeutic use in cardiac arrhythmias, *Drugs* **34:**151–187.
212. Siddoway, L. A. and Woosley, R. L., 1986, Clinical pharmacokinetics of disopyramide, *Clin. Pharmacol.* **11:**214–222.
213. Anon., 1986, Amiodarone, *Med. Lett.* **28:**49–52.
214. Oates, J. A., Wood, A. J. J., and Mason, J. W., 1987, Drug therapy. Amiodarone, *N. Engl. J. Med.* **316:**455–466.
215. Garfinkel, D., Mamelok, R. D., and Blaschke, T. F., 1987, Altered therapeutic range for quinidine after myocardial infarction and cardiac surgery, *Ann. Intern. Med.* **107:**48–50.
216. Harron, D. W. G. and Brogden, R. N., 1987, Propafenone. A review of its pharmacodynamic and pharmacokinetic properties, and therapeutic use in the treatment of arrhythmias, *Drugs* **34:**617–647.
217. Rosansky, S. J. and Brady, M. E., 1986, Procainamide toxicity in a patient with acute renal failure, *Am. J. Kidney Dis.* **7:**502–506.
218. Weisbart, R. H., Yee, W. S., Colburn, K. K., Whang, S. H., Heng, M. K., and Boucek, R. J., 1986, Antiguanosine antibodies: A new marker for procainamide-induced systemic lupus erythematosus, *Ann. Intern. Med.* **104:**310–313.
219. Rocci, M. L., Jr. and Wilson, H., 1987, The pharmacokinetics and pharmacodynamics of newer inotropic agents, *Clin. Pharm.* **13:**91–109.
220. Weber, K. T., Gill, S. K., Janicki, J. S., Maskin, C. S., and Jain, M. C., 1987, Newer positive inotropic agents in the treatment of chronic cardiac failure, *Drugs* **33:**503–519.
221. Oates, J. A., Wood, A. J. J., and Fitzgerald, G. A., 1987, Drug therapy. Dipyridamole, *N. Engl. J. Med.* **316:**1247–1256.
222. Kampmann, J. P., 1987, Pharmacokinetics of various preparations of organic nitrates, *Drugs* **33** (Suppl. 4):5–8.

223. Bogaert, M. G., 1987, Clinical pharmacokinetics of glyceryl trinitrate following the use of systemic and topical preparations, *Clin. Pharmacol.* **12**:1–11.

224. Evers, J., Krakamp, B., Klimkait, W., Dickmans, H. A., Maddock, J., Luckow, V., Cawello, W., and Weib, M., 1986, Pharmacokinetics of isosorbide-5-nitrate in renal failure, *Eur. J. Clin. Pharmacol.* **30**:349–350.

225. Evers, J., Bonn, R., Cawello, W., Luckow, V., Aboudan, F., and Dickmans, H. A., 1987, Pharmacokinetics of isosorbide-5-nitrate during haemodialysis and peritoneal dialysis, *Eur. J. Clin. Pharmacol.* **32**:503–505.

226. Anon., 1987, Drugs that cause sexual dysfunction, *Med. Lett.* **29**:65–70.

227. Anon., 1987, Drugs for hypertension, *Med. Lett.* **29**:1–6.

228. Morrison, G., Spar, B., Walker, B. R., and Goldfarb, S., 1986, The acute and chronic effects of indoramin on renal function, hemodynamics, and transport, *J. Cardiol. Pharm.* **8**(Suppl. 2):S25–S29.

229. Titmarsh, S. and Monk, J. P., 1987, Terazosin. A review of its pharmacodynamic and pharmacokinetic properties, and therapeutic efficacy in essential hypertension, *Drugs* **33**:461–477.

230. Sonders, R. C., 1986, Pharmacokinetics of Terazosin, *Am. J. Med.* **80**(Suppl. 5B):20–24.

231. Jungers, P., Ganeval, D., Pertuiset, N., and Chauveau, P., 1986, Influence of renal insufficiency on the pharmacokinetics and pharmacodynamics of Terazosin, *Am. J. Med.* **80**(Suppl. 5B):94–99.

232. Carlson, R. V., Bailey, R. R., Begg, E. J., Cowlishaw, M. G., and Sharman, J. R., 1986, Pharmacokinetics and effect on blood pressure of doxazosin in normal subjects and patients with renal failure, *Clin. Pharmacol. Ther.* **40**:561–566.

233. Lameire, N. and Gordts, J., 1986, A pharmacokinetic study of prazosin in patients with varying degrees of chronic renal failure, *Eur. J. Clin. Pharmacol.* **31**:333–337.

234. Halstenson, C. E., Opsahl, J. A., Pence, T. V., Luke, D. R., Sirgo, M. A., Plachetka, J. R., Abraham, P. A., and Matzke, G. R., 1986, The disposition and dynamics of labetalol in patients on dialysis, *Clin. Pharmacol. Ther.* **40**:462–468.

235. Lowenthal, D. T., Saris, S. D., Porter, R. S., Bies, C., and Falkner, B., 1987, Pharmacokinetics and pharmacodynamics of transdermal clonidine in renal insufficiency, *Am. Soc. Hypertension* **2**:57a (Abstract).

236. Josselson, J. and Sadler, J. H., 1986, Nephrotic-range proteinuria and hyperglycemia associated with clonidine therapy, *Am. J. Med.* **80**:545–546.

237. Sorkin, E. M. and Heel, R. C., 1986, Guanfacine. A review of its pharmacodynamic and pharmacokinetic properties, and therapeutic efficacy in the treatment of hypertension, *Drugs* **31**:301–336.

238. Gehr, M., MacCarthy, E. P., and Goldberg, M., 1986, Guanabenz: A centrally acting, natriuretic antihypertensive drug, *Kidney Int.* **29**:1203–1208.

239. Kiechel, J. R., 1986, Pharmacokinetics of guanfacine in patients with impaired renal function and in some elderly patients, *Am. J. Cardiol.* **57**:18E–21E.

240. Benfield, P. and Sorkin, E. M., 1987, Esmolol. A preliminary review of its pharmacodynamic and pharmacokinetic properties, and therapeutic efficacy, *Drugs* **33**:392–412.

241. Covinsky, J. O., 1987, Esmolol: A novel cardioselective, titratable, intravenous beta-blocker with ultrashort half-life, *Drug Intell. Clin. Pharm.* **21**:316–321.

242. Reynolds, R. D., Gorczynski, R. J., and Quon, C. Y., 1986, Pharmacology and pharmacokinetics of Esmolol, *J. Clin. Pharmacol.* **26**(Suppl. A):A3–A14.

243. Anon., 1987, Esmolol—A short-acting IV beta-blocker, *Med. Lett.* **29**:57–60.

244. Zech, P., Pozet, N., Labeeuw, M., Laville, M., Hadj-Aissa, A., Arkouche, W., and Poncet, J. F., 1986, Acute renal effects of beta-blockers, *Am. J. Nephrol.* **6**(Suppl. 2):15–19.

245. Paillard, F., Lantz, B., Leviel, F., and Ardaillou, R., 1986, Renal hemodynamic effects of Tertatolol in essential hypertension, *Am. J. Nephrol.* **6**(Suppl. 2):40–44.

246. Bauer, J. H., Reams, G. P., and Lau, A., 1987, A comparison of Betaxolol and Nadolol on renal function in essential hypertension, *Am. J. Kidney Dis.* **10**:109–112.

247. Drayer, D. E., 1987, Lipophilicity, hydrophilicity, and the central nervous system side effects of beta blockers, *Pharmacotherapy* **7**:87–91.

248. Riddell, J. G., Harron, D. W. G., and Shanks, R. G., 1987, Clinical pharmacokinetics of β-adrenoceptor antagonists. An update, *Clin. Pharmacol.* **12**:305–320.

249. Bernard, N., Cuisinaud, G., Pozet, N., Zech, P. Y., and Sassard, J., 1985, Pharmacokinetics of penbutolol and its metabolites in renal insufficiency, *Eur. J. Clin. Pharmacol.* **29**:215–219.

250. Solimon, M., Massry, S. G., and Campese, V. M., 1986, Renal hemodynamics and pharmacokinetics of bevantolol in patients with impaired renal function, *Am. J. Cardiol.* **58**:21E–24E.

251. Van Der Meulen, J., Reijn, E., Heidendal, G. A. K., Donker, O. E., and Donker, A. J. M., 1986, Comparison of the effects of penbutolol and propranolol on glomerular filtration rate in hypertensive patients with impaired renal function, *Br. J. Clin. Pharmacol.* **22**:469–474.

252. Williams, E. M. V., 1987, Bevantolol: A beta-1 adrenoceptor antagonist with unique additional actions, *J. Clin. Pharmacol.* **27**:450–460.

253. Singh, B. N., Deedwania, P., Nademanee, K., Ward, A., and Sorkin, E. M., 1987, Sotalol. A review of its pharmacodynamic and pharmacokinetic properties, and therapeutic use, *Drugs* **34**:311–349.

254. Riddell, J. G., Shanks, R. G., and Brogden, R. N., 1987, Celiprolol. A preliminary review of its pharmacodynamic and pharmacokinetic properties and its therapeutic use in hypertension and angina pectoris, *Drugs* **34**:438–458.

255. Anon., 1986, Enalapril for hypertension, *Med. Lett.* **28**(714):53–56.

256. Bauer, J. H. and Reams, G. P., 1986, Renal effects of angiotensin converting enzyme inhibitors in hypertension, *Am. J. Med.* **83**(Suppl. 4C):19–27.

257. Nelson, E. B., Pool, J. L., and Taylor, A. A., 1986, Pharmacology of angiotensin converting enzyme inhibitors, *Am. J. Med.* **81**(Suppl. 4C):13–18.

258. Packer, M., Lee, W. H., Yushak, M., and Medina, N., 1986, Comparison of captopril and enalapril in patients with severe chronic heart failure, *N. Engl. J. Med.* **315**:847–53.

259. Hockings, N., Ajayi, A. A, and Reid, J. L., 1986, Age and the pharmacokinetics of angiotensin converting enzyme inhibitors enalapril and enalaprilat, *Br. J. Clin. Pharmacol.* **21**:341–348.

260. Fruncillo, R. J., Rocci, J. L., Vlasses, P. H., Mojaverian, P., Shepley, K., Clementi, R. A., Oren, A., Smith, R. D., Till, A. E., Riley, L. J. Jr., Krishna, G., Narins, R. G., and Ferguson, R. K., 1987, Disposition of enalapril and enalaprilat in renal insufficiency, *Kidney Int.* **31**:S117–S122.

261. Creasey, W. A., Funke, P. T., McKinstry, D. N., and Sugerman, A. A., 1986, Pharmacokinetics of captopril in elderly healthy male volunteers, *J. Clin. Pharmacol.* **26**:264–268.

262. Drummer, O. H., Workman, B. S., Miach, P. J., Jarrott, B., and Louis, W. J., 1987, The pharmacokinetics of captopril and captopril disulfide conjugates in uraemic patients on maintenance dialysis: Comparison with patients with normal renal function, *Eur. J. Clin. Pharmacol.* **32**:267–271.

263. Cleary, J. D. and Taylor, J. W., 1986, Enalapril: A new angiotensin converting enzyme inhibitor, *Drug Intell. Clin. Pharmacol.* **20**:177186.

264. Borek, M., Charlap, S., and Frishman, W., 1987, Enalapril: A long-acting angiotensin-converting enzyme inhibitor, *Pharmacotherapy* **7**:133–148.

265. Madeddu, P., Ena, P., Dessi-Fulgheri, P., Glorioso, N., Cerimele, D., and Rappelli, A., 1986, Captopril-induced proteinuria in hypertensive psoriatic patients, *Nephron* **44**:358–360.

266. Donker, Ab. and J. M., 1987, Nephrotoxicity of angiotensin converting enzyme inhibition, *Kidney Int.* **31**:S132–S137.

267. Hogg, K. J. and Hillis, W. S., 1986, Captopril/metolazone induced renal failure, *Lancet* **1**:501–502.

268. Turney, J. H., 1986, Irreversible renal transplant failure after angiotensin converting enzyme inhibition, *Br. Med. J.* **292**:1672.

269. Brown, A. R. and Williams, P. F., 1986, Irreversible renal transplant failure after enalapril therapy, *Br. Med. J.* **292**:732.

270. Hricik, D. E., 1987, Antihypertensive and renal effects of enalapril in post-transplant hypertension, *Clin. Nephrol.* **27**:250–259.

271. Morice, A. H., Brown, M. J., Lowry, R., and Higenbottam, T., 1987, Angiotensin-converting enzyme and the cough reflex, *Lancet* **2**:1116–1118.

272. Inman, W. H. W., 1986, Enalapril-induced cough, *Lancet* **1**:1218.

273. McNally, E. M., 1987, Cough due to captopril, *West. J. Med.* **146**:226–228.

274. Webb, D., Benjamin, N., Collier, J., and Robinson, B., 1986, Enalapril-induced cough, *Lancet* **2**: 1094.

275. Cleland, J. G. F., Dargie, H. J., Pettigrew, A., Gillen, G., and Robertson, J. I. S., 1986, The effects of captopril on serum digoxin an urinary urea and digoxin clearances in patients with congestive heart failure, *Am. Heart J.* **112**:130–135.

276. Debusmann, E. R., Pujadas, J. O., Lahn, W., Irmisch, R., Jané, F., Kuan, T. S, Mora, J., Walter, U., Eckert, H. G., Hajdú, P., and Metzer, H., 1987, Influence of renal function on the pharmacokinetics of ramipril (HOE 498), *Am. J. Cardiol.* **59**:70D–78D.

277. Aurell, M., Delin, K., Herlitz, H., Ljungman, S., Witte, P. U., and Irmisch, R., 1987, Pharmacokinetics and pharmacodynamics of ramipril in renal failure, *Am. J. Cardiol.* **59**:65D–69D.

278. van Schaik, B. A. M., Geyskes, G. G., and Boer, P., 1987, Lisinopril in hypertensive patients with and without renal failure, *Eur. J. Clin. Pharmacol.* **32**:11–16.

279. Rakhit, A., Hurley, M. E., Tipnis, V., Coleman, J., Rommel, A., and Brunner, H. R., 1986, Pharmacokinetics and pharmacodynamics of pentopril, a new angiotensin-converting-enzyme inhibitor in humans, *J. Clin. Pharmacol.* **26**:156–164.

280. Onoyama, K., Kumagai, H., Inenaga, T., Nanishi, F., Okuda, S., Oh, Y., Omae, T., Hayashi, K., and Fujishima, M., 1986, Pharmacokinetic properties of a new angiotensin I-converting enzyme inhibitor in patients with chronic renal failure, *Curr. Ther. Res.* **39**:671–680.

281. Echizen, H. and Eichelbaum, M., 1986, Clinical pharmacokinetics of verapamil, nifedipine and diltiazem, *Clin. Pharmacol.* **11**:425–449.

282. Anderson, P. 1986, Pharmacokinetics of calcium channel blocking agents, *Acta Pharmacol. Toxicol.* **58**:43–57.

283. Boden, W. E., More, G., Sharma, S., Bough, E. W., Korr, K. S., Young, P. M., and Shulman, R. S., 1986, No increase in serum digoxin concentration with high-dose diltiazem, *Am. J. Med.* **81**:425–428.

284. Carrum, G., Egan, J. M., and Abernethy, D. R., 1986, Diltiazem treatment impairs hepatic drug oxidation: Studies of antipyrine, *Clin. Pharmacol. Ther.* **40**:140–143.

285. Edwards, D. J., Lavoie, R., Beckman, H., Blevins, R., and Rubenfire, M., 1987, The effect of coadministration of verapamil on the pharmacokinetics and metabolism of quinidine, *Clin. Pharmacol. Ther.* **41**:68–73.

286. Abernethy, D. R., Schwartz, J. B., Todd, E. L., Luchi, R., and Snow, E., 1986, Verapamil pharmacodynamics and disposition in young and elderly hypertensive patients, *Ann. Intern. Med.* **105**:329–336.

287. Städler, P., Leonardi, L. Riesen, W., Ziegler, W., Marone, C., and Beretta-Piccoli, C., 1987, Cardiovascular effects of verapamil in essential hypertension, *Clin. Pharmacol. Ther.* **42**:485–492.

288. Kleinbloesem, C. H., Van Brummelen, P., Woittiez, A. J., Faber, H., and Breimer, D. D., 1986, Influence of haemodialysis on the pharmacokinetics and haemodynamic effects of nifedipine during continuous intravenous infusion, *Clin. Pharmacol.* **11**:316–322.

289. Tishler, M. and Armon, S., 1986, Nifedipine-induced hypokalemia, *Drug Intell. Clin. Pharm.* **20**: 370–371.

290. Bonadonna, A., Bisetto, F., Munaretto, G., Beccari, A., and Stanic, L., 1987, Agranulocytosis during nifedipine treatment in a hemodialysis patient, *Nephron* **47**:306–307.

291. Van Harten, J., Burggraaf, K., Danhof, M., Van Brummelen, P., and Breimer, D. D., 1987, Negligible sublingual absorption of nifedipine, *Lancet* **1**:1363–1364.

292. Sorkin, E. M. and Clissold, S. P., 1987, Nicardipine. A review of its pharmacodynamic and pharmacokinetic properties, and therapeutic efficacy, in the treatment of angina pectoris, hypertension and related cardiovascular disorders, *Drugs* **33**:296–345.

293. Dow, R. J. and Graham, D. J. M., 1986, A review of the human metabolism and pharmacokinetics of nicardipine hydrochloride, *Br. J. Clin. Pharmacol.* **22:**195S–202S.

294. Baba, T., Ishizaki, T., Murabayashi, S., Aoyagi, K., Tamasawa, N., and Takebe, K., 1987, Multiple oral doses of nicardipine, a calcium entry blocker: Effects on renal function, plasma renin activity, and aldosterone concentration in mild-to-moderate essential hypertension, *Clin. Pharmacol. Ther.* **42:**232–239.

295. Goa, K. L. and Sorkin, E. M., 1987, Nitrendipine. A review of its pharmacodynamic and pharmacokinetic properties, and therapeutic efficacy in the treatment of hypertension, *Drugs* **33:** 123–155.

296. Zeller, F. P. and Spinler, S. A., 1987, Bepridil: A new long-acting calcium channel blocking agent, *Drug Intell. Clin. Pharm.* **21:**487–491.

297. Hirth, C., Federmann, A., and Kazda, S., 1987, The protective effect of the calcium antagonist nisoldipine in glycerol-induced renal failure, in: *Diuretics II Chemistry, Pharmacology and Clinical Applications,* (J. Ruschett and A. Greenberg, eds.), Elsevier, Amsterdam, pp. 490–493.

298. Hertle, L. and Garthoff, B., 1985, Calcium channel blocker nisoldipine limits ischemic damage in rat kidney, *J. Urol.* **134:**1251–1254.

299. Freedman, D. D. and Waters, D. D., 1987, "Second generation" dihydropyridine calcium antagonists, *Drugs* **34:**578–598.

300. Imbs, J. L., Schmidt, M., and Giesen-Crouse, E., 1987, Pharmacology of loop diuretics: State of the art, *Adv. Nephrol.* **16:**137–158.

301. Beermann, B. and Grind, M., 1987, Clinical pharmacokinetics of some newer diuretics, *Clin. Pharmacol.* **13:**254–266.

302. Feig, P. U., 1986, Cellular mechanism of action of loop diuretics: Implications for drug effectiveness and adverse effects, *Am. J. Cardiol.* **57:**14A–19A.

303. Brater, D. C., Anderson, S. A., and Brown-Cartwright, D., 1986, Response to furosemide in chronic renal insufficiency: Rationale for limited doses, *Clin. Pharmacol. Ther.* **40:**134–139.

304. Sherman, L. G., Liang, C. S., Baumgardner, S., Charuzi, Y., Chardo, F., and Kim, C. S., 1986, Piretanide, a potent diuretic with potassium-sparing properties, for the treatment of congestive heart failure, *Clin. Pharmacol. Ther.* **40:**587–594.

305. Walter, U., Röckel, A., Heidland, A., and Heptner, W., 1985, Pharmacokinetics of the loop diuretic piretanide in renal failure, *Eur. J. Clin. Pharmacol.* **29:**337–343.

306. Brater, D. C., Leinfelder, J., and Anderson, S. A., 1987, Clinical pharmacology of torasemide, a new loop diuretic, *Clin. Pharmacol. Ther.* **42:**187–192.

307. Lau, H. S. H., Hyneck, M. L., Berardi, R. R., Swartz, R. D., and Smith, D. E., 1986, Kinetics, dynamics, and bioavailability of bumetanide in healthy subjects and patients with chronic renal failure, *Clin. Pharmacol. Ther.* **39:**635–645.

308. Voelker, J. R., Cartwright-Brown, D., Anderson, S., Leinfelder, J., Sica, D. A., Kokko, J. P., and Brater, D. C., 1987, Comparison of loop diuretics in patients with chronic renal insufficiency, *Kidney Int.* **32:**572–578.

309. Scoble, J. E., Varghese, Z., Sweny, P., and Moorhead, J., 1986, Renal physiology revisited: Amiloride, *Lancet* **2:**326–328.

310. Fairley, K. F., Woo, K. T., Birch, D. F., Leaker, B. R., and Ratnaike, S., 1986, Triamterene-induced crystalluria and cylinduria: Clinical and experimental studies, *Clin. Nephrol.* **26:**169–173.

311. Farge, D., Turner, M. W., Roy, R., and Jothy, S., 1986, Dyazide-induced reversible acute renal failure associated with intracellular crystal deposition, *Am. J. Kidney Dis.* **8:**445–449.

312. Jivraj, K. T., Noseworthy, T. W., Friesen, E. G., Shustack, A. S., Konopad, E. M., and Johnston, R. G., 1987, Spironolactone-induced agranulocytosis, *Drug Intell. Clin. Pharm.* **21:** 974–975.

313. Osborne, R. J., Joel, S. P., and Slevin, M. L., 1986, Morphine intoxication in renal failure: The role of morphine-6-glucuronide, *Br. Med. J.* **292:**1548–1549.

314. Chauvin, M., Sandouk, P., Scherrmann, J. M., Farinotti, R., Strumza, P., and Duvaldestin, P., 1987, Morphine pharmacokinetics in renal failure, *Anesthesiology* **3:**327–331.

315. Säwe, J. and Odar-Cederlöf, I., 1987, Kinetics of morphine in patients with renal failure, *Eur. J. Clin. Pharmacol.* **32:**377–382.

316. Park, G. R., Shelly, M. P., Manara, A. R., and Quinn, K., 1987, Sedation in intensive care: Morphine and renal failure, *Int. Care Med.* **13:**365–366.

317. Woolner, D. F., Winter, D., Frendin, T. J., Begg, E. J., Lynn, K. L., and Wright, G. J., 1986, Renal failure does not impair the metabolism of morphine, *Br. J. Clin. Pharmacol.* **22:**55–59.

318. Moore, R. A., Sear, J. W., Bullingham, R. E. S., and McQuay, H. J., 1986, Morphine kinetics in renal failure, *Adv. Pain Res. Ther.* **8:**65–72.

319. Ratcliffe, P. J., Sear, J. W., Hand, C. W., and Moore, R. A., 1985, Morphine transport in the isolated perfused rat kidney, *Proc EDTA-ERA* **22:**1109–1114.

320. Chan, K., Tse, J., Jennings, F., and Orme, M. L. 'E., 1987, Pharmacokinetics of low-dose intravenous pethidine in patients with renal dysfunction, *J. Clin. Pharmacol.* **27:**516–522.

321. Chan, G. L. C. and Matzke, G. R., 1987, Effects of renal insufficiency on the pharmacokinetics and pharmacodynamics of opioid analgesics, *Drugs Intell. Clin. Pharm.* **21:**773–783.

322. Clissold, S. P., 1986, Paracetamol and phenacetin, *Drugs* **32**(Suppl. 4):46–59.

323. Clissold, S. P., 1986, Aspirin and related derivatives of salicylic acid, *Drugs* **32**(Suppl. 4):8–26.

324. Williams, M. E., Weinblatt, M., Rosa, R. M., Griffin, V. L., Goldlust, M. B., Shang, S. F., Harrison, L. I., and Brown, R. S., 1986, Salsalate kinetics in patients with chronic renal failure undergoing hemodialysis, *Clin. Pharmacol. Ther.* **39:**420–424.

325. Bonney, S. L., Northington, R. S., Hedrich, D. A., and Walker, B. R., 1986, Renal safety of two analgesics used over the counter: Ibuprofen and aspirin, *Clin. Pharmacol. Ther.* **40:**373–377.

326. Brogden, R. N., 1986, Non-steroidal anti-inflammatory analgesics other than salicylates, *Drugs* **32** (Suppl. 4):27–45.

327. Wong, D. G., Spence, J. D., Lamki, L., Freeman, D., and McDonald, J. W. D., 1986, Effect of non-steroidal anti-inflammatory drugs on control of hypertension by beta-blockers and diuretics, *Lancet* **1:**997–1002.

328. Skinner, M. H., Mutterperl, R., and Zeitz, H. J., 1987, Sulindac inhibits bumetanide-induced sodium and water excretion, *Clin. Pharmacol. Ther.* **42:**542–546.

329. Radack, K. L., Deck, C. C., and Bloomfield, S. S., 1987, Ibuprofen interferes with the efficacy of antihypertensive drugs, *Ann. Intern. Med.* **107:**628–635.

330. Toto, R. D., Anderson, S. A., Brown-Cartwright, D., Kokko, J. P., and Brater, D. C., 1986, Effects of acute and chronic dosing of NSAIDs in patients with renal insufficiency, *Kidney Int.* **30:**760–768.

331. Whelton, A., LaFrance, N., Spilman, P. S., Stout, R. L., Drew, H., Watson, A. J., Hermann, J., and Klassen, D., 1986, A prospective, ramdomized, cross-over study of the renal effects of ibuprofen, piroxicam, and sulindac in chronic renal impairment, *Proc. Am. Soc. Nephrol.* **19:**67a (Abstract).

332. Sethi, K., Jain, R., and Malhotra, S., 1986, Effects of long-term sulindac therapy in chronic renal failure, *Proc. Am. Soc. Nephrol.* **19:**60a (Abstract).

333. Gibson, R. P., Dobrinska, M. R., Lin, J. H., Entwistle, L. A., and Davies, R. O., 1987, Biotransformation of sulindac in end-stage renal disease, *Clin. Pharmacol. Ther.* **42:**82–88.

334. Klassen, D., Stout, R. L., Spilman, P. S., and Whelton, A., 1986, Kinetics of sulindac and its metabolites in chronic renal insufficiency, *J. Clin. Pharmacol.* **26:**553.

335. Lynch, S. and Brogden, R. N., 1986, Etodolac. A preliminary review of its pharmacodynamic activity and therapeutic use, *Drugs* **31:**288–300.

336. Shand, D. G., Epstein, C., Kinberg-Calhoun, J., Mullane, J. F., and Sanda, M., 1986, The effect of etodolac administration on renal function in patients with arthritis, *J. Clin. Pharmacol.* **26:**269–274.

337. Verbeeck, R. K., Richardson, C. J., and Blocka, K. L. N., 1986, Clinical pharmacokinetics of piroxicam, *J. Rheumatol.* **13:**789–796.

338. Gonzalez, J. P. and Todd, P. A., 1987, Tenoxicam. A preliminary review of its pharmacodynamic and pharmacokinetic properties, and therapeutic efficacy, *Drugs* **34:**289–310.

339. Horber, F. F., Guenter, T. W., Weidekamm, E., Heizmann, P., Descoeudres, C., and Frey, F. J., 1986, Pharmacokinetics of tenoxicam in patients with impaired renal function, *Eur. J. Clin. Pharmacol.* **29**:697–701.

340. Todd, P. A. and Beresford, R., 1986, Pirprofen. A review of its pharmacodynamic and pharmacokinetic properties, and therapeutic efficacy, *Drugs* **32**:509–537.

341. O'Brien, W. M. and Bagby, G. F., 1987, Carprofen: A new nonsteroidal antiinflammatory drug, *Pharmacotherapy* **7**:16–24.

342. Kantor, T. G., 1986, Ketoprofen: A review of its pharmacologic and clinical properties, *Pharmacotherapy* **6**:93–103.

343. Clissold, S. P. and Beresford, R., 1987, Proquazone. A review of its pharmacodynamic and pharmacokinetic properties, and therapeutic efficacy in rheumatic diseases and pain states, *Drugs* **33**:478–502.

344. Mangan, F. R., Flack, J. D., and Jackson, D., 1987, Preclinical overview of nabumetone, *Am. J. Med.* **83**(Suppl. 4B):6–10.

345. Boelaert, J. R., Jonnaert, H. A., Daneels, R. F., Schurgers, M. L., Thawley, A. R., Undre, N. A., and Cooper, D. L., 1987, Nabumetone pharmacokinetics in patients with varying degrees of renal impairment, *Am. J. Med.* **83**(Suppl. 4B):107–109.

346. Skoutakis, V. A., Acchiardo, S. R., Carter, C. A., Wojciechowski, N. J., Straughn, A. B., and Meyer, M. C., 1986, Dialyzability and pharmacokinetics of indomethacin in adult patients with end-stage renal disease, *Drug Intell. Clin. Pharm.* **20**:956–960.

347. Boiskin, I., Saven, A., Mendez, M., and Raja, R. M., Indomethacin and the nephrotic syndrome, *Ann. Intern. Med.* **106**:776–777.

348. Schwartzman, M. and D'Agati, V., 1987, Spontaneous relapse of naproxen-related nephrotic syndrome, *Am. J. Med.* **82**:329–332.

349. Sennesael, J., Van Den Houte, K., and Verbeelen, D., 1986, Reversible membranous glomerulonephritis associated with ketoprofen, *Clin. Nephrol.* **26**:213–215.

350. Henann, N. E. and Morales, J. R., 1986, Suprofen-induced acute renal failure, *Drug Intell. Clin. Pharm.* **20**:860–862.

351. Henann, J. E., Morales, J. R., 1987, Suprofen-induced acute renal failure revisited, *Drug Intell. Clin. Pharm.* **21**:69–70.

352. Hart, D., Ward, M., and Lifschitz, M. D., 1987, Suprofen-related nephrotoxicity, *Ann. Intern. Med.* **106**:235–238.

353. Wolfe, S. M., 1987, Suprofen-induced transient flank pain and renal failure, *N. Engl. J. Med.* **316**:1025.

354. Snyder, S. and Teehan, B. P., Suprofen and renal failure, *Ann. Intern. Med.* **106**:776.

355. Murrell, G. A. C. and Rapeport, W. G., 1986, Clinical pharmacokinetics of allopurinol, *Clin. Pharmacol.* **11**:343–353.

356. Kuncl, R. W., Duncan, G., Watson, D., Alderson, K., Rogawski, M. A., and Peper, M., 1987, Colchicine myopathy and neuropathy, *N. Engl. J. Med.* **316**:1562–1568.

357. Levin, V. A., 1986, Clinical anticancer pharmacology: Some pharmacokinetic considerations, *Cancer Treatment Rev.* **13**:61–76.

358. Anon., 1987, Cancer chemotherapy, *Med. Lett.* **29**:29–36.

359. Clark, P. I. and Slevin, M. L., 1987, The clinical pharmacology of etoposide and teniposide, *Clin. Pharmacol.* **12**:223–252.

360. D'Incalci, M., Rossi, C., Zucchetti, M., Urso, R., Cavalli, F., Mangioni, C., Willems, Y., and Sessa, C., 1986, Pharmacokinetics of etoposide in patients with abnormal renal and hepatic function, *Cancer Res.* **46**:2566–2571.

361. Belldegrun, A., Webb, D. E., Austin, H. A. III, Steinberg, S. M., White, D. E., Linehan, W. M., and Rosenberg, S. A., 1987, Effects of interleukin-2 on renal function in patients receiving immunotherapy for advanced cancer, *Ann. Intern. Med.* **106**:817–822.

362. Textor, S. C., Margolin, K., Blayney, D., Carlson, J., and Doroshow, J., 1987, Renal, volume, and hormonal changes during therapeutic administration of recombinant interleukin-2 in man, *Am. J. Med.* **83**:1055–1061.

363. Wartha, R., Damjantschitsch, M., Damjanschitsch, V., Kuchl, J., and Gekle, D., 1985, Nephrotoxicity of high dose methotrexate therapy—A long-term follow-up study in five juvenile patients with osteosarcoma, *Proc. EDTA-ERA* **22**:1025–1031.

364. Evans, W. E. and Christensen, M. L., 1985, Drug interactions with methotrexate, *J. Rheumatol.* **12**(Suppl. 12):15–20.

365. Salemans, J., Hoitsma, A. J., De Abreu, R. A., de Vos, D., and Koene, R. A. P., 1987, Pharmacokinetics of azathioprine and 6-mercaptopurine after oral administration of azathioprine, *Clin. Trans.* **1**:217–221.

366. Chan, G. L. C., Canafaz, D. M., and Johnson, C. A., 1987, The therapeutic use of azathioprine in renal transplantation, *Pharmacotherapy* **7**(5):165–177.

367. Reilly, C. S. and Nimmo, W. S., 1987, New intravenous anaesthetics and neuromuscular blocking drugs. A review of their properties and clinical use, *Drugs* **34**:98–135.

368. Mongin-Long, D., Chabrol, B., Baude, C., Ville, D., Renaudie, M., Dubernard, J. M., and Moskovtchenko, J. F., 1986, Atracurium in patients with renal failure, *Br. J. Anaesth.* **58**:44S–48S.

369. Miller, R. D., 1986, Pharmacokinetics of atracurium and other nondepolarizing neuromuscular blocking agents in normal patients and those with renal or hepatic dysfunction, *Br. J. Anaesth.* **58**: 11S–13S.

370. Bencini, A. F., Scaf, A. H. J., Sohn, Y. J., Meistelman, C., Lienhart, A., Kersten, U. W., Schwarz, S., and Agoston, S., 1986, Disposition and urinary excretion of vecuronium bromide in anesthetized patients with normal renal function or renal failure, *Anesth. Analg.* **65**:245–251.

371. Gramstad, L., 1987, Atracurium, vecuronium and pancuronium in end-stage renal failure, *Br. J. Anaesth.* **59**:995–1003.

372. Mujais, S. K., 1986, Transport and renal effects of general anesthetics, *Semin. Nephrol.* **6**(3):251–258.

373. Abu-Romch, S. H., Al-Nakib, B., and Johny, K. V., 1987, Acute renal failure following halothane anesthesia, *Clin. Nephrol.* **27**:213–215.

373a. Ward, A., Chaffman, M. O., and Sorkin, E. M., 1986, Dantrolen. A review of its pharmacodynamic and pharmacokinetic properties and therapeutic use in malignant hyperthermia, the neuroleptic malignant syndrome and an update of its use in muscle spasticity, *Drugs* **32**:130–168.

374. Gupta, S. K., Legg, B., Solomon, L. R., Johnson, R. W. G., and Rowland, M., 1987, Pharmacokinetics of cyclosporine: Influence of rate of constant intravenous infusion in renal transplant patients, *Br. J. Clin. Pharmacol.* **24**:519–526.

375. Öst, L., 1987, Impairment of prednisolone metabolism by cyclosporine treatment in renal graft recipients, *Transplantation* **44**:533–535.

375a. Landgraf, R., Landgraft-Leurs, M. M. C., Nusser, J., Hillebrand, G., Illner, W-D., Abendroth, D., and Land, W., 1987, Effect of somatostatin analogue (SMS201-995) on cyclosporine levels, *Transplantation* **44**:724–725.

376. Balant-Gorgia, A. E. and Balant, L., 1987, Antipsychotic drugs. Clinical pharmacokinetics of potential candidates for plasma concentration monitoring, *Clin. Pharmacol.* **13**:65–90.

377. Benfield, P., Heel, R. C., and Lewis, S. P., 1986, Fluoxetine. A review of its pharmacodynamic and pharmacokinetic properties, and therapeutic efficacy in depressive illness, *Drugs* **32**:481–508.

378. Sommi, R. W., Crismon, M. L., and Bowden, C. L., 1987, Fluoxetine: A serotonin-specific, second-generation antidepressant, *Pharmacotherapy* **7**:1–15.

379. Lieberman, J. A., Cooper, T. B., Suckow, R. F., Steinberg, H., Borenstein, M., Brenner, R., and Kane, J. M., 1985, Tricyclic antidepressant drug and metabolite levels in chronic renal failure, *Clin. Pharmacol. Ther.* **37**:301–307.

380. Goa, K. L. and Ward, A., 1986, Buspirone. A preliminary review of its pharmacological properties and therapeutic efficacy as an anxiolytic, *Drugs* **32**:114–129.

381. Ochs, H. R., Greenblatt, D. J., and Knüchel, M., 1986, Effect of cirrhosis and renal failure on the kinetics of clotiazepam, *Eur. J. Clin. Pharmacol.* **30**:89–92.

382. Mallette, L. W. and Eichhorn, E., 1986, Effects of lithium carbonate on human calcium metabolism, *Arch. Intern. Med.* **146:**770–776.

383. Aquilonius, S. M. and Hartvig, P., 1986, Clinical pharmacokinetics of cholinesterase inhibitors, *Clin. Pharmacokinetics* **11:**236–249.

384. Cedarbaum, J. M., 1987, Clinical pharmacokinetics of anti-parkinsonian drugs, *Clin. Pharmacokinetics* **13:**141–178.

385. Garg, D. C., Baltodano, N., Jallad, N. S., Perez, G., Oster, J. R., Eshelman, F. N., and Weidler, D. J., 1986, Pharmacokinetics of ranitidine in patients with renal failure, *J. Clin. Pharmacol.* **26:** 286–291.

386. Takabatake, T., Ohta, H., Yamamoto, Y., Ishida, Y., Hara, H., Nakamura, S., Ushiogi, Y., Satoh, S., and Hattori, N., 1986, Pharmacokinetics of TZU-0460, a new H_2-Receptor antagonist, in patients with impaired renal function, *Eur. J. Clin. Pharmacol.* **30:**709–712.

387. Campoli-Richards, D. M. and Clissold, S. P., 1986, Famotidine. Pharmacodynamic and pharmacokinetic properties and a preliminary review of its therapeutic use in peptic ulcer disease and Zollinger–Ellison syndrome, *Drugs* **32:**197–221.

388. Halstenson, C. E., Abraham, P. A., Opsahl, J. A., Chremos, A. N., Keane, W. F., and Matzke, G. R., 1987, Disposition of famotidine in renal insufficiency, *J. Clin. Pharmacol.* **27:**782–787.

389. Naesdal, J., Andersson, T., Bodemar, G., Larsson, R., Regårdh, C-G., Skånberg, I., and Walan, A., 1986, Pharmacokinetics of [^{14}C]omeprazole in patients with impaired renal function, *Clin. Pharmacol. Ther.* **40:**344–351.

390. Illingworth, D. R., 1986, Comparative efficacy of once versus twice daily mevinolin in the therapy of familial hypercholesterolemia, *Clin. Pharmacol. Ther.* **40:**338–343.

391. Anon., 1987, Lovastatin for hypercholesterolemia, *Med. Lett.* **29:**99–102.

392. Golper, T. A., Illingworth, D. R., Morris, C. D., and Bennett, W. M., 1989, Lovostatin in the therapy of nephrotic hyperlipemia. *Am. Journ. Kid. Dis.* (in press).

393. Hunninghake, D. B. and Hibbard, D. M., 1986, Influence of time intervals for cholestyramine dosing on the absorption of hydrochlorothiazide, *Clin. Pharmacol. Ther.* **39:**329–334.

394. Monk, J. P. and Todd P. A., 1987, Bezafibrate. A review of its pharmacodynamic and pharmacokinetic properties, and therapeutic use in hyperlipidaemia, *Drugs* **33:**539–576.

395. Chapman, M. J., 1987, Pharmacology of fenofibrate, *Am. J. Med.* **83:**21–25.

396. Blane, G. F., 1987, Comparative toxicity and safety profile of fenofibrate and other fibric acid derivatives, *Am. J. Med.* **83:**26–36.

397. Van Acker, B. A. C., Bilo, H. J. G., Snijders, P., Van Bronswijk, H., Rustemeijer, C., Oe, P. L., and Donker, A. J. M., 1986, Omega-3 polyunsaturated fatty acids improve lipid profile and lower blood viscosity in CAPD patients, *Proc. Am. Soc. Nephrol.* **19:**98a (Abstract).

398. Ferner, R. E. and Chaplin, S., 1987, The relationship between the pharmacokinetics and pharmacodynamic effects of oral hypoglycaemic drugs, *Clin. Pharmacokinetics* **12:**379–401.

399. Pearson, J. G., Antal, E. J., Raehl, C. L., Gorsch, H. K., Craig, W. A., Albert, K. S., and Welling, P. G., 1986, Pharmacokinetic disposition of ^{14}C-glyburide in patients with varying renal function, *Clin. Pharmacol. Ther.* **39:**318–324.

400. Benfield, P., 1986, Aldose reductase inhibitors and late complications of diabetes, *Drugs* **32:**43–55.

401. Brogden, R. N. and Heel, R. C., 1987, Human insulin. A review of its biological activity, pharmacokinetics and therapeutic use, *Drugs* **34:**350–371.

402. Holford, N. H. G., 1986, Clinical pharmacokinetics and pharmacodynamics of warfarin, *Clin. Pharmacokinetics* **11:**483–504.

403. Krstenansky, P. M. and Cluxton, R. J., Jr., 1987, Astemizole: A long-acting, nonsedating antihistamine, *Drug Intell. Clin. Pharm.* **21:**947–952.

404. Ganeval, D., Fischer, A. M., Barre, J., Pertuiset, N., Dautzenberg, M. D., Jungers, P., and Houin, G., 1986, Pharmacokinetics of warfarin in the nephrotic syndrome and effect on vitamin K-dependent clotting factors, *Clin. Nephrol.* **25:**75–80.

405. Ward, A. and Clissold, S. P., 1987, Pentoxifylline: A review of its pharmacodynamic and pharmacokinetic properties, and its therapeutic efficacy, *Drugs* **34**:50–97.

406. Silver, M. R. and Kroboth, P. D., 1987, Pentoxifylline in end-stage renal disease, *Drug Intell. Clin. Pharm.* **21**:976–978.

407. Saltiel, E. and Ward, A., 1987, Ticlopidine: A review of its pharmacodynamic and pharmacokinetic properties, and therapeutic efficacy in platelet-dependent disease states, *Drugs* **34**:222–262.

408. Clissold, S. P., Lynch, S., and Sorkin, E. M., 1987, Buflomedil: A review of its pharmacodynamic and pharmacokinetic properties, and therapeutic efficacy in peripheral and cerebral vascular diseases, *Drugs* **33**:430–460.

409. Gregov, D., Jenkins, A., Siebert, D., Rodgers, S., Duncan, B., Bochner, F., and Lloyd, J., 1987, Dipyridamole: Pharmacokinetics and effects on aspects of platelet function in man, *Br. J. Clin. Pharmacol.* **24**:425–434.

410. Goa, K. L. and Monk, J. P., 1987, Enprostil. A preliminary review of its pharmacodynamic and pharmacokinetic properties, and therapeutic efficacy in the treatment of peptic ulcer disease, *Drugs* **34**:539–559.

411. Gonzalez, J. P. and Brogden, R. N., 1987, Nedocromil sodium. A preliminary review of its pharmacodynamic and pharamcokinetic properties, and therapeutic efficacy in the treatment of reversible obstructive airways disease, *Drugs* **34**:560–577.

412. Cloyd, J. C., Snyder, B. D., Cleeremans, B., and Bundlie, S. R., 1985, Mannitol pharmacokinetics and serum osmolality in dogs and humans, *J. Pharmacol. Exp. Ther.* **236**:301–306.

413. DeBroe, M. E, Van de Vyver, F. L., D'Haese, P. C., Visser, W. J., Elseviers, M. M., and Wedeen, R. P., 1986, Bone lead and the role of lead in renal disease, *Proc. Am. Soc. Nephrol.* **19**:39a (Abstract).

414. Osterloh, J. and Becker, C. E., 1986, Pharmacokinetics of $CaNa_2$ EDTA and chelation of lead in renal failure, *Clin. Pharmacol. Ther.* **40**:686–93.

415. Shusterman, N., Strom, B. L., Murray, T. G., Morrison, G., West, S. L., and Maislin, G., 1987, Risk factors and outcome of hospital-acquired acute renal failure, *Am. J. Med.* **83**:65–71.

416. Lämeire, N., Matthys, E., Vanholder, R., De Keyser, K., Pauwels, W., Nachtergaele, H., Lambrecht, L., and Ringoir, S., 1987, Causes and prognosis of acute renal failure in elderly patients, *Nephrol. Dial. Transplant.* **2**:316–322.

417. Handa, S. P., 1986, Drug-induced acute interstitial nephritis: Report of 10 cases, *Can. Med. Assoc. J.* **135**:1278–1281.

418. Cannon-Babb, M. L. and Schwartz, A. B., 1986, Drug-induced hyperkalemia, *Hosp. Pract.* **99**-127.

419. Cruz, C., Hricak, H., Samhouri, F., Smith, R. F., Eyler, W. R., and Levin, N. W., 1986, Contrast media for angiography: Effect on renal function, *Radiology* **158**:109–112.

420. Taliercio, C. P., Vlietstra, R. E., Fisher, L. D., and Burnett, J. C., 1986, Risks for renal dysfunction with cardiac angiography, *Ann. Intern. Med.* **104**:501–504.

421. Fairley, S. and Ihle, B. U., 1986, Thrombotic microangiopathy and acute renal failure associated with arteriography, *Br. Med. J.* **293**:922–923.

422. Morris, T. W. and Fischer, H. W., 1986, The pharmacology of intravascular radiocontrast media, *Annu. Rev. Pharmacol. Toxicol.* **26**:143–160.

423. Bourin, M., Laporte, V., Guenzet, J., Langlois, S., Pengloan, J., and Rouleau, P., 1986, Pharmacokinetic study of ioxaglate, a low osmolality contrast medium, in patients with renal failure, *Int. J. Clin. Pharmacol. Ther. Toxicol.* **24**:614–621.

424. Albrechtsson, U., Hultberg, B., Lárusdóttir, H, and Norgren, L., 1985, Nephrotoxicity of ionic and non-ionic contrast media in aorto-femoral angiography, *Acta Radiol. Diagnosis* **26**:615–618.

425. Cavaliere, G., Arrigo, G., D'Amico, G., Bernasconi, P., Schiavina, G., Dellafiore, L., and Vergnaghi, D., 1987, Tubular nephrotoxicity after intravenous urography with ionic high-osmolal and nonionic low-osmolal contrast media in patients with chronic renal insufficiency, *Nephron* **46**:128–133.

426. Cedgard, S., Herlitz, H., Geterud, K., Attmam, P-O., and Aurell, M., 1986, Acute renal insufficiency after administration of low-osmolar contrast media, *Lancet* **2:**1281.

427. Evans, J. R. and Cutler, R. E., 1987, Low-osmolar radiocontrast agents and nephrotoxicity, *Dial. Transplant* **16:**504–508.

428. Thompson, W. M., 1986, New intravascular contrast material, *Arch. Intern. Med.* **146:**1688.

429. Schwab, S. J., Hlatky, M., Morris, K., Mark, D., Davidson, C., Skelton, T., and Bashore, T., 1987, Contrast nephrotoxicity: A prospective randomized trial of ionic versus non-ionic radiographic contrast, *Proc. Am. Soc. Nephrol.* **20:**61a (Abstract).

430. Katzberg, R. W., Pabico, R. C., Morris, T. W., Hayakawa, K., McKenna, B. A., Panner, B. J., Ventura, J. A., and Fischer, H. W., 1986, Effects of contrast media on renal function and subcellular morphology in the dog, *Invest. Radiol.* **21:**64–70.

431. Bently, M. D., Vanhoutte, V., Schryver, S. M., Romero, J. C., and Vanhoutte, P. M., 1986, Contraction of isolated canine renal arteries induced by the radiocontrast medium, sodium/meglumine diatrizoate, *Proc. Am. Soc. Nephrol.* **19:**263a (Abstract).

432. Bakris, G. L., Jones, J., and Burnett, J. C., Jr., 1986, Suppression of oxygen free radicals (FR) attenuates the radiocontrast medium (RCM)-induced decline in glomerular filtration rate (GFR), *Proc. Am. Soc. Nephrol.* **19:**206a (Abstract).

433. Humes, H. D., Hunt, D. A., and White, M. D., 1987, Direct toxic effect of the radiocontrast agent diatrizoate on renal proximal tubule cells, *Am. J., Physiol.* **252**(Renal Fluid Electrolyte Physiol. **21**):F246–F255.

434. Scanu, P., de Ligny, H., and Ryckelynck, J. P., 1987, Reversible acute renal insufficiency with combination of enalapril and diuretics in a patient with a single renal-artery stenosis, *Nephron* **45:**321–322.

435. Funck-Brentano, C., Chatellier, G., and Alexandre, J-M., 1986, Reversible renal failure after combined treatment with enalapril and fursemide in a patient with congestive heart failure, *Br. Heart J.* **55:**596–598.

436. Andreucci, V. E., Conte, G., and Dal Canton, A., 1986, The causal role of salt depletion in acute depletion in acute renal failure due to captopril in hypertensive patients with a single kidney and renal artery stenosis, *Postgrad. Med. J.* **62:**43a (Abstract).

437. Cleland, J. G. F., Dargie, H. J., Gillen, G., Robertson, I., East, B. W., Ball, S. G., Morton, J. J., and Robertson, J. I. S., 1986, Captopril in heart failure: A double-blind study of the effects on renal function, *J. Cardiovasc. Pharmacol.* **8:**700–706.

438. Packer, M., Lee, W. H., Medina, N., Yushak, M., and Kessler, P. D., 1987, Functional renal insufficiency during long-term therapy with captopril and enalapril in severe chronic heart failure, *Ann. Intern. Med.* **106:**346–354.

439. Postma, C. T., Hoefnagels, W. H. L., Thien, T. H., and DeBoo, T. H., 1987, ACE inhibitors, atheroma, and renal function, *Lancet* **2:**1080–1081.

440. Michel, J-B., Nochy, D., Choudat, L., Dussaule, J-C., Philippe, M., Chastang, C., Corvol, P., and Menard, J., 1987, Consequences of renal morphologic damage induced by inhibition of converting enzyme in rat renovascular hypertension, *Lab. Invest.* **57:**402–411.

441. Linton, A. L., 1987, AG-ARF, *Renal Failure* **10:**61–62.

442. Editorial, 1986, Aminoglycoside toxicity, *Lancet* **2:**670–671.

443. Kapusnik, J. E. and Sande, M. A., 1986, Novel approaches for the use of aminoglycosides: The value of experimental models, *J. Antimicrob. Chemother.* **17:**7–10.

444. Wood, C. A., Norton, D., Kohlhepp, S., Kohnen, P., Bennett, W., Porter, G., Houghton, D. Brummett, R., and Gilbert, D., 1988, Influence of tobramycin dosing regimen on nephrotoxicity, ototoxicity and antibacterial efficacy in a rat model of subcutaneous abcess, *J. Infect. Dis.* **158:**13–22.

445. DeBroe, M. E., Giuliano, R. A., and Verpooten, G. A., 1986, Choice of drug and dosage regimen. Two important risk for aminoglycoside nephrotoxicity, *Am. J. Med.* **80:**115–118.

446. Bergeron, M. G. and Marois, Y., 1986, Benefit from high intrarenal levels of gentamicin in the treatment of *E. coli* pyelonephritis, *Kidney Int.* **30:**481–487.

447. Meyer, R. D., 1986, Risk factors and comparisons of clinical nephrotoxicity of aminoglycosides, *Am. J. Med.* **80:**119–125.
448. Moore, R. D., Smith, C. R., and Lietman, P. S., 1986, Increased risk of renal dysfunction due to interaction of liver disease and aminoglycosides, *Am. J. Med.* **80:**1093–1097.
449. Sawyers, C. L., Moore, R. D., Lerner, S. A., and Smith, C. R., 1986, A model for predicting nephrotoxicity in patients treated with aminoglycosides, *J. Infect. Dis.* **153:**1062–1068.
450. Bernstein, J. M., Gorse, G. J., Linzmayer, I., Pegram, P. S., Levin, R. D., Brummett, R. E., Markowitz, N., Saravolatz, L. D., and Lorber, R. R., 1986, Relative efficacy and toxicity of netilmicin and tobramycin in oncology patients, *Arch. Intern. Med.* **146:**2329–2234.
451. Lerner, S. A., Schmitt, B. A., Seligsohn, R., and Matz, G. J., 1986, Comparative study of ototoxicity and nephrotoxicity in patients randomly assigned to treatment with amikacin or gentamicin, *Am. J. Med.* **80:**98–104.
452. Mandal, A. K., Mize, G. N., and Birnbaum, D. B., 1987, Transmission electron 8microscopy of urinary sediment in aminoglycoside nephrotoxicity, *Renal Failure* **10:**63–81.
453. Steiner, R. W. and Omachi, A. S., 1986, A Bartter's-like syndrome from capreomycin, and a similar gentamicin tubulopathy, *Am. J. Kidney Dis.* **8:**245–249.
454. Schacht, J. and Van De Water, T., 1986, Uptake and accumulation of gentamicin in the developing inner ear of the mouse *in vitro*, *Biochem. Pharm.* **35:**2843–2845.
455. Tran Ba Huy, P., Bernard, P., and Schacht, J., 1986, Kinetics of gentamicin uptake and release in the rat, *J. Clin. Invest.* **77:**1492–1500.
456. Dulon, D., Aran, J-M., Zajic, G., and Schacht, J., 1986, Comparative uptake of gentamicin, netilmicin, and amikacin in the guinea pig cochlea and vestibule, *Antimicrob. Agents Chemother.* **30:**96–100.
457. Tulkens, P. M., 1986, Experimental studies on nephrotoxicity of aminoglycosides at low doses, *Am. J. Med.* **80:**105–114.
458. Nässaberger, L., Bergstrand, A., and DePierre, J. W., 1987, Biochemical effects of gentamicin on rat kidney cortex. II. Analytical subfractionation after short-term, high-dose treatment, *Exp. Mol. Pathol.* **46:**230–243.
459. Giurgea-Marion, L., Toubeau, G., Laurent, G., Heuson-Stiennon, J. A., and Tulkens, P. M., 1986, Impairment of lysosome–pinocytic vesicle fusion in rat kidney proximal tubules after treatment with gentamicin at low doses, *Toxicol. Appl. Pharmacol.* **86:**271–285.
460. Oshima, M., Hashiguchi, M., Shindo, N., and Shibata, S., 1986, Biochemical mechanisms of aminoglycoside cell toxicity. I. The uptake of gentamicin by cultured skin fibroblasts and the alteration of lysosomal enzyme activities, *J. Biochem.* **100:**1575–1582.
461. Williams, P. S., Hottendorf, G. H., and Bennett, D. B., 1986, Inhibition of renal membrane binding and nephrotoxicity of aminoglycosides, *J. Pharmacol. Exp. Ther.* **237:**919–925.
462. Bennett, W. M., Wood, C. A., Kohlhepp, S. J., Kohnen, P. W., Houghton, D. C., and Gilbert, D. N., 1988, Experimental gentamicin nephrotoxicity can be prevented by polyaspartic acid, *Kidney Int.* **33:**353 (Abstract).
463. Ramsammy, L., Josepovitz, C., Lane, B., and Kaloyanides, G. J., 1986, Polyaspartic acid (PAA) protects against gentamicin (G) nephrotoxicity in the rat, *Proc. Am. Soc. Nephrol.* **19:**217a (Abstract).
464. Ramsammy, L. S., Josepovitz, C., Ling, K-Y., Lane, B. P., and Kaloyanides, G. J., 1985, Effects of diphenyl-phenylenediamine on gentamicin-induced lipid peroxidation and toxicity in rat renal cortex, *J. Pharmacol. Exp. Ther.* **238:**83–88.
465. Marche, P., Olier, B., Girard, A., Fillastre, J-P., and Morin, J-P., 1987, Aminoglycoside-induced alterations of phosphoinositide metabolism, *Kidney Int.* **31:**59–64.
466. Ramsammy, L., Josepovitz, C., and Kaloyanides, G. J., 1987, Gentamicin inhibits generation of inositol phosphates by PTH in primary culture of rabbit proximal tubular cells, *Clin. Res.* **35:**637a (Abstract).
467. Elliott, W. C., Patchin, D. S., and Jones, D. B., 1987, Effect of parathyroid hormone activity on gentamicin nephrotoxicity, *J. Lab. Clin. Med.* **109:**48–54.

468. Ghosh, P. and Chatterjee, S., 1987, Effects of gentamicin on sphingomyelinase activity in cultured human renal proximal tubular cells, *J. Biol. Chem.* **262:**12550–12556.

469. Horio, M., Fukuhara, Y., Orita, Y., Nakanishi, T., Nakahama, H., Moriyama, T., and Kamada, T., 1986, Gentamicin inhibits Na$^+$-dependent D-glucose transport in rabbit kidney brush-border membrane vesicles, *Biochim. Biophys. Acta* **858:**153–160.

470. Mela-Riker, L. M., Widener, L. L., Houghton, D. C., and Bennett, W. M., 1986, Renal mitrochondrial integrity during continuous gentamicin treatment, *Biochem. Pharm.* **35:**979–984.

471. Toubeau, G., Maldague, P., Laurent, G., Vaamonde, C. A., Tulkens, P. M., and Heuson-Stiennon, J. A., 1986, Morphological alterations in distal and collecting tubules of the rat renal cortex after aminoglycoside administration at low doses, *Virchows Arch.* **51:**475–485.

472. Bergeron, M. G., Bergeron, Y., and Marois, Y., 1986, Autoradiography of tobramycin uptake by the proximal and distal tubules of normal and endotoxin-treated rats, *Antimicrob. Agents Chemother.* **29:**1005–1009.

473. Keane, W. F., Welch, R., Gekker, G., and Peterson, P. K., 1987, Mechanism of *Escherichia coli* α-hemolysin–induced injury to isolated renal tubular cells, *Am. J. Pathol.* **126:**350–357.

474. Bernard, A., Viau, C., Ouled, A., Tulkens, P., and Lauwerys, R., 1986, Effects of gentamicin on the renal uptake of endogenous and exogenous proteins in conscious rats, *Toxicol. Appl. Pharmacol.* **84:**431–438.

475. Cronin, R. E., Brown, D. M., and Simonsen, R., 1986, Protection by thyroxine in nephrotoxic acute renal failure, *Am. J. Physiol.* **251:**F408–F416.

476. Pastoriza-Munoz, E., Josepovitz, C., Ramsammy, L., and Kaloyanides, G. J., 1985, Renal handling of netilmicin in the rat with streptozotocin-induced diabetes mellitus, *J. Pharmacol. Exp. Ther.* **241:**166–173.

477. Watson, A. J., Gimenez, L. F., Klassen, D. K., Stout, R. L., and Whelton, A., 1987, Calcium channel blockade in experimental aminoglycoside nephrotoxicity, *J. Clin. Pharmacol.* **27:**625–627.

478. Pattison, M. E., Lee, S. M., and Logan, J. L., 1986, The protective effect of nitrendipine (N) on gentamicin (G) nephrotoxicity in the rat, *Proc. Am. Soc. Nephrol.* **19:**216a (Abstract).

479. Furuhama, K. and Onodera, T., 1986, The influence of cephem antibiotics on gentamicin nephrotoxicity in normal, acidotic, dehydrated, and unilaterally nephrectomized rats, *Toxicol. Appl. Pharmacol.* **86:**430–436.

480. Bryant, T. E., Ohnishi, A., Hamilton, R., and Branch, R. A., 1987, Influence of salt status and a prophylactic effect of ticarcillin during salt depletion in nephrotoxicity induced by gentamicin in the rat, *Clin. Res.* **35:**9a (Abstract).

481. Keniston, R. C., Cabellon, S. Jr., and Yarbrough, K. S., 1987, Pyridoxal 5'-phosphate as an antidote for cyanide, spermine, gentamicin, and dopamine toxicity: An *in vivo* rat study, *Toxicol. Appl. Pharmacol.* **88:**433–441.

482. Reynolds, R. D. and Natta, C. L., 1986, Aminophylline and gentamicin-2, *Am. J. Clin. Nutr.* **43:**636–642.

483. Houghton, D. C., Lee, D., Gilbert, D. N., and Bennett, W. M., 1986, Chronic gentamicin nephrotoxicity. Continued tubular injury with preserved glomerular filtration function, *Am. J. Pathol.* **123:**183–194.

484. Groth, S., Neilsen, H., Sørensen, J. B., Christensen, A. B., Pedersen, A. G., and Rørth, M., 1986, Acute and long-term nephrotoxicity of *cis*-platinum in man, *Cancer Chemother. Pharmacol.* **17:**191–196.

485. Goren, M. P., Wright, R. K., and Horowitz, M. E., 1986, Cumulative renal tubular damage associated with cisplatin nephrotoxicity, *Cancer Chemother. Pharmacol.* **18:**69–73.

486. Metz, U., Kurschel, E., and Graben, N., 1985, Monitoring renal toxicity of *cis*-platinum by urinary enzymes, *Proc. EDTA–ERA* **22:**1087–1090.

487. de Gislain, C., Dumas, M., d'Athis, P., Lautissier, J-L., Escousse, A., and Guerrin, J., 1986, Urinary β2-microglobulin: Early indicator of high dose cisdiamminedichloroplatinum nephrotoxicity? Influence of furosemide, *Cancer Chemother. Pharmacol.* **18:**276–279.

488. Lam, M. and Adelstein, D. J., 1986, Hypomagnesemia and renal magnesium wasting in patients treated with cisplatin, *Am. J. Kidney Dis.* **8**:164–169.

489. De Broe, M. E. and Wedeen, R. P., 1986, Prevention of cisplatin nephrotoxicity, *Eur. J. Cancer Clin. Oncol.* **22**:1029–1031.

490. Nanji, A. A., Stewart, D. J., and Mikhael, N. Z., 1986, Hyperuricemia and hypoalbuminemia predispose to cisplatin-induced nephrotoxicity, *Cancer Chemother. Pharmacol.* **17**:274–276.

491. Reece, P. A., Stafford, I., Russell, J., Khan, M., and Gill, P. G., 1987, Creatinine clearance as a predictor of ultrafilterable platinum disposition in cancer patients treated with cisplatin: Relationship between peak ultrafilterable platinum plasma levels and nephrotoxicity, *J. Clin. Oncol.* **5**: 304–309.

492. Gordon, J. A. and Gattone, V. H. II., 1986, Mitochondrial alterations in cisplatin-induced acute renal failure, *Am. J. Physiol.* **250**(*Renal Fluid Electrolyte Physiol.* **19**):F991–F998.

493. Gordon, J. A., Gattone, V. H., II., and Schoolwerth, A. C., 1986, γ-Glutamyl transpeptidase excretion in cisplatin-induced acute renal failure, *Am. J. Kidney Dis.* **8**:18–25.

494. Magil, A. B., Mavichak, V., Wong, N. L. M., Quamme, G. A, Dirks, J. H., and Sutton, R. A. L., 1986, Long-term morphological and biochemical observations in cisplatin-induced hypomagnesemia in rats, *Nephron* **43**:223–230.

495. Dobyan, D. C., 1985, Long-term consequences of *cis*-platinum–induced renal injury: A structural and functional study, *Anat. Rec.* **212**:239–245.

496. Moel, D. I., Safirstein, R. L., Cohen, R. A., and Penning, J., 1987, The role of prostaglandins in early polyuria induced by cicplatin in the rat, *Nephron* **46**:91–95.

497. Capasso, G., Anastasio, P., Giordano, D., Albarano, L., and DeSanto, N. G., 1987, Beneficial effects of atrial natriuretic factor on cisplatin-induced acute renal failure in the rat, *Am. J. Nephrol.* **7**:228–234.

498. Jones, M. M., Basinger, M. A., Mitchell, W. M., and Bradley, C. A., 1986, Inhibition of *cis*-diamminedichloroplatinum (II)–induced renal toxicity in the rat, *Cancer Chemother. Pharmacol.* **17**:38–42.

499. Bodenner, D. L., Dedon, P. C., Keng, P. C., Katz, J. C., and Borch, R. F., 1986, Selective protection against *cis*-diamminedichloroplatinum (II)–induced toxicity in kidney, gut, and bone marrow by diethyldithiocarbamate, *Cancer Res.* **46**:2751–2755.

500. Von Graffenried, B. and Krupp, P., 1986, Side effects of cyclosporine (Sandimmun) in renal transplant recipients and in patients with autoimmune diseases, *Transplant. Proc.* **18**:876–883.

501. Canadian Multicentre Transplant Study Group, 1988, A randomized clinical trial of cyclosporine in cadaveric renal transplantation, *N. Engl. J. Med.* **309**:809–815.

502. Hall, B. M., Tiller, D. J., Duggin, G. G., Horvath, J. S., Farnsworth, A., May, J., Johnson, J. R., and Shiel, A. G. R., 1985, Post-transplant acute renal failure in cadaver renal recipients treated with cyclosporine, *Kidney Int.* **28**:178–186.

503. Greenberg, A., Egel, J. W., Thompson, M. E., Hardesty, R. L., Griffith, B. P., Bahnson, H. T., Bernstein, R. L., Hastillo, A., Hess, M. L., and Puschett, J. B., 1987, Early and late forms of cyclosporine nephrotoxicity: Studies in cardiac transplant patients, *Am. J. Kidney Dis.* **9**:12–22.

504. Bennett, W., 1985, Basic mechanisms and pathophysiology cyclosporine nephrotoxicity, *Transplant. Proc.* **17**:297–302.

505. Myers, B. D., 1986, Cyclosporine nephrotoxicity, *Kidney Int.* **30**:964–974.

506. Wheatley, H. C., Daltzman, M., Williams, J. W., Miles, D. E., and Hatch, F. E., 1985, Long-term effects of cyclosporine on renal function in liver transplant recipients, *Transplantation* **43**: 641–647.

507. Palestine, A. G., Austin, H. A., Balow, J. E., Antonovych, T. T., Sabnis, S. G., Preuss, H. G., and Nussenblatt, R. B., 1986, Renal histopathologic alterations in patients treated with cyclosporine for uveitis, *N. Engl. J. Med.* **314**:1293–1298.

508. Curtis, J. J., Luke, R. G., Jones, P., Dubovsky, E. V., Whelchel, J. D., and Diethelm, A. G., 1986, Cyclosporine in therapeutic doses increases renal allograft resistance, *Lancet* **2**:477–479.

509. Jackson, N. M., Hsu, C., Visscher, G. E., and Venkatachalam, M. A., and Humes, H. D., 1987,

Alterations in renal structure and function in a rat model of cyclosporine nephrotoxicity, *J. Pharmacol. Exp. Ther.* **242:**749–756.

510. Rogers, T. S., Elzinga, L., Bennett, W. M., and Kelley, V. E., 1988, Selective enhancement of thromboxane in macrophages and kidneys in cyclosporine A induced nephrotoxicity. Dietary protection by fish oil, *Transplantation* **45:**153–156.

511. Keusch, G., Gmür, J., Baumgartner, D., Burger, H. R., Largiader, F., and Binswanger, V., 1986, *De novo* hemolytic uremic syndrome in two renal allograft recipients treated with cyclosporine: Successful therapy with plasmapheresis, *Transplant. Proc.* **18:**1097–1098.

512. Innes, J. T., Cosio, F. G., Mahan, J. D., Nahman, N. S., and Ferguson, R. M., 1986, Cyclosporine enhances endotoxin induced nephrotoxicity in rabbits, *Kidney Int.* **29:**282a (Abstract).

513. Grace, A. A., Barradas, M. A., Mikhailidis, D. P., Jeremy, J. Y., Moorhead, J. F., Sweny, P., and Dandona, P., 1987, Cyclosporine A enhances platelet aggregation, *Kidney Int.* **32:**889–895.

514. Luke, R. G., 1987, Hypertension in renal transplant recipients, *Kidney Int.* **31:**1024–1037.

515. Textor, S. C., Fornan, S. J., Borer, W., and Carlson, J., 1986, Sequential blood pressure hormonal and renal changes during bone marrow transplant recipients with normal renal function, *Clin. Res.* **34:**44a (Abstract).

516. Bellett, M., Cabrol, C., Sassano, P., Leger, P., Corvol, P., and Menard, J., 1985, Systemic hypertension after cardiac transplantation: Effect of cyclosporine on the renin-angiotensin-aldosterone system, *Am. J. Cardiol.* **56:**927–931.

517. Stanek, B., Kovarik, J., Rasoul-Rockenschaub, S., and Silberbauer, K., 1987, Renin–angiotensin–aldosterone system and vasopressin in cyclosporine-treated renal allograft recipients, *Clin. Nephrol.* **28:**186–189.

518. Vellodi, A., Jayatunga, R., and Hugh-Jones, K., 1987, Hemiplegia and focal convulsions as a manifestation of cyclosporine A toxicity, *J. Clin. Pharmacol.* **27:**914–915.

519. Cantarovich, M., Hiesse, C., Lockiec, F., Charpentier, B., and Fries, D., 1987, Confirmation of the interaction between cyclosporine and the calcium channel blocker nicardipine in renal transplant patients, *Clin. Nephrol.* **28:**190–193.

520. Bendz, H., 1985, Kidney function in a selected lithium population, *Acta Psychiatr. Scan.* **72:**451–463.

521. Vaamonde, C. A., Milian, N. E., Magrinat, G. S., Perez, G. O., and Oster, J. R., 1986, Longitudinal evaluation of glomerular filtration rate during long-term lithium therapy, *Am. J. Kidney Dis.* **8:**213–216.

522. Samiy, A. H. and Rosnick, P. B., 1987, Early identification of renal problems in patients receiving chronic lithium treatment, *Am. Psychiatry* **144:**670–672.

523. Jorkasky, D., Amsterdam, J., and Cox, M., 1987, Lithium-induced nephropthy: Final report of a 3-year prospective study, *Proc. Int. Soc. Nephrol.* **10:**17a (Abstract).

524. Walker, R. G., Escott, M., Birchall, I., Dowling, J. P., and Kincaid-Smith, P., 1986, Chronic progressive renal lesions induced by lithium, *Kidney Int.* **29:**875–881.

525. Van Dyke, M., Van Damme-Lombaerts, R., and Proesmans, W., 1985, Neonatal diabetes insipidus due to maternal lithium therapy during pregnancy, *Proc. EDTA–ERA* **22:**1017–1019.

526. Teicher, M. H., Altesman, R. I., Cole, J. O., and Schatzberg, A. F., 1987, Possible nephrotoxic interaction of lithium and metronidazole, *JAMA* **257:**3365–3366.

527. Boton, R., Gaviria, M., and Batlle, D. C., 1987, Prevalence, pathogenesis, and treatment of renal dysfunction associated with chronic lithium therapy, *Am. J. Kidney Dis.* **10:**329–345.

528. Bach, P. H. and Bridges, J. W., 1986, Chemically induced renal papillary necrosis and upper urothelial carcinoma. Part 1, *CRC Crit. Rev. Toxicol.* **15:**217–329.

529. Dubach, U. C., 1985, Analgesic nephropathy, *Proc. EDTA–ERA* **222:**977–983.

530. Burkart, J. M. and Buckalew, V. M., Nephropathy (N) associated with habitual ingestion of acetaminophen (AC), *Proc. Am. Soc. Nephrol.* **19:**33a (Abstract).

531. Segasothy, M., Suleiman, A. B., Puvaneswary, M., and Rohana, A., 1987, Paracetamol: A cause

for analgesic nephropathy (AN) and end-stage renal failure (ESRF), *Proc. Int. Cong. Nephrol.* **10:** 32a (Abstract).

532. Kyle, M. E. and Kocsis, J. J., 1986, The effect of mixed function oxidase induction and inhibition on salicylate-induced nephrotoxicity in male rats, *Toxicol. Appl. Pharmacol.* **84:**241–249.

532a. McCredie, M., Stewart, J. H., Carter, J. J., Turner, J., and Mahony, J. F., 1986, Phenacetin and papillary necrosis: Independent risk factors for renal pelvic cancer, *Kidney Int.* **30:**81–84.

532b. Lornoy, W., Becaus, I., DeVleeschouwer, M., Morelle, V., Fonteyne, E., Thienpont, L., and Mestdagh, J., 1986, Renal cell carcinoma, a new complication of analgesic nephropathy, *Lancet* **1:**1271–1272.

533. Schwartz, A., Kraft, D., Keller, F., Meyer-Sabellek, W., Gawlik, D., and Offermann, G., 1985, Analgesic nephropathy and aluminum toxicity, *Proc. EDTA–ERA* **22:**997–1001.

534. Dunn, M. J. and Patrono, C., eds., 1986, Sympmosium: Renal effects of nonsteroidal antiinflammatory drugs, *Am. J. Med.* **81:**August 25.

535. Epstein, M., ed., 1986, Symposium: Prostaglandins and the kidney. *Am. J. Med.* **80:**January 17.

536. D'Angio, R. G., 1987, Nonsteroidal antiinflammatory drug–induced renal dysfunction related to inhibition of renal prostaglandins, *Drug. Intell. Clin. Pharm.* **21:**954–960.

537. Hart, D. and Lifschitz, M. D., 1987, Renal physiology of the prostaglandins and the effects of nonsteroidal anti-inflammatory agents on the kdiney, *Am. J. Nephrol.* **7:**408–418.

538. L'E Orme, M., 1986, Non-steroidal antiinflammatory drugs and the kidney, *Br. Med. J.* **292:** 1621–1622.

539. Kleinknecht, D., Landais, P., and Goldfarb, B., 1986, Analgesic and nonsteroidal antiinflammatory drug-associated acute renal failure: A prospective collaborative study, *Clin. Nephrol.* **25:**275– 281.

540. Bock, H. A., Frölich, J. C., Ritz, R., and Brunner, F. P., 1986, Effects of intravenous aspirin on prostaglandin synthesis and kidney function in intensive care patients, *Nephrol. Dial. Transplant.* **1:**164–169.

541. Unsworth, J., Sturman, S., Lunec, J., and Blake, D., 1987, Renal impairment associated with non-steroidal antiinflammatory drugs, *Ann. Rheum. Dis.* **46:**233–236.

542. Sipilä, R., Skrifvars, B. O., and Törnroth, T., 1986, Reversible nonoliguric impairment of renal function during azapropazone treatment, *Scand. J. Rhemunatol.* **15:**23–26.

543. Abraham, P. A., Halstenson, C. E., Opsahl, J. A., Matzke, G. R., Ellis, C. L., and Keane, W. F., 1987, Uricosuria: A potential mechanism for suprofen nephropathy, *Proc. Int. Congr. Nephrol.* **10:**448a (Abstract).

544. Segasothy, M., Thyaparan, A., Kamal, A., and Sivalingam, S., 1987, Mefenamic acid nephropathy, *Nephron* **45:**156–157.

545. Ciabattoni, G., Boss, A. H., Patrignani, P., Catella, F., Simonetti, B. M. Pierucci, A., Pugliese, F., Filabozzi, P., and Patrono, C., 1987, Effects of sulindac on renal and extrarenal eicosanoid synthesis, *Clin. Pharmacol. Ther.* **41:**380–383.

546. Swainson, C. P., Griffiths, P., and Watson, M. L., 1986, Chronic effects of oral sulindac on renal haemodynamics and hormones in subjects with chronic renal disease, *Clin. Sci.* **70:**243–247.

547. Mistry, C. D., Lote, C. J., Gokal, R., Currie, W. J. C., Vandenburg, M., and Mallick, N. P., 1986, Effects of sulindac on renal function and prostaglandin synthesis in patients with moderate chronic renal insufficiency, *Clin. Sci.* **70:**501–505.

548. Sethi, K., Jain, R., and Malhotra, S., 1987, Effects of long-term sulindac therapy in chronic renal failure, *Proc. Int. Congr. Nephrol.* **10:**33a (Abstract).

549. Whelton, A., Stout, R. L., Drew, H., LaFrance, N., Spilman, P. S., Crocetti, S. S., Hermann, J., Klassen, D., Delgado, F., and Watson, A. J. 1987, A prospective, randomized, cross-over study of the renal effects of ibuprofen, piroxicam, and sulindac in chronic renal impairment, *Proc. Int. Congr. Nephrol.* **10:**38a (Abstract).

550. Quintero, E., Gines, P., Arroyo, V., Rimola, A., Camps, J., Gaya, J., Guevara, A., Rodamilans, M., and Rodes, J., 1986, Sulindac reduces the urinary excretion of prostaglandins and impairs renal function in cirrhosis with ascites, *Nephron* **42:**298–303.

551. Brater, D. C., Anderson, S. A., and Brown-Cartwright, D., 1987, Reversible acute decrease in renal function by NSAIDs in cirrhosis, *Am. J. Med. Sci.* **294:**168–174.

552. Brater, D. C., Brown-Cartwright, D., Anderson, S. A., and Uaamnuichai, M., 1987, Effect of high-dose etodolac on renal function, *Clin. Pharmacol. Ther.* **42:**283–289.

553. Ruilope, L. M., Garcia-Robles, R., Paya, C., Alcazar, J. M., Miravalles, E., Sancho-Rof, J., Rodicio, J., Knox, F. G., and Romero, J. C,. 1986, Effects of long-term treatment with indomethacin on renal function, *Hypertension* **8:**677–684.

554. Nicholls, A. J., Shortland, J. R., and Brown, C. B., 1985, Mefenamic acid nephropthy—A spectrum of renal lesions, *Proc. EDTA–ERA* **22:**991–996.

555. Schneider, P. D., 1986, Nonsteroidal antiinflammatory drugs and acute cortical necrosis, *Ann. Intern. Med. 105:*303–304.

556. Moss, A. H., Riley, R., Murgo, A., and Skaff, L. A., 1986, Over-the-counter ibuprofen and acute renal failure, *Ann. Intern. Med.* **105:**303.

557. Justiniani, F. R., 1986, Over-the-counter ibuprofen and nephrotic syndrome, *Ann. Intern. Med.* **105:**303.

558. Tolins, J. P. and Seel, P., 1989, Ibuprofen induced interstitial nephritis and the nephrotic syndrome, *Nephron* (in press).

559. Artinano, M., Etheridge, W. B., Stroehlein, K. B., and Barcenas, C. G., 1986, Progression of minimal-change glomerulopathy to focal glomerulosclerosis in a patient with fenoprofen nephropathy, *Am. J. Nephrol.* **6:**353–357.

560. Alavi, N., Lianos, E. A., Venuto, R. C., Mookerjee, B. K., and Bentzel, C. J., 1986, Reduction of proteinuria by indomethacin in patients with nephrotic syndrome, *Am. J. Kidney Dis.* **8:**397–403.

561. Laurent, J., Belghiti, D., Bruneau, C., and Lagrue, G., 1987, Diclofenac, a nonsteroidal antiinflammatory drug, decreases proteinuria in some glomerular diseases: A controlled study, *Am. J. Nephrol.* **7:**198–202.

562. Netter, P., Bannworth, B., Pere, P., and Nicolas, A., 1987, Clinical pharmacokinetics of D-penicillamine, *Drugs* **13:**317–333.

563. Ntoso, K. A., Tomaszewski, J. E., Jimenez, S. A., and Neilson, R. G., 1986, Penicillamine-induced rapidly progressive glomerulonephritis in patients with progressive systemic sclerosis: Successful treatment of two patients and a review of the literature, *Am. J. Kidney Dis.* **8:**159–163.

564. Feehally, J., Wheeler, D. C., Mackay, E. H., Oldham, R., and Walls, J., 1987, Recurrent acute renal failure with interstitial nephritis due to D-penicillamine, *Renal Failure* **10:**55–57.

565. Rehan, A. and Johnson, K., 1986, IgM nephropathy associated with penicillamine, *Am. J. Nephrol.* **6:**71–74.

566. Matthey, F., Perrett, D., Greenwood, R. N., and Baker, L. R. I., 1986, The use of D-penicillamine in patients with rheumatoid arthritis underoing hemodialysis, *Clin. Nephrol.* **25:**268–271.

567. Blocka, K. L. N., Paulus, H. E., and Furst, D. E., 1986, Clinical pharmacokinetics of oral and injectable gold compounds, *Clin. Pharmacol.* **11:**133–143.

568. Hall, C. L., Harrison, P. R., McKenzie, J. C., Tribe, C. R., and McIvor, A., 1987, The natural history of gold nephropathy: A long term study of 21 patients, *Proc. Int. Congr. Nephrol.* **10:**65a (Abstract).

569. Pitts, T. O., Spero, J. A., Bontempo, F. A., and Greenberg, A., 1986, Acute renal failure due to high-grade obstruction following therapy with ε-aminocaproic acid, *Am. J. Kidney Dis.* **8:**441–444.

570. Wilson, C., Azmy, A. F., Beattie, T. J., and Murphy, A. V., 1986, Hypermagnesemia and progression of renal failure associated with renacidin therapy, *Clin. Nephrol.* **25:**266–267.

571. Davis, M. C. E., Jr., Carpenter, Col. J. L., Ognibene, A. J., and McAllister, C. K., 1986, Rifampin-induced acute renal failure, *South. Med. J.* **79:**1012–1015.

572. Murray, A. N., Cassidy, M. J. D., and Templecamp, C., 1987, Rapidly progressive

glomerulonephritis associated with rifampicin therapy for pulmonary tuberculosis, *Nephron* **46:** 373–376.

573. Leighton, J. D., Walker, R. J., and Lynn, K. L., 1986, Trimipramine-induced acute renal failure, *NZ Med. J.* **99:**248.

574. Björck, S., Westberg, G., and Svalander, C., 1987, Hydralazine-induced glomerulonephritis: A serious complication to long-term treatment, *Proc. Int. Congr. Nephrol.* **10:**51a (Abstract).

575. Skinner, R. and Ferner, R. E., 1986, Acute renal failure without acute intravascular haemolysis after nomifensine overdosage, *Hum. Toxicol.* **5:**279–280.

576. Addo, E. and Poon-King, T., 1986, Leucocyte suppression in treatment of 72 patients with paraquat poisoning, *Lancet* **1:**1117–1120.

577. Turk, J., Morrell, L., and Avioli, L. V., 1986, Ethylene glycol intoxication, *Arch. Intern. Med.* **146:**1601–1603.

578. Gabow, P. A., Clay, K., Sullivan, J. B., and Lepoff, R., 1986, Organic acids in ethylene glycol intoxication, *Ann. Intern. Med.* **105:**16–20.

579. Weaver, A. N. and Sica, D. A., 1987, Mannitol-induced acute renal failure, *Nephron* **45:**233–235.

580. Giménez, A. and Mampaso, F., 1986, Characterization of inflammatory cells in drug-induced tubulointerstitial nephritis, *Nephron* **43:**239–240.

581. Boucher, A., Droz, D., Adafer, E., and Noël, L-H., 1986, Characterization of mononuclear cell subsets in renal cellular interstitial infiltrates, *Kidney Int.* **29:**1043–1049.

582. Toll, L. L., Lee, M., and Sharifi, R., 1987, Cefoxitin-induced interstitial nephritis, *South. Med. J.* **80:**274–276.

583. Geller, R. J., Chevalier, R. L., and Spyker, D. A., 1986, Acute amoxicillin nephrotoxicity following an overdose, *Clin. Toxicol.* **24:**175–182.

584. Nolan, C. R., Anger, M. S., and Kelleher, S. P., 1986, Eosinophiluria—A new method of detection and definition of the clinical spectrum, *N. Engl. J. Med.* **315:**1516–1519.

585. Sacks, P. and Fellner, S. K., 1987, Recurrent reversible acute renal failure from amphotericin, *Arch. Intern. Med.* **147:**593–595.

586. Tolins, J. P. and Rai, J. L., 1986, Amphotericin B: Pathophysiology of adverse renal hemodynamic effects in the rat, *Clin. Res.* **34:**558a (Abstract).

587. McCarthy, J. T. and Staats, B. A., 1986, Pulmonary hypertension, hemolytic anemia, and renal failure, *Chest* **89:**608–610.

588. Cantrell, J. E., Phillips, T. M., and Schein, P. S., 1985, Carcinoma-associated hemolytic–uremic syndrome: A complication of mitomycin C chemotherapy, *J. Clin. Oncol.* **3:**723–734.

589. Desablens, B., Fievet, P., Pruna, A., Claisse, J. F., Westeel, P. F., Tolani, M., and Fournier, A., 1986, Hemolytic–uremic syndrome after cancer chemotherapy without mitomycin C, *Nephron* **42:** 343–344.

590. Bertani, T., Cutillo, F., Zoja, C., Broggini, M., and Remuzzi, G., 1986, Tubulointerstitial lesions mediate renal damage in Adriamycin glomerulopathy, *Kidney Int.* **39:**488–496.

591. Mimnaugh, E. G., Trush, M. A., and Gram, T. E., 1986, A possible role for membrane lipid peroxidation in anthracycline nephrotoxicity, *Biochem. Pharm.* **35:**4327–4335.

592. Reid, G. M. and Muther, R. S., 1987, Nitroprusside-induced acute azotemia, *Am. J. Nephrol.* **7:** 313–315.

593. Wright, L. F. and DuVal, W., Jr., 1987, Renal injury associated with laxative abuse, *South. Med. J.* **80:**1304–1306.

Index